Diagnostic Radiology in Paediatrics

POSTGRADUATE PAEDIATRICS
SERIES

Under the General Editorship of

JOHN APLEY
C.B.E., M.D., B.S., F.R.C.P.

Emeritus Consultant Paediatrician, United Bristol Hospitals

Diagnostic Radiology in Paediatrics

I. R. S. Gordon, MD, FRCP, FRCR(London)
Consultant Radiologist

F. G. M. Ross, FRCR(London), FFR(RCSI)
Consultant Radiologist

*Bristol Royal Hospital for Sick Children,
Bristol Health District (Teaching)*

Butterworths
LONDON BOSTON
Sydney—Wellington—Durban—Toronto

THE BUTTERWORTH GROUP

ENGLAND

Butterworth & Co. (Publishers) Ltd
London: 88 Kingsway, WC2B 6AB

AUSTRALIA

Butterworths Pty Ltd
Sydney: 586 Pacific Highway,
   Chatswood, NSW 2067
Also at Melbourne, Brisbane, Adelaide
and Perth

SOUTH AFRICA

Butterworth & Co. (South Africa) (Pty) Ltd
Durban: 152–154 Gale Street

NEW ZEALAND

Butterworths of New Zealand Ltd
Wellington: 26–28 Waring Taylor Street, 1

CANADA

Butterworth & Co. (Canada) Ltd.
Toronto: 2265 Midland Avenue,
   Scarborough, Ontario, M1P 4S1

USA

Butterworth (Publishers) Inc
Boston: 19 Cummings Park,
   Woburn, Mass. 01801

First published 1977

ISBN 0 407 00121 2

Library of Congress Cataloging in Publication Data

Gordon, Ian Ronald Simson.
   Diagnostic radiology in paediatrics.
   (Postgraduate paediatrics series)
   Bibliography: p.
   Includes index.
   1. Pediatric radiology. I. Ross, Francis George
Mabyn, joint author. II. Title. III. Series.
RJ51.R3G6   618.9′2007′572   76-9080
ISBN 0-407-00121-2

Typeset By Butterworths Litho Preparation Department
Printed in England by Wm Clowes & Sons Ltd. Beccles

CONTENTS

FOREWORD

The authors' intent and scope are clear: to provide a text for doctors who diagnose childrens' disorders. Judging as a paediatrician, it appears to me that they have scored a notable success. Their book would enhance the diagnostic effectiveness of any childrens' doctor, whether still in training or of good experience.

Like any of the intertwining branches of Medicine, radiology can be approached from various aspects. The clinician need not encumber himself with its physics and electronics and technicalities; but he will make the most of what it has to offer when he appreciates what the expertise of radiologists can reasonably be expected to achieve, which investigations are difficult or dangerous, what they aim to demonstrate, how reliable be their results. Such considerations are prominent in this book. It advises diagnosticians what to expect and not to expect, what to ask for and not to ask for. It gives answers clearly and it discusses and illustrates them in depth and satisfying detail.

What does the practising radiologist need in order to contribute most effectively to paediatrics? He has no need to be deeply versed in the minutiae of clinical examination, in aetiology or theoretical background, in details of treatment or social adaptation; but he does need to share an awareness of these. Experience shows that the partnership is most alert to the Daedalian possibilities of differential diagnosis, and it is most happy, when the radiologists mix with paediatricians, when they are exposed to the same climate of thinking and doing, and when both can get down on hands and knees to play with the patients.

The daily routine of the two authors has, I know, been intimately shared with clinicians for many years, to their mutual enrichment. They speak the same language— and understand baby-talk! Both authors are very experienced teachers. I find their exposition simple and clear. It is a refreshing relief from that not uncommon professional addiction, *ignotum per ignotius*, the explanation that is obscurer than the thing it is meant to explain.

Yes, the daily bread and butter tasks of radiology must be processed safely, quickly and accurately; but one of the ingredients of a good radiology department is curiosity, to ensure that the spirit of enquiry acts as a leavener. In research Dr Ross has contributed handsomely in cardiology and ultrasonics. Dr Gordon has contributed most fundamentally in measurement, and, as I have remarked before, 'The paediatrician is a measuring doctor' because he deals always with growth and change. It is not surprising that the diagnostic radiology department in which they work (and unmistakeably enjoy their work) has been a focus and a magnet attracting difficult problems and enthusiastic problem solvers.

This book is an extension of Dr Gordon's and Dr Ross's personal teaching and discussions both with clinicians and radiologists over many years. I have no doubt that sharing the authors' great experience with a wider circle will prove of value to doctors in many countries. From this book they will obtain up-to-date and practical information, to enable them to make the best use of diagnostic radiology for the benefit of their patients.

John Apley

PREFACE

In recent years there has been a considerable expansion in the variety of radiological methods and they have been extended to cover more disease patterns. There is therefore a place for a text which presents these developments in a reasonably concise form for the guidance of all doctors who care for children. This book is derived from the experience of two radiologists who work in a childrens' hospital, and the emphasis given to various diseases is dictated not merely by their personal interests but reflects the type of work which is requested from them by the clinical staff of that hospital.

Considerations of size have necessitated a degree of selection, and in particular it was not thought that a detailed account of fractures was essential to our purpose in this book.

One of the authors has a special interest in bone tumours and in cardiology and the space allotted to these topics expresses the considerable experience gained in these fast expanding fields. Similarly, the other author has a special interest in skeletal dysplasias enhanced by the recently established Bristol Registry of Bone Dysplasias. It is their firm conviction that, even though the study of these mostly very rare conditions may seem somewhat academic, it is only by increased familiarity with all their aspects—radiological, clinical, biochemical and histological—that progress towards more effective prevention and cure will be achieved. This author has also been interested in the application of quantitative measurements to the radiographs of children.

In the adult the abnormal can be compared with a relatively fixed normal and the deviations (from the latter seen in the former) can be analysed. In the child the normal comprises a transient process rather than a fixed state and in order to detect abnormalities a knowledge of the manner and rate at which the normal appearances alter with the age of the child is necessary. This can, it is emphasized, be facilitated by the possession of reliable radiographic parameters; accordingly the final chapter is devoted to indicating where such data can be obtained.

In addition to being of assistance to the paediatrician, it is hoped that this book may also provide postgraduate doctors training in Radiology and in Paediatrics with a succinct account of the subspeciality of Paediatric Radiology. There is still a shortage of trained radiologists and it is the belief of the authors that Radiology in

xi

general, and Paediatric Radiology in particular, is about to undergo a period of expansion of knowledge resulting from the exploitation of new techniques. These will afford great opportunities for radiologists and paediatricians to attain a wider variety of information than is currently available. To that end this book may hope to make some contribution by providing a foundation upon which future advances can be securely based. On the other hand, in the financial climate prevailing in so many parts of the world at the present time, it is most important that the value of the information gained by each

diagnostic method, radiological or otherwise, should be assessed in the light of the cost of performing that examination. In short, the cost-effectiveness of each examination must be examined critically. There is an undoubted misuse of radiology in many quarters and it is hoped that this text may play a small part in assisting in such an assessment of radiological examination as applied to children.

I.R.S. Gordon
F.G.M. Ross

Acknowledgements

The authors enthusiastically acknowledge the assistance they have had from the radiographic staff of the Teaching Hospital without which this book would not have been possible.

The majority of the reproductions of the radiographs were produced by Ilford Ltd. and the others by Mr. J. E. Hancock at the Bristol Royal Infirmary. The authors are indebted to both for the high standards they have set and for their willingness and tolerance in meeting their requirements. The line drawings result from the expertise of Mr. E. J. Turnbull, S.E.N., Department of Radiodiagnosis, Bristol Royal Infirmary, to whom the authors are particularly grateful. Mrs. Joyce Andrews cheerfully typed most of the manuscript and the staff of Butterworths have been helpful, courteous and tolerant. Finally, the authors wish to thank their wives for the help and support they have received over many months.

1 SKELETAL DYSPLASIAS

CLASSIFICATION

The dysplasias comprise a group of disorders of the skeletal system of congenital origin. Most of them are hereditary and therefore are likely to be due basically to a biochemical defect which interferes with the normal processes of growth and development of bone. Unfortunately in only a few dysplasias is there any detailed knowledge of such aetiological factors; in the remainder the differentiation of one condition from another depends upon a topographical and morphological description of its features, together with its natural history and type of inheritance.

As a result, the classification of the numerous syndromes which have been defined by the use of such criteria is a matter of some complexity. A number of skeletal dysplasias are known in which a common cause has been identified, for instance those in which excessive amounts of mucopolysaccharides are excreted in the urine. Such diseases share many common clinical and radiological features and can logically be considered together.

Rubin (1964) has made an attempt to bring some order into the methods by which these disorders are arranged, by relating them, firstly, to the part of the bone predominantly involved and, secondly, to whether the condition is a hypoplasia or hyperplasia or what he terms a dystrophy or dysostosis.

It is proposed here to adopt a primarily topographical arrangement to allow a discussion of common radiological features without the necessity of too much repetition, but such a grouping should not be considered to imply any necessary relationship between the various conditions which are placed together. This arrangement allows a subdivision into Generalized and Localized Dysplasias as suggested by Jaffe (1937), and into Epiphyseal, Metaphyseal and Diaphyseal Dysplasias as originally proposed by Jansen (1934). There may be a problem in assigning any individual case to one or other of these categories and this is made more difficult by the existence of intermediate types, and of cases which show features characteristic of more than one entity. Attempts to do this on the basis of one particular characteristic, clinical, radiological, histological or biochemical, or on the features observed at the age of presentation may lead to difficulty. It is important to take into account all aspects of the case, including those affecting systems other than the skeleton. When the diagnostic problem is particularly difficult, the development of the case over a period of time should be watched in order to assess the effect of increasing growth and maturation. This may allow signs to become manifest which may be of great help in determining the nature of the condition.

EPIPHYSEAL DYSPLASIAS

DYSPLASIA EPIPHYSEALIS MULTIPLEX

This condition, described by Fairbank (1946), is an example of a purely skeletal dysplasia of congenital origin, which involves a limited area of the skeleton. Both the clinical and radiological features reflect the fact that the abnormality is mainly one of epiphyseal development. It presents most commonly at the age of 3 or 4 years, reaching a peak of severity in early adolescence and thereafter improving to such a degree that the disease can re regarded as self-limiting. There is however a tendency to the early development of degenerative arthritis in adult life.

Radiological features

In this condition ossification of an individual epiphysis occurs, not from one centre, but from multiple centres,

1

2

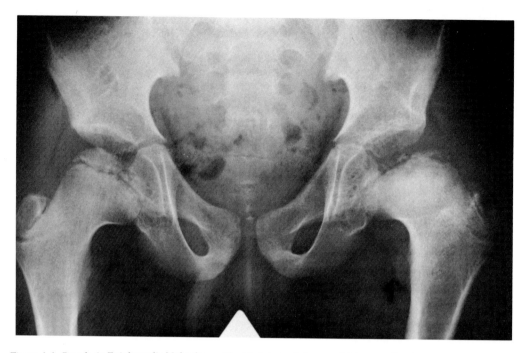

Figure 1.1. Dysplasia Epiphysealis Multiplex: The hip joints of a boy aged 14 years. The femoral capital epiphyses have ossified from several centres which have not yet united especially on the left. The epiphyses are both flattened and widened and corresponding widening of the femoral necks is also present

which ultimately fuse to form a homogeneous but permanently deformed epiphysis (*Figure 1.1*). Most of the epiphyses in the skeleton are affected in this way. The resultant deformity may take various forms; flattening, wedging or irregularity of the articular surface being commonly seen. The carpal and tarsal bones are similarly affected. They may be hypoplastic or deformed and may be fused to one another, especially in the tarsus. The metaphyses of the long bones, although they may be widened and deformed, are not primarily affected and growth is only slightly impaired. In spite of the abnormality in the development of the epiphyses and round bones, there is no delay in ossification or in fusion, and the skeletal age is in most cases within the normal range. Deformities such as coxa vara and genu valgum are frequently present. The abnormalities are bilaterally symmetrical and most commonly occur in the epiphyses at the hips and knees. Ödman (1959) states that homologous joints in the upper and lower limbs tend to be affected together, such as the elbows and knees, or the metacarpophalangeal and metatarsophalangeal joints. In some cases the peripheral joints are predominantly affected and in others the changes are confined to a single site. Although the skull and spine are characteristically normal, variants have been described in which spinal abnormalities are present which resemble those of Scheuermann's disease. There is anterior wedging of the vertebral bodies and fragmentation and irregularity of the epiphyses at their anterior angles. These changes may lead to kyphosis and scoliosis.

The condition may resemble other diseases in which the epiphyses are primarily involved, especially hypothyroidism (*see* page 8). In Perthes' disease changes in the hips may result in a very similar appearance, but these are most commonly only on one side. If such changes are bilateral, the possibility of this type of dysplasia should be suspected.

SPONDYLO-EPIPHYSEAL DYSPLASIA

Under this term are grouped a number of conditions which have been recently confirmed as separate genetic entities. There are three distinct types:
  (1) Spondylo-epiphyseal dysplasia congenita, arising soon after birth and inherited as a dominant.
  (2) Spondylo-epiphyseal dysplasia tarda, with an onset in later childhood and inherited as an X-linked recessive condition occurring only in males.
  (3) Pseudo-achondroplasia in which there is a late onset and a marked degree of shortening of the peripheral bones of the limbs. This feature is in contrast to the other types in which dwarfism is less marked and it is predominantly due to shortening of the trunk.

In all these types epiphyseal changes resembling those of dysplasia epiphysealis multiplex described above, occur but with the additional of spinal lesions, which consist of flattening or other abnormalities in the shape of the vertebral bodies. The skull and facial bones are normal throughout this group. The three types form a continuous spectrum at one end of which is the tarda form; at the other end is pseudo-achondroplasia with spondylo-epiphyseal dysplasia congenita being intermediate between the two.

Spondylo-epiphyseal dysplasia tarda

In this condition the changes are almost confined to the spine and the hips. The limbs are of normal length and show relatively minor epiphyseal irregularities, but there is a tendency to the development of premature osteoarthritis. Weinfeld *et al.* (1967) consider the shape of the vertebral bodies to be the hallmark of the disease, but this feature is not fully manifest until early adolescence. All the vertebrae are affected. Their bodies are reduced in height anteriorly but they are increased in height in the posterior half due to dense mounds of bone which form localized bulges of both the upper and lower end-plates. The intervertebral disc spaces are in consequence narrowed posteriorly and a moderate thoracic kyphosis is usually present. The odontoid process is sometimes hypoplastic. The resultant generalized platyspondyly resembles that of Morquio's disease, but the late onset and relatively normal limbs are useful differentiating features.

Pseudo-achondroplasia

In this condition the limb-shortening overshadows the spinal changes and gives rise to severe short-limbed dwarfism with a superficial resemblance to achondroplasia. The hands and feet show the most severe abnormalities, which consist of fragmentation and irregularity of the carpal and tarsal bones and of the epiphyses of the metacarpals, metatarsals and phalanges. These latter bones are all markedly shortened (*Figure 1.2b*). The metaphyses are irregular, and flared. Similar changes occur in the proximal long bones. In the spine the vertebral bodies show step-like defects at their upper and lower angles, and a central beak-like protrusion from the anterior surface (*Figure 1.2a*). A severe scoliosis may ensue in later childhood. In distinction to true achondroplasia the interpedicular distances are of normal width and the pelvis is small; the acetabular margins are irregular, the sacrosciatic notches are wide and there is a tendency to protrusio acetabuli (Ford *et al.*, 1961).

Spondylo-epiphyseal dysplasia congenita

In this condition both spinal and limb changes occur, and the latter decrease in severity in the distal parts of the limb. The vertebral bodies are compressed and abnormal in shape, though in this type, the height of the posterior part of the body is reduced to a greater extent than that of the anterior part and this results in the body being pear-shaped in the lateral projection. A severe thoracic kyphosis and lumbar lordosis ensue in later adolescence. The epiphyses, the carpal and tarsal bones ossify late and irregularly. The epiphyses of the heads of the humeri and femora are often absent. This type of spondylo-epiphyseal dysplasia is associated with abnormalities of other systems and there may be a cleft palate, talipes equinovarus and, most notably, visual defects, due to a high degree of myopia and retinal detachment. Fraser *et al.* (1969), analysing a large series of children with ocular handicaps, found several cases of this type of

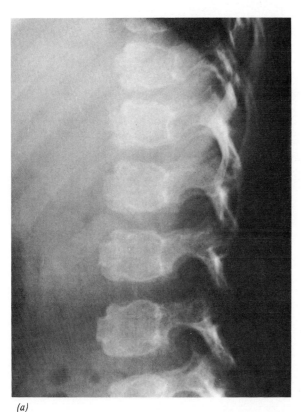

(a)

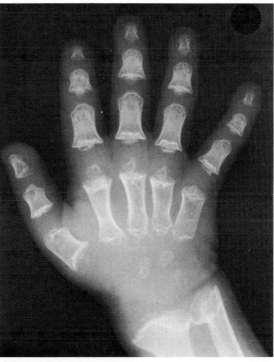

(b)

Figure 1.2. Pseudo-achondroplasia: (a) Lateral view of the lumbar spine. The vertebral bodies are characterized by an apparent central projection of the anterior surface due to the step-like defects above and below it. (b) The bones of the hand are markedly shortened with irregular dense metaphyses and deformity of the epiphyses and carpal bones

4

skeletal dysplasia; most of these were also deaf and two appeared to be mentally retarded. Recognition of the skeletal abnormalities may be possible at a relatively early age—even at birth. This may be of considerable importance, as it may allow measures to be instituted which will prevent the onset of blindness in later life.

DYSPLASIA EPIPHYSEALIS CALCIFICANS (CONRADI'S DISEASE)

In this dysplasia, also, the abnormalities are not confined to the skeletal system, but the radiological appearances of the bones in the first year or two of life are so striking that they may overshadow the extraskeletal features. The former consist of dense, stippled calcifications within the cartilaginous parts of every bone undergoing endochondral ossification (*Figure 1.3*). These calcifications are prominent in the region of the epiphyses of the long bones, especially in the hips and shoulders, but they also occur in the carpus and tarsus, in the spine and in the tracheal and laryngeal cartilages. They are separate from, and precede, the epiphyseal ossification centres. The latter can develop normally, though they are usually deformed and flattened. The calcification gradually disappears during the second year of life, after which the radiological picture is one of a short-limbed type of dwarfism. The metaphyses of the long bones are widened

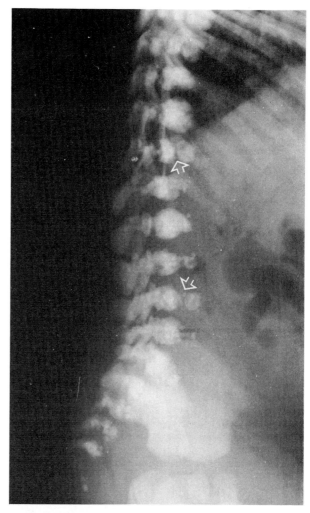

(a)

Figure 1.3. Dysplasia Epiphysealis Calcificans: (a) The vertebral bodies are irregular and deformed with a coronal cleft in many of them (arrowed); stippled calcification is present in the cartilage surrounding the primary centres of ossification. (b) In the foot, the secondary ossification centres are small and multicentric and are surrounded by stippled calcifications which also occur within those tarsal bones, such as the cuneiforms, which have not yet begun to ossify

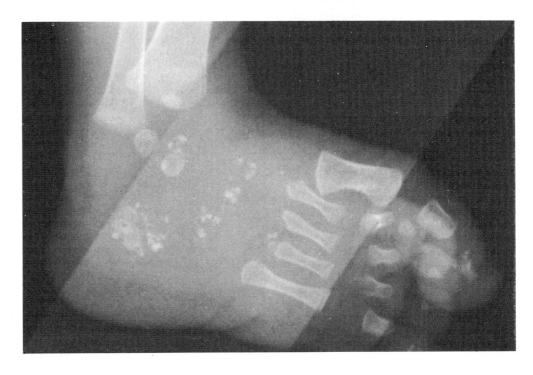

(b)

and irregular, resembling those of achondroplasia, but less symetrically distributed on the two sides of the body. Deformities are common, due partly to a disparity in length between the paired bones of the limbs, but there is also a severe scoliosis. The latter is often preceded by 'coronal cleft' vertebral bodies in which two ossification centres are present, one anterior to the other (see page 31 and Figure 1.3). It follows therefore that if these children present in the first year of life, the radiological picture is diagnostic. However, they do not do well and many of them die early from intercurrent infections. Some cases do survive and present in later childhood when the diagnostic problem may be more difficult. Comings et al. (1968) have pointed out that the overall pattern of abnormalities constitutes a fairly characteristic syndrome which allows a diagnosis to be made even though the stippled calcifications are no longer present. In addition to the short limbs and deformities the following features may be seen in dysplasia epiphysealis calcificans in older children: cataracts; optic atrophy; mental retardation; skin lesions of various types; cleft palate; micrognathos; flexion contractures at various joints; congenital dislocation of the hips; syndactyly and polydactyly; congenital heart disease; genito-urinary abnormalities. Some of these features can be demonstrated by appropriate radiological investigations.

MUCOPOLYSACCHARIDOSES

This group of diseases is included here, although the skeletal system is not involved alone and the bony abnormalities are not confined to the epiphyses. The pattern of skeletal involvement, however, shows some analogies with the other epiphyseal dysplasias, in particular the spondylo-epiphyseal group. The most striking feature common to these conditions is an abnormality in the basic biochemistry of the skeletal system, as a result which an excessive amount of acid mucopolysaccharide is excreted in the urine and deposited in the cells of different tissues. Because it is likely that genetically determined abnormalities of the skeletal system have biochemical or enzymatic defect as their underlying cause, a consideration of the nature of the abnormal mucoplysaccharide affords a rational method of classification. In practice, the conditions defined by variations in the type of chemical substance excreted have characteristic clinical and radiological features. It should, however, be noted that very similar radiological appearances can occur in cases without any demonstrable abnormality in mucopolysaccharide metabolism (Spranger and Schuster, 1969).

Hurler's syndrome

The recognition of this condition is usually easy from the abnormal facies, mental impairment and corneal opacities. The radiological appearance of the skeleton is quite distinctive and affects all parts, though the extent to which individual regions are involved is variable. It is also usual for these changes to be recognized only during the second or third year of life.

The skull vault is large and often abnormally dense and there is premature fusion of the sutures, especially the sagittal suture. The anterior fontanelle is large and closes late. These features do not necessarily imply any degree of hydrocephalus, but in a few cases the cerebrospinal fluid may be obstructed due to deposition of mucopolysaccharides in the meninges. In others the ventricles may be dilated as a result of cerebral atrophy. The pituitary fossa is abnormal in shape in a proportion of cases, either being unusually deep or else elongated in its anteroposterior diameter, with a 'J'-or omega-shaped outline. This latter deformity is due to a deepening of the chiasmatic sulcus lying anterior to the tuberculum sellae and is not confined to cases of Hurler's syndrome (Figure 1.4a and 9.15). The mandible is widened from side to side and the teeth are small, widely spaced and poorly formed. The symphysis menti is prolonged forwards into a sharp point; the condyle is deformed and shortened with a flat or even concave and notched articular surface which is best seen in the lateral projection (Figure 1.4a). The ribs are narrowed posteriorly and widen gradually in their anterior half. The latter part of the ribs is often turned upward, and these ribs are described as resembling palm fronds or scythe blades. In the spine there is a localized kyphosis at the thoracolumbar junction. The body of the first or second lumbar vertebra is deformed. There is a hook-like projection of the lower half and a defect of the upper half of the anterior aspect of the body (Figure 1.4b). The shape of the pelvis is usually very characteristic. The acetabula are shallow. Their roofs slope upwards at a normal or slightly increased angle and form a straight line with the lateral border of the ilium, such that the acetabular and iliac angles (see page 355) are approximately equal. As a result the ilia are wide and they have a prominence of the lateral part of the iliac crest (Figure 1.4d). The pelvis at the acetabular level is relatively narrowed. There is deformity of the epiphyses of the heads of the humeri and femora with some degree of coxa valga. There is also a loss of constriction in the long bones which results in the shafts having a rectangular shape; the cortices are thinned. The metaphyses often lie obliquely to the long axes of the bones. The hands and feet are more abnormal than the rest of the limbs. There is considerable irregularity of the carpal and tarsal bones and delay in epiphyseal ossification. A characteristic tapering of the proximal ends of the metacarpals and of the distal ends of the phalanges gives a somewhat claw-like aspect to the hands, a feature which is aggravated by the flexed and contracted joints of the fingers (Figure 1.4c). Bone growth is impaired and skeletal maturation is retarded.

Other types of mucopolysaccharidosis

The radiological picture described above is shared to some extent by all the conditions in which evidence of abnormal mucopolysaccharide metabolism is present and has been referred to by the term 'dysostosis multiplex'. However, many of the other types of mucopolysaccharidosis have their own characteristic features which, together with clinical and biochemical differences, allow differentiation one from the other. Thus the X-linked recessively inherited 'Hunter's syndrome' lacks the

6

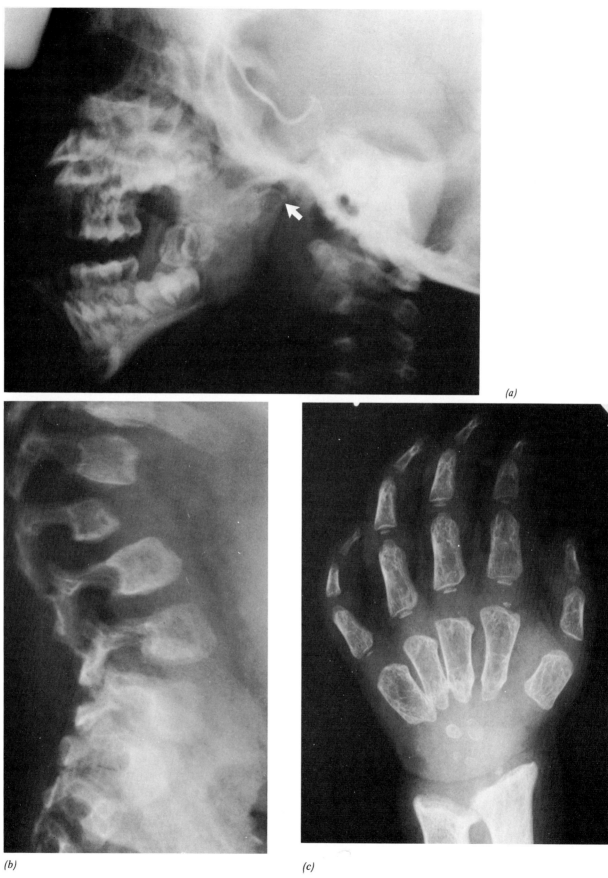

(a)

(b)

(c)

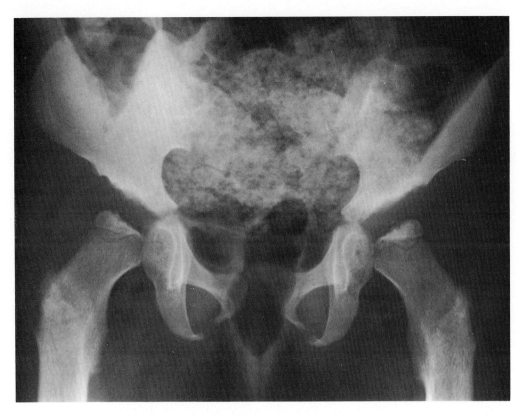

(d)

Figure 1.4. Mucopolysaccharidoses – Hurler's Syndrome: (a) The base of the skull and jaws show charac-teristic abnormalities. The pituitary fossa is elongated in its antero-posterior dimension due to an exaggeration of the chiasmatic sulcus lying above the tuberculum sellae with an elevation of the anterior clinoid process (see also Figure 9.15). The condyle of the mandible is short (arrowed) with blunting and flattening of its articular surface. (b) An acute kyphosis has developed in the upper part of the lumbar spine in association with a small deformed vertebral body at LV2. (c) In the hand, the metacarpals and phalanges are widened and shortened with a coarse, open trabecular pattern, tapering of the distal ends of the metacarpals, obliquity of the distal radial and ulnar metaphyses and flexion deformities of the fingers; the carpal bones are small and of an abnormal shape. (d) The pelvis is abnormal in shape due to the lateral projection of the ilia, the lateral border of which continues the line of the acetabular roofs. The femoral heads are flattened with dense, slightly fragmented epiphyses and a degree of coxa valga is present

dorsolumbar kyphosis but shows a particular liability to precocious osteoarthritis of the hip. In the *'Sanfilippo syndrome'*, in which mental impairment is especially severe, there is a less abnormal radiological appearance; thickening of the cranial vault and a uniformly ovoid shape of the vertebral bodies, with no localized kyphosis, are characteristic features. In the *Scheie syndrome* a spondylolisthesis of the lumbosacral spine, deformed vertebral bodies and arthritic-like changes in the joints of the hands are particularly characteristic.

The most distinctive skeletal abnormalities occur in *Morquio's disease,* in which abnormal mucopolysac-charides have been identified in the urine in some cases. It is still uncertain whether all the cases which show the radiological features originally described by Morquio and by Brailsford are biochemically abnormal. It has been suggested that Morquio's disease may be a symptom complex due to several different causes. The skeletal abnormalities consist of the following features. Wide-spread flattening of all the vertebral bodies, which have a tongue-like projection of the middle third of the anterior surface (*Figure 1.5*). This may be preceded by a stage where the deformity predominantly affects the

dorsolumbar junction and thereby approximates more closely to the appearances in Hurler's syndrome. The odontoid process is small or absent. The ilia are square with broad, swollen iliac crests; the acetabula are deep and irregular. Their roofs are flat and fragmented and the pelvic cavity is increased in height and narrowed from side to side. The epiphyses, carpal and tarsal bones ossify in an irregular manner from multiple centres, especially those of the heads of the femora, which are particularly small and deformed and often show lateral subluxation and coxa valga. Growth is quite severely impaired but, owing to the generalized platyspondyly and thoracic kyphosis, the resultant dwarfism tends to be of the 'short trunk' type. The limb bones are shorter than normal, and the irregular metaphyses are set obliquely to the long axis of the bone, resulting in pro-gressive deformity.

In addition to these well-recognized types of mucopolysaccharidosis, each with its own characteristic genetic, clinical, radiological and biochemical findings, abnormal mucopolysaccharides have been reported in a number of other skeletal dysplasias, notably Marfan's syndrome, diaphyseal aclasis and the nail—

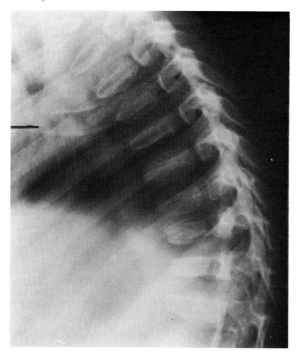

Figure 1.5. Mucopolysaccharidoses – Morquio's Disease: There is characteristic flattening of all the vertebral-bodies, the anterior borders of which are pointed in many cases

patella syndrome. Finally, it has become recognized recently that patients may show radiological changes indistinguishable from typical Hurler's syndrome in the absence of any evidence of abnormal mucopolysaccharide metabolism. These cases have been termed *pseudo-Hurler's syndrome* or *neurovisceral lipidosis* and it has been suggested that they belong to a group of conditions in which abnormalities of lipoid storage occur analogous to that in Niemann–Pick's disease (Spranger and Schuster, 1969). The bones are usually normal in the latter condition, but in other members of this group such as *I-cell disease* or *generalized gangliosidosis*, involvement of both the skeleton and the central nervous system may occur.

HYPOTHYROIDISM

The bone changes observed in children with hypothyroidism (Astley, 1958) are in many ways very similar to those seen in the dysplasias already described in this section. The most obvious effect of a lack of thyroid hormone on bone development is retardation in the process of conversion of the cartilaginous skeleton to bone; and because the effect is only manifested relatively late in intra-uterine life, or even after birth, it is the secondary centres, the epiphyses and the carpal and tarsal bones which are affected to the greatest extent.

The assessment of retardation of skeletal maturation has been discussed elsewhere (*see* page 344), but it must be emphasized that in hypothyroidism skeletal maturation is affected to a greater extent than bone growth, so that the bone age tends to fall below the height age, unlike most other causes of defective growth in which the reverse is the case. Within the first few months of

life, retardation of skeletal maturation may be the only abnormal radiological findings, the bones being otherwise normal. This is because the specific signs of abnormal bone formation are confined to the secondary centres of ossification, most of which do not become visible on a radiograph until after the first 6 months of postnatal life. In most cases of congenital hypothyroidism (cretinism), the condition will be diagnosed and treated before this and the radiological appearances of the bones may show no further abnormality.

In unrecognized or untreated cretins, however, and even more strikingly in cases of juvenile myxoedema, in which the hypothyroidism comes on after birth or during early childhood, the effect of lack of thyroid on ossification may be much more apparent. In particular, the epiphyses may ossify from several separate centres (*epiphyseal dysgenesis*). This produces an appearance of epiphyseal fragmentation, which is often accompanied by deformity, particularly in sites subject to weight-bearing, such as the heads of the femora or spine (*Figure 1.6a*). In the latter site, it may be associated with a local kyphosis at the thoracolumbar junction, a 'hook-shaped' vertebra in which the lower half of the body projects anteriorly (*Figure 1.6b*). This is very similar to that seen at a slightly later age in Hurler's syndrome. It is suggested that epiphyseal dysgenesis results from delay in ossification, which allows a more extensive maturation of the cartilage cells to occur. When the supply of thyroid hormone eventually allows ossification to proceed it does so throughout the whole of the epiphysis simultaneously, and not in a regular, progressive manner as occurs in normal bone growth.

Although in hypothyroidism growth is impaired to a relatively less marked degree than in those types of dysplasia in which the metaphysis or growth plate is primarily involved, the limbs tend to be disproportionately short and the long bones appear to be relatively wide with a thickened cortex. Transverse bands of osteosclerosis are also commonly seen on the diaphyseal side of the metaphyses and in the periphery of the carpal and tarsal bones or of the larger epiphyses. A more diffuse increase in bone density sometimes occurs, even approaching that of the sclerosing types of dysplasia, such as osteopetrosis. It is usually more localized in its distribution, and it may be limited to one region of the body, such as the base of the skull and facial bones. The increase in bone density is reversible with thyroid administration and it appears to result from a temporary positive calcium balance leading to storage of the excess in the bones. Rarely this may also result in deposition of calcium in the soft tissues or in the kidney, producing nephrocalcinosis. The development of the paranasal sinuses and of the mastoid air cells may be retarded in older children with hypothyroidism. A delay in the ossification of membrane bones may result in the sutures or fontanelles being abnormally wide for the age of the child, often with multiple Wormian bones. This feature may lead to confusion with osteogenesis imperfecta or cleidocranial dysostosis.

Treatment with thyroxine results in the resolution of these changes and a return to normal radiological appearances. Serial estimations of the degree of skeletal maturation may be made during the course of treatment. This affords an indication of the effectiveness of treatment. in restoring the bone age to a normal

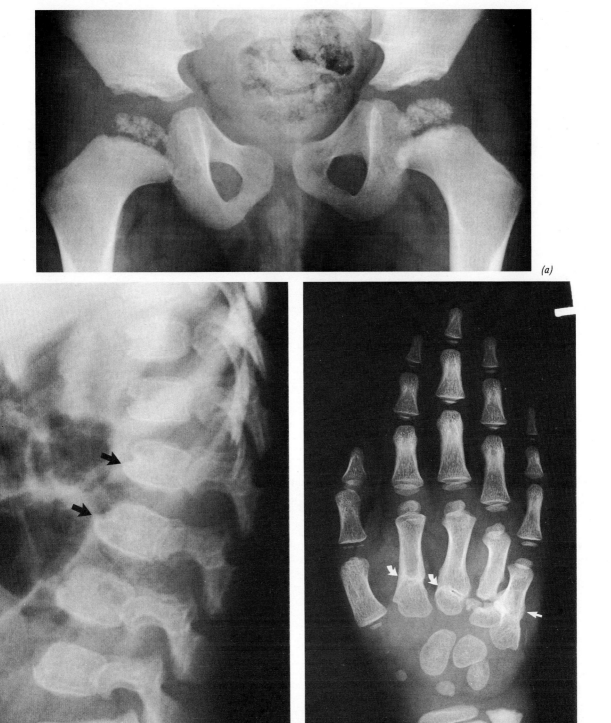

Figure 1.6. Hypothyroidism: (a) The epiphyses for the femoral heads have ossified from a large number of separate centres which have not yet fused together; the epiphyses are flattened and the femoral necks are widened with a prominent 'beak-like' projection of their medial ends. (b) The kyphosis at the thoracolumbar junction is associated with a hook-like projection of the lower part of the anterior border of the bodies of LV1 and LV2 (arrowed). (c) The hand of a boy aged 8½ years with juvenile myxoedema shows considerable delay in skeletal maturation, the bone age being estimated at 6.0 years (Tanner and Whitehouse method). There are fractures of the metacarpals resulting from a previous injury (arrowed). The fracture of the ring finger metacarpal has not united due to the lack of thyroxine

value. It will also give evidence of overdosage, with may result in an acceleration of skeletal maturation together with other symptoms of hyperthyroidism.

METAPHYSEAL DYSPLASIAS

ACHONDROPLASIA

This condition is the commonest of the skeletal dysplasias, and it produces a severe short-limbed type of dwarfism which is easily recognizable clinically. Nevertheless, the radiological features may help to confirm the diagnosis, and may indicate the likelihood of complications due to the abnormal bone growth. The long bones present the most striking abnormalities. Their longitudinal growth is severely restricted by the basic defect which predominantly involves the growth plate and the adjacent metaphysis. The metaphysis is widened due to the unimpeded apposition of periosteal new bone at the periphery of the growth cartilage and at the sites of muscle attachments. The distal surface of the metaphysis is abnormal in shape and it envelops the epiphysis within a concave socket. This appearance derives from the fact that the growth of the metaphysis is most severely impaired in its central part (*Figure 1.7a*). Metaphyseal growth is retarded to a greater extent in the proximal limb bones than in the distal ones and may be unequal in extent in the paired bones. These features lead to bowing of the shafts of the long bones and other deformities such as coxa vara and genu varum. The epiphyses are relatively unaffected and, although the appearance of ossific centres at the knee may be delayed until after birth, the skeletal age in the older child is usually normal. The skull is characteristically abnormal in shape. This is due to the combination of diminished growth of the base arising from defective endochondral ossification at the spheno-occipital synchondrosis and normal growth of the cranial vault. The latter therefore appears to be relatively large. The middle portion of the base of the skull is especially shortened, the clivus is steep and the foramen magnum is small. The basal angle is reduced, ranging from 85–120 degrees. These features may lead to serious neurological sequelae due to obstruction to cerebrospinal fluid flow, and in consequence to a true hydrocephalus. Cohen *et al.* (1967) reviewing the neurological complications of achondroplasia, advocate careful attention to the rate of growth of the cranial vault. They point out that a sudden increase in size is to be regarded seriously. Some degree of ventricular dilatation, without reduction in the thickness of the cerebral cortex, can be present in achondroplasia even without obstruction. The small size of the foramen magnum may also contribute to pressure on the spinal nerves or long tracts.

Abnormalities occur in the size and shape of the spinal canal. It is characteristically narrowed from front to back due to defective growth of the pedicles, and also from side to side. This occurs especially in the lumbar region, where the interpedicular distances become smaller from the upper lumbar vertebrae to the lumbosacral junction, instead of having the normal increase at this level (*see Figure 9.22 page 353*). There is often localized thoracolumbar kyphosis associated with a central beaking of the anterior aspect of the bodies of the twelfth thoracic and first or second lumbar vertebrae (*Figure 1.7b*). This feature is similar to that already described in Hurler's syndrome and in hypothyroidism. Both these features are much less evident in the first year of life (Langer *et al.*, 1967). The most helpful feature in the diagnosis of achondroplasia at this age is the shape of the pelvis, which is always abnormal. This results from a failure of growth of the ilium at the margins of the acetabular cartilage. The 'handle' of the ilium is in consequence almost absent and the sacrosciatic notch forms a narrow cleft instead of the normal wide sweep. The sacrum articulates low on the ilium and comes to lie almost horizontally, resulting in exaggeration of the normal lumbar lordosis. The roof of the acetabulum is flat and the acetabular angle is reduced to zero or may become negative. The blade of the ilium is square in outline. The shape of the pelvic cavity is flattened from above downwards. Caffey (1958) has likened it to a champagne glass rather than the wine glass shape seen in spondylo-epiphyseal dysplasia or Hurler's syndrome, in which conditions the pelvis is narrowed from side to side. The difference between the acetabular and iliac angles is markedly increased in contrast to Hurler's syndrome (*Figure 1.7c*). The ratio between the height of the disc spaces and that of the vertebral bodies is abnormal in achondroplasia, the disc–body ratio being increased from a normal value of 0.33 to about 1.0.

The abnormalities of the spine and pelvis may lead to complications in later life, at which time the flattening of the pelvic cavity, and in particular of the inlet, may lead to dystocia in females. The combination of the narrow anteroposterior diameter of the spinal canal and the thoracolumbar kyphosis, which becomes more severe with increasing age, may lead to paraplegia. Serial radiography of the spine or myelography may assist in assessing an increase in the severity of these deformities and in indicating the need for treatment.

DYSPLASIAS ALLIED TO ACHONDROPLASIA

It has long been recognized that the extent and severity of the features of achondroplasia are variable from case to case, the abnormalities occasionally being limited to one side fo the body, to one limb or even to one bone. There has been an increasing tendency to separate these variants from classic achondroplasia, as distinct genetic entities. Some of these newly described conditions deserve a brief mention.

Hypochondroplasia

Beals (1969) has described cases which differ from classical achondroplasia in the following features. They present at a later age, they show a less severe degree of dwarfism, though this is still characteristically of the short-limbed type, and they do not exhibit the characteristic cranial, spinal and pelvic abnormalities of achondroplasia.

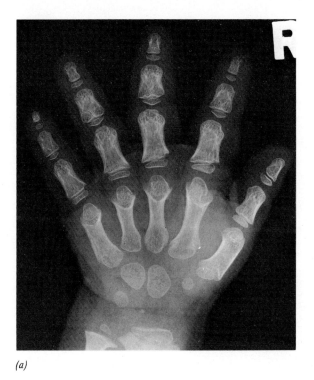

(a)

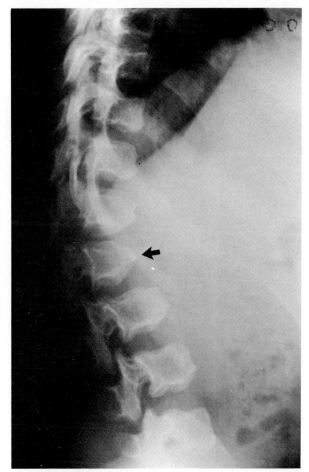

(b)

Figure 1.7. Achondroplasia: (a) The hand of a child aged 4½ years. The metacarpals and phalanges are abnormally short but of normal width. The epiphyses of the metacarpals are enveloped by the concave metaphyses. The epiphyseal and carpal bone ossification centres have developed normally and the bone age is estimated as 5.2 years (Tanner and Whitehouse method). (b) A kyphosis is present at the thoracolumbar junction associated with deformity of the body of LV2 (arrowed), the anterior surface of which is pointed. The posterior surface of the lumbar vertebrae are concave. (c) The shape of the pelvis is very characteristic with a small sacrosciatic notch (arrowed) and an acute angle between the vertical lateral borders of the ilia and the horizontal roof of the acetabula. The reduction of the interpedicular distance in the lower lumbar vertebrae, the horizontal sacrum and the short femora with exaggeration of the trochanters and muscle attachments are also notable features

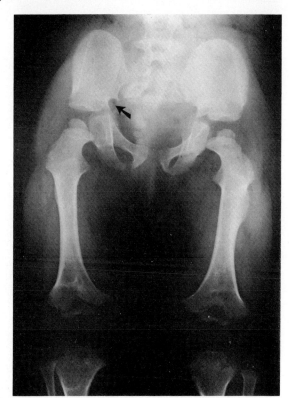

(c)

12

Achondrogenesis and thanatophoric dwarfism

Infants suffering from these conditions die early, either *in utero* or within the first weeks of postnatal life. The cause of this is still not certain, but it may be related to the defective growth of the ribs which prevents or impedes the onset of normal respiration. Compression of the medulla or of the cervical cord has also been suggested as a cause of death. Such cases have formerly been regarded as severe forms of achondroplasia, which they may resemble closely both clinically and radiologically. However, the fatal outcome contrasts with the course of patients with achondroplasia, who are usually strong and have a normal life span. The radiological features also differ. There is more marked shortening of the limb bones and ribs and a greater reduction in the height of the vertebral bodies (*Figure 1.8*). The latter may be completely unossified in achondrogenesis. The metaphyses, though irregular in shape with sharp spikes of periosteal bone at their periphery, are not flared to so great an extent as in achondroplasia. The skull is often abnormal: either it has a short base and a relatively large vault or a severe form of craniostenosis described as a 'cloverleaf skull' (*see* page 27 and *Figure 1.24*). Although very rare, these two dysplasias may be recognized *in utero*; which may be an important observation in view of their prognostic implications (Keats *et al.*, 1970).

Infantile thoracic dystrophy

A number of other conditions are known in which respiratory difficulty, arising from failure of the ribs to grow normally may be a prominent feature (*Figure 1.9*). These conditions have been well reviewed by Hull and Barnes (1972), who stress that surgical reconstruction of the thorax may allow the lungs to expand adequately on inspiration. This applies especially to cases of infantile thoracic dystrophy in whom in addition to the short

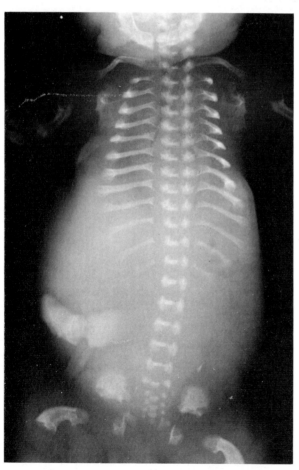

(a)

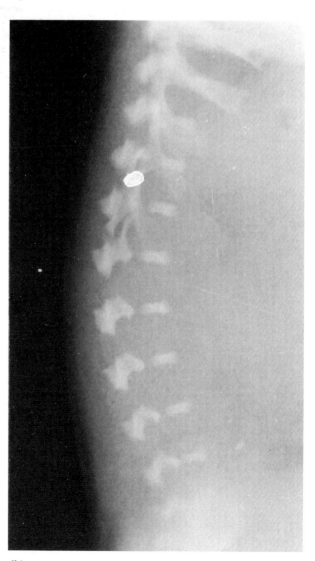

(b)

Figure 1.8. Thanatophoric Dwarfism: (a) This infant died shortly after birth. The thorax is long and narrow with very short ribs and the abdomen relatively protruberant. The vertebral bodies are grossly flattened with wide disc spaces between them and the limbs are very short with bowing of the shafts of the long bones. (b) Lateral view of the lower thoracic and lumbar spine which emphasises the flat vertebral bodies and the shortness of the ribs (By courtesy of Dr. J. M. Sheach, City Hospital, Exeter)

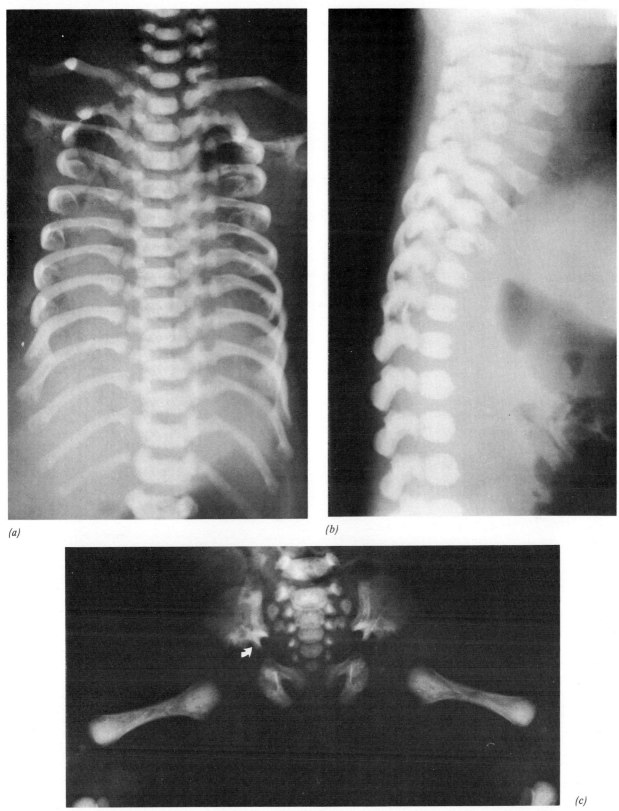

(a)

(b)

(c)

Figure 1.9. Infantile Thoracic Dystrophy: (a) The thorax is long and narrow due to the shortening of the ribs whose anterior ends are widened and cup shaped. (b) Lateral view of the thoracolumbar spine showing the very short ribs but relatively normal vetebrae. (c) The pelvis is flattened from above downwards with a characteristic trident shape of the lower border of the ilia (arrowed). The femora are short with a convexity of the metaphyses

14

ribs and consequent narrowing of the thoracic cage, the ilia are characteristically trident shaped, due to elongation of the anterior and inferior iliac spines (*Figure 1.9c*). There is also shortening of the metacarpals, metatarsals and phalanges, often with cone-shaped epiphyses as in peripheral dysostosis. If affected children survive infancy, the ribs may grow to an extent which permits fairly good respiratory function, but stature is usually diminished. The length of the limbs is less disproportionate to that of the rest of the body than in achondroplasia; the skull and spine are normal.

Diastrophic dwarfism

In this condition the presence of a severe short-limbed dwarfism may lead to confusion with achondroplasia. There is a distinctive 'constellation' of abnormalities. In addition to the shortening of the long bones there are deformities of the hands and feet in which the thumbs and big toes are short and project at right angles to the long axis of the limb ('hitch-hikers' thumb), deformed ears, a cleft palate and progressive scoliosis. The shape of the long bones, and in particular of the metaphyses, resembles achondroplasia quite closely. The spinal changes are more widespread than in achondroplasia and there is a progressive scoliosis rather than a kyphosis. In addition, the lower lumbar interpedicular distances are narrowed. The joints are often subluxated and show flexion contractures, leading to progressive deformity. The epiphyses ossify late and this is in contrast to the carpal and tarsal bones, which, though they are deformed, may ossify earlier than usual. The deformities, which are among the most striking features of this dysplasia, should enable it to be easily differentiated from achondroplasia, particularly as the child grows beyond infancy. The condition has recently been reviewed (Wilson *et al.*, 1969).

METAPHYSEAL DYSOSTOSIS

Among the skeletal dysplasias whose effects are confined to the metaphysis, a number of conditions have been grouped together under this term. These conditions have radiological features which resemble those of rickets, but they lack the characteristic biochemical abnormalities. Rarely, the disorganization of the metaphyses may be so severe as to suggest enchondromata of the type occurring in Ollier's disease. Much commoner are the cases in which widened growth plates and sclerotic, irregular metaphyses are the predominant features (*Figure 1.10*). Flaring of the metaphyses, similar to that seen in achondroplasia, and also deformities, especially at the hips and knees, may also occur and they are associated with bowing of the shafts of the long bones. The epiphyses are usually normal, although recently cases have been described in which the epiphyses are also deformed and resemble those in dysplasia epiphysealis multiplex. Similarly, the spine is commonly normal, though a variant has been described in which there is a widespread flattening of vertebral bodies, in association with metaphyseal changes, identical with other cases of metaphyseal dysostosis. Affected children present because of short stature and abnormal gait. It is important to distinguish them from cases of rickets, because they will not benefit from the administration of vitamin D. In fact, attempts to treat them as cases of vitamin D resistant rickets may easily lead to the development of toxic effects, including nephrocalcinosis and renal failure.

Certain additional abnormalities have been reported in association with the radiological picture of metaphyseal dysostosis. McKusick *et al.* (1965) has noted fine rather sparse hair, megacolon and malabsorption as in coeliac disease. He regards this as a well-defined genetic entity, which has been termed 'cartilage-hair hypoplasia'. Steatorrhoea, due to pancreatic insufficiency and

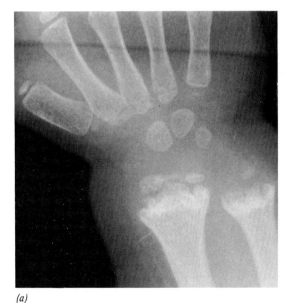 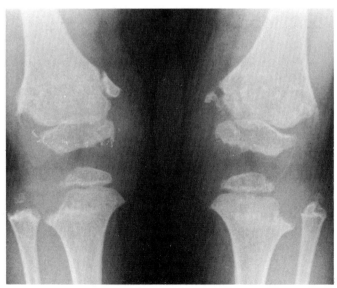

(a)   *(b)*

Figure 1.10. Metaphyseal Dysostosis: (a) The metaphyses at the distal ends of the radius and ulna are irregular and sclerotic; the epiphyses also show irregularity of ossification in this case, but in general tend to be normal. (b) The knees of the same case with irregular defects and fragmentation of the femoral and tibial metaphyses

neutropenia, forms yet another combination of abnormalities associated with metaphyseal dysostosis (Taybi *et al.*, 1969). In this variant dwarfism is often quite marked and the hips are particularly severely involved. These cases may be mistaken for fibrocystic disease, but they do not develop lung changes.

DIAPHYSEAL ACLASIS AND OLLIER'S DISEASE

These two conditions are sometimes grouped together as different expressions of a single disease process, under the term dyschondroplasia. It is, however, a matter of controversy whether they should be regarded as a form of neoplasm or as a skeletal dysplasia, in view of the fact that a common feature of both is the occurrence of multiple benign cartilage tumours. However, both conditions may be due to fragments of the growth plate becoming displaced during embryonic development. In *diaphyseal aclasis* these fragments continue to undergo endochondral ossification, but in an inappropriate situation, and characteristic osteochondromata are formed. These are composed of a stalk of bone, the cortex and trabeculation of which are continuous with those of the parent bone, and there is a cap of growth cartilage. In *Ollier's disease*, the abnormal fragment of growth cartilage lies within the central portion of the parent bone and fails to undergo ossification; it then persists as an enchondroma. However, the growth of the bone as a whole is often defective, and there may be considerable shortening and deformity. Diaphyseal aclasis is a hereditary condition and therefore would seem logically to be regarded as a skeletal dysplasia. Ollier's disease, on the other hand, is not familial or hereditary. It is however sometimes associated with other malformations, such as haemangiomata (a combination known as Maffucci's syndrome), vitiligo or melanomata.

The radiological features of diaphyseal aclasis are quite distinctive and unlikely to be confused with those of any other type of dysplasia. The osteochondromata are multiple and they may arise from the metaphyseal regions of most of the long bones, in which position they project obliquely with their apices directed away from the end of the bone. Their base may be narrow or wide. They may also originate in the spine, ribs, scapulae and pelvis. The region from which the osteochondroma arises, especially in the long bones, is frequently widened and deformed due to the interference which occurs in the normal process of modelling (*Figure 1.11*). Linear growth is not often impaired. The osteochondroma may lead to pressure effects on adjacent structures such as other bones, nerves, blood vessels or the spinal cord. Chondrosarcomas have been reported in a small proportion of cases and this complication may be detected by a change in the radiological appearances of the lesions.

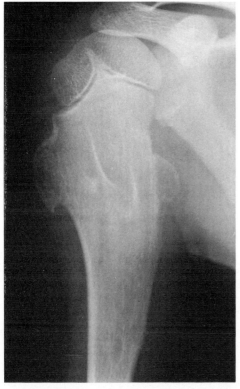

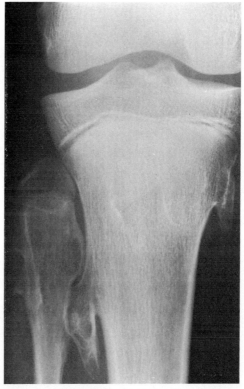

(a)   *(b)*

Figure 1.11. Diaphyseal Aclasis: (a) The upper end of the humerus with broad-based osteochondromata arising from the medial and lateral aspects; the widening of the shaft due to lack of normal modelling ('aclasis') is well shown. (b) Upper ends of tibia and fibula with several osteochondromata; one of those arising from the tibia has produced a pressure defect on the adjacent fibula. The apices of the tumours project towards the centre of the shaft

16

In Ollier's disease enchondromata appear as well-defined, translucent areas in the bone and characteristically contain dense, speckled or streaky areas of calcification within the limits of the lesion. If large enough they cause expansion of the bone and thinning of the cortex. The affected bones are often markedly shortened and sometimes bowed (*Figure 1.12*). The chondromata in the small bones of the hands and feet may grow to a considerable extent, producing gross deformities, but continued enlargement often ceases after the growth of the body comes to an end (*see Figure 2.7*). The epiphyses are unaffected in the early stages, but may be involved later. The lesions are often situated on one side of the body only, a distribution which is similar to that seen in fibrous dysplasia with which Ollier's disease can sometimes be confused clinically. Pathological fracture, though relatively uncommon, may be a presenting symptom. The haemangiomata of Maffucci's syndrome, while usually obvious clinically, may give radiological signs in the form of small calcified thrombi visible as phleboliths within the soft tissues. As in diaphyseal aclasis, sarcomatous change may sometimes occur.

CHONDROECTODERMAL DYSPLASIA (ELLIS–VAN CREVELD SYNDROME)

Although this is a very rare type of skeletal dysplasia it is of interest in that there are characteristic radiological

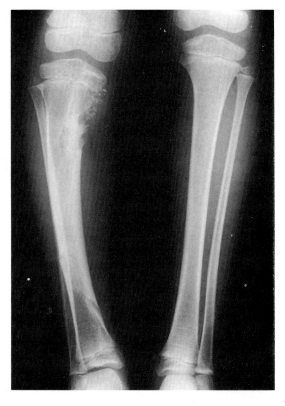

Figure 1.12. Ollier's Disease: Chondromata are present at both ends of the tibia, which is shortened and bowed laterally

features which enable it to be recognized fairly easily. The bone lesions are associated with anomalies of many other tissues and organs. Of the latter the most striking are the abnormalities of the hair, nails and teeth resembling those of ectodermal dysplasia, but more serious abnormalities occur in the heart and lungs. A single atrium giving rise to a cor triloculare is the commonest of the cardiac anomalies, though septal defects, aortic valve lesions and transposition of the great arteries have also been reported. Such heart lesions occur in just over half the cases and to a large extent determine the chance of survival. Pulmonary function and development may also be defective; in this respect the ribs are very short and the thorax in consequence very small (*see Infantile thoracic dystrophy, page 12*).

The skeletal dysplasia results in a short-limbed type of dwarfism superficially resembling achondroplasia, but it affects the distal segments of the limbs, especially the hands and feet. The metacarpals, metatarsals and phalanges are short and wide. The metaphyses of the long bones are irregular, but show a curious variability in shape, some being widened and others narrowed and tapered. The appearances at the proximal end of the tibia are, according to Caffey (1952), particularly characteristic. The metaphysis is wide and slopes obliquely on either side of the midpoint and there is a small eccentrically placed epiphysis on its medial aspect. Fusion of carpal bones, especially the capitate and hamate, and polydactyly of the hands are also characteristic features.

DIAPHYSEAL DYSPLASIAS

OSTEOGENESIS IMPERFECTA

This is one of the commonest of skeletal dysplasias and, in spite of a considerable degree of variation in severity, is one of the most easily recognizable. Multiple and recurrent fractures are prominent features and this condition should be considered in any child presenting with fractures which occur after inadequate trauma (Levin, 1964). The frequency of fracture and their sites vary considerably from case to case, but if numerous, they will often lead to marked deformity of the long bones which become thickened and shortened as the fractures heal.

Deformities, however, also arise because of the effect of weight-bearing and other stresses acting on the relatively soft bones, which may become bent into grotesque shapes. Together with an excessive tubulation of the shafts this gives rise to a characteristic appearance of abnormally thin, severely bowed long bones (*Figure 1.13c*). The spine and pelvis are also deformed, there being severe kyphosis or double scoliosis and protrusio acetabuli, the latter possibly leading to a triradiate pelvis (*Figure 1.13b*) The vertebral bodies resemble those of osteoporosis with concavity of the end-plates due to the bulging of the intervertebral discs into the adjacent vertebral bodies. The skull also shares in the effects of bone-softening, and this process results in basilar invagination and an outward bulging of the vault over the skull-base to give an appearance similar to a 'tam o'shanter'. This, together with the multiple Wormian bones and relatively poor bone density, produces a characteristic appearance (*Figure 1.13a*). The facial

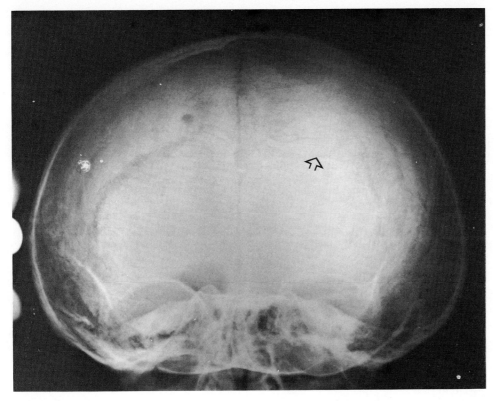

(a)

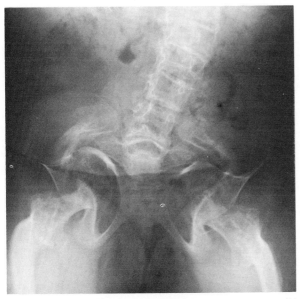

(b)

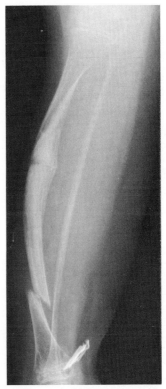

(c)

Figure 1.13. Osteogenesis Imperfecta: (a) Anteroposterior view of the skull in which the vault is flattened and widened and the base protrudes upwards in the midline ('basilar invagination'). The presence of numerous sutural bones (arrowed) is a common feature ('mosaic skull'). (b) Softening of the spine and pelvis has resulted in a scoliosis and a severe protrusio acetabuli (triradiate pelvis). (c) Multiple fractures and bowing of the tibia; the bones are decalcified and over-constricted (except where callus has formed in relation to the healing fracture)

bones are relatively small and hypoplastic, so that the skull in the postero-anterior projection has the appearance of an inverted triangle. The teeth are abnormal in that the pulp canal is absent, but the enamel layer is normal. The lamina dura, though it is often preserved, may disappear.

The bony trabecular pattern may be abnormal, not only from the effects of the healing fractures, but also owing to the development of a peculiar 'whorled' appearance of the spongiosa of the ends of the shafts of the long bones. The cortex is thinner than normal and the middle thirds of the shafts narrower than normal. The joints are hypermobile due to laxity of the ligaments and capsular attachments, and there may be dislocations, especially affecting the head of the radius. This feature serves to emphasize the fact that this disease is one of connective tissue generally and its effects are not confined to the skeletal system. Bone formation as such is not deficient, and this is confirmed by the manner in which some of the fractures heal. The production of callus may at times be so abundant as to lead to suspicion of the presence of a malignant tumour, not only from the radiological appearances but also from the clinical and histological features. However, the structure of such bone is abnormal and recent opinion is in favour of a defect in the bone matrix, and in particular collagen production, as the basic lesion in this condition.

The variation in the severity of this disease may be reflected in the radiological appearance. On the one hand the condition may be very mild, consisting of little more than an increased liability of fractures; on the other hand it may be severe, with a considerable growth defect and deformities which are so gross as to lead to a bizarre and unmistakeable picture. In severe cases, the disease may be recognized radiologically from the appearances of the fetus *in utero*. The density of the bones may be so poor as to make it difficult to detect a fetus at all. The petrous temporal bones may however stand out by contrast and be mistaken for calcification in the maternal mesenteric glands (Aitken *et al.*, 1965). Usually, however, sufficient detail can be detected to reveal the presence of a fetus which has abnormally short limbs and deformities of the spine and thorax. These fetuses not infrequently fail to survive the stress of labour and are stillborn.

The differential diagnosis of cases of osteogenesis imperfecta is not usually difficult. The short limbs in the severely affected cases resemble achondroplasia, but the other radiological features are very different. The appearances of the cranial vault are similar to cleidocranial dysostosis and pyknodysostosis, but again the features elsewhere in the skeleton should be distinctive.

FIBROUS DYSPLASIA

It is possible that this term includes several disease entities, which are characterized by the presence of a common histology. Certainly the radiological appearances are variable and correspond to differences in the natural history and course of the condition. An accepted classification of cases of fibrous dysplasia is into monostotic and polyostotic forms, according to whether a single bone or several bones are affected. Craniofacial lesions do not easily fit into this classification and have a different radiological appearance from those in the long bones. Clinically, also, there are cases in which a polyostotic type of fibrous dysplasia is associated with skin pigmentation and sexual and skeletal precocity; these cases are commonly separated from the others as the McCune—Albright syndrome.

Monostotic fibrous dysplasia

This type of the disease presents relatively late in childhood in most cases (Gibson and Middlemiss, 1971). However, Turner *et al.* (1963) have described cases resembling in most respects those of a monostotic fibrous dysplasia in newborn infants (*Figure 1.14b).*

The commonest bones to be affected in the monostotic type are the femur and tibia. Radiologically the lesions are shown as osteolytic areas which are usually eccentrically placed in relation to the cortex and medulla of the long bones, and they have a dense margin which is well defined on its inner surface, but fades more gradually into the surrounding bone. The central part of the lesion may contain a few coarse trabeculae and show a diffuse increase in bone density. The cortex over the lesion may be thinned and expanded (*Figure 1.14*). If this feature is not present at the first examination serial films reveal that the condition undergoes slow expansion, at least until after puberty, at which time growth of the skeleton as a whole ceases. Pathological fracture, though not uncommon is often responsible for bringing the condition to the notice of the patient. Healing of such fractures occurs normally. There may also be a recurrence of the condition after incomplete surgical excision and bone grafting.

Polyostotic fibrous dysplasia

This is also most commonly seen in the femur and tibia, but it may involve the other limb bones, the pelvis, the skull and facial bones, the ribs, spine and scapulae. When the possibility of this type of fibrous dysplasia is suspected, a radiograph of the pelvis and thighs is the most generally useful examination and will show the presence of an abnormality in over 90 per cent of cases. The radiological appearances differ considerably from those of the monostotic type (*Figure 1.15*). Though commonest in the metaphyses of the long bones, the disease tends to spread throughout the whole length of the bone instead of remaining as a localized lesion. Furthermore, the cortex is directly involved in the disease process instead of being merely thinned and expanded by a predominantly medullary lesion. The whole architecture of the bone is disturbed. The differentiation between cortex and medulla is lost and the trabecular pattern of the spongiosa replaced by a confusion of shadows of differing density, mixed up together to give an appearance which is well described by Falconer and Cope (1942) as being like slowly ascending columns of smoke. Areas of translucency occur, but they have ill-defined margins and are very variable in size and shape. There is no generalized decalcification of the bones. Areas of increased density occur, either giving an amorphous 'ground glass' appearance, or sometimes a coarsely

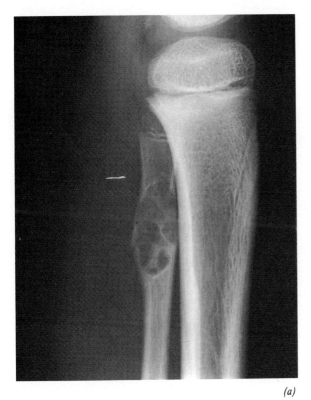

(a)

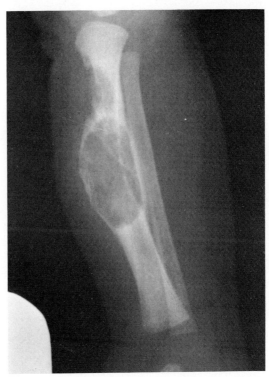

(b)

Figure 1.14. Monostotic Fibrous Dysplasia: (a) A lesion of the upper end of the fibula, through which a pathological fracture has occurred. (b) Lesions in the tibia of an infant in the first month of life; one has expanded and thinned the cortex. The condition is very unusual in a child as young as this and such cases have been described as 'neonatal fibrous dysplasia'

granular pattern resembling the skin of an orange. Increased bone density is particularly characteristic of fibrous dysplasia of the skull base and facial bones, to much an extent that they have been described as a separate variant (*Figure 1.15c*).

Deformities, mostly due to softening of the bones, occur commonly in the later stages and are associated with considerable thickening of the shafts of the affected bones. Coxa vara is one of the most frequent types of deformity. It may be severe and associated with bowing of the femoral shaft, giving rise to the type of deformity described as the shepherd's crook femur. Scoliosis, kyphosis and contraction of the pelvic cavity are also not uncommon. In cases of the *McCune–Albright syndrome*, the radiological appearances of the bones do not differ from those of other types of polyostotic disease, but the bone age may be accelerated due to the skeletal precocity. The rate of spread of polyostotic lesions is very variable and can sometimes be quite slow. A progressive course is, however, the rule and it is likely that in some, if not all, cases, it continues after the cessation of normal growth.

The diagnosis of polyostotic fibrous dysplasia is usually easy, the appearances being distinctive. Although historically the condition was for some time confused with hyperparathyroidism, under the general term of 'osteitis fibrosa', the presence of diffuse decalcification of bone and of cortical erosions should enable this condition to be distinguished from fibrous dysplasia. Paget's disease may resemble polyostotic fibrous dysplasia radiologically, but it is not a disease of childhood and differs in its clinical features. Monostotic fibrous

dysplasia, on the other hand, may be much more difficult to diagnose because the radiological appearances are in no way pathognomonic. Confusion with bone systs, fibrous cortical defects, congenital pseudarthrosis, and enchondromata may readily occur and the distinction may not be possible radiologically.

SCLEROSING DIAPHYSEAL DYSPLASIAS

Osteopetrosis

This condition is relatively easily diagnosed from the characteristic radiological appearances and is often discovered as an incidental finding in patients who are examined for some other purpose. The condition is known to exist in two forms, which are genetically distinct. One form is inherited as a dominant and presents in adolescence, or even in adult life, with few symptoms other than a liability to fracture easily (*Figure 1.16*). The other form is inherited as a recessive and presents soon after birth with severe symptons and a bad prognosis due to a progressive anaemia, hydrocephalus, cranial nerve involvement and an increased liability to infection.

In both forms radiographs of any part of the skeleton reveal a diffuse increase in bone density without significant changes in morphology (*Figures 1.16 and 1.17*). The individual bones retain their recognizable shape, but there is a slight tendency towards defective modelling in the shafts of the long bones. The normal distinction between cortex and medulla may be lost and the bone

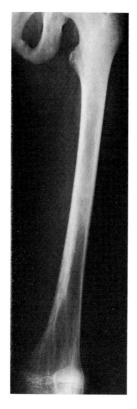

(a)

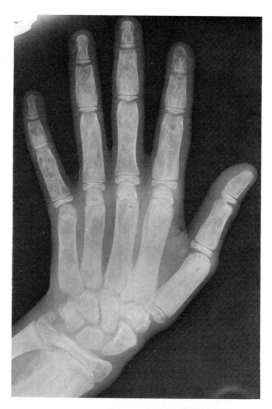

(b)

(c)

Figure 1.15. Polyostotic Fibrous Dysplasia: (a) Areas of increased bone density involving both the cortex and medulla are present in the femur of this girl aged 9 years who also had pigmented spots and sexual precocity. She is thus an example of the McCune—Albright syndrome. (b) The hand of another case showing increased bone density, coarse trabeculation and expansion of the central portion of the diaphyses. (c) A third case in which the skull base is thickened and abnormally dense. Evidence of fibrous dysplasia was present elsewhere in the skeleton

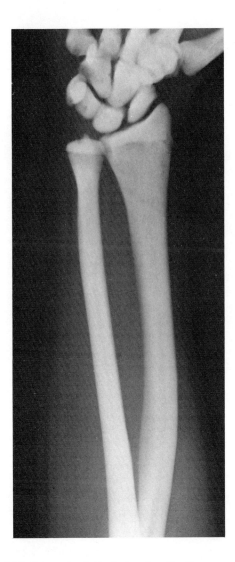

Figure 1.16. Osteopetrosis (tarda form): The forearm and wrist of an adolescent boy with the dominant form of the disease. The bones show a uniform increase in density but are normal in shape and size

therefore appears uniformly dense throughout. It is not uncommon, however, especially in the severe recessive type, for local variations in density to occur (*Figure 1.17c*). These may take the form either of transverse striations or of an endobone in which the outline of the bone as it originally was at an earlier stage in development can be seen within it, separated from the rest of the bone by a zone of lesser density. These effects are the result of variations in the amount of bone laid down at different times. Changes which may occur at the metaphyses resemble rickets in their radiological appearance; the exact nature of these changes is not known. The presence of fractures resulting from the abnormal brittleness of the bones has been mentioned, and these heal rapidly, but some delay in subsequent remodelling is likely. The teeth are often abnormal and they have small underdeveloped roots and absent pulp cavities. An increased thickness of the lamina dura has been described, but it is difficult to detect owing to tne density of the surrounding bone. Trapnell (1968)

points out that it may be a useful distinguishing sign in patients in whom osteomyelitis of the mandible has developed. Osteomyelitis is liable to occur in osteopetrosis, and this sign may help to separate these cases from those in whom osteomyelitis produces sclerosis in otherwise normal bone.

Pyknodysostosis

This uncommon dysplasia exhibits features which are characteristic both of osteopetrosis (uniformly increased bone density and a tendency to multiple fractures from insufficient cause) and of cleidocranial dysostosis (defective ossification of the cranial vault and clavicles). These features are combined with a short-limbed type of dwarfism. In addition, there are widened sutures with multiple Wormian bones, hypoplasia of the jaws with an increased mandibular angle and frequent mandibular fractures. Vertebral fusion may occur especially between the atlas and axis and at the lumbosacral junction. The teeth are abnormally shaped and the deciduous teeth tend to persist. The bones of the hands, especially the distal phalanges, are abnormal and show a progressive shortening and tapering, with absent distal tufts.

Progressive diaphyseal dysplasia (Englemann's disease)

This dysplasia is often familial and is, at least when considered over a period of years, fairly easily recognized from its radiological appearance. It presents in early childhood with a fusiform or cylindrical expansion of the central part of the diaphyses of the long bones, and this is due to progressive thickening of the cortex on both its endosteal and periosteal aspects (*Figure 1.18*). The distribution of the abnormal bone is symmetrical on the two sides of the body and at first is sharply demarcated from the normal metaphyses and epiphyses. The changes spread towards the metaphyses, involving bone that was previously normal. (Neuhauser *et al.*, 1948) (*Figure 1.18c*). The periosteal thickening is often laminated at first, but as the condition progresses this is less apparent. The distinction between cortex and medulla becomes blurred. The cortical bone is irregularly converted into cancellous bone and this leads to the development of areas of lesser density, particularly in the vicinity of the foramina for the nutrient artery. The progressive nature of the condition is one of its important features. As the child matures more of each individual bone and more of the skeleton as a whole becomes involved in the disease. No bone is exempt, although the extremities and spine are likely to be involved late in the disease. The skull and facial bones show marked thickening and increase in density which may lead to facial deformity of the leontiasis ossea type and also to deafness and optic atrophy.

CHROMOSOMAL DYSPLASIAS

TRISOMY

This type of chromosomal abnormality results in a wide spectrum of development defects, among which the

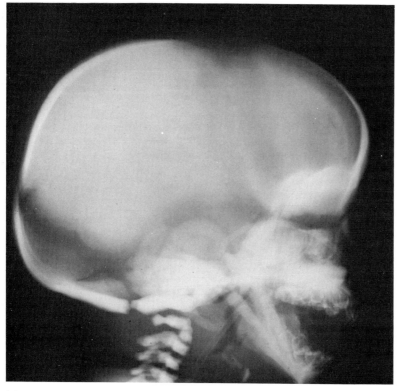
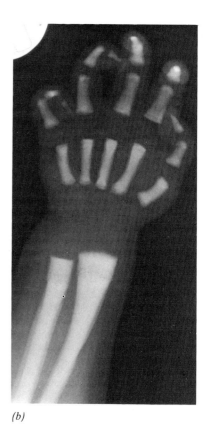

(a)   (b)

Figure 1.17. Osteopetrosis (congenita form): (a) The skull of an infant aged 1 month with the recessive type. The increased bone density is associated with some degree of thickening especially of the skull base and the sutures appear unusually prominent by contrast. (b) The hand and wrist of the same infant as in Figure 1.17a. The metaphyses are slightly ill-defined and there is a transverse lucent zone crossing the diaphysis and less dense periosteal new bone along the shaft of the radius and ulna

skeletal lesions comprise only a relatively minor part. However, from the radiological point of view, bone lesions present characteristic features which may help in the recognition of affected infants, particularly when the clinical signs are indefinite.

Trisomy of the 13–15 group (Patau's syndrome) and Trisomy of the 17–18 group (Edwards' syndrome)

In these two diseases the clinical signs are usually severe and sufficiently characteristic to allow recognition of the condition. The radiological features are nevertheless of some interest and have been well reviewed by Astley (1966). In Trisomy 17–18, the most constant signs are in the thorax, which is wide in its transverse diameter, with ribs which are slender and irregular and clavicles which are thin and defective. In the hands and feet, the thumbs and big toes are characteristically hypoplastic and there are V-shaped gaps between the first and second toes and between the fingers. The phalanges and metacarpals are small and poorly ossified and, in the lateral view of the feet, the forefoot is dorsiflexed relative to the talus and calcaneum, resulting in the rocker-bottom type of deformity. The pelvis is small and the ilia are rotated upwards and medially so that the acetabular and iliac angles are increased. There is a high incidence of cardiac, gastrointestinal and genito-urinary anomalies which may also give rise to radiological abnormalities. Cases of Trisomy 13–15 give a somewhat similar radiological picture, but the abnormalities are not so extensive. They have certain features, such as polydactyly, severe microcephaly and midline clefts in the skull which are characteristic.

Trisomy 21–22 (Down's syndrome)

The radiological features are less striking than in the types described above. The shape of the pelvis is, however, often characteristic and is due to an outward and downward rotation of the ilia which appear flared with decreased iliac and acetabular angles (*see* page 355). Astley (1963), using the iliac index (Caffey and Ross, 1956), found that, although there was some overlap with a series of normal controls, an iliac index of below 60 was very suggestive of Trisomy 21–22, whereas a value of over 78 probably excluded it. The shape of the skull has also been considered to be abnormal but this is not easy to recognize radiologically, apart from orbital hypotelorism leading to an abnormally small interorbital distance. Clinodactyly, brachymesophalangia of the little fingers and a V-shaped gap between the first and second toes are features which are not uncommon but they are by no means diagnostic. In the spine, dislocation of the atlas relative to the axis and irregularities of the vertebral bodies resembling those in Scheuermann's disease are seen in older children or young adults with this syndrome.

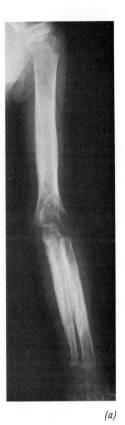 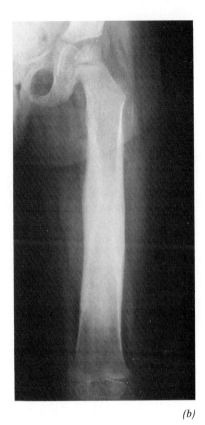 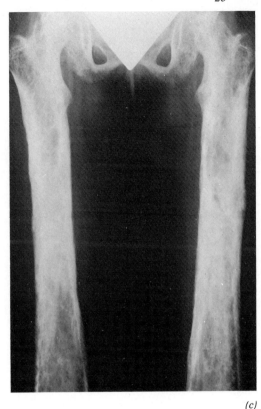

(a)   *(b)*   *(c)*

Figure 1.18. Progressive Diaphyseal Dysplasia: (a) The left arm of a girl aged 2½ years with increased width and density of the central part of the diaphyses; the cortex is thickened and the corticomedullary junction ill defined. The metaphyses and epiphyses are relatively unaffected. (b) The left femur of the same case with similar diaphyseal thickening. (c) The femora of the same case at the age of 13½ years, by which time the increased bone density and cortical thickening are more widespread and extend further along the shaft towards the metaphyses

ABNORMALITIES OF THE SEX CHROMOSOMES

Turner's syndrome

In this condition there is only a single X chromosome and there is no development of the gonads. These abnormalities are associated with a well-recognized pattern of somatic anomalies, of which the short stature and webbing of the neck are familiar features. These are accompanied in a proportion of cases by an equally characteristic pattern of radiological features of the bones (Astley, 1963; Haddad and Wilkins, 1959). There is loss of bone density and a coarse trabecular pattern in the hands and around the major joints of the limbs; these features are probably related to the deficiency in oestrogens. The thorax is widened and there are irregularities in the outline of the ribs and widening of the intercostal spaces (*Figure 1.19a*). Scoliosis, kyphosis and lordosis are occasionally present, but more striking are irregularities of the angles of the vertebral bodies, which resemble those in Scheuermann's disease. They may be associated with flattening of the vertebral body as a whole. Partial fusion of the cervical vertebrae or hypoplasia of the atlas has also been described in association with the short, webbed neck. Clinically, cubitus valgus is a common feature, but radiologically the appearances of the wrist joint and metacarpals are more striking. The distal ends of the radius and ulna

may be deformed and the ulnar styloid process absent. The proximal carpal bones may be misshapen and they are often fused. There may also be a decrease in the carpal angle (*see* page 39). The fourth metacarpal is relatively short, both in relation to the third metacarpal and to the phalanges, and the bones of the hand are abnormally slender, apart from the tufts of the distal phalanges which are large, producing a drumstick deformity (*Figure 1.19b*). There is also a deformity of the medial condyles of the tibiae which are large, depressed and protrude to the medial side of the knee. These appearances to some degree resemble Blount's disease (*see* page 32 and *Figure 1.19c*). The skeletal abnormalities, together with the presence of cardiac and renal lesions, form a distinctive and diagnostic combination which assists in differentiation from other types of growth defect. The relation of the skeletal maturation to bone growth is also distinctive in that, before puberty, the two are associated as in constitutional or primordial dwarfism, the bone age being that of a normal female child. However, after puberty the pattern changes with progressive slowing of maturation, related to the absence of gonadal hormones. Epiphyseal fusion may not be completed until 25 years of age or even older.

It is recognized that radiological and somatic abnormalities similar to those in Turner's syndrome occur in both boys and girls with normal sex chromosomes and such cases are referred to a *Noonan's syndrome* or the *Turner phenotype*. In general, these conform to the

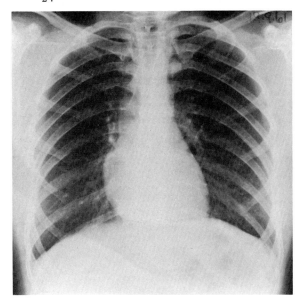

(a)

Figure 1.19. Turner's Syndrome: (a) In the thorax, the anterior ends of the ribs are narrow and widely separated. The heart in this case was normal, but in a proportion of cases signs of coarctation of the aorta may be present (see Chapter 4). (b) The bones of the hand are lacking in density with a coarse open trabecular pattern; the lunate and triquetral bones are fused and the fourth metacarpal is short relative to the adjacent meta-carpals and phalanges. (c) The medial tibial condyle is deformed with an obliquity of the articular surface

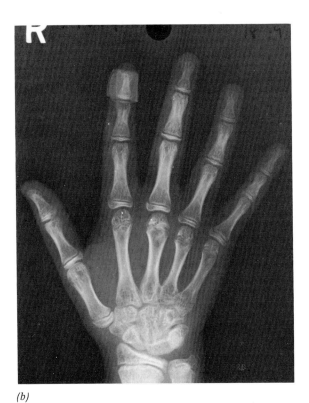

(b)

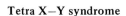

(c)

same pattern as in Turner's syndrome, but there are certain differences of emphasis. In Noonan's syndrome there is a greater degree of craniofacial involvement, including microcephaly, hypoplasia of the mandible and dental malocclusion. Other features are sternal deformity, either depression or increased convexity, and a higher incidence of fusion of the vertebrae and carpal bones.

Tetra X—Y syndrome

Radiological anomalies are also common in this con-dition (Houston, 1967). The cranial capacity is markedly reduced and there is an increase in the thickness of the bones of the vault. There are small or absent paranasal sinuses and hypertelorism with the interorbital distance exceeding 30 mm. Kyphosis also occurs and it is occasionally accompanied by scoliosis and vertebral fusion. Deformities of the humerus, radius and ulna at the elbows, together with either radio-ulnar synostosis or dislocation of the head of the radius, are particularly characteristic. Other less common deformities are elongation of the distal end of the ulna, irregularity or absence of carpal bones, a shallow intercondylar fossa of the femur and short, wide distal phalanges of the big toes which are separated from the other toes by a wide gap. Skeletal maturation is retarded, especially after puberty, as in Turner's syndrome, and growth may be excessive due to delayed epiphyseal fusion.

CRANIOFACIAL DYSPLASIAS

This group includes a number of skeletal dysplasias in which the predominant changes involve the skull and facial bones, either alone or in combination with anomalies of other parts of the skeleton or of various organs.

CRANIOSTENOSIS

Premature fusion of the sutures of the cranial vault may result in a variety of bizarre deformities of the head, depending on which sutures are involved. There are three common types:

(1) That in which the sagittal suture fuses early, resulting in a long, flat, narrow head.

(2) That in which one or both coronal sutures are fused and in which the head is tall and short.

(3) That in which multiple sutures are fused. In this type the head is often less abnormal in shape than in the others, but there is an increase in intracranial pressure due to the overall reduction in cranial capacity (*Figure 1.20*).

The relation between the abnormality in the shape of the head and the sutures which are affected is defined by Virchow's law, which states that growth of the cranial vault is prevented from occurring in a direction at right angles to the affected suture, but that to compensate for this, excessive growth can occur parallel to it (*Figure 1.21*). In skull radiographs the fused sutures are no longer visible, or they may be narrower than would be expected in a normal child of a comparable age. Sometimes they have a dense or heaped-up margin. The effects of increased intracranial pressure are similar to those seen in cerebral tumours or hydrocephalus, but they occur in a skull in which the vault is of normal or reduced size. An increase in the depth and extent of the normal 'convolutional' indentations of the inner table is a particularly prominent feature, but erosion of the dorsum sellae and of other prominences of the skull base may also occur. Assessment of the cranial capacity from radiographs may be especially useful in this condition, because when only one suture is

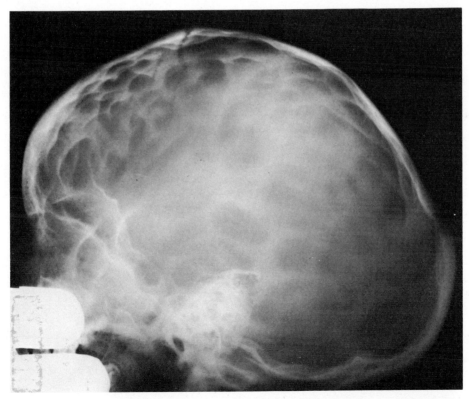

Figure 1.20. Craniostenosis — Multiple Sutural Fusion: The skull of a child with premature fusion of both the sagittal and coronal sutures. The shape of the vault is not grossly abnormal, but there is evidence of a rise in intracranial pressure. This has produced a marked increase in convolutional markings on the inner table especially over the vertex and frontal regions. The anterior part of the base of the skull is shortened with backward prolongation of the occipital bones

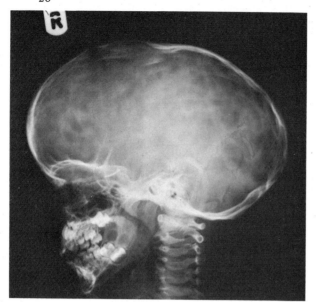

(a)

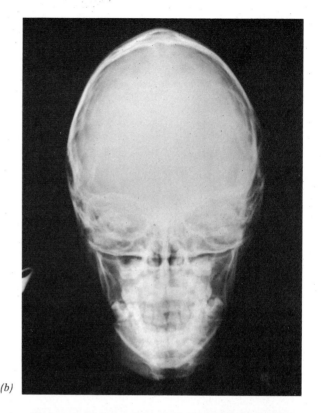

(b)

Figure 1.21. Craniostenosis – Sagittal Fusion: (a) Fusion of the sagittal suture alone results in considerable deformity of the cranial vault which is long and relatively diminished in height ('scaphocephaly'). (b) Anteroposterior view showing that the sagittal suture is not visible

involved, the compensatory growth at the open sutures may be sufficient to allow normal brain growth to occur, whereas this may not be the case when multiple sutures are fused. Head circumference measurements may be misleading when considerable abnormalities in the shape of the vault are present.

An interesting and very characteristic radiographic pattern may be produced when only one coronal suture fuses prematurely. The cranial vault in such a case becomes asymmetrical, with reduction in the size of the hemicranium on the side of the fused suture. The floor of the anterior fossa and the lesser wing of the sphenoid on this side are both elevated, but paradoxically, the petrous bone and the temporomandibular joint are depressed due to compensatory growth at the unfused temporoparietal suture. The orbit on the abnormal side is elliptical in shape and its upper and outer angle is drawn out to an acute angle. The point of junction of the sagittal and lambdoid sutures is deviated to the abnormal side. This appearance, and especially the shape of the orbit, is very characteristic (Figure 1.22). Conversely, the appearance in the more serious cases of craniostenosis with multiple sutural fusions may be much less abnormal, at least until severely raised intracranial pressure has occurred with irreversible brain damage. In some cases early diagnosis will enable this to be prevented, but it has become increasingly apparent that many cases of craniostenosis are accompanied by cerebral hypoplasia, which arises as an associated feature, unaffected by the extent or severity of the craniostenosis.

Other congenital anomalies are often associated with craniostenosis, particularly in relation to the rest of the skeleton. Synostoses have been described between many individual bones. Syndactyly of the hands and feet,

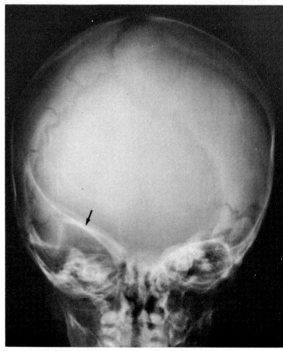

Figure 1.22. Craniostenosis – Hemicoronal Fusion: Anteroposterior view of the skull of a child with fusion of the right coronal suture only. The cranial vault is asymmetrical with a reduction in the size of the right hemicranium, and elevation of the roof of the right orbit (arrowed), which is elliptical in shape. The other sutures are abnormally wide and the right petrous temporal bone lies at a lower level than the left owing to the compensatory downward expansion of the middle and posterior fossae

distinctive in that the digits are joined by the distal phalanges, constitute a characteristic entity, known as acrocephalosyndactyly or Apert's syndrome (*Figure 1.23*). Synostoses have also been described involving the vertebrae, radius, ulna and humerus at the elbow and the tarsal bones, suggesting that there may be an overall tendency throughout the skeletal for contiguous bones to fuse with one another.

Craniostenosis, combined with hypoplasia of facial bones, small nasal cavities and defects of the sinuses and palate, occurs in Crouzon's disease (*Figure 1.24*). A severe deformity of the head, which is trilobed in shape, can result when craniostenosis is combined with a failure of normal growth of the base of the skull. This can be associated with shortening of the limb bones and bony ankylosis of the elbows and is termed the cloverleaf skull (*Figure 1.24*). The outlook is poor and most affected children die in early infancy. Duggan *et al.* (1970) have compiled a list of the conditions with which craniostenosis may be associated and in most of these it is clearly part of the congenital abnormality. There is, however, a condition in which the craniostenosis follows the performance of a ventricular shunt procedure for the treatment of hydrocephalus (*see Figure 8.29*, page 318). There is evidence to suggest that this occurs when the valve used operates at too low a pressure, and allows too rapid a reduction in the intracranial pressure. The effect of this is to allow the bones of the cranial vault to become contiguous, which results in rapid sutural fusion. There is evidence to suggest that the shape which results from such fusion may be of a distinctive type: the skull is relatively tall and narrow (Andersson, 1966).

CLEIDOCRANIAL DYSOSTOSIS

In this dysplasia the abnormalities predominantly affect bones ossified in membrane. The appearance of the cranial vault has some resemblance to that seen in osteogenesis imperfecta. There are wide fontanelles and multiple sutural bones. The base of the skull is unaffected and there is little or no deformity due to bone softening. The association of these skull changes with defective ossification of the clavicles and of the symphysis pubis enables this condition to be recognized easily (*Figure 1.25*).

MANDIBULOFACIAL DYSOSTOSIS ('FIRST ARCH SYNDROME')

This is a syndrome in which the abnormalities are localized to the facial bones, jaws and ears. It can be recognized by the facial appearance. The jaws are small the malar bones absent or defective and there is an

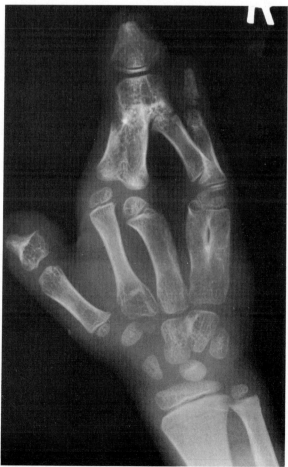

(a)

(b)

Figure 1.23. Craniostenosis – Acrocephalosyndactyly (Apert's Syndrome: (a) Lateral view of the skull. The cranial vault is abnormally tall and relatively short from front to back (turricephaly). This occurs with fusion of both coronal sutures. Treatment has been undertaken by the construction of artificial sutures with strips of metal foil to prevent subsequent fusion and to allow expansion of the cranial cavity. (b) The hand of the same child with the characteristic fusion of the distal and middle phalanges; the proximal phalanx of the thumb is absent

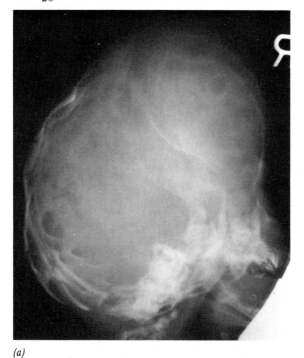

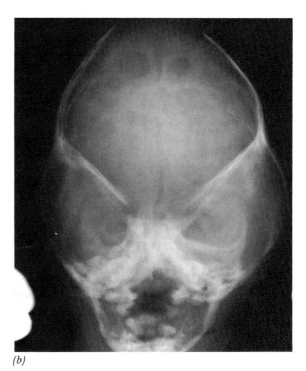

(a)   (b)

Figure 1.24. Craniostenosis – Crouzon's Disease: (a) Lateral view of the skull of an infant born with a severely deformed cranial vault due to fusion of the lower ends of the coronal and of the sagittal sutures; the base of the skull is severely shortened and the facial bones are hypoplastic. (b) Anteroposterior view of the same infant showing the striking 'trilobed' appearance of the cranial vault. This child shows the features both of Crouzon's disease and of the cloverleaf skull

antimongoloid slant to the eyes. Radiology is of importance in demonstrating the extent of the abnormalities of the ear, especially the presence or absence of ossicles and the fact that the inner ear structures are normally developed (Stovin *et al.*, 1960). This may indicate whether surgical treatment can alleviate the deafness from which these children suffer. It has been suggested that a developmental error in the formation of the first and second branchial arches and of the cleft between them is responsible for this condition.

CRANIOLACUNIA

Defects in the cranial vault may occur in the newborn infant, associated with hydrocephalus and meningomyelocoele. These are of little practical importance and disappear rapidly as the child grows. They may, however, be recognized *in utero* and should not be confused with the convolutional markings resulting from increased intracranial pressure. The margins of the defects in craniolacunia are much more sharply defined (*Figure 1.26*).

OTHER TYPES

A number of congenital syndromes have been described in which craniofacial abnormalities are combined with growth defects and with anomalies of the vertebrae and of the hands and feet. In some of these conditions, radiology of affected areas may suggest the diagnosis and delineate the extent and cause of the disabilities. This is particularly the case in the following conditions.

Hallermann-Streiff syndrome

The cranial vault is large and poorly ossified, the mandible is hypoplastic, there are spinal anomalies and the bone age is retarded.

Oropalatal digital syndrome

The base of the skull is dense and the sutures are wide. The hips and radial heads are dislocated and the carpal and tarsal bones of the phalanges of the toes are deformed.

Rubinstein-Taybi syndrome

There are dental abnormalities, microcephaly, short broad thumbs and big toes, the distal phalanges of which are displaced outwards.

Oculo-auriculo-vertebral dysplasia (Goldenhar syndrome)

Defects in development of the ears occur and there are deformed or fused vertebral bodies, agenesis of sacrum, hemivertebrae and spina bifida.

De Lange's syndrome

There is microcephaly, brachycephaly, dysplasia of the head of the radius often with dislocation, short first metacarpals, clinodactyly, brachymesophalangia of the

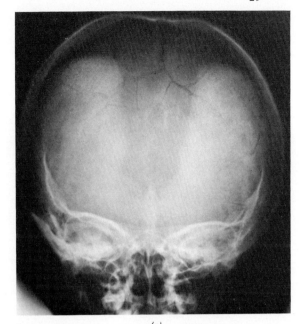

Figure 1.25. Cleidocranial Dysostosis: (a) Anteroposterior view of the skull showing the defective ossification of the bones of the vault with a very enlarged anterior fontanelle and several sutural bones. (b) Orthopantomogram of the jaws of the same case showing irregularity of dentition. (c) Chest film showing the characteristic defects in the ossification of both clavicles

(a)

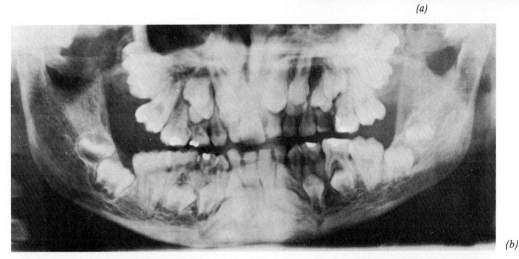

(b)

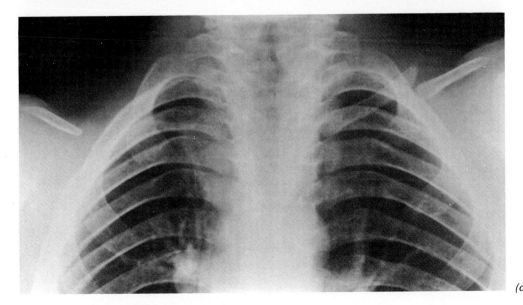

(c)

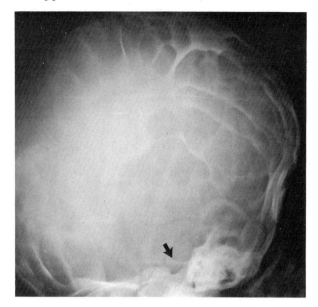

Figure 1.26. Craniolacunia: The cranial vault shows multiple areas of thinning separated by sharply defined bars in which the bone is of normal thickness. Compare this appearance with the increased convulutional markings shown in Figure 1.21. The pituitary fossa is arrowed

little fingers, and absence of the carpals, metacarpals and phalanges of the ulnar aspect of the hand. Skeletal maturation is markedly retarded corresponding to the considerable growth defect.

SPINAL DYSPLASIAS

Most types of skeletal dysplasias affect the spine to a greater or lesser extent. There are a number of conditions of congenital origin in which the lesions are localized to certain parts of the vertebral column. These are conveniently discussed together under this heading.

KLIPPEL-FEIL SYNDROME

The classic triad of a short neck with painless limitation of movement and a low hairline is shown radiologically to be the result of fusion of some or all of the cervical vertebrae. Demonstration of the correct number of intervertebral foramina through which the cervical nerve roots emerge will indicate whether all seven vertebrae are present; in some cases one or more vertebrae may be absent (*Figure 1.27*).

The diagnosis of the basic abnormality presents no difficulty, but there are many associated abnormalities, some of which are of radiological importance. Among these are:

Sprengel's deformity, which consists of elevation of the scapula on one or both sides, often with the development of bony elements connecting its superomedial angle with the cervical spine, is well recognized.

Congenital heart lesions, usually ventricular septal defect, but occasionally other types as well, especially in girls.

Hearing loss. This is also very common and in about half of these cases the external ears are abnormal. In

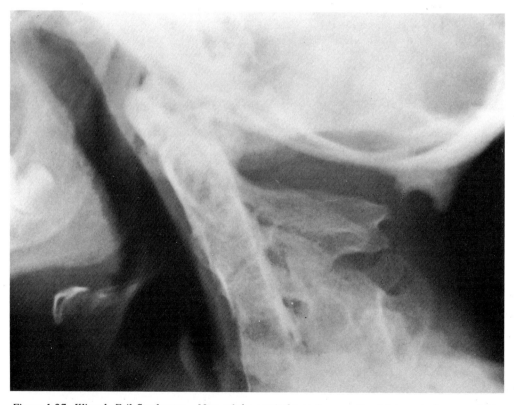

Figure 1.27. Klippel–Feil Syndrome: Most of the cervical vertebrae are fused into a single mass of bone

these cases radiology may be of particular importance in demonstrating the presence or absence of the inner ear. In particular, the internal auditory canals may be abnormally short and fail to reach the vestibule, and the semicircular canals may be absent.

Other spinal lesions, such as spina bifida and scoliosis, defects in the occipital bones, craniostenosis, micrognathos and abnormalities of dentition may also be demonstrated.

Fusion of individual vertebrae occurs not uncommonly elsewhere in the spine, but it is of less importance than in the Klippel-Feil syndrome. Such lesions can sometimes be difficult to distinguish from narrowing of the disc space which has resulted from inflammatory disease or trauma of the adjacent vertebrae.

VERTEBRAL CLEFTS: SPONDYLOLYSIS AND SPONDYLOLISTHESIS

A cleft between the two halves of the neural arch (spina bifida) is as a rule of little significance and is referred to elsewhere (*see* page 306). A cleft may occur in the body of a vertebra, dividing it into two lateral masses and giving rise to a deformity known as butterfly vertebra. Less common is the coronal cleft, which results when the vertebral body forms from two ossific centres, one behind the other (*see Figure 1.3a*). This anomaly, like the former, is of little clinical significance, though it is of interest from its association with dysplasia epiphysealis calcificans (*see* page 4).

A cleft which may be unilateral or bilateral may also occur in the pars interarticularis of the lumbar vertebrae (spondylolysis) in association with spondylolisthesis.

This deformity is of particular importance when the body of the fifth lumbar vertebra is allowed to slide forward upon the sacrum by virtue of the discontinuity between the upper and lower articular facets (*Figure 1.28*). This is because it results in pain and disability, and may lead to dystocia in women of childbearing age. Considerable controversy has existed over the question of whether the spondylolysis of the pars interarticularis is of congenital origin or arises as the result of repeated minor trauma. Several cases have been recently reported in which previous radiographs have shown an intact isthmus at an earlier age, which would support the latter hypothesis. The familial incidence in some cases, on the other hand, suggests the presence of a congenital dysplasia predisposing to the development of the actual cleft.

SACRAL AGENESIS

This anomaly occurs in relation to spinal dysraphism and anterior meningocele (*see* page 309). In this latter condition the sacrum is only unilaterally deficient and it is shown as a very characteristic sickle-shaped bony mass encircling the oval defect through which the sac of the meningocoele protruded. Complete absence of the sacrum produced an abnormally shaped pelvis. It is associated with small, cone-shaped or tapered lower limbs and with talipes equinovarus or calcaneovarus. Symmetrical, but less extensive, defects of the sacrum may be difficult to detect unless looked for carefully; but they are important because they may be associated with deformities in the lower limbs, bladder dysfunction and anorectal atresia.

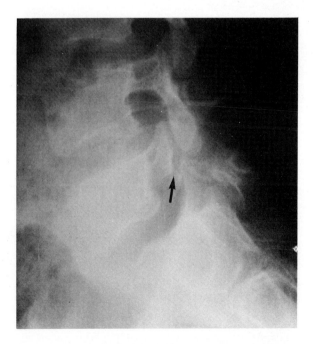 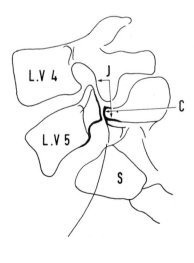

Figure 1.28. Spondylolysis: There is a cleft (C) in the pars interarticularis of the fifth lumbar vertebra (arrowed). This has allowed the body of LV5 to slide forwards relative to the sacrum (S) producing a spondylolisthesis

LOCALIZED DYSPLASIAS PREDOMINANTLY AFFECTING THE LIMBS

PERIPHERAL DYSOSTOSIS

Although this condition was first described by Brailsford (1953), it has proved difficult to establish as an entity since many, if not all of its features may occur either in normal children or in other well-established types of dysplasia. However, Newcombe and Keats (1969) consider that it is a genetically distinct condition inherited as an autosomal dominant. The most striking radio-locical feature is a disproportionate shortening of the metacarpals, metatarsals and phalanges, which is due to early fusion of the epiphyses. These have a distinctive 'cone shape' which is produced by central portions of the epiphyses projecting into the adjacent metaphyses (*Figure 1.29*). These appearances are most commonly found in the proximal and middle phalanges. They are of more significance in the hands than in the feet, where they occur in 7 per cent of otherwise normal girls, though less commonly in boys (Giedion, 1967). Other minor epiphyseal anomalies, such as 'pseudo-epiphyses'

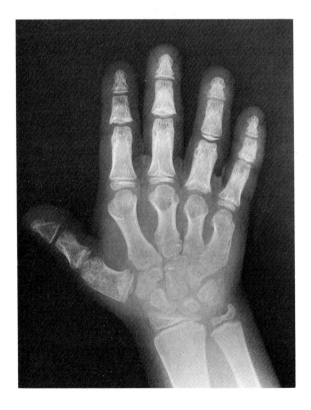

Figure 1.29. Peripheral Dysostosis: Marked brachydactyly is present affecting all the digits. This has occurred due to premature fusion of the metacarpal and some of the phalangeal epiphyses; a number of epiphyses show the characteristic 'cone shape' with fusion between the apex of the cone and the diaphysis, e.g. in the phalanges of the thumb, the proximal phalanx of the ring finger, the middle phalanges of the index and middle fingers and in most of the distal phalanges

at the proximal end of the metacarpals and at the distal ends of the phalanges and abnormally dense epiphyses, have been recorded. These non-specific epiphyseal anomalies are accompanied by some degree of general growth defect, an accelerated bone age (due to premature epiphyseal fusion), shortening of the ulnae, changes in the femoral heads resembling Perthes' disease, defective ossification of the distal ends of the tibiae and fibulae and absence or dislocation of the patellae. The thorax, spine, pelvis and skull are normal. Congenital renal defects in association with peripheral dysostosis have recently been described (Saldino and Mainzer, 1972). The differential diagnosis is very wide and must be made from chondro-ectodermal dysplasia, Turner's syndrome, pseudohypoparathyroidism and many other conditions in which short metacarpals and phalanges occur.

DYSCHONDROSTEOSIS (LERI-WEILL SYNDROME)

A localized disturbance in the growth of part of the epiphyseal plate is probably responsible for the deformities which are present in this condition. These present relatively late in childhood, probably because they are made more obvious by the prepubertal growth spurt. They are most commonly localized to the elbow and wrist. There is shortening of the long bones and as this affects the legs the children are short in stature. The shortening is characteristally 'mesomelic' in distribution, with the radius and ulna, tibia and fibula affected more markedly than the other limb bones (Langer, 1965). In addition the radius is bowed both laterally and dorsally, and there is a defect in the ulnar aspect of the distal metaphyses; the epiphysis is triangular in shape. The distal end of the ulna is dislocated dorsally and the head of the bone is abnormally dense (*Figure 1.30*). A similiar deformity may also occur as an isolated finding and be due to local injury or osteomyelitis. Occasionally it is part of other dysplasias such as diaphyseal aclasis, Ollier's disease or Turner's syndrome.

Blount's disease, which affects one side of the proximal end of the tibia, may be related to dyschond-rosteosis. It is likely that local trauma, pressure or osteitis may play a greater part in its aetiology. Nevertheless, the fact that Blount's disease has a higher incidence in some parts of the world than in others would point to a congenital dysplasia as a basis for some cases of this condition. The deformity, usually genu varum, is produced by the obliquity of the articular surface of one of the tibial condyles.

DYSMELIA

Anomalies of the limbs, in which one or more bones are either hypoplastic or absent, form an important group because of the marked disability that results from the more severe grades. It is a group of conditions in which radiological assessment of the exact nature and degree of the abnormality is of value in determining the type and efficacy of remedial measures when these are

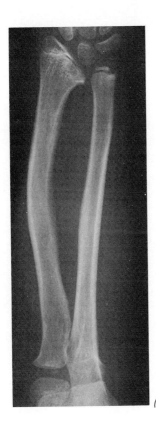

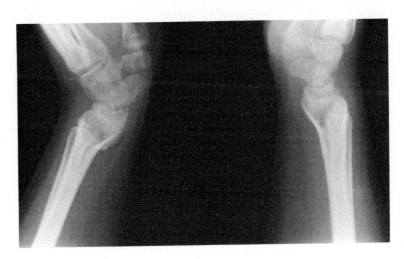

Figure 1.30. Dyschondrosteosis: (a) Forearm showing bowing of the radial shaft; the epiphysis is triangular and there is a medial defect at the distal end of the radius. The carpal bones project between the radius and ulna. (b) Lateral view of both wrists showing the dorsal displacement of the head of the ulna

(a)

(b)

required. The classification of these lesions has recently been clarified by Henkel and Willert (1969). They consider that there is a pattern of anomalies involving an axis through the humerus, radius and thumb in the upper limb, some or all of these bones being hypoplastic or completely absent according to the severity of the condition. This pattern is constant whether the cause is genetically determined or due to an acquired embryopathy. They contrast this type of anomaly with aplasia of the ulna and fibula, cleft hand and foot, and congenital amputation of the distal part of the limb, conditions which they consider to arise by a different mechanism.

The results of the administration of thalidomide to mothers during the early months of pregnancy have been well documented by Grainger *et al.* (1962) and by Cuthbert and Spiers (1963). In the most severely affected cases there is a phocomelia, in which the hands and feet are directly attached to the trunk and there is aplasia of all the other limb bones. In other less severely affected cases the radius, thumb and big toes are absent and there is manus varus, or triphalangy of the thumbs and big toes (*Figure 1.31*). Pelvic defects in the region of the symphysis pubis, cleft sternum and cervicodorsal spina bifida have also been described. The incidence of skeletal deformities has been estimated as 20 per cent of all infants born to mothers taking thalidomide during pregnancy, all four limbs being involved in three-quarters of these infants. Anomalies of other systems may also be present, notably atresias of the alimentary tract, including imperforate anus, and congenital heart lesions; both of these conditions can be usefully investigated radiologically. The presence of congenital heart lesions

has led to difficulty in differentiating cases of thalidomide embryopathy from cases which are primarily congenital in origin, an entity which has been referred to as the Holt—Oram syndrome (Holt and Oram, 1960). Originally the syndrome was described as a combination of atrial septal defect with dysmelia of the upper limbs only. This consisted of an aplasia of the radius and thumb, or relatively minor anomalies of the carpal bones and thumbs (*Figure 1.32*). It is now becoming recognized that there is a much wider spectrum in which other cardiac malformations and anomalies of parts of the skeleton, other than the radius and thumb, may be present. There is also an association between congenital heart disease and a large number of other skeletal dysplasias, of which the trisomy group, especially Down's syndrome, the sex chromosome anomalies, such as Turner's syndrome and tetra X—Y syndrome, chondro-ectodermal dysplasia, Marfan's syndrome and Fanconi's anaemia are well established examples.

CONGENITAL BOWING OF THE LONG BONES, CONGENITAL COXA VARA AND PSEUDARTHROSIS

Areas of defective ossification, in which the normal bone is replaced by fibrous tissue, or by tissue with a histological appearance similar to that found in monostotic fibrous dysplasia, are present in all these conditions. These may occur either in conjunction with each other or independently. In such cases bending of the shafts of the long bones may be

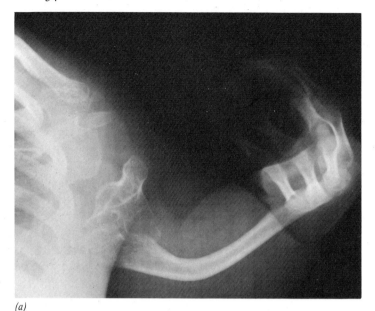

(a)

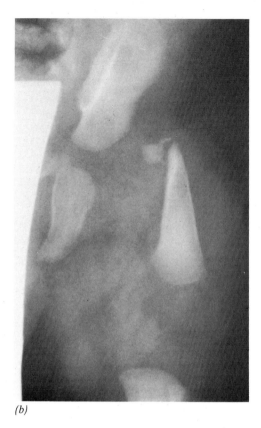

(b)

Figure 1.31. Dysmelia: (a) The upper limb of a child born to a mother who had taken thalidomide during early pregnancy. The humerus is represented by a small triangular fragment which does not articulate with the glenoid fossa. The radius and thumb are absent and there is manus varus. (b) The thigh of another case in which thalidomide resulted in limb deformity. In this case the proximal part of the femur is hypoplastic with severe coxa vara and dislocation of the hip

present at birth and may affect several bones. Commonly there is thickened cortex along the concave side of the curved segment (*Figure 1.33*). In other cases the bone may be hypoplastic or there may be a gap which is either present initially, resulting in a congenital pseudarthrosis, or develops later from a fracture at the site of the bowing which fails to heal. Lloyd-Roberts and Shaw (1969) consider that the presence of segmental bone sclerosis, cystic changes within the bone or an hour-glass contracture indicate that a pseudarthrosis is likely to ensue. The commonest single bone to be affected is the tibia, in which the curvature can be convex anteriorly or posteriorly. It is often associated with other congenital defects, particularly talipes equinovarus or calcaneovalgus, absent fibulae, congenital dislocation of the hips, rib or spinal anomalies, cleft palate and micrognathos. In some cases several bones are involved, chiefly the humeri, femora and fibulae, and often symmetrically on the two sides of the body.

Bowing of the neck of the femur is present in congenital coxa vara and there is commonly an irregular defect or hypoplasia of the proximal end of the bone, the capital epiphysis being either absent or ossifying late. In the latter case it is misshapen or displaced. An associated dislocation of the hip or acetabular dysplasia is not uncommon. Ring (1961) has reviewed these femoral lesions and states that they range from simple hypoplasia or coxa vara to complete aplasia of the femur. Coxa vara is a relatively common deformity with a varied aetiology, often due to trauma, epiphysiolysis of the femoral head, osteomyelitis, tuberculosis, rickets, Perthes' disease, cysts or tumours of the femoral neck and a

large number of the generalized skeletal dysplasias already described. Most of these types may be distinguished by their characteristic radiological appearance. The congenital type shows a wide, irregular epiphyseal growth plate at the proximal end of the femur. This lies in a vertical plane and often shows a characteristic triangular bony fragment at either the upper or the lower end, giving it a Y or λ shape.

CONGENITAL DISLOCATION OF THE HIPS

If treatment is to be effective in ensuring the development of normal hip structure and function in children born with congenital dislocation, it is essential that the diagnosis should be made in the neonatal period. It is generally agreed that radiology is not the most reliable method for this purpose. At birth, the abnormal hip joint is unstable and is not permanently dislocated, so that it is a matter of chance whether or not dislocation is present at the time the radiograph is taken. Even if it is dislocated, the cartilaginous nature of both the head of the femur and the rim of the acetabulum, and also the fact that the femoral head is displaced predominantly backwards, makes it difficult to assess the true relationship of the femur to the acetabular socket (*Figure 1.34*). For these reasons, it is generally agreed that it is preferable to rely on clinical signs in the detection of the condition in the newborn infant and to reserve radiological examination to confirm that treatment has been effective in maintaining the hip in a reduced position. After 3 or 4 months, the ossific centre for the femoral head starts to appear and this allows the position of the head to be assessed more accurately. Nevertheless, in cases in which the clinical signs are equivocal, it may be justifiable to employ radiography to help in reaching a positive diagnosis. Attempts have therefore been made to determine criteria which will overcome the disadvantages referred to above. It has been accepted that one of the primary features of the condition is a dysplasia of the hip joint, and that this is manifested by defective ossification of the acetabular roof. It has been suggested that this may be detected by an increase in the acetabular angle (*see* page 355), and by delay or irregularity in the ossification of the epiphysis for the head of the femur. Unfortunately, as both Coleman (1956) and Caffey *et al.* (1956) have shown, on the basis of a survey of large numbers of newborn infants, the range of variation in the value of the acetabular angle is so wide (15–39 degrees), that its use in diagnosis is very limited. However, when it is over 40 degrees and markedly unequal on the two sides the acetabular angle may serve to confirm other signs of the abnormality. The angle may, however, be normal in the presence of instability. Wilkinson

and Carter (1960) have used it in older children to assess the likelihood that conservative treatment will be successful. A good result is to be anticipated in those cases where the acetabular angle initially is below 25 degrees at 1 year of age.

Various measurements which relate the position of the neck of the femur to the pelvis have been devised. Of these, the present authors consider that Perkins' line is the most useful. Coleman (1956) found that part of the femoral neck lay medial to it in all but one of 300 normal hips but was lateral to it in 58 per cent of clinically abnormal hips; he regards that and other such measurements (*see Figure 9.28* page 357) mainly as corroborative evidence and finds that they are positive in about 70 per cent of neonates with congenital dislocation. On the other hand, a negative result in this respect should be ignored.

Andren and Von Rosen (1958) have devised a technique which they claim will help to differentiate normal from unstable hips in the newborn infant. This technique depends on the premise that internal rotation of the femur when it is abducted to 45 degrees will force the head more securely into the socket if

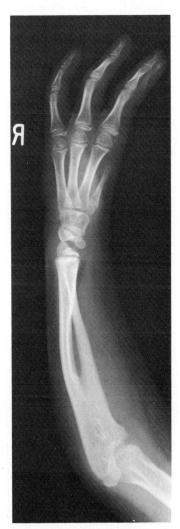

(a)

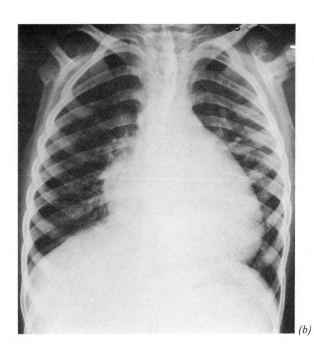

(b)

Figure 1.32. Holt–Oram Syndrome: (a) The right hand and forearm showing radio-ulnar synostosis and absence of the thumb and much of the index finger; the carpal bones are defective with fusion of the bones in the distal row. (b) The chest of the same case showing right-sided cardiac enlargement and pleonaemic lung fields due to an atrial septal defect

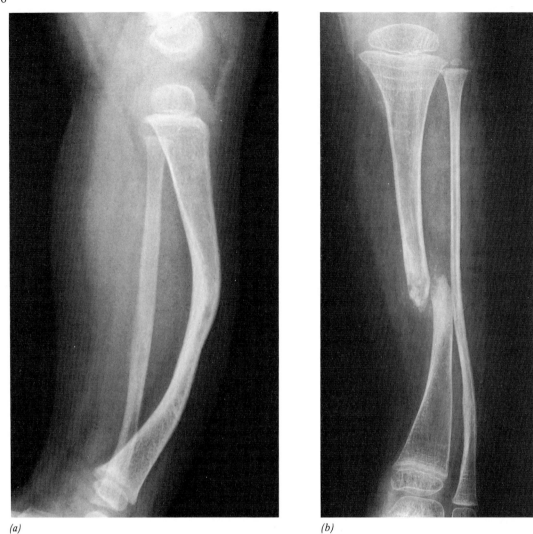

(a)   (b)

Figure 1.33. Congenital Bowing of the Long Bones with Pseudarthrosis: (a) Lateral view of the tibia of a girl aged 20 months which is bowed anteriorly with thickening of the posterior cortex on the concavity of the curve. This deformity had been present since birth. (b) Anteroposterior view of the same case 2 years later following a fracture at the site of the bowing, which has failed to unite leading to a pseudarthrosis

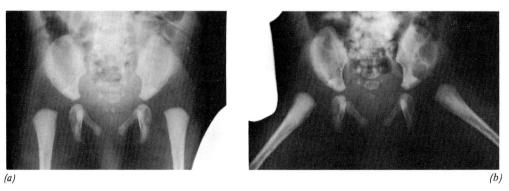

(a)   (b)

Figure 1.34. Congenital Dislocation of the Hips: The hip joints of an infant aged 2 days with bilateral congenital instability of the hip joints. These films illustrate well the difficulty in detecting the malposition of the femoral heads before the capital epiphyses have ossified and where the condition is bilateral. The Andren–Von Rosen view (b) with the femora abducted to 45 degrees and internally rotated may be helpful in demonstrating upward displacement of the long axis of the femur. The dysplasia of the acetabula is also apparent in the loss of a sharp distinction between the roof of the acetabula and the lateral border of the ilia

it is in its normal relation to the acetabulum. However, this technique will exaggerate the degree of displacement if the head is dislocated. The direction in which the long axis of the femur is pointing either in relation to the margins of the acetabulum or to the lumbosacral joint will allow the displacement to be recognized. When the femur is dislocated, the prolongation of its long axis passes outside the acetabular margin and cuts the lumbar spine above the lumbosacral joint. Clearly this technique relies very much on absolute accuracy in positioning the infant and in abducting the leg to exactly 45 degrees, neither of which can be assured in practice. If this method is to be used with any prospect of accurate results, the radiologist must supervise the examination. Even so, the method may well be unreliable unless steps are taken to ensure that an unstable hip is actually dislocated at the time the examination is carried out.

Tomography and arthrography have also been used to assist in an accurate determination of the position of the head of the femur. The former may be expected to give information as to the presence of posterior displacement but not until the centre for the head of the femur is ossified; at this stage, however, it may have a place, especially when the hip is examined through a plaster cast. Arthrography carries a slight risk of subsequent avascular necrosis of the head of the femur and it is not advocated as a method for initial diagnosis in the newborn. However, arthrography has some value in the investigation of older children in whom the hip will not stay reduced following conservative treatment (*Figure 1.35*). In such cases it may reveal some of the causes for failure, such as an hour-glass contracture of the capsule and a hypertrophy of the ligamentum teres, or the presence of a reflexed cartilaginous labrum, lying between the head of the femur and the floor of the acetabulum. In the normal hip arthrogram, the labrum is outlined by a small pointed projection of the synovial cavity lying on the outer or upper surface of the head of the femur.

Other radiological features have been described in congenital dislocation of the hip. Among these is a small pit or depression normally present on the roof of the acetabulum, as described by Doberti and Manhood (1968). When this is displaced outside the limits of the acetabulum it may occasionally be a useful confirmatory sign. The development of anteversion of the femoral neck may be a cause of continued instability, and this can readily be qualitatively assessed by radiological means. Quantitative measurement of its degree requires a more sophisticated technique (Dunlap *et al.*, 1953) (*see* page 357). Similarly, the development of sequelae, such as avascular necrosis and deformities of the femoral head (*Figure 1.36*), and the need for control of the results of surgical treatment necessitate repeated radiographic examination. In such cases the problem of gonad protection and the assessment of radiation dosage are important factors which must be kept in mind by both radiologist and clinician.

OSTEO-ONYCHO DYSPLASIA—NAIL-PATELLA (FONG) SYNDROME

This is a hereditary condition which affects both ectodermal and mesodermal tissues and which affords a striking combination of abnormalities many of which are demonstrable by radiology. These include:

(1) Bilateral dislocation of the heads of the radii with associated deformity both of the radial heads and of the capitellum and lateral epicondyles of the humerus.

(2) An abnormal shape of the ilia in which the lateral borders are concave and the anterior superior spines unusually prominent. In addition there is a bony exostosis capped by a layer of cartilage projecting from the posterior aspect of both ilia ('iliac horns'). The latter may not be visible before the age of 3 years.

(3) Absent or abnormally shaped patellae which have a tendency to dislocate laterally in association with deformity of the lateral femoral condyles.

(4) Dysplasia of the nails.

DYSPLASIAS OF CONNECTIVE TISSUE WITH SKELETAL INVOLVEMENT

MARFAN'S SYNDROME

It is well established that this condition is due to a generalized defect in connective tissue. It is manifested by laxity of joints, abnormalities in the eyes, especially of the lens and cornea and of the cardiovascular system. Changes in the medial coat of the aorta and pulmonary artery may lead to dilatation or even rupture and produce a dissecting aneurysm. It is also associated with characteristic abnormalities in the proportions between trunk and limbs and between the width and length of the metacarpals, metatarsals and phalanges (*Figure 1.37*). The latter feature, clinically presenting as 'arachnodactyly', may be confirmed radiologically by the use of the metacarpal index devised by Sinclair *et al.* (1960) and extended to cover the paediatric age range by Joseph and Meadow (1969) (*see* page 358).

Other abnormalities which are of radiological interest are dolichocephaly associated with deformity of the pituitary fossa, kyphoscoliosis, spondylolisthesis, widening of the spinal canal, a funnel sternum or, occasionally, anterior bowing of the sternum, femoral epiphysiolysis, displaced patellae, dysplasia of the hips with 'congenital dislocation'.

ARTHROGRYPOSIS MULTIPLEX CONGENITA

Contractures of the joints and gross diminution in the size of the muscle bundles, the latter being represented by thin, string-like cords, are the most constant radiological features of this condition but are not specific signs. They may occur in diseases of the spinal cord or peripheral nerves, particularly meningomyelocele and the Werdnig–Hoffman type of motor neurone disease (Poznanski and La Rowe, 1970). The abnormalities in arthrogryposis are however usually widespread. They affect both upper and lower limbs and to a lesser extent the trunk. Contractures of the elbows and wrists with ulnar deviation of the hands are common (*Figure 1.38*). Adduction of the hips, often with dislocation and resultant deformity of the acetabulum, produces a stiff joint and this resists attempts to reduce the dislocation. The phenomenon is in contrast to the condition present

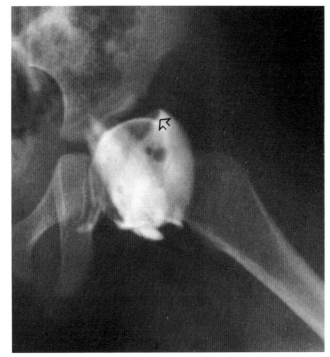

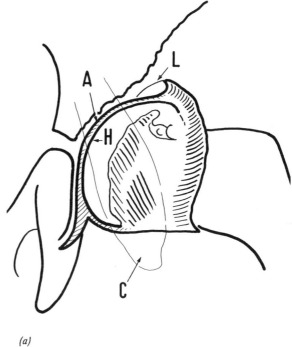

(a)

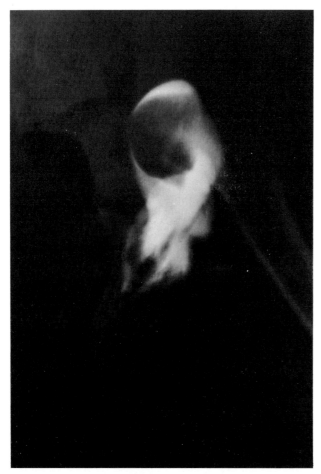

Figure 1.35. Arthrography of the Hip Joint in Infancy: (a) Normal left hip joint. There is only a thin layer of contrast medium between the femoral head (H) and the acetabular floor (A). The position of the cartilaginous portion of the acetabular roof or labrum (L) (arrowed) on the upper surface of the femoral head is well demonstrated. Leakage of contrast medium into the psoas muscle has occurred during the procedure and overlies the medial part of the cartilaginous femoral head (C). (b) Dislocation of the hip. There is stretching and distortion of the capsule of the joint with probable constriction below the femoral head which may prevent closed reduction of the dislocation. (c) (next page) Subluxation of the hip with failure to reduce the head of the femur completely as shown by the relatively large pool of contrast medium lying between the head of the femur (H) and the floor of the acetabulum (A). The cause of this is likely to be due to reflection of the acetabular labrum (L) between the femoral head and the acetabular floor. The orbicular ligament (0) forms a transverse defect in the contrast medium around the femoral neck

(b)

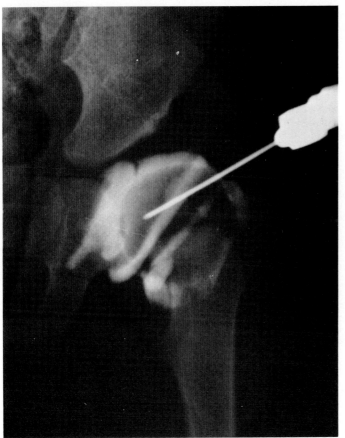

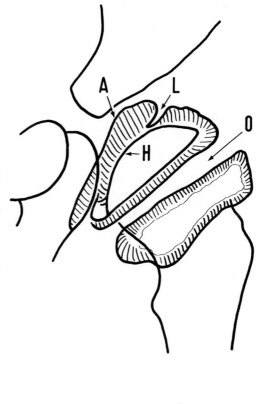

(c)

when the hip is congenitally dislocated: It is then lax and easily reduced. The knees are commonly flexed and they may show tibia recurvatum. Various deformities of the feet, including talipes equinovarus, vertical talus and congenital amputations of the toes, may be present. The bones are generally small, slender and decalcified and, as a result, may fracture easily. The carpal bones are frequently fused, either involving the whole carpus, or only those on the radial side. The carpal angle may also be increased and the average value may be 161 degrees (compared with the normal value of 131 degrees), the effect of which is that the proximal carpal bones are in a straight line (Poznanski *et al.*, 1976). Syndactyly and polydactyly and radio-ulnar synostosis may also occur.

In the spine there is scoliosis or torticollis, hemivertebrae and fusion of vertebrae, often of the Klippel—Feil type (*see* page 30). The skull is small and the sutures narrowed. The vault is frequently deformed and asymmetrical. This is due to the fact that the child is relatively immobile and as a result adopts a fixed abnormal posture. This may lead to pressure deformities. Fusion of the temporomandibular joints may be present and this may lead to hypoplasia of the mandible.

Differential diagnosis of this condition may be difficult, and indeed the exact nature and definition of the disease has been a matter of controversy. However, it is likely that it represents a generalized mesenchymal defect, which may result in joint contractures and deformities and these may arise early in intra-uterine life. Alternatively it has been suggested that the joint contractures and the abnormal attitude of the fetus *in utero* may be the result of an amyoplasia, a primary failure of the muscles to develop, or to an abnormality of the anterior horn cells in the spinal cord. However, whatever the cause, the radiological picture may resemble closely dysplasias such as osteogenesis imperfecta, diastrophic dwarfism, trisomy 17—18, the nail—patella syndrome, as well as that in diseases of the nervous system.

MYOSITIS OSSIFICANS PROGRESSIVA

This severely disabling and generally fatal condition begins during the first decade of life, with the development of areas of heterotopic bone. These arise in response to trauma in the first instance, but they progress until so much of the muscle and connective tissue is converted to bone that the victim becomes immobilized and dies from respiratory infection. Its recognition is not difficult because of the characteristic bony masses, particularly in the sterno-mastoid muscle and around the shoulder girdle, upper arm and back muscles. There is also an almost universal incidence of reduction in the size of the big toes and absence of the proximal phalanx (*Figure 1.39*). Synostoses of the phalanges of the other toes is common and the thumbs are also occasionally abnormal. Illingworth (1971) has also reported abnormally wide femoral necks and bony exostoses (presumably due to areas of ossification in muscle attachments) and dental

40

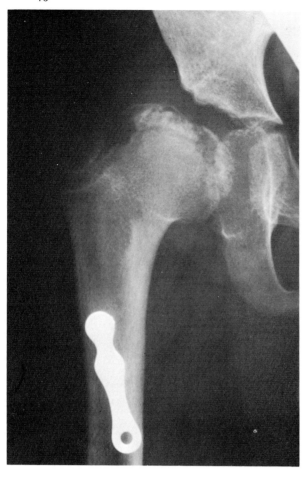

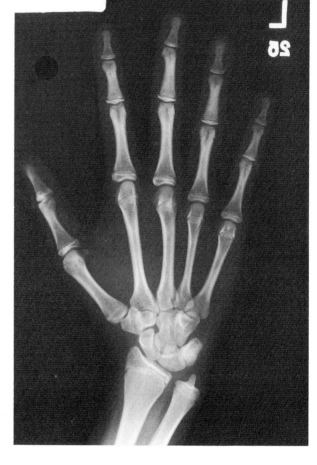

Figure 1.36. Congenital Dislocation of the Hip — Late Sequelae: The epiphysis for the head of the femur has become flattened and fragmented due to avascular necrosis following unsuccessful attempts at reduction. A metal plate has been inserted at the site of a previous osteotomy

Figure 1.37. Arachnodactyly: Long slender metacarpals and phalanges in a girl with Marfan's syndrome. The metacarpal index in this case was 11.1. (normal range 5.0 – 7.5)

anomalies. The development of osteosarcoma in the abnormal bony masses may rarely occur.

PROGERIA (HUTCHINSON—GILFORD SYNDROME)

The predominant features of this condition are loss of subcutaneous fat, muscle atrophy and bone resorption. Clinically, premature and progressive ageing give rise to a highly characteristic picture, and the radiological features may be equally striking and distinctive. The skull is apparently large, this appearance being due to craniofacial disproportion with hypoplasia of the maxilla and mandible and not to a true enlargement of the vault. The sutures are wide and the fontanelles remain open. Ozonoff and Clemett (1967) report strips of unossified membrane parallel to the grooves for the lateral sinuses. The teeth are crowded and malplaced. There is progressive resorption of the clavicles starting at the outer ends and resulting in a complete disappearance of these bones; occasionally the posterior ends of the upper four ribs are also resorbed. In the limbs, the distal phalanges undergo progressive resorption and become tapered. The long bones are generally slender but because the cortex remains locally dense they are disproportionately thick and the medullary cavity becomes progressively narrowed. Growth is retarded after the first year or two, but skeletal maturation is usually within the normal range. The soft tissues are all thin, but the atrophy of the subcutaneous tissue is particularly marked.

The conditions most likely to be confused radiologically are acro-osteolysis (disappearing bone disease) and cleidocranial dysostosis, but the clinical features are so distinctive that the diagnosis should not be difficult.

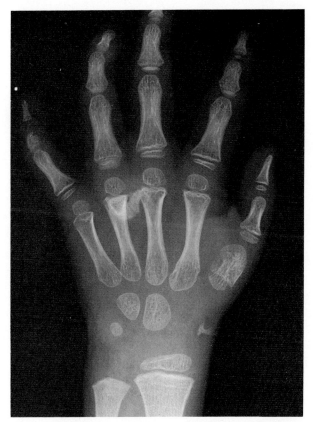

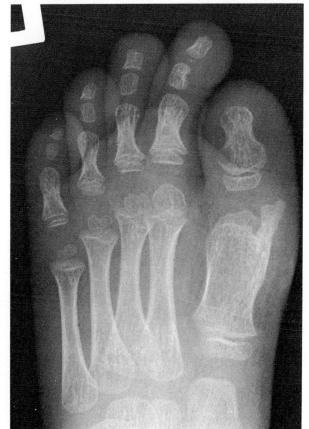

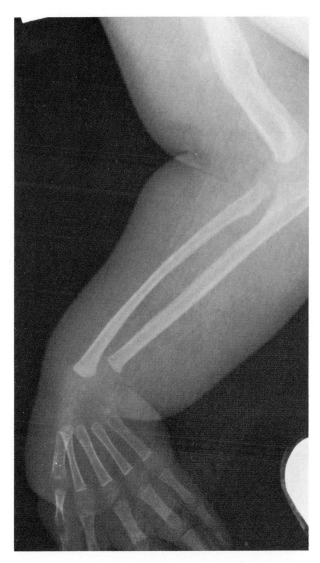

(a)

(b)

Figure 1.38. (above) Arthrogryposis Multiplex Congenita: The bones appear decalcified and reduced in width; the deformities (flexion of the elbow and ulnar deviation of the wrist) result from contractures of the soft tissues, notably the muscles which are just visible as thread-like densities within the widened subcutaneous tissues. There is a healed fracture of the shaft of the humerus

Figure 1.39. (right) Myositis Ossificans Progressiva: (a) The hand showing heterotopic bone formation in relation to the neck of the fourth metacarpal and on the radial aspect of the carpus. The first metacarpal and the middle phalanx of the little finger are abnormally short. (b) The foot of the same case. The big toe is shortened due to absence of the proximal phalanx; heterotopic bone is present on the medial aspect of the head of the short first metatarsal

42

REFERENCES

Aitken, G. W. E., Cohen, A. and Verco, P. W. (1964). 'Osteogenesis imperfecta; a case discovered *in utero*.' *J. Fac. Radiol.* **6**, 62

Andersson, H. (1966). 'Craniosynostosis as a complication after operation for hydrocephalus.' *Acta Paediat. Scand.* **55**, 192

Andren, L. and Von Rosen, S. (1958). 'The diagnosis of dislocation of the hip in newborns and the primary result of immediate treatment.' *Acta Radiol.* **49**, 89

Astley, R. (1958). 'Hypothyroidism in children.' *Br. J. Radiol.* **31**, 346

— (1963). 'Chromosomal abnormalities in childhood, with particular reference to Turner's syndrome and mongolism.' *Br. J. Radiol.* **36**, 2

— (1966). 'Trisomy 17/18.' *Br. J. Radiol.* **39**, 86

Beals, R. K. (1969). 'Hypochondroplasia; a report of five kinddreds.' *J. Bone Jt Surg.* **51A**, 728

Brailsford, J. F. (1953). *The Radiology of Bones and Joints* (5th edn). London; Churchill

Caffey, J. (1952). 'Chondroectodermal dysplasia (Ellis–van Creveld disease). Report of three cases.' *Am. J. Roentgl.* **68**, 875

— (1958). 'Achondroplasia of pelvis and lumbrosacral spine; some roentgenographic features.' *Am. J. Roentgl.* **80**, 449

and Ross, S. (1956). 'Mongolism (mongoloid deficiency) during early infancy–some newly recognised diagnostic changes in the pelvic bones.' *Pediatrics, Springfield* **17**, 642

— Ames, R., Silverman, W. A., Ryder, C. T. and Hough, G. (1956). 'Contradiction of the congenital dysplasia–Predislocation hypothesis of congenital dislocation of the hip through a study of the normal variation in acetabular angles at successive periods in infancy.' *Pediatrics, Springfield* **17**, 632

Cohen, M. E., Rosenthal, A. D. and Matson, D. D. (1967). 'Neurological abnormalities in achondroplastic children.' *J. Pediat.* **71**, 367

Coleman, S. S. (1956). 'Diagnosis of congenital dysplasia of the hip in the newborn infant.' *J. Am. med. Ass.* **162**, 548

Comings, D. E., Papazian, C. and Schoene, H. R. (1968). 'Conradi's disease; chondrodystrophia calcificans congenita, congenital stippled epiphyses.' *J. Pediat.* **72**, 63

Cuthbert, R. and Speirs, A. L. (1963). 'Thalidomide induced malformations–a radiological survey.' *Clin. Radiol.* **14**, 163

Doberti, A. and Manhood, J. (1968). 'A new radiological sign for early diagnosis of congenital hip dysplasia.' *Annls Radiol.* **11**, 276

Duggan, C. A., Keener, E. B. and Gay, B. B. (1970). 'Secondary craniosynostosis.' *Am. J. Roentgl.* **109**, 277

Dunlap, K., Shands, A. R. Hollister, L. C., Gaul, J. S. and Streit, H. A. (1953). 'A new method for determination of torsion of the femur.' *J. Bone Jt Surg.* **35A**, 289

Fairbank, H. A. T. (1946). 'Dysplasia epiphysealis multiplex.' *Proc. R. Soc. Med.* **39**, 315

Falconer, M. A. and Cope, C. L. (1942). 'Fibrous Dysplasia of bone with endocrine disorders and cutaneous pigmentation (Albright's disease).' *Q. J. Med. N.S.* **11**, 121

Ford, N., Silverman, F. N. and Kozlowski, K. (1961). 'Spondyloepiphyseal dysplasia (Pseudoachondroplastic type).' *Am. J. Roentgl.* **86**, 462

Fraser, G. R., Friedmann, A. I., Maroteaux, P., Glen-Bott, A. M. and Mittwoch, U. (1969). 'Dysplasia spondylo-epiphysaria congenita and related skeletal dysplasias among children with severe visual handicaps.' *Archs Dis. Childh.* **44**, 490

Gibson, M. J. and Middlemiss, J. H. (1971). 'Fibrous Dysplasia of Bone.' *Br. J. Radiol.* **44**, 1

Giedion, A. (1967). 'Cone shaped epiphyses of the hands and their diagnostic value. The tricho-rhino-phalangeal syndrome.' *Annls Radiol.* **10**, 322

Grainger, R. G., Morris, A. H. and Ward, P. (1962). 'Phocomelic deformity and maternal thalidomide administration, a report of four cases.' *Br. J. Radiol.* **35**, 687

Haddad, H. M. and Wilkins, L. (1959). 'Congenital anomalies associated with gonadal asplasia; Review of 55 cases.' *Pediatrics, Springfield* **23**, 885

Henkel, L. and Willert, H–G. (1969). 'Dysmelia. A classification and a pattern of malformation in a group of congenital defects of the limbs.' *J. Bone Jt Surg.* **51B**, 399

Holt, M. and Oram, S. (1960). 'Familial Heart Disease with skeletal malformations.' *Br. Heart J.* **22**, 236

Houston, C. S. (1967). 'Roentgen findings in the XXXXY chromosome anomaly.' *J. Can. Ass. Radiol.* **18**, 258

Hull, D. and Barnes, N. D. (1972). 'Children with small chests.' *Archs Dis. Childh.* **47**, 12

Illingworth, R. S. (1971). 'Myositis ossificans progressiva (Munchmeyer's disease).' *Archs Dis. Childh.* **46**, 264

Jaffe, H. L. (1937). Quoted by Hirsch, I. S. (1937). 'Generalised Osteochondrodystrophy. The eccentrochondroplastic form.' *J. Bone Jt Surg.* **35**, 297

Jansen, M. (1934). 'Uber atypische Chondrodystrophie (Achondroplasie) und über eine noch nicht beschriebene angeborene Wachstumsstörung des Knochensystems: Metaphysäre Dysotosis.' *Z. orthop. Chir.* **61**, 253

Joseph, M. C. and Meadow, S. R. (1969). 'The metacarpal index of infants.' *Archs Dis. Childh.* **44**, 515

Keats, T. E. Riddervold, H. O. and Michaelis, L. L. (1970). 'Thanatophoric Dwarfism.' *Am. J. Roentgl.* **108**, 473

Kozlowski, K. (1964). 'Metaphyseal dysostosis; report of five familial and two sporadic cases of a mild type.' *Am. J. Roentgl.* **91**, 602

Langer, L. O. (1965). 'Dyschondrosteosis; a heriditable bone dysplasia with characteristic roentgenographic features.' *Am. J. Roentgl.* **95**, 178

— Baumann, P. A. and Gorlin, R. J. (1967). 'Achondroplasia.' *Am. J. Roentgl.* **100**, 12

Levin, E. J. (1964). 'Osteogenesis imperfecta in the adult.' *Am. J. Roentgl.* **91**, 973

Lloyd-Roberts, G. C. and Shaw, N. E. (1969). 'The prevention of pseudarthrosis in congenital kyphosis of the tibia.' *J. Bone Jt Surg.* **51B**, 100

McKusick, V. A., Eldridge, R., Hostetler, J. A., Ruangwit, U. and Egeland, J. A. (1965). 'Dwarfism in the Amish. II. Cartilage–hair hypoplasia.' *Bull. Johns Hopkins Hosp.* **116**, 285

Neuhauser, E. B. D., Schwachman, H., Wittenborg, M. and Cohen, J. (1948). 'Progressive diaphyseal dysplasia.' *Radiology* **51**, 11

Newcombe, D. S. and Keats, T. E. (1969). 'Roentgenographic manifestations of hereditary peripheral dysostosis.' *Am. J. Roentgl.* **106**, 178

Odman, P. (1959). 'Hereditary enchondral dysostosis; twelve cases in three generations mainly with peripheral locations.' *Acta Radiol.* **52**, 97

Ozonoff, M. B. and Clemett, A. R. (1967). 'Progressive osteolysis in progeria.' *Am. J. Roentgl.* **100**, 75

Poznanski, A. K. and La Rowe, P. C. (1970). 'Radiographic manifestations of the arthrogryposis syndrome.' *Radiology* **95**, 353

— Garn, S. M. and Shaw, H. A. (1976). 'The carpal angle in the congenital malformation syndromes.' *Ann. Radiol.* **19**, 141

Ring, P. A. (1961). 'Congenital abnormalities of the femur.' *Archs Dis. Childh.* **36**, 410

Rubin, P. (1964). *Dynamic Classification of Bone Dysplasias*. Chicago; Year Book Medical Publishers

Saldino, R. M. and Mainzer, F. (1971). 'Cone shaped epiphyses (CSE) in siblings with hereditary renal disease and retinitis pigmentosa.' *Radiology* **98**, 39

Sinclair, R. J. G., Kitchin, A. H. and Turner, R. W. D. (1960). 'The Marfan syndrome.' *Q. Jl Med. N.S.* **29**, 19

Singleton, E. B., Daeschner, C. W. and Teng, C. T. (1960). 'Peripheral Dysostosis.' *Am. J. Roentgl.* **84**, 499

Spranger, J. and Schuster, W. (1969). 'Classifiable and nonclassifiable mucopolysaccharidoses.' *Annls Radiol.* **12**, 365

Stovin, J. J., Lyon, J. A. and Clemmens, R. L. (1960). 'Mandibulofacial dysostosis.' *Annls Radiol.* **12**, 365

Taybi, H., Mitchell, A. D. and Friedman, G. D. (1969). 'Metaphyseal dysostosis and the associated syndrome of pancreatic insufficiency and blood disorders.' *Radiology* **93,** 563

Trapnell, D. H. (1968). 'Periodontal manifestations of osteopetrosis.' *Br. J. Radiol.* **41,** 669

Turner, A. F., Mikity, V. G. and Meyers, H. I. (1963). 'Neonatal fibrous dysplasia.' *J. Pediat.* **62,** 936

Weinfeld, A., Ross, M. W. and Sarasohn, S. H. (1967). 'Spondylo-

epiphyseal dysplasia tarda; a cause of premature osteoarthritis.' *Am. J. Roentgl.* **101,** 851

Wilkinson, J. and Carter, C. O. (1960). 'Congenital dislocation of the hip; the results of conservative treatment.' *J. Bone J. Surg.* **42B,** 669

Wilson, D. W., Chrispin, A. R. and Carter, C. O. (1969). 'Diastrophic dwarfism.' *Archs Dis. Childh.* **44,** 48

2 TUMOURS AND TUMOUR-LIKE LESIONS IN BONE

INTRODUCTION

The occurrence of tumours in bone is relatively rare and in a lifetime it is unlikely that any one practitioner will see a sufficient number to make him an expert in the subject. If however he is known to make a special study of them, cases will be referred to him and he can become experienced in their diagnosis and management. Experience will be even more fruitful if he can be associated with colleagues of different specialities who can each study the cases from his own diagnostic point of view, thus forming a panel of interested specialists. The panel might well consist of orthopaedic surgeons, pathologists, diagnostic radiologists, radiotherapists, paediatricians, histochemists, and the like; several successful Bone Tumour Registries, for instance those at Bristol and Leeds, have been set up on these lines.

It must be emphasized that it is important to make a correct diagnosis of bone tumours because different tumours have different prognoses. Correct diagnosis can be made only as a result of a multidisciplinary approach, each discipline making its own contribution to the final diagnosis. If any discipline is at variance with the final diagnosis then the whole diagnosis must be reconsidered in case a mistake is being made.

The function of diagnostic radiology is to detect the presence of the tumour, locate its site, determine its extent within the bone and outside it, and decide whether the tumour arises outside the bone and secondarily invades it. Radiology may also determine whether the tumour is solitary or whether multiple tumours are present, it may demonstrate a tumour's vascularity and, if thought advisable, its progress with time or under treatment. It may also show whether pulmonary metastases are present. Radiology must in addition try to differentiate the tumour from inflammatory and other lesions, determine whether the tumour is benign or malignant and suggest differential diagnoses in order of preference. Both for the radiologist and the pathologist different lesions may appear indistinguishable but they are not

necessarily identical. This dilemma can usually be resolved by combining the two approaches.

In a work of the scope of this book, the subject cannot be covered in very great detail and readers who are particularly interested are referred to the more detailed works: Coley (1972); Greenfield (1969); Dahlin (1967); Graham (1966); Murray and Jacobson (1971); Price and Ross (1973); Lichtenstein (1965); Spjut *et al.* (1971). However, sufficient information is given here to provide paediatricians with a working knowledge of those tumours which occur in children.

The classification of the histological typing of primary bone tumours and tumour-like lesions, which was adopted by the World Health Organisation (Schajowicz *et al.*, 1972) is used; only those tumours affecting children will be described. The definitions of the individual tumours used in the text are those given in the above-mentioned classification. Secondary or metastatic tumours will be dealt with at the end of the chapter.

BONE-FORMING TUMOURS

BENIGN

Osteoma

Definition: A benign lesion consisting of well-differentiated mature bone tissue, with a predominantly lamellar structure, and showing very slow growth.

Osteomata almost exclusively involve the skull and face bones and predominate in the paranasal sinuses, especially the frontal sinuses. They are mostly asymptomatic. They have been reported from the age of 10 years but are commonest in the fourth and fifth decades.

Radiologically an osteoma shows as a well-defined dense opacity arising on a broad base from the wall of one of the paranasal sinuses, most frequently the frontal or ethmoid sinuses.

Osteoid osteoma

Definition: A benign osteoblastic lesion characterized by its small size (usually less than 1 cm), its clearly demarcated outline and by the usual presence of a surrounding zone of reactive bone formation. Histologically it consists of cellular, highly vascularized tissue made up of immature bone and osteoid tissue.

The term osteoid osteoma was suggested to describe this lesion which previously has been thought to be inflammatory in origin (Jaffe, 1935). Osteoid osteoma has been reported in almost every bone in the body with the exception of skull, sternum and clavicle. It is most common in the bones of the lower limbs, especially the femur and tibia. Byers (1968) collected 431 cases from the literature between 1935 and 1965, 87 per cent of which occurred between the ages of 5 and 24 years. Osteoid osteoma is two or three times commoner in males than in females. It causes pain which is characteristically more severe at night.

Osteoid osteomata may be cortical, cancellous or subperiosteal in site. The cortical type is the classic lesion, producing extensive dense periosteal new bone and sclerosis with a central, usually translucent, nidus (*Figure 2.1*). The nidus is small, as a rule no more than 1 cm in diameter, rounded or oval and it may have a dense, calcified centre. The density of the bone is greatest just around the nidus. If the lesion is in cancellous bone, relatively little sclerosis is produced and this may be at a distance from the lesion. This type may be located in the neck of the femur or in the vertebrae or small bones of the hand or foot. The subperiosteal osteoid osteoma may be in similar locations. It may cause pressure erosion of the underlying cortex, with little sclerosis; periosteal new bone may be formed and occasionally there is a joint effusion. Tomography may be necessary to show the lesion and to define the central nidus. On arteriography the nidus is vascular (Lindbom *et al.*, 1960). An osteoid osteoma may lead to an increase in length of the affected bone (Spjut *et al.*, 1971).

Osteoblastoma

Definition: A benign lesion with a histological structure similar to that of osteoid osteoma, but characterized by its larger size (usually more than 1 cm) and by the usual absence of any surrounding zone of reactive bone formation.

Most of the affected patients are between 10 and 35 years of age. The tumour frequently occurs in a vertebra (neural arches, spinous processes and body). In the long bones it occurs in the metaphysis or diaphysis and is frequently located in the femur and tibia,

Radiologically the lesion is well circumscribed; it may consist of a central translucency, larger than that of an osteoid osteoma, surrounded by an area of sclerosis and with periosteal new bone formation overlying it. It may produce expansion of the bone. In a long bone the tumour tends to show central destruction over an area of about 2 or more centimetres diameter in which there may be an irregular, dense nidus, and the lesion may be surrounded by some sclerosis or periosteal new bone. If the lesion grows rapidly it may be purely destructive.

MALIGNANT

Osteosarcoma

Definition: A malignant tumour, characterized by the direct formation of bone or osteoid tissue by the tumour cells.

Cell and matrix differentiation may occur in several directions producing five histological types (*see* Table):

TABLE

Histological type of osteosarcoma	Differentiating towards cell type
Osteoblastic	Osteoblasts and bone
Fibroblastic	Fibroblasts and fibres
Chondroblastic	Chondroblasts and cartilage
Anaplastic	Mixture of above types
Pleomorphic	Spheroidal and spindle cells

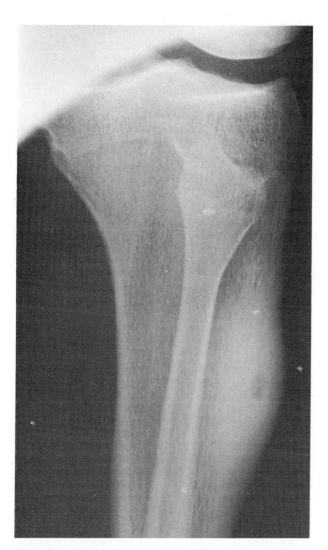

Figure 2.1. Osteoid Osteoma of Left Tibia: Dense cortical new bone is present causing thickening of the upper end of the tibia. A small oval translucency lies within the area of increased density

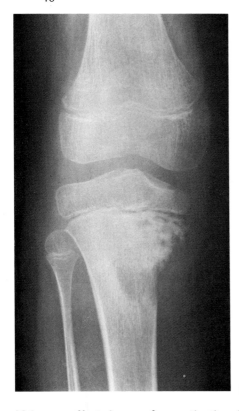

(a)

Figure 2.2. Metaphyseal Osteosarcoma of Right Tibia: An area of destruction is present on the medial side of the upper tibia, extending downwards from the metaphysis and involving the cortex on the posteromedial aspect of the bone. Ill-defined areas of increased bone density are present within the lesion. (a) Anteroposterior projection. (b) Lateral projection

(b)

Males are affected more frequently than females. Most osteosarcomata arising in otherwise normal bone occur between the ages of 10 and 25 years. Of these the tumours may originate in any bone including the small bones of the hands and feet but are commonest around the knee joint in the lower end of the femur and upper end of the tibia (Ross, 1964) (*Figure 2.2*) The next commonest site is in the upper end of the humerus. Osteosarcoma may be metaphyseal or diaphyseal in origin in the long bones (*Figure 2.4*). The tumour most frequently arises eccentrically in the metaphyseal region of a long bone. It spreads along the shaft and through the cortex into the surrounding soft tissues, raising the periosteum as it progresses. Some tumours arise more superficially in the cortex and some parosteally (*see below*). Osteosarcoma may arise in bone that is already pathological, but this seldom occurs in childhood. Cases have been reported of osteosarcoma complicating fibrous dysplasia. Osteosarcomata metastasize early by the bloodstream to the lungs and also to the other bones. Multicentric tumours occur very rarely.

The radiological appearances vary considerably, emphasizing the pleomorphic nature of the tumour. The osteoblastic or chondroblastic type of tumour may produce plentiful, dense new bone. Apart from this it is not possible to forecast the histological type from the radiological appearance. Osteosarcoma produces wither destruction or new bone but most frequently a combination of these features. The destruction is predominantly intramedullary but the cortex may be involved or more frequently both medulla and cortex. The destruction may be uniform or patchy and the margins of the affected area are usually fairly well defined. The surrounding bone is normal or sclerotic. New bone formation is shown as sclerosis within the medulla and this may be either uniform or patchy in appearance, most frequently the latter. Interspersed between the areas of sclerosis may be areas of destruction, giving the bone a spotty appearance. The spread of the sclerosis and destruction is limited by the epiphyseal plate. Other evidence of bone formation is shown by the production of periosteal new bone on the surface, and this may be layered, spiculated or amorphous in type. The periosteal new bone central to the tumour extension may be destroyed and this feature produces the well-known Codman's triangle (*Figure 2.6*). When the tumour extends outside the bone, a mass may be seen displacing the normal translucent soft tissue planes away from it. Amorphous and spiculated tumour bone is frequently seen in the soft-tissue mass. Pathological fracture may occur through the lesion. Cannon ball metastases sometimes containing new bone may be seen in the lung. If the tumour is cortical in origin intramedullary destruction may be absent or minimal. On arteriography, most osteosarcomata show a pathological circulation (*Figure 2.3*). Under radiation therapy the tumour may regress within the bone and the extra-osseous component become better defined (*Figure 2.6*).

Juxta-cortical (parosteal) osteosarcoma

Definition: A distinct type of osteosarcoma, characterized by an origin on the external surface of a bone and a high degree of structural differentiation. These tumours grow relatively slowly and have a better prognosis than the ordinary type of osteosarcoma.

Osteosarcoma of this type have been described as being attached to the parent bone cortex by part of their broad base, and they tend to encircle the bone in a mushroom fashion, leaving a clear space a few millimetres thick between this and the tumour at its periphery. The tumour usually consists of dense bone, and periosteal new bone is absent. It arises most commonly in the third, fourth and fifth decades but may also occur in children. The importance of this type of tumour lies in the fact that its prognosis (65 per cent five-year survival rate) is so much better than that of osteosarcoma.

Extraskeletal osteosarcomata in the soft tissues of the extremities have been reported in children over 3 years of age but are commoner in adults.

CARTILAGE-FORMING TUMOURS

BENIGN

Chrondroma

Definition: A benign tumour characterized by the formation of mature cartilage but lacking in the histological

characteristics of chondrosarcoma (high cellularity, pleomorphism and presence of large cells with double nuclei or mitoses).

This tumour is relatively common. It may be single or multiple. When multiple and predominantly unilateral, the condition is described as Ollier's disease and if accompanied by haemangiomata, Maffucci's syndrome (*see page 15 and Figure 3.12*). Children with chondromata present after the second decade. This tumour may arise within the medulla where it is described as an enchondroma or more superficially in the cortex or beneath the periosteum where it is known as an ecchondroma. It is considered to arise from a cartilage rest and is therefore seen in the first place in the metaphyseal region of the bone.

Radiologically an enchondroma is seen as a well-defined area of destruction, usually with a thin dense rim around it, in the medulla of a long bone (*Figure 2.7*). It erodes the cortex from within and may expand the bone. Areas of calcification may be seen within it.

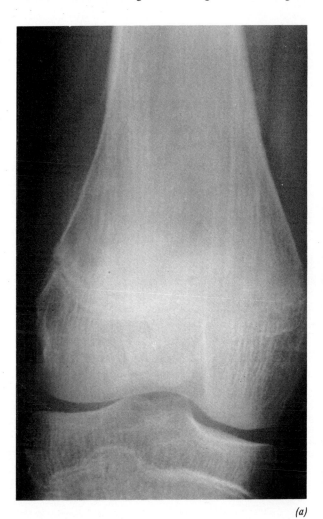

(a)

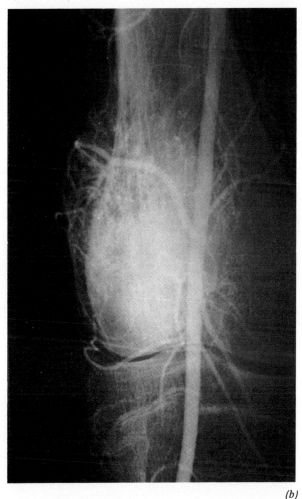

(b)

Figure 2.3. Metaphyseal Osteosarcoma of Femur: (a) Plain film of the lower end of the right femur. There is an area of increased bone density in the lateral side of the metaphysis with subcortical destruction. The lateral cortex of the bone is intact but there is a soft tissue mass visible on its outer aspect within which there are faint opacities due to new bone formation. (b) A femoral arteriogram of the same case reveals the extent of the tumour both within the bone and the adjacent soft tissues. This is apparent from the large number of arterial branches supplying the highly vascular lesion which shows a pathological circulation and a tumour blush

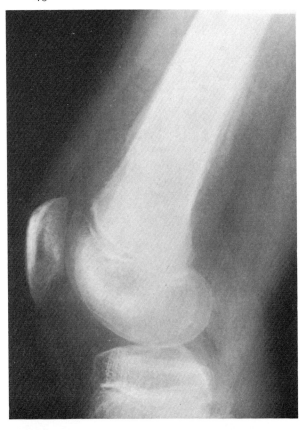

Figure 2.4. Diaphyseal Osteosarcoma of Femur: Lateral projection of the lower end of the femur. There is a diffuse area of increased bone density obscuring the corticomedullary junction. A soft tissue swelling surrounds both aspects of the bone and there is extensive periosteal new bone on the anterior and posterior surfaces. The new bone has been destroyed distally to give the appearance of a 'Codman's triangle'

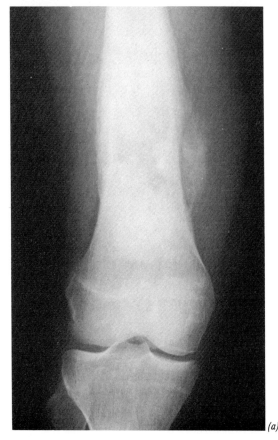

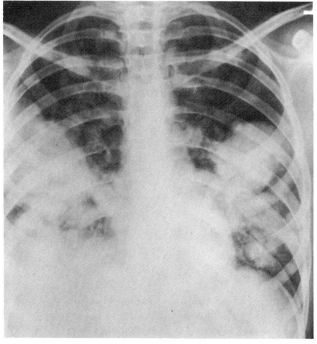

Figure 2.5. Diaphyseal Osteosarcoma of Femur: (a) Plain film of the lower end of the femur showing extensive medullary osteosclerosis in the diaphysis. Within the sclerosis there is an irregular area of bone destruction. Periosteal new bone and an amorphous density within the soft tissue mass on the medial aspect of the bone are also present. (b) Chest film of the same case showing multiple pulmonary metastases of variable size and density; some of them are bone forming

(a)

(b)

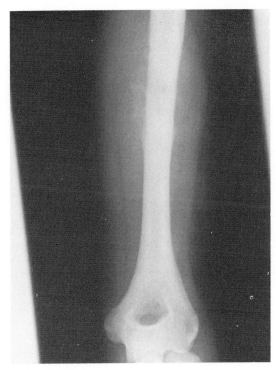
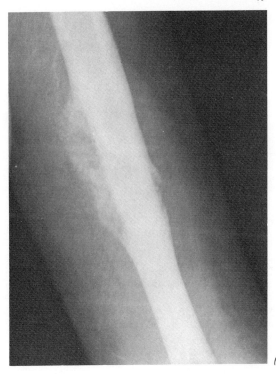

(a)   *(b)*

Figure 2.6. Diaphyseal Osteosarcoma of Humerus: (a) An anteroposterior view of the left humerus demonstrating an ill-defined, partly productive lesion of the midshaft. Opacities are present within the soft tissue mass on the medial aspect of the bone and there are well marked 'Codman's triangles' present distally. (b) The same case following radiotherapy showing a considerable increase in the extent of the ossification in the soft tissue mass

Fracture may take place through the lesion. Multiple enchondromata may be present. In Maffucci's syndrome, the intra-osseous lesions are accompanied by phleboliths in the soft tissues.

If the chondroma is superficial, the destruction will occur in the cortex, which may be deficient or expanded, and there may be some organized periosteal new bone bridging the angle between the expanded tumour and the cortex.

Osteochondroma

Definition: A cartilage-capped bony projection on the external surface of a bone.

This lesion is common and occurs in any bone preformed in cartilage. It may be solitary or multiple, the latter being known as diaphyseal aclasis (*see* page 15). The tumour is sited most commonly at the metaphyseal end of a long bone, and the sites of predilection are the lower end of the femur (*Figure 2.8*), the upper end of the tibia and the upper end of the humerus. The tumour may have either a narrow pedunculated or broad sessile base on the parent bone. This tumour is frequent in children and its growth will cease when skeletal maturity is reached. As the parent bone increases in length, the osteochondroma comes to be sited further away from the growing end of the bone.

Radiologically, the tumour appears as a bony outgrowth from the surface of the bone, sharply defined and with either a narrow or a wide base. The trabeculation of the parent bone is continuous into the stalk

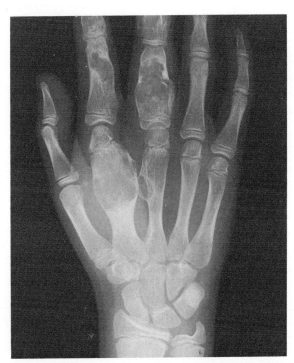

Figure 2.7. Multiple Enchondromata of the Right Hand: Several irregular translucent areas are present in the metacarpals and phalanges of the index, middle and ring fingers due to enchondromata. They have caused expansion of the bone and thinning of the cortex. There is a recent fracture through the lesion in the proximal phalanx of the middle finger

and the cortex of the parent bone extends out as the cortex of the osteochondroma (*Figure 2.8; see also Figure 1.11*). The tumour is usually directed away from the end of the bone. In children the cartilage cap is not visible but in adult life it becomes irregularly calcified. If large, the osteochondroma will displace surrounding soft-tissue planes. When the tumour is broad-based and near the end of the long bone, the outline of the long bone is disturbed and there will be failure of modelling. It may produce pressure erosion of adjacent bones, i.e. a tibial osteochondroma may produce pressure erosion of the fibula. Occasionally an osteochondroma may be fractured by trauma.

Chondroblastoma

Definition: A relatively rare benign tumour, characterized by highly cellular and relatively undifferentiated tissue made up of rounded or polygonal chondroblast-like cells with distinct outlines, together with multinucleated giant cells of osteoclast type arranged either singly or in groups. On the whole, little intercellular material is seen, but in the presence of small amounts of cartilaginous intercellular matrix with areas of focal calcification is typical.

This tumour is very rare. It is commoner in males than in females in the ratio of 2 to 1. It almost invariably arises in the epiphysis of a long bone and it is commonest in the femur, tibia and humerus. The majority are recognized in the second decade of life.

The tumour shows radiologically as a well-defined area of destruction, often with a thin sclerotic rim, in the epiphysis, but it may expand to involve the metaphysis (*Figure 2.9*). It may have hazy calcification in it producing a cotton-wool appearance. Periosteal reaction is unusual. On arteriography the tumour may be highly vascular.

Chondromyxoid fibroma

Definition: A benign tumour characterized by lobulated areas of spindle-shaped or stellate cells, with abundant myxoid or chondroid intercellular material, separated by zones of more cellular tissue rich in spindle-shaped or rounded cells with a varying number of multinucleated giant cells of different sizes. Large pleomorphic cells may be present and can result in confusion with chondrosarcoma.

This tumour is uncommon, It arises predominantly between the ages of 10 and 30 years but seldom before the age of 5 years. It occurs equally in males and females. The commonest site is in the upper end of the tibia and about 75 per cent occur in the lower limbs.

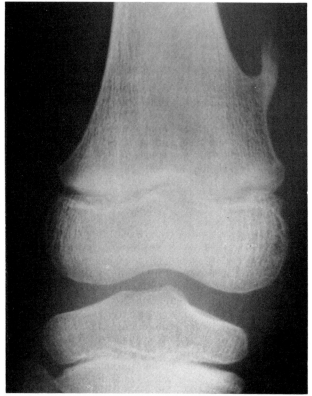

(a)

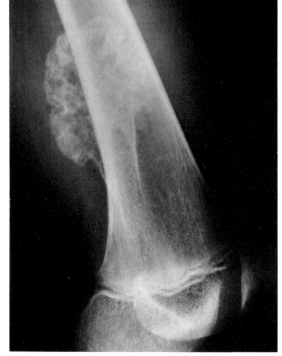

(b)

Figure 2.8. Osteochondromata of Femora: (a) There is a small osteochondroma arising from the medial aspect of the lower end of the femur. Its tip is characteristically directed towards the centre of the shaft. Its base is broad and merges into the cortex on either side. There is some loss of the normal modelling of the bone in the neighbourhood of the tumour. (b) There is a larger pedunculated osteochondroma which also arises from the lower end of the femur and which is seen in the lateral projection. The cap of cartilage at the apex of the tumour is irregularly calcified and shows a lobulated outline

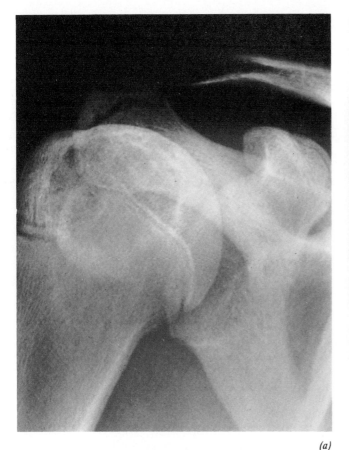
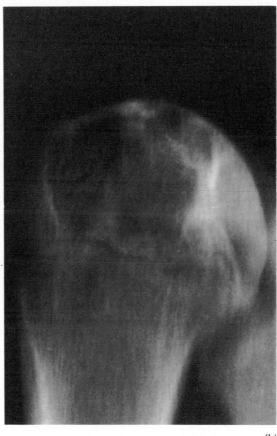

(a)   *(b)*

Figure 2.9. Chondroblastoma of Humerus: *(a) A destructive tumour of the proximal epiphysis of the humerus showing a well-defined sclerotic margin and ill-defined densities within it. (b) A tomogram of the same case showing that the tumour is confined to the epiphysis*

Radiologically, the tumour presents as a sharply defined area of destruction, rounded, oval or lobulated in outline and sometimes with a thin sclerotic rim (*Figure 2.10*). It may be subcortial in position and produce localized expansion with organized periosteal new bone around it and endosteal sclerosis. There is seldom calcification in the tumour.

MALIGNANT

Chondrosarcoma

Definition: A malignant tumour characterized by the formation of cartilage, but not of bone, by the tumour cells. It is distinguished from chondroma by the presence of more cellular and pleomorphic tissue, and by appreciable numbers of plump cells with large or double nuclei. Mitotic cells are infrequent.

The literature on chondrosarcoma is difficult to assess because there has been failure in the past in many series to differentiate between the true chondrosarcoma and chondroblastic osteosarcoma. The latter conforms to the familiar pattern of osteosarcoma, being most common in the second and third decades. True chondrosarcoma is, in fact, rare before the age of 20 years. Only 10 of the 288 cases of chondrosarcoma reported by Henderson and Dahlin (1963) were under the age of 20 years. It is most frequent in the fourth, fifth and sixth decades. Chondrosarcoma is commonest in the bones of the pelvis and shoulder girdle, femur, scapula, humerus and ribs. In the pelvis and shoulder girdle the tumour tends to be peripheral in type in that it grows out from the bone; in the tubular bones the tumours tend to be central in position. Chondrosarcoma may be primary or secondary. The secondary tumour arises in a pre-existing cartilaginous lesion and the primary one arises *de novo*.

The tumour presents radiologically as a fairly well defined area of medullary destruction which erodes the inner aspect of the overlying cortex. Periosteal new bone is also laid down so that the bone becomes expanded. There may be some subcortical or medullary sclerosis and areas of calcification may be seen within the lesion. Some chondrosarcomata, however, may be purely destructive and their margins not so well defined. Secondary chondrosarcoma arising from a pre-existing central chondroma appears as alteration and lack of definition in the outline of the original lesion and destruction of the cortex overlying it perhaps with some periosteal new bone formation. If secondary chondrosarcoma arises in a pre-existing osteochondroma, the cap of the osteochondroma will increase rapidly in size, producing a soft tissue mass and the areas of calcification already in the cap may be destroyed by the chondrosarcoma. Other areas of calcification may develop in the

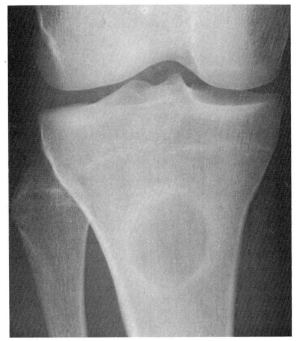

(a)

Figure 2.10. Chondromyxoid Fibroma of Right Tibia: There is a well-defined spherical translucent area with a dense margin in the anterior aspect of the upper end of the tibia. There is some expansion and thinning of the cortex overlying the tumour (a) Anteroposterior projection. (b) Lateral projection (There is an artefact overlying the posterior aspect of the tibia)

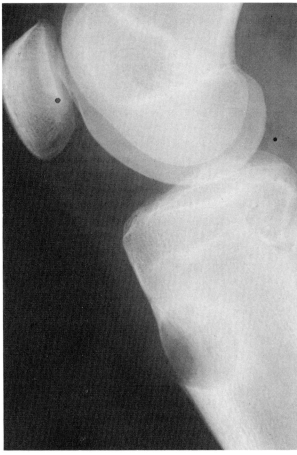

(b)

soft tissue mass. In the same way, the stalk of the osteo-chondroma may be destroyed. Rapid increase in size of a pre-existing chondromatous lesion which is frequently associated with the onset of pain is a strong reason for suspecting the development of malignancy. On arteriography chondrosarcomata are avascular. This tumour is rare in childhood (Middlemiss, 1964).

GIANT-CELL TUMOUR
(OSTEOCLASTOMA)

Definition: An aggressive tumour, characterized by richly vascularized tissue consisting of rather plump, spindle-shaped or ovoid cells and by the presence of numerous giant cells of osteoclast type, which are uniformly distributed throughout the tumour tissue. Relatively little collagen is present.

Giant-cell tumour is commonest between the ages of 20 and 40 years and it is rarely seen before the age of epiphyseal fusion, though well documented cases have occurred in teenagers (Dahlin, 1967).

Radiologically, the tumour produces · eccentric destruction in the epiphysis or metaphysis which leads to thinning and expansion of the overlying cortex (*Figure 2.11*). The junction between tumour destruction and surrounding normal bone is not well defined. The cortex over the tumour may be destroyed and a tumour mass extend into the soft tissues. Pathological fracture may

occur and as it heals periosteal new bone may be seen. Apparent septa may be shown crossing the radiolucent area—these are due to ridges on the bony edge of the tumour. After treatment with radiotherapy or surgery, the lesion will fill in with irregular bone.

MARROW TUMOURS

Ewing's sarcoma

Definition: A malignant tumour characterized by tissue with a rather uniform histological appearance made up of densely packed small cells with round nuclei but without distinct cytoplasmic outlines or prominent nucleoli. Often the tumour tissue is divided into irregular masses by fibrous septa. The intercellular network of reticulin fibres which is a feature of reticulosarcoma is not seen.

The majority of these tumours contain intracellular glycogen (Schajowicz, 1959). There has been much controversy over the origin and nature of this tumour. The discussion has centred round the difficulties of the differential diagnosis of malignant round-cell tumours of bone and the separation of the specific tumours, Ewing's sarcoma, reticulosarcoma and metastatic neuroblastoma.

Ewing's sarcoma is a very malignant tumour and it arises between the ages of 5 and 20 years with a peak

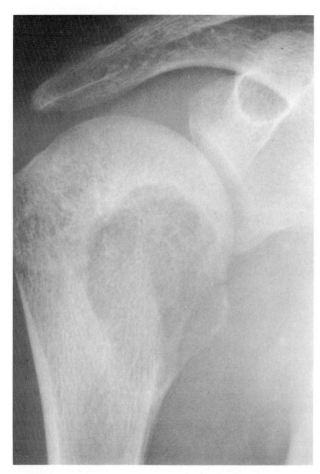

Figure 2.11. Giant Cell Tumour of the Humerus: There is an eccentric area of bone destruction in the medial side of the upper metaphysis of the humerus with a slightly lobulated outline. Ridges of bone are shown crossing the area of the tumour. The cortex though thinned and expanded is intact

incidence between 10 and 20 years of age. It is commonest in the diaphysis of a long bone but it also occurs in the flat bones particularly in the ilium and ribs. Radiologically, the tumour produces ill-defined medullary and central destruction which when first seen is usually extensive within the long bone (*Figure 2.12*). Widespread periosteal new bone, particularly of the onion-peel type, may be apparent; spiculated new bone may also be produced. Patchy intramedullary sclerosis may occur. It may produce diffuse soft tissue swelling and it may metastasize to other bones. Ewing's sarcoma has to be differentiated from osteosarcoma, reticulosarcoma, metastatic neuroblastoma and infections.

Reticulosarcoma of bone

Definition: A malignant lymphoid tumour with a rather varied histological structure. The tumour cells are usually rounded and rather pleomorphic and may have well-defined cytoplasmic outlines; many of their nuclei are indented or horseshoe-shaped and have prominent nucleoli. In most cases numerous reticulin fibres are present and are distributed uniformly between the tumour cells.

Reticulosarcoma of bone may occur at any age but it is more common after the age of 20 years. It may occur as a primary neoplasm in the bone or the bone may be involved in systematized reticulosarcoma. The former condition is the only one considered here. Reticulosarcoma has been reported in almost every bone but it is commonest in the long tubular bones of the upper and lower limbs. Nearly half the cases occur in the lower end of the femur and upper end of the tibia. It is three times commoner in males than in females.

Radiologically, the tumour produces patchy ill-defined destruction in the medulla and cortex with some periosteal new bone over the lesion (*Figure 2.13*). There may be some sclerosis but it is usually not marked except in the upper end of the tibia. A soft tissue tumour may be seen. On treatment with radiotherapy the lesion rapidly regresses and the bone may return almost to normal texture.

Lymphosarcoma of bone

Definition: A malignant lymphoid tumour characterized by well-differentiated (lymphocytic) or poorly differentiated (lymphoblastic) cells.

It is indistinguishable radiologically from reticulosarcoma.

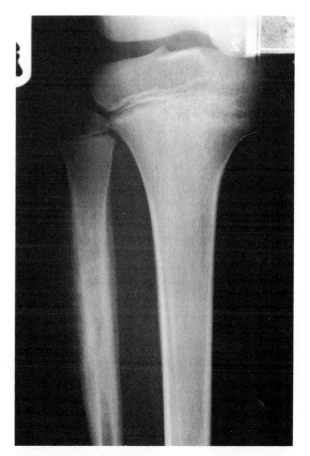

Figure 2.12. Ewing's Sarcoma of Fibula: There is a tumour of the upper part of the fibula producing widespread periosteal new bone and patchy sclerosis of the medulla. The corticomedullary junction is ill defined

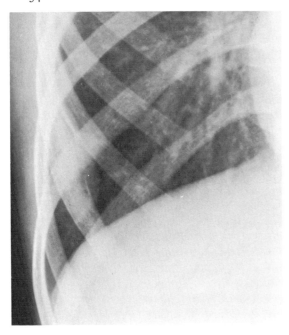

Figure 2.13. Reticulosarcoma of Rib: There is a tumour of the right seventh rib, which has caused expansion of the bone with periosteal new bone formation and ill-defined sclerosis. A soft tissue mass can also be seen extending medially from the affected area of bone

VASCULAR TUMOURS

BENIGN

Haemangioma

Definition: A benign lesion consisting of newly formed blood vessels, either of capillary or cavernous type.

This lesion occurs typically in a vertebra or in the vault of the skull. It may be seen at any age but it is most common in middle-aged females.

Radiologically vertebral haemangiomata produce coarse vertical striation of the body, and there may also be a coarse trabecular pattern extending into the neural arch and transverse processes. The bone is not enlarged. In the skull the area of destruction may contain a stellate central density, the so-called 'sunburst appearance'. Multiple haemangiomata may occur involving one or several bones. A soft-tissue haemangioma may also involve bone. This is shown by increased growth in length and expansion of the bone with a coarse mottling. Phleboliths may be seen in the surrounding soft tissues in the extra-osseous part of the haemangioma.

Vanishing bone disease or haemangiomatosis is a very rare abnormality which affects patients of all ages but is more frequent in adults than children.
The radiological appearances show progressive disappearance of bone, usually of the axial skeleton, but it may also affect the long bones. Arteriography fails to show any abnormality to account for the appearances. Lymphangiomatosis may produce a similar lesion.

INTERMEDIATE OR INDETERMINATE

Haemangio-endothelioma

Haemangiopericytoma

MALIGNANT

Angiosarcoma

All these lesions are exceedingly rare and the histology is not clear-cut. Though they may occur in children, a discussion of them is outside the scope of this book.

OTHER CONNECTIVE TISSUE TUMOURS

BENIGN

Desmoplastic fibroma

Definition: A benign tumour characterized by the formation of abundant collagen fibres by the tumour cells. The tissue is poorly cellular and nuclei are ovoid or elongated. The cellularity, pleomorphism and mitotic activity that are features of fibrosarcoma are lacking.

The term desmoplastic fibroma was introduced to describe a rare group of fibrous tissue lesions in bone which were distinct from fibrosarcoma and other benign fibrous lesions (Jaffe, 1958). They are histologically like the desmoid tumours in soft tissue. They occur in adolescents and young adults and affect the long bones, vertebrae and pelvis. Radiologically, there is destruction in the medulla, erosion of the cortex and expansion, the lesion giving an appearance of aggressiveness. There may be some sclerosis and periosteal new bone formation.

MALIGNANT

Fibrosarcoma

Definition: A malignant tumour characterized by the formation by the tumour cells of interlacing bundles of collagen fibres and by the absence of other types of histological differentiation, such as the formation of cartilage or bone.

Undoubtedly many fibrosarcomata of bone in the past have been diagnosed as fibroblastic osteosarcomata and parosteal fibrosarcomata, but the existence of primary fibrosarcoma of bone as a separate entity is now accepted. There are histochemical differences between osteosarcoma and fibrosarcoma (Jeffree and Price, 1965) and the 5- and 10-year survival rate of fibrosarcoma is slightly better than that of osteosarcoma. In a series of 50 cases of fibrosarcomata reported by Eyrebrook and Price (1969), 15 had an established predisposing cause (previous cartilage lesions, Paget's disease or previous radiotherapy) but none of these occurred in children. Fibrosarcoma is rare in children and in the same series only 3 arose in patients below the age of 20 years. The age incidence contrasts with that of osteosarcoma which has its peak incidence in the second decade. Fibrosarcoma is commonest in the long bones in

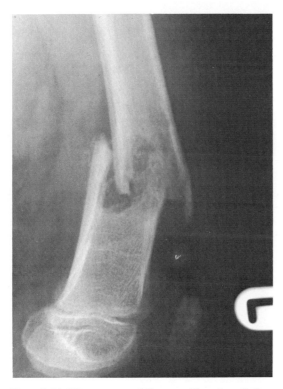

Figure 2.14. Fibrosarcoma of Femur: There is medullary destruction in the lower half of the femur. A pathological fracture has occurred through the tumour. (By courtesy of the Editor of Journal of Bone and Joint Surgery*)*

the femur, in the humerus and tibia, in that order. It tends to arise in the diaphysis and its origin may be central in the medulla or more superficial.

Radiologically, destruction predominates and is most extensive in the medulla (*Figure 2.14*). It may be uniform or patchy over a circumscribed area. Its margins are ill defined. Though the cortex is breached reactive new bone may be laid down on the surface, producing expansion. However, Codman's triangle may be produced. Occasionally medullary sclerosis occurs, either within the area of destruction or in the surrounding bone. Cases do occur in which medullary sclerosis predominates. Pathological fracture through the lesion is common. A soft tissue mass may develop around the affected bone. On arteriography fibrosarcomata tend to be avascular and therefore failure to demonstrate a pathological circulation on arteriography does not exclude the presence of a fibrosarcoma.

OTHER TUMOURS

Adamantinoma of bone

Definition: A malignant, or at least locally malignant, tumour characterized by the presence of circumscribed masses of apparently epithelial cells surrounded by spindle-shaped tissue. The peripheral cells of the supposed epithelial formations are columnar and palisaded, while the central cells have a stellate arrangement and are separated by spaces; this gives the lesion some degree of

resemblance to the ameloblastoma ('adamantinoma') of the jaw, and to other epithelial tumours of basal-cell type.

The term adamantinoma implies that the tumour has or can produce enamel, but none is ever shown histologically. It probably arises from congenital cell rests. Patients are usually about 35 years old but the tumour has been reported at the age of 8 years. It is very rare and is most frequently situated in the shaft of the tibia. Radiologically the tumour produces destruction of bone and appears as a well-demarcated area of translucency with a lobulated outline. It has a multiloculated appearance and may cause expansion. Occasionally it can lead to the development of sclerosis.

Neurofibroma

The term neurofibroma is sometimes used for certain benign tumours of nerves that do not have the distinctive histology of neurilemmoma. The name has been applied to multiple nerve and soft tissue lesions in neurofibromatosis (von Recklinghausen's disease). No cases of intra-osseous neurofibromata appear to have been authenticated (Schajowicz *et al.*, 1972). Other types of skeletal change, including scoliosis, growth disorders, congenital bowing and pseudarthrosis are common in neurofibromatosis but they are not due to neurofibromatous tissue actually in the bones. These changes are:

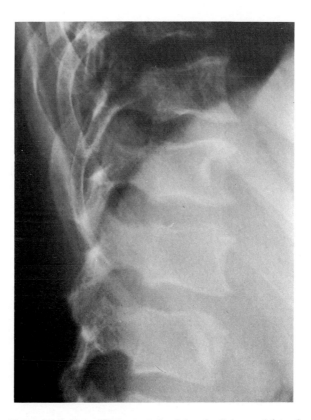

Figure 2.15. Neurofibromatosis Involving the Spine: A lateral view of the thoracolumbar spine showing well-marked anterior 'scalloping' of the vertebral bodies due to pressure erosion by neurofibromatous tissue

56

(1) Disturbances of growth which may produce unequal limb lengths, enlargement and asymmetrical development of the skull.

(2) Erosion of bone, which may occur from pressure by a neurofibroma arising in a nerve close to the bone. This tumour usually arises from the cells of the nerve sheath. It is likely to be clinically significant when it arises in an enclosed space such as in the spinal canal or internal auditory canal.

(3) Kyphoscoliosis, which most frequently occurs in the cervical and thoracic regions. Posterior scalloping of the vertebral bodies is due to internal meningoceles rather than neurofibromata. However, anterior scalloping may also occur (*Figure 2.15*) and this is produced by neurofibromatous tissue.

(4) Pseudarthrosis which may start in young children as a bowing of the tibia and which leads to actual resorption with pointing of the ends of the bones (*see* page 00). In some cases this is considered to be due to neurofibromatosis.

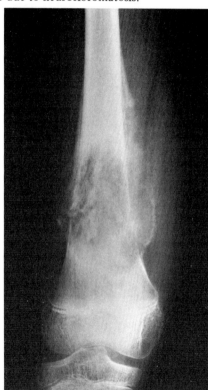

Figure 2.16. Unclassified Bone Tumour of Femur: An area of bone destruction in the lower end of the shaft of the femur which has destroyed the cortex and extended into the soft tissues. There is abundant periosteal new bone formation over the lesion which has also produced some bone expansion. (This lesion was unclassified by the Bristol Bone Tumour Registry)

UNCLASSIFIED TUMOURS

Occasionally tumours are encountered the nature of which is uncertain, though they are clearly of osseous origin. In such cases the diagnosis may remain in doubt in spite of full and competent radiological and pathological opinion (*Figure 2.16*). It may even be impossible to decide whether the lesion is benign or malignant.

TUMOUR-LIKE LESIONS

SOLITARY BONE CYST (SIMPLE OR UNICAMERAL BONE CYST)

Definition: A unicameral cavity filled with clear or sanguineous fluid and lined by a membrane of variable thickness, which consists of loose vascular connective tissue showing scattered osteoclast giant cells and sometimes areas of recent or old haemorrhage or cholesterol clefts.

About three-quarters of solitary bone cysts occur in the upper ends of the humerus and femur. The cyst arises in the metaphysis and frequently extends to the epiphyseal line. As the bone grows the cyst migrates along the shaft so that in older children the lesion may be seen at a distance from the epiphyseal plate. It may arise in other bones such as the radius, ulna, tibia, calcaneum, ilium, pubic bone or in a metatarsal or rib. The vast majority of bone cysts are solitary but patients

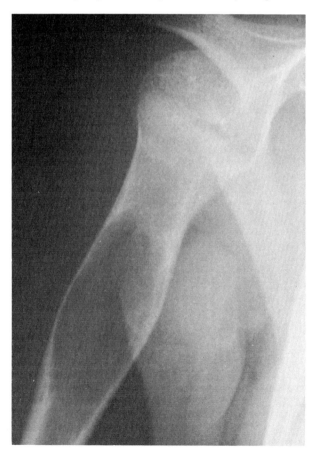

Figure 2.17. Simple Bone Cyst of Humerus: There is an expanding, uniformly translucent area of bone destruction in the upper end of the right humerus. The cortex is thinned and the margins of the lesion are well defined

with two cysts have been reported (Sadler and Rosenhain, 1964). The development of a cyst has been reported between the ages of 1½ and 72 years but most arise in childhood. They are three times more common in males than in females. Cysts may cause pain but patients frequently present for the first time with a fracture through the cyst.

Radiologically the cyst causes a well-defined area of bone destruction (*Figure 2.17*), which may have a thin condensed margin, in the metaphysis of a long bone. It is frequently smooth in outline but may have a wavy outline and an appearance of septa across it due to ridges of bone on the edges of the lesion. The cortex over the lesion may be thinned from within and expansion may take place. Fractures through the cyst are common, after which some periosteal new bone may form. After fracture the lesion may fill in with bone and resolve but this is unusual. Even after the cyst has been curretted and filled with bone chips, recurrence is fairly frequent.

Aneurysmal bone cyst

Definition: An expanding osteolytic lesion consisting of blood-filled spaces of variable size separated by connective tissue septa containing trabeculae of bone or osteoid tissue and osteoclast giant cells.

This lesion was stabilised as a pathological entity by Lichtenstein (1950), before which the lesions were usually regarded as giant-cell tumours. This lesion most frequently arises in patients in the second and third decades but has been reported between the ages of 6 years and 61 years. Pain and swelling are the presenting symptoms. The rate of growth is very variable, some enlarging rapidly in a matter of months and others remaining stationary for years. The shaft of the long bones, especially of the lower limbs, is the commonest location for the lesion. It may arise eccentrically within the bone. It may occur in the flat bones, especially in the appendages of the vertebral bodies.

Radiologically, an aneurysmal bone cyst is a destructive lesion, producing an area of well-defined radiolucency with thinning of the overlying cortex and frequently considerable expansion of the bone. There may be a condensed rim to the lesion. The cortex over the lesion may be completely destroyed but before this happens portions of the cortex will remain intact. Fracture through the lesion is common and healing of the fracture may lead to the development of periosteal new bone. New bone may also form in the recess between the expanded part of the lesion and the adjacent cortex of the parent bone. In the flat bones and in the appendages of the vertebrae the lesion produces similar radiological appearances. After the insertion of bone chips, the lesion

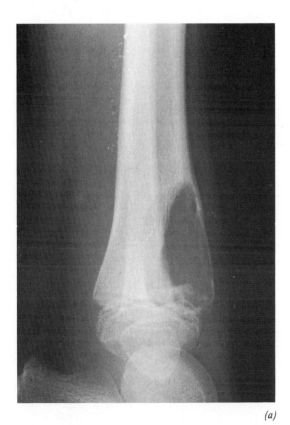 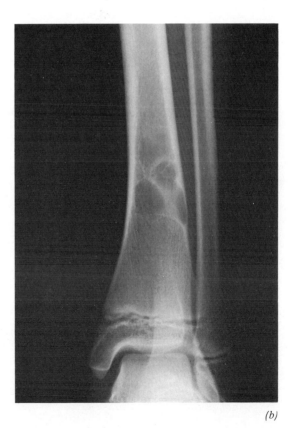

(a)   (b)

Figure 2.18. Aneurysmal Bone Cyst of Tibia: (a) An eccentrically placed well-defined translucent lesion on the anterior aspect of the distal metaphysis of the tibia. The cortex over the lesion is thinned and slightly expanded. (b) The same lesion 5 years later. Not only is the lesion rather smaller but growth during the interval has separated it from the distal metaphysis

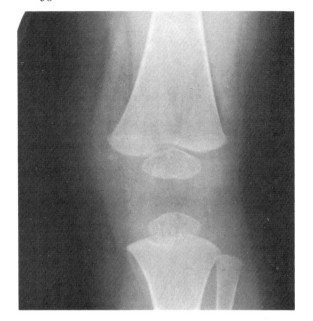

(a)

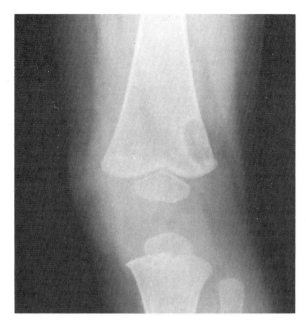

(b)

Figure 2.19. *Fibrous Cortical Defect of Femur: A well-defined oval area of bone destruction has developed on the lateral aspect of the lower end of the femur adjacent to the metaphysis. Healing occurs by a gradual obliteration of the lesion and by thickening of the sclerotic margin. (a) Knee of a child aged 17 months before the lesion has developed. (b) Established fibrous cortical defect 5 months later. (c) Healing stage 18 months later*

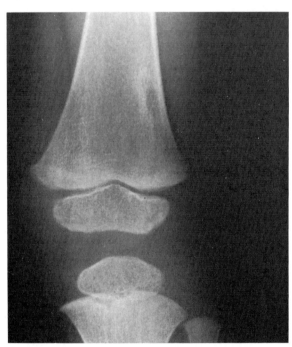

(c)

may fill in with regenerated bone (*Figure 2.18*). If arteriography is performed, the area of destruction produced by the tumour may take up the contrast medium, producing a blush at its site.

Metaphyseal fibrous defect (non-ossifying fibroma)

Definition: A non-neoplastic bone lesion of obscure aetiology, characterized by the presence of fibrous tissue with a whorled pattern containing multinucleated giant cells, haemosiderin pigment and lipid-bearing histocytes. It usually involves the metaphyseal region of long bones, in children or adolescents.

There has been much debate as to the pathogenesis of metaphyseal fibrous defect and non-ossifying fibroma. The authors believe that they are the same lesion, the metaphyseal fibrous defect being a small version of the non-ossifying fibroma. The lesion occurs in children in the lower end of the femur (*Figure 2.19*) and at the upper and lower ends of the tibia but it may also occur in other bones. According to Caffey (1955) this lesion will be found in 35 per cent of children. There is a definite familial tendency and there may be multiple lesions. Radiologically non-ossifying fibroma appears as a well-defined lobulated outlined radiolucent lesion with a fine condensed margin, occurring in the metaphysis of a long bone (*Figure 2.20*). The site of origin of the lesion is superficial or cortical and it frequently produces localized expansion with some involvement of the underlying medulla. The cortical defect is smaller than the non-

ossifying fibroma but both lesions are cortical in site. Caffey has shown that the lesions may regress within a year, but some recur. Others may heal with sclerosis (*Figure 2.19c*).

Histiocytosis

Definition: A non-neoplastic lesion of unknown aetiology, characterized by an intense proliferation of reticulo-histiocytic elements with varying numbers of eosinophilic leucocytes, neutrophilic leucocytes, lymphocytes, plasma cells and multinucleate giant cells.

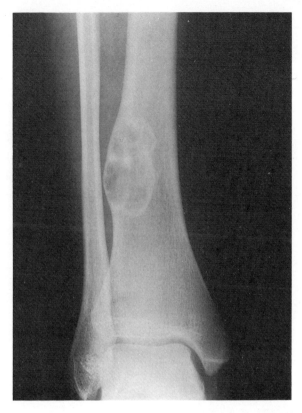

Figure 2.20. Non-ossifying Fibroma of Tibia: An eccentric lesion in the lower end of the tibia causing expansion of the medial cortex. The margin is well-defined, sclerotic and lobulated in outline, especially where it projects into the medulla

Eosinophil granuloma, Hand–Schüller–Christian disease and Letterer–Siwe disease are now classified as histiocytosis X or reticulo-endotheliosis. The three conditions form a spectrum of disease from the benign eosinophil granuloma through the chronic Hand–Schüller–Christian disease to the more malignant Letterer–Siwe disease (Ennis *et al.*, 1973). The common pathological condition is the proliferation of histiocytes with secondary deposits in them of lipids. However, one form may transform to another.

EOSINOPHIL GRANULOMA

This is the commonest of the lesions and it occurs most frequently in the second and third decades but it may occur even in middle age. Between one-half and three-quarters of the lesions are solitary (*Figure 2.21a*). The cases with multiple lesions usually have two or three, but they may number as many as five or six (*Figure 2.21b*). Eosinophil granuloma is commonest in the long bones, pelvis, skull and the flat bones. The typical lesion is one of well-defined bony destruction with sharp edges which in the flat bones may be undermined and serrated. The lesion may have a sclerotic rim which is usually thin. Sequestra within the lesion are seen and appear as densities within the main area of lysis. Sometimes the lesion does not have a sharp outline and its appearance suggests aggressiveness, especially as it may have an over-

lying periosteal reaction. It may, however, heal in 12 to 18 months and will respond to radiotherapy. The lesion may occur anywhere in the spine and it commonly produces marked collapse (vertebra plana) and this may be associated with a paravertebral shadow which is most likely to be due to haematoma. The ability of the vertebral bodies to reconstitute in time is noteworthy. Pathological fracture may occur through the lesions in long and flat bones. Abnormality in the lungs in the form of interstitial infiltration may be seen on chest radiographs and this occurs in less than 10 per cent of cases.

HAND–SCHÜLLER–CHRISTIAN DISEASE

In Hand–Schüller–Christian disease there may be lymphadenopathy, hepatosplenomegaly, diabetes insipidus and exophthalmos as well as the bone lesions, the latter being usually multiple and widely distributed. The radiological appearances of the individual bone lesions are the same as in eosinophil granuloma. In the skull there may be destruction in the base, and also lesions in the vault; the latter may coalesce to form the classical 'geographical skull' (*Figure 2.21c*). The lesions are slow in development and usually produce little new bone unless a fracture develops through the lesion. Pulmonary infiltration occurs in this variant as well.

LETTERER–SIWE DISEASE

Letterer–Siwe disease is the acute fulminating type of histiocytosis X arising usually in a child under 2 years of age, who is very ill. There is hepatosplenomegaly, lymphadenopathy, fever, a sore mouth, mediastinal lymphadenopathy and pulmonary infiltration. The bone lesions are not so common as in the other variants but they may be multiple. The lesion is not so well-defined as in eosinophil granuloma and it is seen most frequently in the diaphyseal ends of the long bones.

Fibrous dysplasia

A benign condition, presumably developmental in nature, characterized by the presence of fibrous connective tissue with a characteristic whorled pattern and containing trabeculae of immature non-lamellar bone. This condition is discussed in detail elsewhere (*see* page 18).

Myositis ossificans

A non-neoplastic condition, sometimes associated with trauma. The lesion may occur on the external surface of a bone or in soft tissues at a distance from the periosteal surface. The abnormal tissue is characterized by proliferation of fibrous tissue and by formation of large amounts of new bone. Cartilage may also be present. This condition is discussed further elsewhere (*see* page 39).

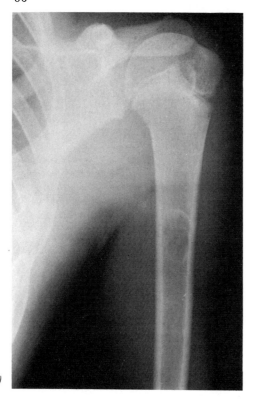

(a)

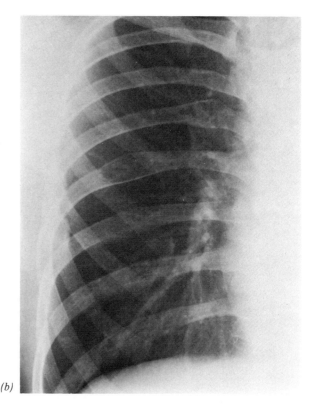

(b)

Figure 2.21. Histiocytosis X: (a) There is a centrally placed oval destructive lesion in the shaft of the humerus. The edge is well defined with a thin sclerotic margin. (b) Lesions in several ribs of the same child. The cortex is expanded and thinned. (c) The skull of the same case showing a number of round translucent destructive lesions in the cranial vault

METASTATIC OR SECONDARY TUMOURS IN BONE

Metastatic neoplasm in bone is rare in childhood, the best-known examples being neuroblastoma and leukaemia but other rarer conditions do exist. The latter will not be discussed in this work.

Metastatic neuroblastoma

Metastatic neuroblastoma, when first seen, is usually widely disseminated in bone and soft tissue but a lesion which appears to be solitary may present on occasions. Metastatic neuroblastoma produces medullary and cortical destruction which tends to have a spotty or speckled appearance. The destruction may occur anywhere in the long or flat bones but it has a predilection for the ends of the long bones. Layered periosteal new bone formation is usually present; it may extend a long distance up the shaft indicating extensive subperiosteal neoplasm. The new bone may also be spiculated and this may on occasions be the most conspicuous feature. Patchy sclerosis may develop within the bone. The appearance of patchy and extensive destruction of the vault bones of the skull with widening of the sutures, particularly the coronal suture, is well known (*see*

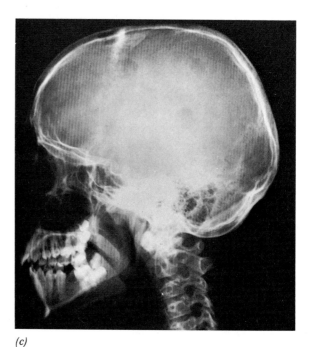

(c)

page 270). Large soft tissue masses may be present in association with the bone lesions and these may be particularly apparent on the chest radiograph in relation to the ribs. The plain radiograph of the abdomen may show speckled calcification in the suprarenal tumour mass and intravenous urography may show downward displacement of the kidney.

Metastases from Ewing's tumour and osteosarcoma

These two tumours are liable to metastasize to bones other than the bone in which the tumour originates. In osteosarcoma this occurs in 10 per cent of cases (Ross, 1964). The radiological appearance of the metastases is usually similar to that of the primary tumour.

Leukaemia

Leukaemia is a malignant state which primarily affects the medulla of the bone. There are two main types—myelogenous and lymphatic—depending on the type of cell which proliferates. It occurs in acute and chronic forms and in childhood the commonest form is acute lymphoblastic leukaemia. The radiological appearances of this conditions are discussed on page 76.

REFERENCES

GENERAL

Coley, B. L. (1972). *Neoplasms of Bone and Related Conditions* (3rd edn). New York; Hoeber

Dahlin, D. C. (1967). *Bone Tumours. General Aspects and an Analysis of 2,276 Cases* (2nd edn). Springfield; Thomas

Graham, W. D. (1966). *Bone Tumours.* London; Butterworths

Greenfield, G. B. (1969). *Radiology of Bone Diseases.* Philadelphia; Lippincott

Lichtenstein, L. (1965). *Bone Tumours* (3rd edn). Saint Louis; Mosby

Murray, R. O. and Jacobson, H. G. (1971). *The Radiology of Skeletal Disorders.* Edinburgh; Churchill-Livingstone

Price, C. H. G. and Ross, F. G. M. (1973). 'Bone: certain aspects of neoplasia.' Proceedings of the 24th Symposium of the Colston Research Society, held in Bristol, 1972 (Colston Papers, No. 24). London; Butterworths

Schajowicz, F., Ackerman, L. V. and Sissons, H. A. (1972). 'Histological typing of bone tumours.' In *International Histological Classification of Tumours No. 6.* Geneva; World Health Organisation

SPECIFIC LESIONS

Byers, P. D. (1968). 'Solitary benign osteoblastic lesions of bone: osteoid osteoma and osteoblastoma. *Cancer,* **22,** 43

Caffey, J. (1955). 'On fibrous defects in cortical walls of growing tubular bones.' *Adv. Pediat.* **7,** 13

Dahlin, D. C. (1967). 'Giant cell tumour (osteoclastoma).' In *Bone Tumours* (2nd edn), pp. 78–89. Springfield; Thomas

Ennis, J. T., Whitehouse, G., Ross, F. G. M. and Middlemiss, J. H. (1973). 'The radiology of the bone changes in histiocytosis X.' *Clin. Radiol.* **24,** 212

Eyre-Brook, A. L. and Price, C. H. G. (1969). 'Fibrosarcoma of bone. Review of fifty consecutive cases from the Bristol Bone Tumour Registry.' *J. Bone Jt Surg.* **51B,** 20

Henderson, E. D. and Dahlin, D. C. (1963). 'Chondrosarcoma of bone—a study of two hundred and eighty-eight cases.' *J. Bone Jt Surg.* **45A,** 1450

Jaffe, H. L. (1935). 'Osteoid-osteoma.' A benign osteoblastic tumor composed of osteoid and atypical bone.' *Archs Surg. Chicago* **31,** 709

— (1958). 'Desmoplastic fibroma and fibrosarcoma.' In *Tumors and Tumorous Conditions of the Bones and Joints.* pp. 298–303. Philadelphia; Lea and Febiger

Jeffree, G. M. and Price C. H. G. (1965). 'Bone tumours and their enzymes.' *J. Bone Jt Surg.* **47B,** 120

Lichtenstein, L. (1950). 'Aneurysmal bone cyst. A pathological entity commonly mistaken for giant-cell tumor and occasionally for hemangioma and osteogenic sarcoma.' *Cancer,* **3,** 279

Lindbom, A., Lindvall, N., Söderberg, G. and Spjut, H. J. (1960). 'Angiography in osteoid osteoma.' *Acta Radiol.* **54,** 327

Middlemiss, J. H., (1964). 'Cartilage tumours.' *Br. J. Radiol.* **37,** 277

Price, C. H. G. (1974). Personal communication

Ross, F. G. M. (1964). 'Osteogenic sarcoma.' *Br. J. Radiol.* **37,** 259

Sadler, A. M. and Rosenhain, F. (1964). 'Occurrence of two unicameral bone cysts in the same patient.' *J. Bone Jt Surg.* **46A,** 1557

Schajowicz, F. (1959). 'Ewing's sarcoma and reticulum cell sarcoma of bone, with special reference to the histochemical demonstration of glycogen as an aid to differential diagnosis.' *J Bone Jt Surg.* **41A,** 349

Schajowicz, F., Ackerman, L. V. and Sissons, H. A. (1972). 'Histological typing of bone tumours.' In *International Histological Classification of Tumours No. 6,* p. 45 Geneva; World Health Organisation

Spjut, H. J., Dorfman, H. D., Fechner, R. E. and Ackerman, L. V. (1971). 'Tumors of bone and cartilage.' In *Atlas of Tumor Pathology 2nd Series, Fascicle 5,* p.123. Washington D.C.; Armed Forces Institute of Pathology

3 SKELETAL SYSTEM

METHODS

PLAIN FILMS

In the investigation of diseases of the skeletal system, the inherent contrast supplied by the mineral content of the bone allows direct radiological visualization of changes in its structure and form. Nevertheless, there are limitations imposed by the very fact that the bones absorb x-rays; in consequence they cast a dense shadow in the film which can obscure much of the detail of the changes arising from disease processes. A good example of this is afforded by the early signs of trabecular destruction resulting from disease such as osteomyelitis or tumours. Because this process takes place deep within the substance of the bone, the signs do not become apparent on a radiograph until nearly half of the bone mass has been destroyed. Because of this the presence of disease is not revealed until many days after its onset.

Much of the finer structure of bone, in particular the pattern of the trabeculae in the medulla, is difficult to visualize clearly unless the technique employed is very accurate. This applies especially to factors such as immobilization, contrast and exposure. The faster and more sensitive types of films and the use of intensifying screens will impair fine detail because of the large grain size. Even with young children, however, it may be possible to use a fine grain film which does not need intensifying screens, without increasing the length of the exposure to such an extent that detail is lost through movement. Detail is also enhanced by ensuring that the focal spot from which the x-rays originate is as small as possible. In the case of the child's forearm, hand or foot, the thickness of the tissues is small enough to allow the exposure to be reduced to the degree necessary for the use of a small focal spot.

TOMOGRAPHY

The disadvantages referred to above, which result from the absorption of x-rays by those parts of the bone lying in front of or behind the area affected by disease and so obscuring it, can be offset by the use of tomography. By its capacity to blur out such unwanted shadows, tomography may reveal the lesion at an earlier stage, or show more completely its full extent. For this reason it may afford a very useful adjunct to conventional radiography, where this has failed to demonstrate a lesion as completely as possible, always provided that adequate immobilization can be assured. This is essential to achieve the best results and is not always easy to attain in small infants.

MACRORADIOGRAPHY

Macroradiography is a technique by which a magnified image of the part is produced. This is achieved by increasing the distance between the part to be radiographed and the film. This requires the use of a tube with a fine focal spot. Although it may not show anything which cannot be detected on the conventional film, it does so more clearly and may lessen the possibility of overlooking features which depend on appreciation of very fine detail.

TECHNIQUES INVOLVING THE USE OF CONTRAST MEDIA

The value of the use of contrast media in relation to diseases of bones or joints is less than in other systems.

It is limited to arthrography and arteriography, neither of which has a very extensive application in the paediatric field.

Arthrography

The injection of water-soluble, positive-contrast medium into the synovial cavity of a joint is used chiefly as an aid to the management of hip diseases such as congenital dislocation or Perthes' disease. It has little place in the diagnosis of such conditions. In the knee, it may be useful in elucidating the nature of injuries which give equivocal clinical signs and fail to respond to treatment. The introduction of air as well as positive contrast medium to produce 'double contrast' films, may enhance the value of the technique. The method is simple and is free of serious sequelae provided strict aseptic precautions are taken.

Arteriography

The injection of contrast medium into an artery can occasionally be useful in clarifying the nature of swellings in the limbs where it is uncertain whether they are inflammatory or neoplastic in nature or, if the latter, whether the lesion is benign or malignant.

ISOTOPE SCANNING

The use of radioactive isotopes, which are taken up selectively by tumour tissue, also has a place in the investigation of bone tumours.

INFLAMMATORY DISEASE OF BONES AND JOINTS

OSTEOMYELITIS

This condition, in spite of the introduction of anti-biotics, is still an important disease in childhood. The latent period of a week to 10 days separating the onset of the clinical signs and symptoms and the development of radiological abnormalities is well recognized. It is equally well known that in many cases the early use of antibiotics can prevent or minimize the development of these signs, and that, as a result, the radiological appearances can be unusual and atypical; or, alternatively, they may appear more extensive and striking than would be expected from the relatively mild and insidious symptoms.

Radiology is nevertheless useful as a means of diagnosis, in the assessment of the extent and course of the disease and in detecting the development of sequestra. Areas of bone destruction, often ill defined and patchy in nature, occur classically in the metaphyseal region of the long bones, whence the disease may extend towards the diaphysis (*Figure 3.1a*); It is rare for it to cross the growth plate and involve the epiphysis, unlike tuberculosis osteitis (*see* page 64). Periosteal new bone formation is commonly an associated feature and indicates spread of the infection beneath the periosteum (*Figure 3.1c*). Sometimes, if the destructive lesions are not

extensive or situated deep within the bone, the periosteal reaction may be the earliest or even the only sign of osteomyelitis. The inflammatory process may cause a pathological fracture or necrosis of a portion of bone. Such a sequestrum is shown as an isolated fragment which is often denser than the bone surrounding it (*Figure 3.1a*); Again, if it is deeply situated, it can be hidden by overlying structures, in particular by the dense sclerotic bone which forms around the inflammatory focus as healing begins to occur. The radiological appearances in the later stages are dominated by the processes of healing and there is an irregular thickening and sclerosis of the bone so that much of the normal architecture may be obscured (*Figure 3.1b* and *Figure 3.2*).

These appearances may be modified in cases where osteomyelitis develops in unusual sites, such as the spine or the jaws, or in the epiphyses of the long bones. In very young infants, the clinical signs may be initially those of septicaemia; these can mask the signs of the local bone lesion which is sometimes first revealed on radiography. Because of this mode of origin, the osteomyelitis is not infrequently multifocal, though it is not symmetrically distributed as is the case with other inflammatory bone disease.

Epiphyses

Epiphyseal osteomyelitis commonly occurs around the knee or hip joints (Roberts, 1970). It may be associated with septic arthritis (*see* page 64). The bone destruction characteristically involves the peripheral part of the epiphysis, and the central part remains intact (*Figure 3.3*). Restoration of the areas of destroyed bone and articular surface may occur up to several years after the initial infection. Damage to the growth plate is an important accompaniment of such cases and may result in shortening of a limb or asymmetry of a bone such as the mandible. The resulting deformity may be a source of severe disability.

Spinal lesions

Osteomyelitis of the spine is a relatively rare disease but one which may give rise to misleading symptoms such as abdominal or hip pain. The radiological changes do not differ materially from those elsewhere, but the intervertebral disc spaces are usually narrowed. Paraspinal abcesses are shown by the presence of a soft tissue shadow alongside the spine in the thoracic region. In the lumbar region, they may cause a bulging of the psoas shadow.

Phalanges

Osteomyelitis of the phalanges occurs in children as a result of infection by a number of different organisms of which tuberculosis and syphilis are well recognized. They are also characteristically involved in chronic granulomatous disease (*see* page 191).

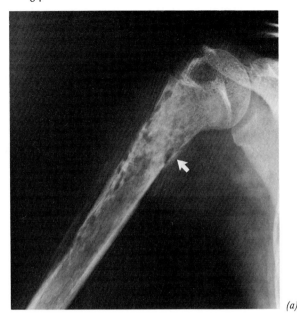

(a)

Figure 3.1. Osteomyelitis: (a) Humerus showing patchy areas of bone destruction with a pathological fracture and separation of a sequestrum (arrowed). (b) The same case after 2 months' treatment showing healing of the destructive lesions and incorporation of the dense new bone into the underlying cortex. (c) A lesion in the shaft of the femur where surgery has been carried out to evacuate the subperiosteal abcess leaving a 'cuff' of periosteal new bone (arrowed) resembling the 'Codman's triangle' seen in malignant bone tumour (see page 46)

Tuberculosis of bone

Osteitis due to tuberculosis is much less common that it used to be. The radiological appearances differ little from those resulting from pyogenic osteomyelitis, apart from the greater liability to spread across the growth plate, to involve the epiphysis and to infect the joint (*Figure 3.4*). There is a less marked degree of bone reaction and consequent bone sclerosis in the healing stage.

Viral osteitis

Bone lesions in viral infections are rare but have been described following smallpox, after vaccination due to infection of the bones by vaccinia virus and in rubella (*see* page ·67). The smallpox lesions are strikingly symmetrical in distribution, affecting the elbows and the small bones of the hands and feet.

SEPTIC ARTHRITIS

Pyogenic inflammation of the joints may be a primary infection or associated with osteomyelitis, particularly where this involves the epiphyses. The radiological signs tend to be common to both conditions, though the sequence in which they appear may be different. Thus, the earliest features are soft tissue swelling, with obliteration of the tissue planes around the affected joint, and subluxation of the bones forming the joint (*Figure 3.5*). The latter is due to the presence of pus under

(b)

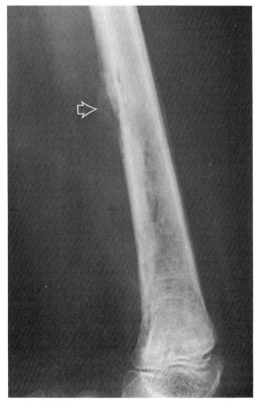

(c)

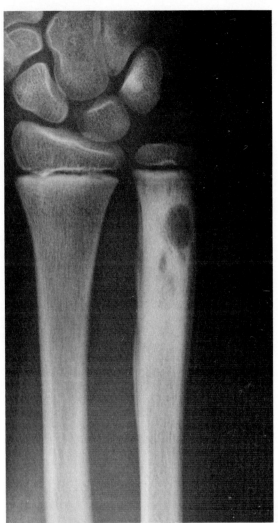

tension within the capsule. Later, periosteal new bone formation and erosion of the juxta-capsular bone may occur. The hip is the commonest joint to be involved in infancy, but in older children, the knee is much more frequently affected. Radiology is of value, not only in making the original diagnosis, but even more in detecting the existence of complications such as necrosis of the femoral head and the deformities arising as a result of it (Eyre-Brook, 1960). There may be enlargement of the articular portions of the bone due to hyperaemia. Failure of the epiphysis of the head of the femur to ossify or, if the ossific centre has begun to develop, displacement relative to the shaft of the bone, affords evidence of epiphyseal necrosis and damage to the growth plate. Arthrography in such cases can occasionally be useful in determining the degree to which the joint has been damaged and in assisting the surgeon to plan reparative treatment.

SYPHILIS

Congenital syphilis can affect the bones both during the perinatal period and in later childhood. It seems likely that these two types are different in nature (Cremin and Fisher, 1970).

The perinatal lesions are characteristically polyostotic and symmetrical, and occur most frequently during the

Figure 3.2. 'Brodie's Abcess'. Osteomyelitis of the Distal End of the Ulna. Such a bone abcess may arise either where the original infective focus is deep seated, where the inflammatory process is relatively low grade or treatment has been ineffective in completely eradicating it. The abcess cavity has a smooth dense wall and growth of the affected bone has been stimulated so that the ulna is slightly longer than the radius

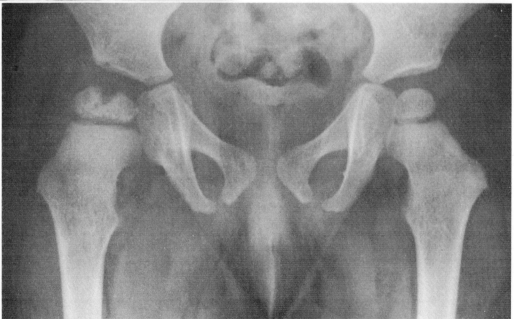

Figure 3.3. Epiphysitis of the Right Femur: Bone destruction affects only part of the epiphysis, the ossified portion being larger than that of the normal left hip, with concomitant widening of the femoral neck

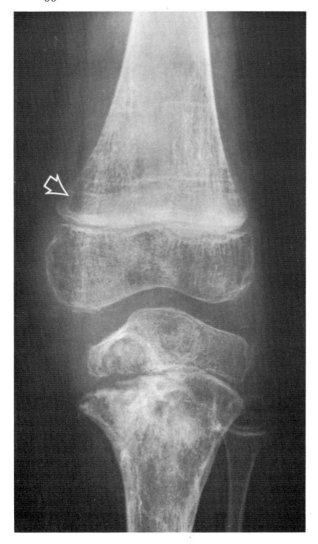

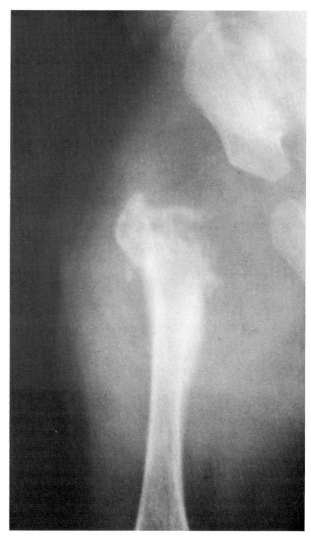

Figure 3.4. Tuberculosis of Bone: A lesion of the right tibia with the characteristic spread across the growth plate. There is marked decalcification of the bones, with narrowing of the joint space and cortical erosion at the lower end of the femur (arrowed) indicative of spread of the inflammatory process to involve the knee joint

Figure 3.5. Septic Arthritis of the Right Hip: Extensive bone destruction, periosteal new bone formation around the shaft of the femur and massive soft tissue swelling indicate the extent and severity of the inflammatory reaction. The femur is displaced out of the acetabulum and the subsequent progress indicated that necrosis of the head of the femur had occurred

first 2 months of life. There is a zone of increased bone density across the metaphysis with a zone of translucency on its diaphyseal aspect. The area of increased density has an irregular border with tooth-like projections and longitudinal bands of dense bone directed towards the epiphyseal plate. In the region of the translucent zone, the cortex may be destroyed, but often only on one side of the bone. This is particularly frequent on the medial side of the proximal end of the tibia, where it is known as Wimberger's sign (*Figure 3.6a*), but this can also occur in other bones. Erosion of the sigmoid notch of the ulna is a sign which is particularly characteristic (Levin, 1970). Periosteal new bone is formed in one or more layers or as a homogeneously dense band of new bone along the shafts of most of the long bones, but stopping short of the metaphyses (*Figure 3.6b*). Fractures with impaction and displacement of the metaphyseal plates are not uncommon. Ill-defined bone defects may be present in the skull. These radiographic signs are of value in the differential diagnosis of infants who present with misleading clinical features, which may cause them to be regarded as cases of pneumonia or gastroenteritis, or in infants who fail to thrive. These signs may also help in assessing the efficacy of treatment, since unequivocal evidence of healing may be seen 2 weeks after starting treatment. Reossification, union of fractures and incorporation of periosteal new bone into the cortex with remodelling may be complete, on an average, in 3 months.

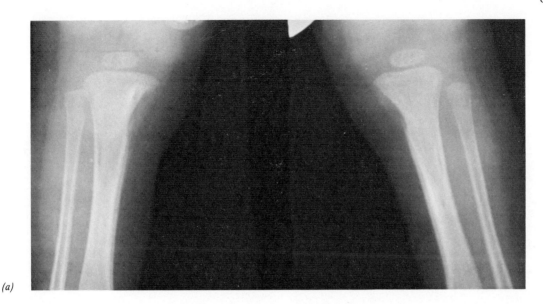

(a)

Figure 3.6. Congenital Syphilis (perinatal lesions): (a) Symmetrical areas of bone destruction on the medial aspects of both tibiae with associated periosteal new bone (Wimberger's sign). (b) More extensive destructive lesions of the distal metaphyses of the radius and ulna with soft tissue swelling and extensive periosteal new bone formation

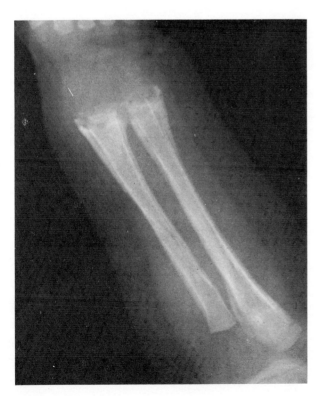

(b)

The lesions seen in later childhood are rare, especially with modern treatment. They consist of bilateral symmetrical thickening of the cortex of the tibia and fibula ('Sabre tibia'). Arthropathy (Clutton's joints) also occurs and may show little except soft tissue swelling. There may also be erosion of the articular surface and ankylosis, especially in the knee joint. Gummata present as well-defined circumscribed areas of bone destruction with associated periosteal reaction (*Figure 3.7*).

These latter lesions are due to a granulomatous inflammatory process. The perinatal lesions on the other hand are non-specific and confined to the growing part of the bones without involving the epiphyses, joints or soft tissues. It has been suggested that they may be basically dystrophic rather than inflammatory in nature, and are similar in type to the bony lesions of rubella and eythroblastosis fetalis, which they tend to resemble.

RUBELLA OSTEOPATHY

Among the widespread effects of maternal rubella on the fetus during intra-uterine life are lesions occurring in the bones. These comprise alternating longitudinal bands of increased and diminished bone density at the ends of the diaphysis. The metaphysis may show a transverse band of diminished bone density and appear irregular and ill defined. These changes are commonest in the distal femora and proximal tibiae (*Figure 3.8*). They may also occur in the anterior ends of the ribs and in the pelvis. They are symmetrical and resemble the metaphyseal changes seen in congenital syphilis, but periosteal new bone does not occur. They are present in about half the cases and can be visible at birth, though more often appearing by the age of 7 days. Spontaneous regression then takes place and the bones appear normal in 2 to 3 months. If the child fails to thrive they can persist for a longer time. Enlargement of the anterior fontanelle and widening of the sutures in the skull have been described.

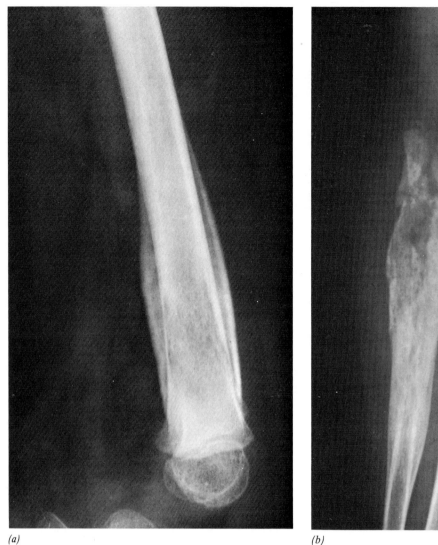
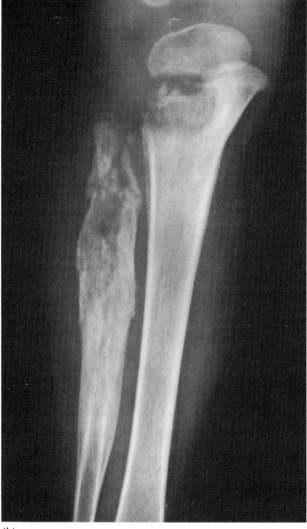

(a)   *(b)*

Figure 3.7. Congenital Syphilis (late childhood lesions): (a) Lesion of lower femur in a child aged 6 years, resembling pyogenic osteomyelitis in its combination of patchy destructive lesions and localized periosteal new bone around it. (b) Lesion of the tibia and fibula of the same child, showing more extensive and well-defined areas of bone destruction probably of a gummatous nature

INFANTILE CORTICAL HYPEROSTOSIS
(Caffey's syndrome)

This disease usually affects infants under 5 months of age. It gives rise to striking and distinctive radiological features, which accompany the swellings with which the child presents clinically.

The radiological features of the syndrome comprise extensive periosteal new bone which extends along the whole of the diaphysis of affected bones, either in the form of multiple thin layers or as more massive thickening of the cortex (*Figure 3.9*). This occurs predominantly on the outer surface. New bone is also laid down on the endosteal aspect of the cortex and produces an alteration in the texture of the shaft. Destructive bone lesions are not present and the epiphyses are not involved. The mandible, ulna, clavicles and ribs are the most common sites. Almost any bone may be affected but the lesions are rare in the cranial vault, spine and pelvis. The mandible is always involved at some stage, though not necessarily initially (*Figure 3.10a*) (Caffey and Silverman, 1945). The condition is self-limiting, and the radiological signs disappear entirely in most cases by the age of 3 years. A few instances have been recorded where the changes are more persistent or have recurred. Cross-union between the radius and ulna has been reported (Padfield and Hicken 1970). Occasionally, a pleural effusion may be formed when the ribs are involved (*Figure 3.10b*).

The radiological appearances of infantile cortical hyperostosis resemble many types of inflammatory bone disease such as osteomyelitis (which is often multifocal in infants), syphilis and viral infections of bone such as smallpox. Differential diganosis is not however difficult because of the highly distinctive distribution of the lesions, the age incidence and the absence of any evidence of bone destruction.

Figure 3.8. Rubella Osteopathy: Transverse bands of reduced bone density and loss of definition of the femoral and tibial metaphyses combined with longitudinal dense striations extending into the diaphysis in a neonate with a history of maternal rubella (By courtesy of Dr. G. R. Airth, Southmead Hospital)

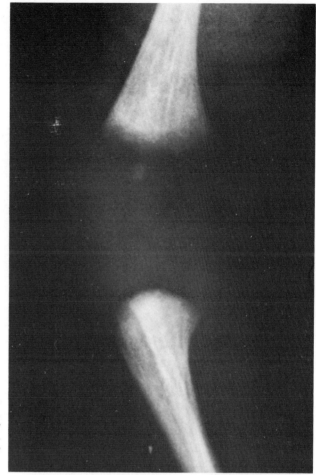

Figure 3.9. (Below) Infantile Cortical Hyperostosis: (a) Symmetrical thickening of the shafts of the long bones due to apposition of periosteal new bone to the outside of the cortex and to a lesser extent on its endosteal aspect. (b) Lateral view of same case showing that the thickening occurs symmetrically all round the shaft

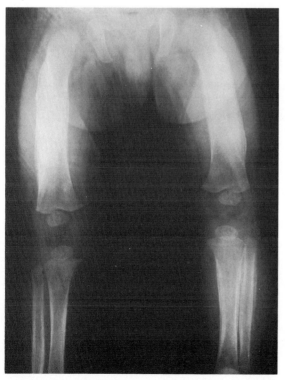

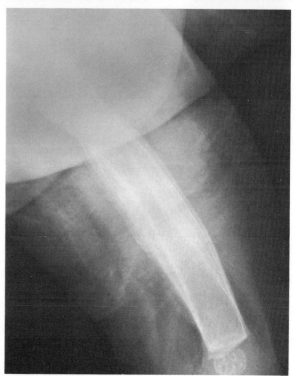

(a)

(b)

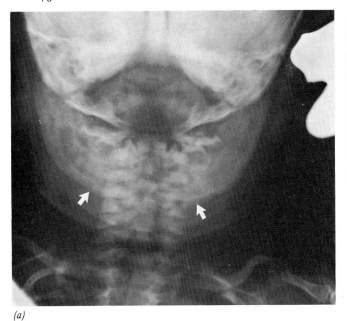

(a)

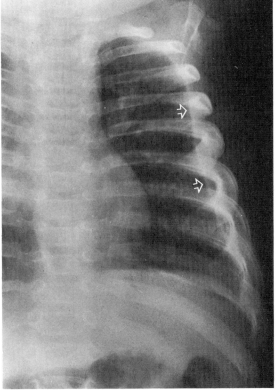

(b)

Figure 3.10. Infantile Cortical Hyperostosis: (a) Symmetrical periosteal new bone on the external aspect of the mandible (arrowed) a very characteristic site. (b) Periosteal new bone on the upper and lower cortices of the ribs. A thin lamellar pleural effusion is present along the lateral chest wall in association with these lesions (arrowed)

RHEUMATOID ARTHRITIS (Still's disease)

Rheumatoid arthritis presents a different pattern in children from that seen in adults and this applies equally to the radiological features (Martel *et al.*, 1962). These differences comprise:

(1) a predilection for joints which are related to the site of most active bone growth (knees, wrists and ankles) in contrast to the small joints of the hands and feet;

(2) a greater tendency for only one joint to be involved;

(3) the presence of certain radiological signs such as periosteal new bone formation and alterations in skeletal growth and maturation which are only seen in children.

The radiological features of the established disease are:

(a) narrowing of the joint spaces due to destruction of the articular cartilage;

(b) marginal erosions of bone at the site of the attachment of the capsule;

(c) severe generalized and juxta-articular osteoporosis (*Figure 3.11*).

However, it is important to note that these signs in children may occur several years after the onset of symptoms. This is especially true where the disease is monarticular. During the period of radiological latency the appearances are non-specific, and they consist of little more than periarticular soft tissue swelling and a slowing of bone growth. This is one of the most salient features of rheumatoid arthritis in children. It takes the form of a reduction in the diameter and length of the

long bones. The carpal and tarsal bones are abnormally small; together with the narrowing of the intercarpal joint spaces, this produces a shrivelled appearance which is very distinctive. Growth of the mandible is also defective where the temporomandibular joints are affected (in about 20 per cent of cases). This results in a symmetrical micrognathos, out of all proportion to the morphological changes in the joints themselves. Skeletal maturation is usually accelerated and the combination of small, but excessively mature epiphyses and carpal bones is characteristic. In addition to the bones, the soft tissues of a limb undergo atrophy even when only one joint is involved.

Osteoporosis may be very marked in the advanced stage of the disease; it may lead to compression fractures of the epiphyses and metaphyses around the weight-bearing joints, increasing the degree of deformity. The use of steroids in treatment tends to accentuate the severity of this osteoporosis and may be associated with multiple crush features of the vertebral bodies. Sometimes the osteoporosis takes the form of transverse zones of radiolucency across the metaphyses of long bones in proximity to affected joints.

Periosteal new bone, seen in about 25 per cent of cases, affects the metacarpals, metatarsals and phalanges and is only rarely seen in other bones (*Figure 3.11a*). It is often a relatively early sign. Bony ankylosis may occur as a result of rheumatoid arthritis. New bone formation in combination with the immobility of the patient may contribute to this, Soft tissue calcification may be present either around involved joints or in the wall of the peripheral arteries.

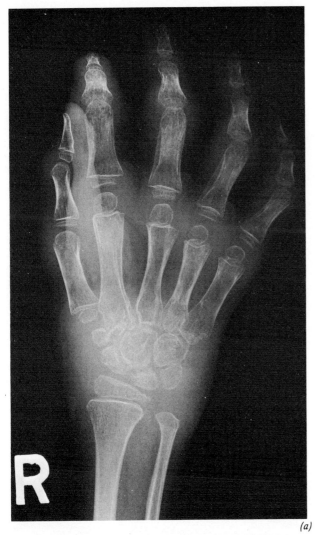

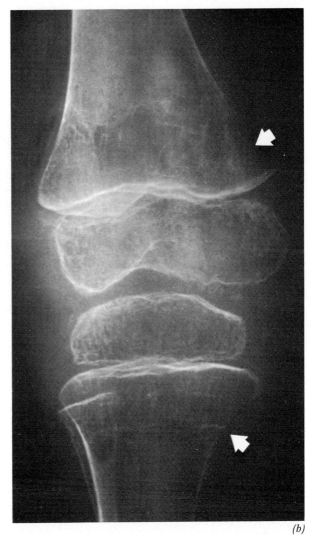

(a)

(b)

Figure 3.11. Juvenile Rheumatoid Arthritis: (a) In the bones of the hand the combination of severe decalcification especially adjacent to the affected joints with periosteal new bone formation around the shafts of the 2nd matacarpal and proximal phalanges is distinctive. The joint spaces between the radius, the individual carpal bones and the metacarpals are markedly narrowed with considerable soft tissue swelling around the carpus and many of the smaller joints of the fingers. (b) In the knee joint the decalcification is even more marked and is associated with destruction of the cortex of the medial aspect of the femur and tibia at the site of the capsular attachment (arrowed)

The relative frequency of monarticular lesions, especially in the early stages of the disease, has been mentioned and in such cases the knee is the most common joint to be involved. This form of the disease is difficult to diagnose radiologically because of the late appearance of erosions, and the consequent discrepancy between the clinical and radiological signs. In some cases there may never be involvement of other joints. Rosberg and Laine (1967) consider that in most cases other joints are ultimately affected. In such cases the disability may be considerable.

Involvement of the cervical spine occurs in about 25 per cent of cases. Radiological examination is desirable in any child with pain and stiffness of the neck. This may demonstrate narrowing of the disc spaces and subluxation, particularly at the atlanto-axial joints. The odontoid process may be displaced backwards relative to the anterior arch of the atlas. Fusion may occur between the posterior apophyseal joints, or between the atlas and the base of the skull or the odontoid process.

Heart involvement is not very common in rheumatoid arthritis but, when present, usually takes the form of pericarditis, leading to an enlarged globular heart shadow and diminished cardiac pulsation on screening.

Rheumatoid arthritis can be confused with a number of conditions affecting the joints. It is difficult to diagnose with certainty in the early stages before specific signs have developed and in the monarticular form of the disease. The distinction between pyogenic, tuberculous and other specific infective types of arthritis may be particularly difficult. The early development of bone destruction is in favour of all these conditions.

When the spine is predominantly involved, rheumatoid arthritis has to be distinguished from ankylosing spondylitis, which is not unknown in children. Ankylosing spondylitis affects the thoracolumbar rather than the cervical region of the spine and, although the hip and knee joints can be affected, the smaller joints of the hands and feet are not involved. The sacro-iliac joints are almost always affected. In the early stages the radiological signs are slight and difficult to distinguish from the normal appearance of the sacro-iliac joint.

NON-SPECIFIC SPONDYLITIS (discitis)

This condition has usually been regarded as inflammatory, although in most instances blood culture and bone biopsy have not yielded any organisms (Brass and Bowler 1969). It may be precipitated by minor trauma to the back and Alexander (1970) has recently made out a case for regarding it as primarily traumatic. He considers that it is due to a shear stress which leads to a disruption between the end-plate of the vertebral body and the intervertebral disc.

The condition occurs most commonly in early childhood and is localized to the lower lumbar spine. Pain, often following minor injury, is the usual presenting symptom but its distribution may be misleading and may suggest disease in the hip or abdomen. Radiology is therefore the method most likely to lead to the diagnosis. The radiological appearances consist of narrowing of a disc space together with loss of definition and destruction of the adjacent parts of the vertebral bodies (*Figure 3.12a*). This can involve the whole surface of the body adjacent to the disc or may be more localized and resemble a Schmorl's node (*Figure 3.12b*). When the condition begins to heal a zone of bone sclerosis develops deep to the area of destruction. Complete recovery occurs in 3 to 4 months and complications are rare. The intervertebral discs most frequently affected are those between L3 and L5. The condition is indistinguishable radiologically from spondylitis due to specific infections such as staphylococcal osteitis, tuberculosis or brucella. The self-limiting course and absence of permanent deformity or ankylosis may assist in this distinction.

HYPERTROPHIC PULMONARY OSTEO-ARTHROPATHY

Bilateral, symmetrical periosteal new bone along the shafts of the tibia, fibula, radius and ulna, metacarpals and metatarsals, together with clubbing of the fingers and toes, occurring in chronic pulmonary or cardiac disease, is occasionally seen in childhood, though less commonly than in adults (*Figure 3.13*). Arthropathy of the knees, wrists and ankles can also be a feature of the condition and one which may lead to confusion with rheumatoid arthritis. Bronchiectasis, tuberculosis and empyema are no longer the most prevalent primary diseases which give rise to hypertrophic pulmonary osteoarthropathy in childhood. Cyanotic congenital heart disease and fibrocystic disease affecting the lungs are now more frequent causes. Biliary cirrhosis is also a rare cause in children.

The bone lesions are completely reversible if the underlying condition can be alleviated but it is unusual for this to occur. Rarely, the syndrome can occur as a primary condition with no apparent cause. Such cases may be hereditary and appear usually after puberty. In addition in these cases there may be defects in the ossification of the cranial vault and multiple Wormian bones. Some cases are associated with thickened, fur-

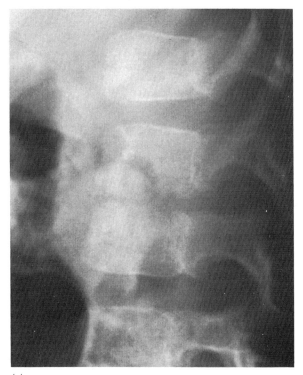
(a)

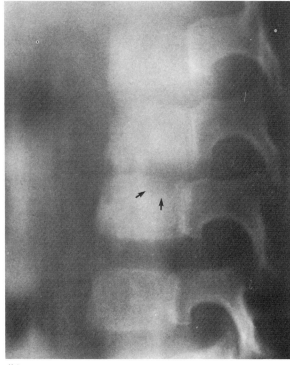
(b)

Figure 3.12. Discitis: (a) A lesion of the intervertebral disc between LV2 and LV3 has resulted in narrowing of the disc space and destruction of the end-plates of the adjacent vertebral bodies. (b) Tomography of the same child reveals a more extensive area of bone destruction extending into the body of LV3 (arrowed)

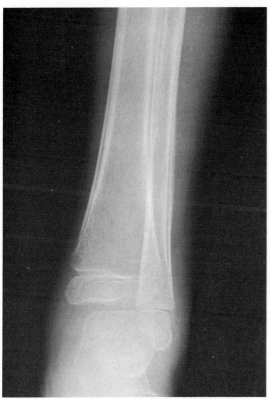

(a)

rowed skin over the face and forehead and with hyper-hidrosis. They are then referred to as pachydermoperiostosis: hereditary clubbing of the fingers and toes may be an incomplete form of this condition.

BONE LESIONS IN BLOOD DISEASES

ANAEMIA

Bone lesions in children with anaemia occur more commonly in certain types than in others, and they are produced by a variety of different mechanisms. In some cases they are due to an increase in haemopoiesis, with a resultant expansion of the marrow spaces or development of extramedullary haemopoietic tissue. In others there may be a disturbance in the process of endochondral ossification, with a resultant growth defect or disturbed bone architecture. The anaemia may predispose to infection or infarction of bone. Finally, certain anaemias may be associated with a characteristic pattern of congenital anomalies.

Thalassaemia

This disease is due to an abnormality in the protein component of the haemoglobin molecule. It is characterized by a severe chronic haemolytic anaemia and

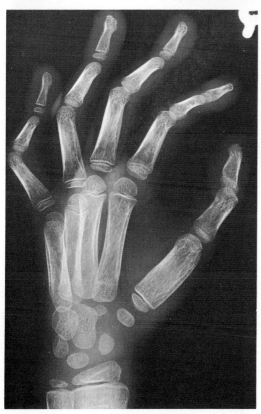
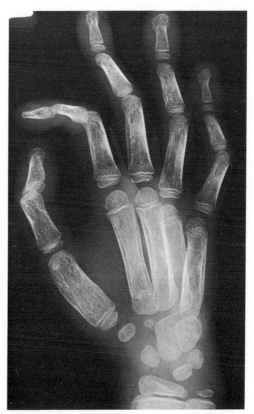

(b)

Figure 3.13. Hypertrophic Pulmonary Osteoarthropathy: (a) Periosteal new bone along the shafts of the tibia and fibula with soft tissue swelling around the ankle joint in a child with bronchiectasis. (b) The hands of the same child; the symmetrical periosteal new bone along the shafts of the metacarpals and phalanges is associated with soft tissue swelling of the terminal segments of the digits and to a lesser extent of the tufts of the distal phalanges ('clubbing')

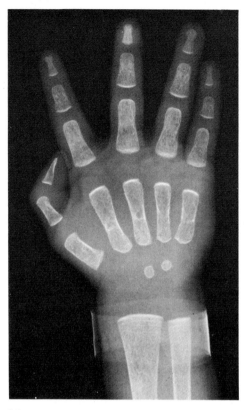

(a)

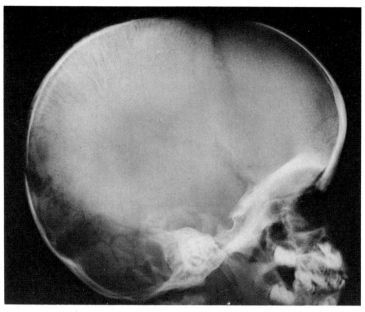

(b)

Figure 3.14. Bone Changes in Thalassaemia: (a) Sparse trabeculae in the medulla and thinning of the cortex of the metacarpals and phalanges due to hypertrophy of the red marrow. This is a response to a long continued haemolytic anaemia. (b) In the skull, there is a characteristic thickening of the diploe of the parietal bones with thickened trabeculae giving a 'striated' appearance

extensive skeletal abnormalities, most of which arise as a result of the compensatory increase in haemopoietic tissue (Caffey, 1957).

The medullary cavities of the long bones and the diploic spaces of the calvarium are widened with a reduction in the number and thickness of the trabeculae and thinning of the cortical bone, the inner margin of which is scalloped (*Figure 3.14a*). Occasionally pathological fractures may occur, especially in the femora. In the long bones, the normal constriction of the shaft is replaced by a square or fusiform appearance. Sometimes the hypertrophy of the marrow tissues is localized and suggests a 'tumour'. This occurs especially in the ribs. In this situation a thin shell of bone may surround a mass of red marrow or haemorrhagic fluid. Such a mass may appear to project into the thoracic cavity, and is termed a 'costal osteoma'. The distribution of such bone lesions varies with the age of the child. They are common in the small bones of the hands in early childhood. After puberty changes may also occur in the skull, spine, ribs and pelvis. The appearances in the vault of the skull in which bony trabeculae are arranged at right angles to the surface of the thickned bone giving a 'hair-on-end' appearance are very striking (*Figure 3.14b*). The part of the occipital bone below the external occipital protuberance, however, does not show this widening. The paranasal sinuses, especially the antra and the mastoid air cells, may be poorly developed. The maxilla is sometimes enlarged relative to the mandible, resulting in dental malocclusion.

In addition to these signs of marrow hyperplasia, the anaemia causes a profound disturbance in bone development. Premature fusion of the epiphyses may also occur

from about the age of 10 years and leads to shortening and deformity of the affected bones, especially when it involves only a part of the growth plate. This is most commonly seen in the humerus, femur and tibia, and does not appear to be related to the severity of the anaemia. Gallstones may be present due to the excessive amounts of bile pigment excreted.

Iron deficiency anaemias

Children with anaemia due to lack of iron can occasionally show bone changes in the skull vault and in the long bones similar to, but less well marked than, those described in thalassaemia. These changes are not well correlated with the severity of the anaemia, but show a definite relation to low birth weight and prematurity.

Sickle-cell disease

This type of anaemia is, like thalassaemia, due to an abnormality of haemoglobin, resulting not only in a haemolytic anaemia and marrow hyperplasia but in changes in the shape of the red blood cells when they are exposed to low oxygen tensions. This latter feature results in blockage of small blood vessels with the production of infarcts which occur in bone as well as in other tissues.

The radiological changes produced are a combination of two features: expansion of the medulla of the long bones and the diploic spaces of the cranial vault as described in thalassaemia, and the effects of bone in-

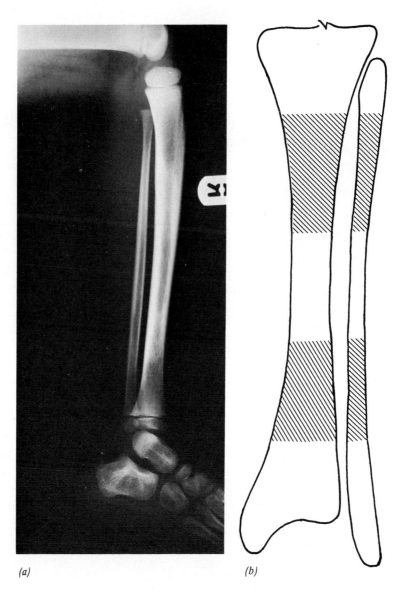

Figure 3.15. Sickle-cell Disease: (a) Bands of increased bone density are present at the junction of the upper and middle thirds and of the middle and lower thirds of the shaft. (b) Diagram of zones of increased bone density in long bones

(a) (b)

farction and infection. The former changes are somewhat less marked in sickle-cell anaemia. The cortex and trabeculae may be thinned and the intertrabecular spaces are widened throughout the skeleton. The appearance of vertical spiculation is rare in the skull.

Those bone lesions which result from infarction may take the form of areas of diffuse sclerosis of the cortex and are especially distinctive (Bohrer, 1970) (*Figure 3.15*). They may also appear as dense calcified lesions at the ends of the long bones. Localized ischaemic lesions occur also in the hips. The appearances are then those of avascular necrosis of the capital epiphysis of the femur, which undergoes fragmentation and progressive deformity. In the small bones of the hands and feet, deposition of periosteal new bone along the shaft is combined with irregular areas of translucency within the substance of the bone. The whole bone may be involved. These changes are symmetrical and can be completely reversible (*Figure 3.16*); such a 'hand—foot' syndrome

may be confused with low-grade osteomyelitis due to organisms of the salmonella group. Both are characteristic of sickle-cell anaemia. The osteomyelitis is not, however, so symmetrical in distribution and is not necessarily confined to the hands and feet. The symptoms can be relatively mild, so that a pathological fracture may occur, with consequent shortening and deformity (Middlemiss and Raper, 1966).

Interference with bone growth, probably related to deficiency in blood supply or to infection, can be generalized as in thalassaemia. Alternatively it may affect local sites such as the metaphyses of the long bones, which become 'cupped', or the end-plates of the vertebral bodies, which assume a characteristic biconcave shape. This is more angular and less regularly curved than the 'cod-fish' type of vertebra occurring in osteoporosis. These local disturbances of growth are probably mainly related to deficiency in blood supply or to infection.

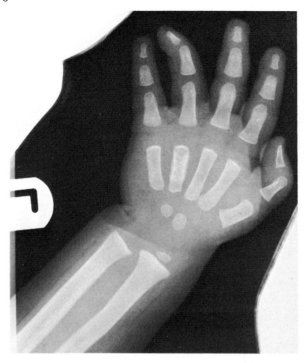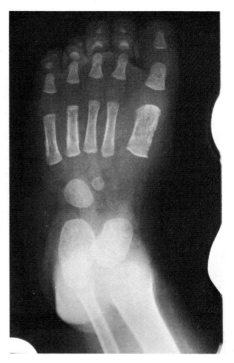

Figure 3.16. Sickle-cell Disease ('hand-foot syndrome'):   Irregularity of the trabecular pattern of the medulla and periosteal new bone around the shaft is present in the 4th metacarpal and in the 1st and 4th metatarsals

Erythroblastosis fetalis

Bone changes have been described in children with this type of anaemia (Brenner and Allen, 1963). These have been described as due to a disturbance of endochondral bone formation. Radiologically this is seen as a translucent zone at the distal end of the long bones, especially the radius. A generalized increase in bone density has also been described and it has been claimed that this feature may enable the diagnosis to be made *in utero*.

Congenital hypoplastic anaemia

It is recognized that skeletal anomalies involving the spine and limbs may be associated with erythrogenesis imperfecta or with Fanconi's anaemia. In the former condition, the defect in blood formation is confined to the red cell series and is associated with polydactyly and shortened, abnormally shaped phalanges. Other congenital anomalies may be present, including ventricular septal defect, dysplastic or hydronephrotic kidneys, mental retardation and dwarfism.

Fanconi's anaemia is a pancytopenia in which the pattern of associated anomalies is different from erythrogenesis imperfecta. There is absence or hypoplasia of the radius and of the radial carpal and metacarpal bones. The distal phalanges may also be absent with syndactyly of the toes, congenital dislocation of the hips and talipes equinovarus. Fused vertebrae or hemivertebrae can occur. The bone age is retarded and there may be microcephaly and renal anomalies.

LEUKAEMIA

Bone changes may occur in all forms of leukaemia but are commoner in lymphatic leukaemia than in the other types.

Areas of diminished bone density are the commonest finding, but one which is non-specific. These may take the form of single discrete lesions resembling cysts or benign tumours, or of multiple punctate lesions. Transverse bands occur across the metaphyses of the ribs and especially at the wrists and knees which are the sites of most rapid bone growth (Willson, 1959) (*Figure 3.17a*). The latter has been considered to be one of the most frequent and characteristic bone lesions, but in one large series it was found to occur in only 14 per cent (Silverman, 1948). Similar appearances may occur in the spine, where they can be associated with collapse of the anterior part of the vertebral bodies,

Periosteal new bone formation may occur along the shafts of the long bones or in the vicinity of discrete osteolytic lesions (*Figure 3.17b*). In addition there may occasionally be a diffuse bone sclerosis. None of these changes is diagnostic of leukaemia, but the combination is often suggestive. The presence of the metaphyseal zones of diminished bone density is particularly characteristic, but it should be remembered that in infants under the age of 2 years such zones are not uncommon in any chronic illness or in septicaemia, which can simulate leukaemia clinically.

HAEMOPHILIA

Haemophilia and other disorders of the clotting processes

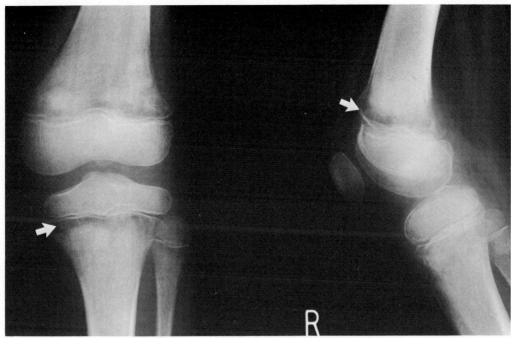

(a)

Figure 3.17. Bone Lesions in Leukaemia: (a) A transverse band of diminished density is present at the femoral, tibial and fibular metaphyses (arrowed). (b) In the upper femur the band of diminished bone density at the upper femoral metaphysis is accompanied by patchy translucent areas and periosteal new bone around the upper shaft

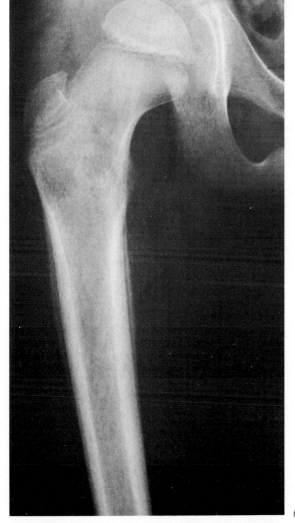

(b)

Figure 3.18. Bone Lesions in Leukaemia: A localized discrete area of bone destruction in the shaft of the femur associated with periosteal new bone overlying it (arrowed)

lead to recurrent haemorrhage as a result of injuries which are often relatively minor, Such haemorrhages can occur in many parts of the body other than the bones and joints. An intussusception resulting from a haemorrhage into the wall of the small intestine may produce diagnostic radiological appearances (*see* page 228). Haemorrhages into the retroperitoneal tissues may produce a scoliosis and cause obliteration of the psoas and renal outlines and even displacement of the bowel or ureter.

Recurrent haemarthroses lead to swelling around the joints which radiologically appear denser than the surrounding soft tissues. This is partly due to thickening of the capsule and synovial membrane and partly to the deposition of haemosiderin within the haematoma accentuated by the associated atrophy of the surrounding muscles. With each successive episode of bleeding, progressive degenerative changes occur and these result in narrowing of the joint space, the development of

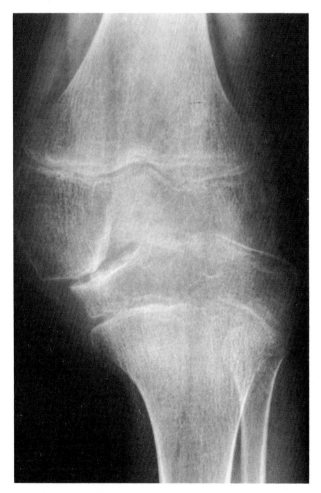

Figure 3.19. Haemophilia – Joint Lesions: Subluxation of the knee joint with severe loss of joint space due to recurrent haemarthroses. The femoral and tibial condyles are disproportionately enlarged compared to the shafts of the bones

osteophytes and sclerosis and cyst formation in the subchondral bone (*Figure 3.19*). These changes closely resemble the changes of osteoarthritis in later life. An inflammatory reaction is also provoked which can be reflected in the radiological appearances. These comprise juxta-articular osteoporosis, marginal bone erosions and periosteal new bone and resemble those seen in rheumatoid arthritis. Enlargement of the epiphyses and acceleration of skeletal age are a result of the hyperaemia which develops in this condition. Scalloping of the intercondylar notch of the distal end of the femur and enlargement of the head of the radius are also features particularly characteristic of haemophilia.

Local haemorrhage into the substance of the bone may occur and results in the development of cystic spaces which, although similar to the subchondral cysts due to degenerative arthrosis, tend to be larger and more numerous and to occur in unusual sites such as the elbow. Bleeding when it occurs into the growth plate may result in shortening of the long bones due to premature epiphyseal fusion or in deformity from displacement of the epiphysis. Deformity may also result from avascular necrosis which may be caused by interruption of the blood supply by a haematoma. This is particularly likely to occur in the head of the femur, the head of the radius and the talus. It produces an appearance very similar to that seen in Perthes' disease, but tends to be progressive with very little attempt at repair.

Finally, haemorrhage under the periosteum although surprisingly uncommon in haemophilia, may produce a very striking and distinctive radiological picture. Elevation of the periosteum followed by calcification within the haematoma and new bone formation beneath it results in the formation of prominent spurs of bone projecting from the edge of the lesion. In addition, repeated subperiosteal bleeding can generate such a degree of pressure on the underlying bone that progressive bone destruction results. This lesion may closely resemble a bone tumour but it is important that its true nature be recognized, since attempts to biopsy such a 'pseudo-tumour' can have fatal results from uncontrollable haemorrhage. Such lesions are seen particularly in the ilium, the femur and the calcaneum, their site presumably being related to weight-bearing and liability to minor trauma. Fortunately they are relatively rare, with an incidence estimated to be about 2 per cent of all cases of haemophilia.

METABOLIC BONE DISEASE

OSTEOPOROSIS

This term is frequently used loosely to include all types of demineralization of bone, especially where it has proved difficult to determine the exact cause. However, in view of the many conditions in which true osteoporosis may occur, it may be important to recognize osteoporosis and differentiate it from other types of demineralization, if correct treatment is to be applied. Such osteoporosis may be generalized or localized.

In true osteoporosis the diminution in radiographic bone density is due to a reduction in the amount of bone tissue present, and in children this can be due to the following causes:

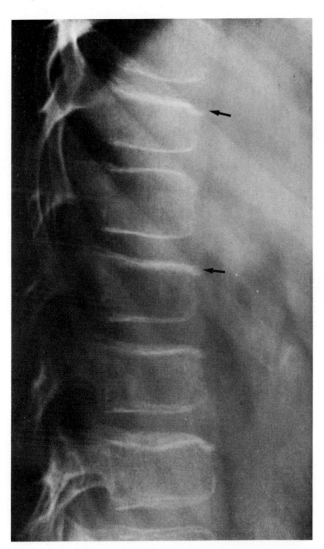

Figure 3.20. Osteoporosis of Spine: There are fractures of several vertebral bodies which are reduced in height with a linear band of increased bone density at their upper borders due to crushing and compression of the trabeculae (arrowed)

(1) Congenital, as in osteogenesis imperfecta.
(2) Deficiencies, especially of protein or vitamin.
(3) Endocrine disorders.
   (a) Deficiency of anabolic steroids.
   (b) Hypopituitary or hypogonadal disease.
   (c) Excess of katabolic steroids.
   (d) Hyperthyroidism.
(4) Liver disease.
(5) Prolonged immobility, such as occurs after fractures or with Still's disease.

Apart from the widespread lack of density in the bones, there are certain features, which if not diagnostic, are at least suggestive of true osteoporosis. (1) The cortical bone may be thinned, but paradoxically appears relatively dense, compared to the medulla where the trabeculae are reduced in number. This results in the characteristic pencilled outline to the bones, with an open, rather coarse trabecular pattern. (2) Pathological fractures may occur, especially in the bones of the lower limbs and in the spine. The vertebral bodies are reduced in height with a dense zone of compressed bone parallel to their upper and lower surfaces (*Figure 3.20*). The intervertebral disc spaces are relatively wide and bulge into the adjacent vertebrae, producing a 'codfish' spine. These spinal changes are particularly prominent in children who have been on long-term steroid therapy.

Idiopathic juvenile osteoporosis

In addition to the types listed above in which osteoporosis is present as part of a primary disease or as a result of therapy, cases have been described in children between 8 and 11 years of age in which the osteoporosis appears to have no identifiable cause (Dent and Friedman, 1965). Radiologically this condition may be indistinguishable from other types of osteoporosis, especially osteogenesis imperfecta, but it lacks the features of the primary disease. The diagnosis is therefore made largely by exclusion. It can however be a matter of some importance since the condition is sometimes persistent and may result in considerable impairment of growth with deformity and disablement.

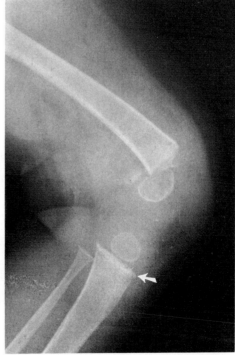

Figure 3.21. Scurvy — early stage in the knee joint of an infant aged 10 months: there is displacement of the distal epiphysis of the femur with a fracture of the adjacent metaphysis. A well marked Fränkel's line (arrowed) is present at the proximal metaphysis of the tibia but the rest of the bones are decalcified

VITAMIN DEFICIENCIES

Scurvy

Deficiency of vitamin C leads to a true osteoporosis since ascorbic acid is essential for the formation of collagen. The matrix of both bone and cartilage is consequently deficient in quantity.

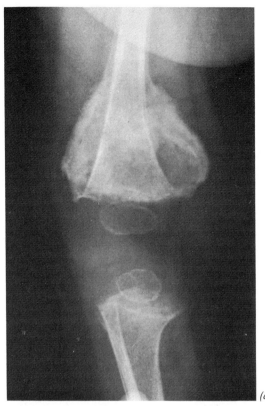
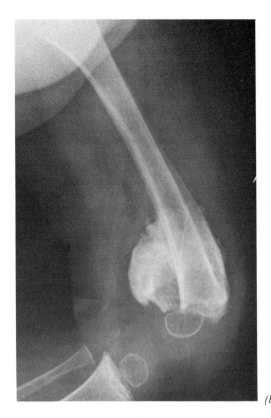

(a)

(b)

Figure 3.22. Scurvy – Late Stage: (a) The same child as in Figure 3.21 several months later with a massive calcified subperiosteal haematoma and metaphyseal spurs. (b) A lateral view taken at the same time shows that the epiphyseal displacement persists and that a dense outline has developed around the margin of the femoral epiphysis

Radiologically a severe degree of diminution in bone density affecting the whole skeleton is one of the cardinal features. In addition, the zone of provisional calcification at the junction of the growth plate and the metaphysis becomes wider than normal. This appears on the radiographs as a well-defined dense border at the growing ends of the long bones (Fränkel's line). It is seen around the margins of the epiphyses and also of the carpal and tarsal bones, an appearance which becomes more prominent during the early stages of healing. The abnormal brittleness of this zone leads to the production of microfractures. These are responsible for the formation of characteristic metaphyseal spurs and also for displacement of the epiphysis (*Figure 3.21a*). Due to the effect of the lack of ascorbic acid on the capillary endothelium, haemorrhage beneath the periosteum occurs in response to relatively minor injury with the production of large subperiosteal haematomas around the shafts of the long bones. These calcify rapidly and this calcification can be shown on the radiograph (*Figure 3.22*). Ultimately these haematomas become incorporated into the underlying cortex which may become thickened and irregular as a result.

The classical radiological appearances are sufficiently distinctive, especially in conjunction with the clinical features, to make the diagnosis without difficulty in most cases. It is, however, necessary to avoid confusing scurvy with the effects of repeated trauma in infancy (*see* page 88); in this latter condition the bones are usually of normal density. It is curious that abnormalities in the spine which are so prominent in other types of osteoporosis such as that due to steroids, are rare in scurvy. However, flattening and biconcavity of the vertebral bodies have been described, in particular in scurvy affecting older children and adults.

Rickets

The effects of lack of vitamin D, due either to unsuitable diet or to malabsorption from the intestine, are familiar. The bones generally lack density. The metaphyses are widened and cupped with a loss of the normal sharply defined border adjacent to the growth plate which takes on an irregular 'frayed' appearance. The distance between the metaphysis and the epiphysis is increased because the interval is occupied not only by the cartilage of the growth plate itself but also by a zone of uncalcified osteoid (*Figure 3.23a*). Correspondingly, the diaphysis appears abnormally short and may be bowed due to bending of the relatively soft osteoid and a consequent change in the direction of bone growth. These changes depend for their production on active growth and are most conspicuous where growth is most rapid, as at the wrists, knees and ankles and the anterior ends of the ribs (*Figure 3.23b*). For the same reason the epiphyseal border of the growth plate is commonly well defined and any loss of sharp outline is confined to the surface of the epiphysis underlying the articular cartilage where growth is most active. Some retardation of skeletal maturation may occur but is seldom severe. In the absence of active growth the abnormal appearances may

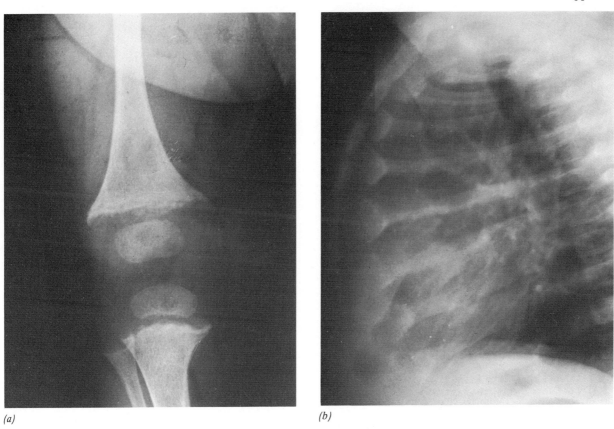

(a)

(b)

Figure 3.23. Rickets: (a) The metaphyses of the femur and tibia are flared and concave at the periphery. The spaces between the metaphyses and the epiphyses are widened representing zones of uncalcified osteoid tissue. The edges of the ossified portions of the metaphyses are ill-defined and irregular. (b) The anterior ends of the ribs at the costochondral junctions are widened, ill-defined and concave

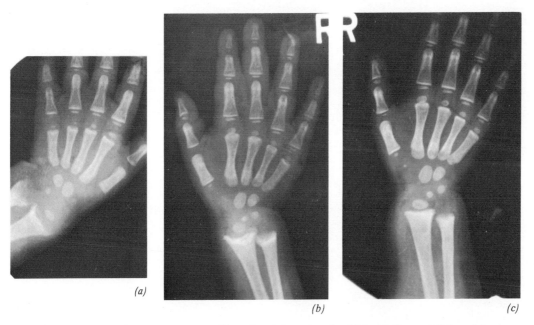

(a)

(b)

(c)

Figure 3.24. Healing Rickets: Successive radiographs of the wrist of a child with dietary deficient rickets over a period of 2 months following administration of vitamin D. The zone of uncalcified osteoid becomes calcified so that the growth plate returns to its normal width. The metaphyses of the radius and ulna become straight and well-defined. The density of the metaphyses of the metacarpals and phalanges becomes increased in the final film, (a) April (b) May (c) July

be confined to a generalized lack of bone density, with or without fractures and deformities. These features are entirely unspecific and may be impossible to distinguish from osteoporosis. Changes in the skull are in general less evident than would be expected from the clinical signs, but in severe infantile rickets the sutures and fontanelles are widened and their edges are ill defined. These changes are particularly marked in the oculo-cerebro-renal syndrome (*see* page 83).

The radiographic signs of healing may be expected to occur within 1 or 2 weeks after treatment has been started. The zone of osteoid becomes calcified and this is often manifested as a dense line at the metaphyseal aspect of the growth plate, with a translucent zone still present between it and the main part of the diaphysis. Similarly, uncalcified osteoid which has accumulated beneath the periosteum of the long bones, may calcify, giving rise to a layer of 'periosteal new bone' along the shaft. The density of the newly calcified osteoid may often appear excessive by contrast with the demineralized bone adjacent to it, but if this increased density persists or continues to increase, it may be an indication of overdosage (*Figure 3.24*).

The appearances of florid rickets are distinctive and easy to detect. The milder degrees can be more difficult, especially if the positioning of the limb is faulty so that the metaphysis is not lying exactly at right angles to the x-ray beam. The obliquity thus produced can mimic the slight lack of definition which results from early rickets.

DISORDERS OF CALCIUM AND PHOSPHORUS METABOLISM

Renal tubular disease

A large number of conditions are known in which the constituents of the glomerular filtrate fail to be reabsorbed in the renal tubules due to deficiency of the specific enzymes or to toxic or infective damage to the tubule cells. Most of these conditions cause rickets in the growing child or osteomalacia in later life because the tubules are unable to reabsorb phosphate. This is therefore lost to the body ('hypophosphataemic rickets or phosphate diabetes'). The signs of the resulting rickets can be detected on radiography of the bones. It is to be noted that such renal rickets is to a greater or lesser degree resistant to the therapeutic effects of vitamin D, though most cases will show healing if enough vitamin D is given over long periods. Renal tubular disorders also inhibit bone growth to a variable extent and in the cases where this is a marked feature the rachitic changes may be absent and the bones merely appear demineralized.

The radiological appearances of the growth plate and metaphyses in patients with renal rickets differ little from those in cases arising from dietary deficiency rickets (Rose, 1964). However, the age of presentation in renal tubular disease is likely to be higher and there may be areas of increased bone density, particularly in the form of transverse bands parallel to the growth plate. These dense lines alternating with translucent lines reflect the tendency to alternate healing and reactivation (*Figure 3.25*). This is a characteristic feature (Steinbach and Noetzli, 1964). It is not uncommon for

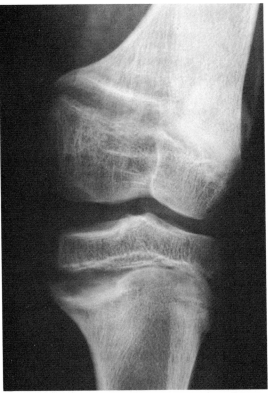

Figure 3.25. Renal Tubular (vitamin D-resistant) Rickets: The knee joint of a child aged 9 years. The zone of uncalcified osteoid is only present in the medial parts of the metaphyses and is associated with transverse lines of increased bone density on the diaphyseal aspect due to partial healing

the rachitic changes to involve only the medial half of the femoral and tibial metaphyses at the knee.

High doses of vitamin D may be needed for long periods before healing occurs. This entails a risk of overdosage with the production of toxic effects from hypercalcaemia. Therefore, assessment of the effects of treatment is of particular importance in this group of diseases. In this context, the radiographic evidence of healing of the rickets will enable treatment to be stopped or dosage to be reduced (*Figure 3.26*). Metaphyseal lines of increased bone density or nephrocalcinosis are signs indicative of hypervitaminosis D. Nephrocalcinosis which is unrelated to high doses of vitamin D may occur together with rickets in renal tubular acidosis. This condition results from an inability of the renal tubular cells to reabsorb base. This causes a mobilization of calcium from the skeleton and results in hypercalciuria. The alkalinity of the urine favours precipitation of calcium in the renal tubular cells. Children with this condition tend to develop multiple renal calculi in later life.

Although in the majority of cases of renal tubular disease the bone changes are those of generalized demineralization or of rickets, some cases may show bone changes which are due to secondary hyperparathyroidism (*see below*). This may be the case in patients who have the severe type of Fanconi syndrome. These children who have cystinosis, are markedly dwarfed and their prognosis is poor. Detection of cortical erosions, particularly on the medial aspect of the proximal ends of

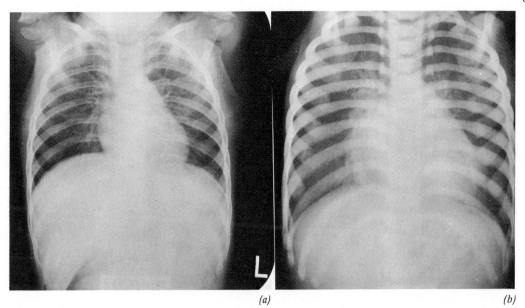

(a)   *(b)*

Figure 3.26. Hypervitaminosis D: Radiographs of the thorax of a child with Fanconi syndrome (a) at presentation and (b) after an interval of 1 year, during which period high doses of vitamin D had been given continuously. In (b) the uniform density of the ribs with loss of the distinction between the cortex and the medulla is indicative of overdosage

the tibiae, may herald the onset of renal failure from glomerular disease.

Very florid rickets, with pathological fractures, and localized thickening of the cranial vault in the parietal regions occurs in about half the cases of oculo-cerebro-renal (Lowe's) syndrome. In this condition renal tubular rickets is accompanied by glaucoma and severe mental retardation.

Craniostenosis has been described in several types of rickets, most commonly in hypophosphataemic rickets, but the cause of this is not understood (Reilly *et al.*, 1964).

Other types of rickets

Children are occasionally seen in whom rickets occurs in spite of an adequate intake of vitamin D and in the absence of demonstrable renal tubular defects. Some of these (Dent *et al.*, 1970) have been on long term anti-convulsant therapy which is thought to disturb the liver enzyme systems concerned with steroid metabolism. Urinary diversion undertaken for ectopia vesicae or other diseases of the lower urinary tract may also result in the development of rickets several years later. Finally, a group of children has been described under the term 'vitamin D dependent rickets'. It has been suggested that this is an inherited disorder in which rachitic changes, indistinguishable from deficiency rickets, develop in spite of adequate amounts of vitamin D in the diet. The rachitic changes are associated with a severe myopathy and both of these features respond well to moderate amounts of vitamin D. It is stated that in this type of rickets skeletal maturation is severely retarded and that the carpal and tarsal bones, when they appear, are markedly deformed (Dent *et al.*, 1968). Flattening of the vertebral bodies (platyspondyly) with a central tongue of bone projecting from their anterior surfaces

may occur and simulate Morquio's disease or spondylo-epiphyseal dysplasia. These bone changes appear to respond well to treatment.

Hyperparathyroidism

This condition may result either from an adenoma or hyperplasia of the parathyroids, or it may be secondary to chronic renal failure. In the latter condition the retention of phosphate and the consequent lowering of the serum calcium level stimulates the parathyroids to overactivity.

The radiological appearances of the direct effects of parathyroid overaction on the skeleton are similar in the two types. However, hyperparathyroidism due to renal disease will be accompanied by rickets or osteo-malacia and by a patchy increase in bone density. This complex bone picture is known as 'renal osteodystrophy'.

Primary hyperparathyroidism is very rare in child-hood, but it can cause an acute illness in infants which may be fatal. It is accompanied by cortical erosions, which leave the subcortical trabeculae projecting freely on the surface of the bone in a manner which is charac-teristic (*Figure 3.27*). Such erosions can readily be detected in certain sites, notably the medial aspect of the proximal ends of the tibiae, the clavicles, the thenar aspect of the middle phalanges, the humeral and femoral necks, the calcaneum, the ribs and ischial tuberosities. The lamina dura of the teeth is defective, but often this may be patchy. Pathological fractures may occur in the region of the metaphyses of the long bones and these may result in the ends of the bones forming an oblique angle with the long axis (*Figure 3.27b*). Small 'cystic' areas, which are mainly endosteal in type, are less obvious than in adults (Rajasuriya *et al.*, 1964). The cranial vault may be slightly widened and have a mottled, granular rather 'fuzzy' appearance. Soft tissue calcification,

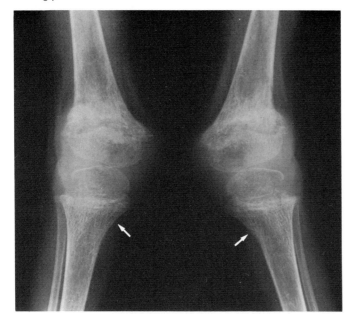

Figure 3.27. Hyperparathyroidism in Renal Osteodystrophy: (a) The knees of a child suffering from renal failure due to obstructive uropathy. There is a severe genu valgum due to tilting of the femoral and tibial metaphyses. Destruction of the cortex is evident along the medial side of the tibia (arrowed). Although the bones are generally decalcified, there are patchy areas of increased density in the region of the metaphyses. (b) The wrists of the same child. The obliquity and irregularity of the metaphyses of the radius and ulna are particularly striking

(a)

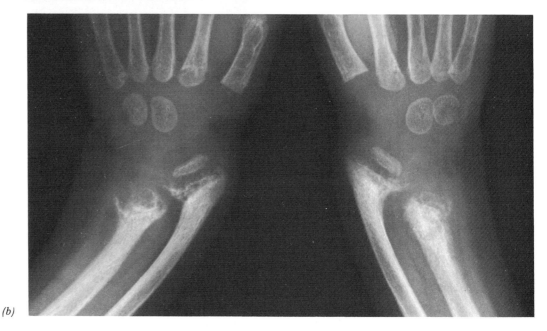

(b)

nephrocalcinosis and renal calculi occur but it is stated that these features are relatively less common in children than in adults (Du Bois *et al.*, 1969).

The radiological features described above are all present in 'renal osteodystrophy' (*Figure 3.27*), but rachitic changes often precede the development of secondary hyperparathyroidism. Osteosclerosis develops later than the other changes and takes at least 3 years to appear. It is most commonly seen in the spine, where it takes the form of transverse bands at the upper and lower edges of the vertebral bodies ('rugger-jersey spine'); it also commonly occurs in the metaphyses of the long bones, especially the humeri and femora, and in the ribs, pelvis, clavicles and skull. It may present as a uniform granular density or a more open reticular pattern due to

thickening of individual trabeculae. The latter is a hyperostosis rather than a true osteosclerosis, the bone being present in an excessive quantity but without an abnormally high mineral content. It has been suggested that excess of calciton could be responsible for the production of the hyperostosis. A recent theory is that the rachitic changes may be due to an acquired resistance to the normal action of vitamin D.

Hypoparathyroidism

Tetany due to failure of parathyroid function is of rare occurrence in infancy. It is however an important diagnosis to make since it can masquerade as 'fits' or epilepsy.

The associated skeletal abnormalities are helpful in the differential diagnosis.

The radiological features are often inconspicuous. Transverse bands of increased bone density, particularly at the metaphyses of the long bones, may occur and be associated with abnormalities in the development and eruption of the teeth. These may either be hypoplastic or be lost early due to caries. The jaws may be abnormally short and wide. Calcification may occur in the soft tissues, as in hyperparathyroidism, but the distribution is different in the two conditions, being common in the basal ganglia of the brain or around the major joints in hypoparathyroidism.

A striking pattern of skeletal abnormalities occurs in some cases of hypoparathyroidism. In these cases the fault is thought to lie in a failure of the target organ to respond and not in a failure of the parathyroid glands to secrete enough hormone. Such cases are for this reason termed 'pseudohypoparathyroidism'. The skeletal changes comprise: (1) brachydactyly, due to shortening of the metacarpals, metatarsals and phalanges, the result of premature epiphyseal fusion. The shortening of the bones in the hands and feet occurs in the ring and little fingers and in the third and fourth digits of the feet more frequently than in the other digits (*Figure 3.28*); (2) bowing of the long bones with exostoses; (3) localized osteoporosis around the joints; (4) thickening of the cranial vault (Steinbach and Young, 1966). There is also mild mental retardation and some reduction in stature, the affected children being recognizable from their thick-set, obese body habitus and round face. It is known that these skeletal features can also occur without hypoparathyroidism, either independently or in relatives of cases of pseudohypoparathyroidism. It is likely therefore that they represent an associated genetic entity which is sometimes, but not always, accompanied by renal tubule cells which do not respond to parathormone.

Brachydactyly due to short metacarpals, metatarsals and phalanges can occur in other types of skeletal dyplasia, particularly peripheral dysostosis, chondro-ectodermal dysplasia, Turner's syndrome and myositis ossificans progressiva. Difficulties in diagnosis can therefore result. In cases of hypoparathyroidism the characteristic biochemical abnormalities should indicate the diagnosis.

HYPOPHOSPHATASIA

This rare inborn error of metabolism becomes manifest usually in newborn infants, but milder cases are described which present later in childhood. The skeletal changes which are produced in this condition resemble those of severe florid rickets, but occur at a much earlier age as a rule. The diagnosis can readily be confirmed by the abnormally low level of serum alkaline phosphatase and by the presence of an abnormal metabolite, phospho-ethanolamine, in the urine.

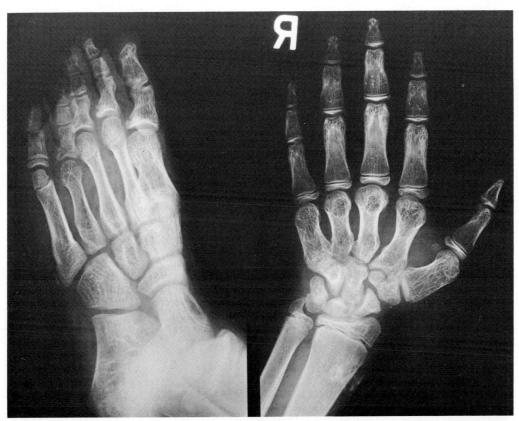

Figure 3.28. Pseudohypoparathyroidism: Shortening of the metacarpals and metatarsals and of some of the phalanges is associated with a coarse open trabecular pattern and with soft tissue calcification around the distal end of the radius

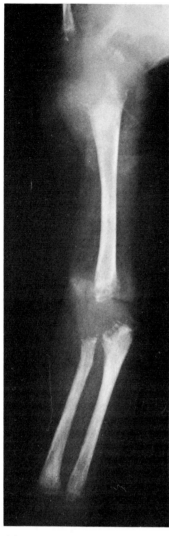

(a)

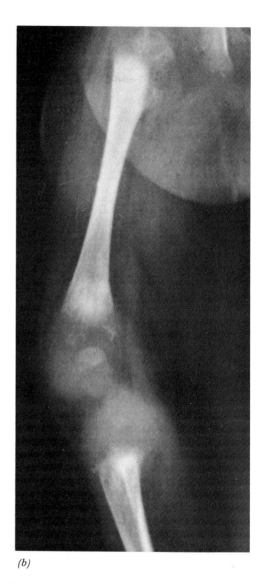

(b)

Figure 3.29. Hypophosphatasia: (a) There is marked irregularity and 'fraying' of all the metaphyses of the humerus, radius and ulna. (b) Similar changes are present in the femur and tibia with a very wide zone of uncalcified osteoid between the metaphyses and the epiphyses (By courtesy of Dr. P. P. Franklyn, Bradford Children's Hospital)

It is considered that the basic defect is deficient production of alkaline phosphatase by the hypertrophic cartilage cells and proliferating osteoblasts at the site of normal bone growth (James and Moule, 1966). Radiologically, the metaphyses of all the long bones are markedly abnormal, being frayed and irregular in outline. There is a wide zone of unossified bone between the diaphysis and the epiphysis which causes the long bones to appear to be very short. Longitudinal tongues or clefts of unossified bone extend into the diaphysis from the growth plate, and the latter is often angled relative to the long axis of the bone. The trabecular pattern in the metaphyses may be coarse and irregular; recalcified osteoid produces islands of bone sclerosis within areas of decreased density. Periosteal new bone may be present and lead to thickening of the cortex. Deformities are common, particularly bowing of the shafts (*Figure 3.29*). The skull may also be abnormal with defective ossification of the vault producing wide sutures and fontanelles. The wide sutures may be deceptive, since fusion may occur prematurely resulting in reduction in the size of the cranial cavity and signs of increased intracranial pressure. The deciduous teeth appear abnormal

due to wide pulp spaces and resorption of the apices of tooth roots which results in their premature loss.

Usually the diagnosis of hypophosphatasia is not difficult, but a low serum alkaline phosphatase can occasionally occur in other conditions, notably scurvy, hypothyroidism, idiopathic hypercalcaemia and osteogenesis imperfecta. In rickets, however, the phosphatase is always markedly increased and this, together with the difference in age incidence, should prevent confusion between the two conditions.

AMINO-ACIDURIAS

Some of the conditions in which abnormal amino acids appear in the urine are associated with radiological changes in the skeleton.

Cystinosis and the Fanconi syndrome

These conditions have already been considered in relation to renal tubular disorders (*see* page 82) and are associated with rickets.

Tyrosinosis

This condition shows similar skeletal abnormalities, in addition to which there is enlargement of the liver, spleen and kidneys. The appearance of the latter on urography may suggest polycystic disease or conditions such as leukaemia and glycogen storage disease. The occurrence of hypophosphataemic rickets may suggest the diagnosis and enable treatment to be started before irreversible hepatic dysfunction ensues.

Homocystinuria

This is a relatively rare disease, which is sometimes accompanied by radiological changes in the bones. The overall picture resembles that of Marfan's syndrome, with excessive growth and bowing of long bones, long slender fingers and toes, scoliosis and a thickening of the cranial vault. Large facial bones are associated with prognathism and overdeveloped paranasal sinuses. There is generalized demineralization. The metaphyses are irregular and dense and the epiphyses, carpal and tarsal bones abnormally large. Focal calcification occurs in the growth plate of the wrists, either as separate dots or as spicules projecting into it from the metaphyses (Morreels *et al.*, 1968). Intravascular thromboses are common; these may be a cause of death, and for this reason angiography is to be avoided. A means of differentiating homocystinuria from Marfan's syndrome lies in the metacarpal index which is usually normal in homocystinuria, since both the length and the width of the metacarpals are increased.

Phenylketonuria

Bone changes occur in some cases of this disease. The metaphyses may be cupped, superficially resembling rickets. There may be dense calcified spicules extending longitudinally across the epiphyseal plate. They may persist in later childhood as striations of dense bone within the diaphysis. These features are associated with retardation of skeletal growth and maturation and it has been suggested they could be related to the restricted diet employed in the treatment of the condition and not to the disturbance in tyrosine metabolism. However, similar changes can occur in other types of aminoaciduria (Holt and Allen, 1967).

WILSON'S DISEASE

Changes in the bones, resembling those described in the previous section, are known to occur in adolescents with this condition (Mindelzun *et al.*, 1970). These changes are similar to those of vitamin D resistant type of rickets or osteomalacia, but are accompanied by spinal deformity which consists of irregularity of the end-plates and anterior wedging of the vertebral bodies. Fractures of the articular surfaces of the knee and ankle joints similar to osteochondritis dissecans may occur and there may be fragmentation and sclerosis of subchondral bone in the wrists, elbows and small joints of the hands and feet. It is uncertain whether these bone changes are due to a direct effect of the disturbances of copper metabolism on the bones, or occur indirectly as a result of deposition of copper in the renal tubular cells. They have little relationship to the severity of the hepatic cirrhosis or of the abnormal signs in the central nervous system.

TRAUMATIC BONE DISEASE

The value of radiological examination in cases of injury is recognized to be as great in children as it is in adults; it may perhaps be more important, as clinical examination and history-taking may not be so easy. There is usually no difficulty in recognizing fractures and dislocations, provided adequate views which have been taken in two planes, preferably at right angles to each other, are available. It is not proposed therefore to discuss this subject further in general terms. Certain specific aspects merit a closer examination and these will be described in more detail (*Figure 3.30*).

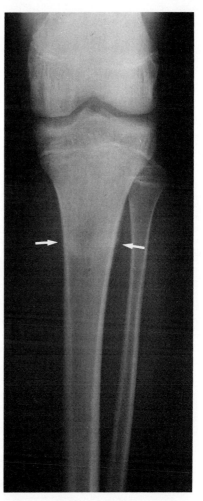

Figure 3.30. Stress Fracture: A horizontal line of increased density is present at the site of an undisplaced and healing fracture (arrowed). Such lesions may sometimes occur in the absence of a clear history of injury

THE 'BATTERED BABY' SYNDROME

It has become increasingly apparent in recent years that small infants can be the victims of non-accidental violence. When this is the case a history of injury may not be obtained, or the facts related may be misleading. In these cases the radiological appearances may be very characteristic and may afford a valuable part of the evidence which establishes the nature and causes of the injuries inflicted. There may be simple straightforward fractures or epiphyseal displacements, particularly when a child has been struck or thrown (*Figure 3.31b*). Such lesions should always be looked for in any suspected case. Particular attention should be given to the time that is likely to have elapsed after the fractures were sustained, since a discrepancy between the date of the injuries, as suggested by the radiological evidence, and that alleged in the history may give an indication of their true nature. The radiological appearances may however consist only of irregularity of the metaphyses of the long bones with fragments of bone, partially or completely separated from them. These fragments may either comprise the whole of the zone of provisional calcification, when they form part of an epiphyseal separation, or be confined to the outer angles of the metaphyses. Such metaphyseal fragmentation is very suggestive of trauma and is usually followed after 7 to 14 days by calcification along the outside of the cortex of the adjacent diaphysis (Silverman, 1953; Caffey, 1957). The younger the child the more rapid is the development of this calcification.

It is most extensive near the metaphyses, though not infrequently it extends along the whole length of the shaft. It is due to subperiosteal haemorrhage with calcification within the haematoma. Subsequently the calcified haematoma becomes united with the underlying cortical bone, widening it and giving it an irregular outline (*Figure 3.31a*).

There is a constant sequence of changes during the healing phase of this type of injury, during which the metaphyseal avulsion fractures heal and unite to the subjacent bone. The original slight displacement leads on healing to a very characteristic appearance of the metaphyses, which become 'squared', often with small spurs at the outer angles (*Figure 3.31a*). If the growth plate is displaced at an angle to the long axis of the bone, deformity may be produced as a result of further growth; together with the irregularly thickened cortex, these appearances make it possible to recognize old injuries many years after they have been sustained. The lesions just described result from shaking or twisting the child's limbs as well as from direct blows to the periosteal surface of the long bones. They should however be regarded as only one part of a continuous spectrum. This ranges from the effects of neglect and deprivation on the nutrition and general development of the child with retardation of growth, to more extensive injuries to other organs such as the brain, the spinal cord and the abdominal organs as well as the skeleton. Among the soft tissue injuries a particular type of abdominal lesion is found in 'battered babies' which differs from those sustained in road traffic accidents (Gornall *et al.,* 1972). In the latter the spleen and kidney are the organs chiefly at risk, whereas in non-accidental injury it is the liver and the small intestine which are most often damaged.

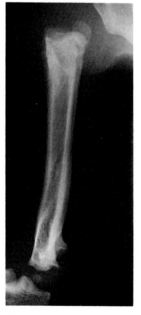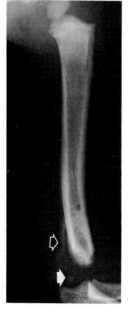

(a)

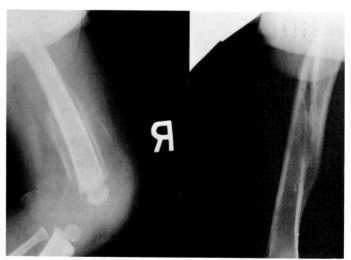

(b)

Figure 3.31. The 'Battered Baby' Syndrome: These radiographs show the presence of bony injuries at different sites and at several different times. (a) Both humeri of an infant aged 21 months taken at the same time. On the left side there is evidence of a fairly recent injury with displacement of the epiphysis for the capitellum (solid white arrow), metaphyseal fragmentation and localized calcification in a subperiosteal haematoma (outline white arrow). On the right side there is evidence of a much older injury of the same type in which the cortex is thickened and irregular due to organized subperiosteal new bone and where metaphyseal spurs are present at both ends of the humerus due to healed avulsion injuries. (b) Lateral films of both femora of the same child. The right femur (on left) was examined at the age of 9 months and shows a calcifying subperiosteal haematoma. The left femur (on right) examined at 17 months of age shows a healing fracture of the shaft

These injuries result in perforation, intramural haematoma of the bowel or in avulsion of the common bile duct. Fractures of vertebrae and narrowing of the disc spaces with anterior notching of the vertebral bodies are produced by hyperflexion of the spine. Evidence of haematomata due to associated injury of the spinal cord may be found on myelography in a number of these cases. Fractures of the long bones are sometimes associated with chronic subdural haematoma in infancy (Caffey, 1946). The limb fractures in such cases are often more recent than the subdural haematomata and it has been suggested that they are due to repeated trauma even where there is no clear history.

The incidence of the 'battered baby syndrome' is hard to estimate because it is often difficult to establish the diagnosis with certainty. It is estimated that it accounts for 10–15 per cent of all trauma in the first 3 years of life in Denver, Colorado (Kempe, 1971). The incidence may not be quite so high in this country but it is certainly not infrequent in most paediatric units. It is a condition, however, which it is very important to detect because the patient and his siblings may be at risk from subsequent injury. On the other hand, bony injuries occurring from a trivial force are known in a number of conditions such as osteogenesis imperfecta, osteopetrosis and scurvy; but most of these give evidence of their presence by other bony abnormalities which are easily recognizable on radiography. However, fractures can occur in bones which are radiologically normal. Immobilization, or the presence of paralysis, weakens the resistance of the bones to injury. The absence of a normal perception of pain may also allow the patient to injure himself. In all these cases the effect may appear to be disproportionate to the apparent cause and they can be confused with the 'battered baby' syndrome.

EPIPHYSEAL INJURIES

Injuries to the epiphyses are of particular importance because of the possibility of damage to the growth plate either directly from the trauma or from secondary ischaemia. These injuries may lead to deformity, consequent upon arrest of growth or development in an abnormal direction, due to displacement of the growth plate. Such injuries are relatively common, comprising 10–15 per cent of all trauma to the long bones in children (Salter and Harris, 1963). They occur predominantly in males and in late childhood or adolescence. Their occurrence as part of the 'battered baby' syndrome has been referred to already.

Most cases are not difficult to recognize radiologically, although errors can arise in certain cases. Firstly, when displacement is absent or has been spontaneously reduced. In such cases the presence of a thin lamella of metaphyseal bone which is usually attached to a separated epiphysis may be a valuable indication of injury. Secondly, when the epiphyseal ossification centre has not yet ossified, as is often the case in the newborn infant. Such injuries, though rare, may occur as a result of birth trauma at the proximal ends of the humerus or femur. Local soft tissue swelling and an abnormal position of the metaphysis may be the only radiological signs, although early evidence of repair in the form of callus or metaphyseal bony fragments can be useful additional

features. The femoral lesions in particular can easily be confused with congenital dislocation of the hip, though there is no associated acetabular dysplasia. The displacement may be more marked in the lateral than in the anteroposterior view.

Where the normal epiphyseal growth plate has a complex arrangement, such as at the elbow, a film of the uninjured side should be taken for comparison. In the rare type of injury, in which the growth plate is crushed without any associated epiphyseal or metaphyseal fractures, the only radiological evidence of the lesion may be premature fusion of the epiphysis with arrest of growth. In such cases, serial measurement of the length of the long bones on the two sides of the body may be required to assess the need for, and also the effectiveness of, surgical treatment designed to lengthen the bones on the injured side or to shorten those on the opposite side.

Epiphyseal injuries may result in avascular necrosis which becomes apparent as a diffuse increase in bone density. If only part of the growth plate is damaged angulation between the shaft and the epiphysis may result in incomplete arrest of growth. This also accounts for the metaphyseal 'cupping' which may occur if the arrest of the growth is in the central segment of the growth plate, and the peripheral part continues to grow normally (Caffey, 1970). The ends of the bones become splayed laterally with the epiphyses appearing to sink into the concave metaphysis.

Slipped femoral epiphysis

Epiphyseal injuries, like other fractures, may be 'pathological', and associated with generalized bone disease such as scurvy, osteomyelitis or renal osteodystrophy. In such cases the underlying condition is usually obvious. Slipped femoral epiphyses (adolescent coxa vara) should probably be included in the 'pathological' group in view of the generally accepted opinion that it is related to hormonal changes occurring at, or just before, puberty.

Both anteroposterior and lateral films are essential to diagnose the condition. Displacement of the epiphysis of the femoral head is predominantly backwards and it may give little evidence of its presence on the anteroposterior film. However, absence of the normal projection of the capital epiphysis beyond the line of the upper surface of the neck, prolongation of the lower angle of the epiphysis into a downward-directed 'beak' and exclusion of the most medial part of the femoral metaphysis from the confines of the acetabulum are useful clues in the anteroposterior view (*Figure 3.32*). Comparison with the opposite hip should also be helpful except when the condition is bilateral, which is rarely the case. In the majority of cases of slipped femoral epiphysis, the bone age is retarded and such slowing of skeletal and sexual maturation is associated with an increased susceptibility to epiphyseal injury (Morscher, 1967). The degree of retardation is however slight and has little diagnostic value.

Apophyseal injuries

Epiphyses at the sites of muscle attachment are often

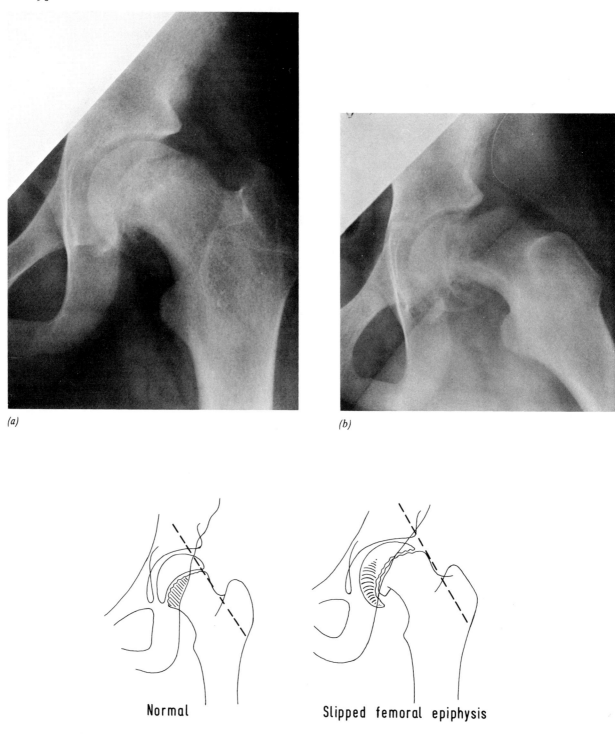

(a)

(b)

Normal

Slipped femoral epiphysis

(c)

Figure 3.32. Slipped Femoral Epiphysis: *(a) Anteroposterior view showing loss of the normal projection of the upper angle of the epiphysis beyond the line of the upper surface of the neck, prolongation of the lower angle of the epiphysis into a 'beak' and loss of the clearly defined border of the metaphysis, the medial part of which is displaced out of the acetabulum. (b) Lateral view of the femur showing the posterior direction of epiphyseal displacement, the neck of the femur being displaced correspondingly forwards. (c) Diagram illustrating the relationship between the head and neck of the femur and the acetabulum in the anteroposterior view of a normal child and in a case of slipped femoral epiphysis*

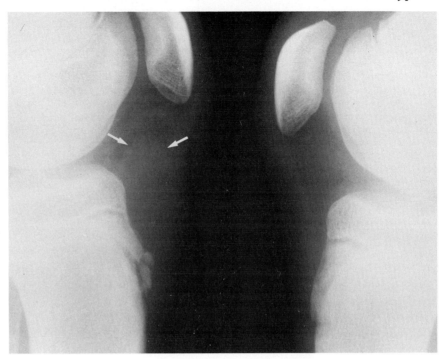

Figure 3.33. Osgood–Schlatter's Disease: Comparison of the abnormal knee (left) with the opposite side which is normal. There is displacement of the bony fragment separated from the tibial tubercle and encroachment upon the infrapatellar fat pad by soft tissue swelling associated with the injury (arrowed)

referred to as traction epiphyses or apophyses. These can also be the site of avulsion injury. Such injuries have in the past been grouped with lesions which are predominantly ischaemic in nature, as examples of 'osteochondritis'. An example of this type of lesion is Osgood–Schlatter's Disease. This is an avulsion injury of the tibial tubercle, the epiphysis for which is at the site of attachment of the ligamentum patellae. The radiological signs of this condition are displacement and fragmentation of the epiphysis with swelling of the adjacent soft tissues (*Figure 3.33*). The diagnosis is often rendered difficult by the fact that ossification normally occurs from several centres in variable sequence. This difficulty is even more marked in the case of an analogous lesion at the attachment of the tendo Achillis to the epiphysis for the tubercle of the calcaneum. It is thought likely that the radiological signs, which have been described in this condition as Sever's disease, are wholly due to normal variations in the mode of ossification of this epiphysis.

OSTEOCHONDRITIS DISSECANS

Separation of a part of the articular surface of a joint, usually including both articular cartilage and the underlying subchondral bone, differs from simple fractures involving joint surfaces by the fact that the former fail to unite. This is due in part to the instability of the detached fragment and in part to ischaemic necrosis. These lesions result in a defect in the articular surface and the detached fragment of bone and cartilage persists as a loose body within the joint. Radiology enables such lesions to be diagnosed, provided that the site of the defect can be visualized in profile (*Figure 3.34*). This may not always be achieved in the standard projections and special views have to be taken to visualize it adequately. The knee joint is a frequent site of this lesion.

It occurs on the posterior part of the medial femoral condyle, bordering on the intercondylar fossa. Special radiographic views with angulation of the central beam through the intercondylar fossa are needed to allow the defect to be seen in profile. Other sites in which this lesion may arise are the articular surface of the patella, the lateral femoral condyle, the head of the femur, the capitellum of the humerus, the talus and the heads of the metatarsals. Lesions occurring in the latter site (Freiberg's disease) are peculiar in that females are more often affected than males, whereas males are affected twice as often as females when the condition occurs elsewhere (*Figure 3.35*).

Recognition of osteochondritis dissecans on radiographs is usually not difficult, but confusion may arise from the fact that irregularities of the articular surfaces may occur normally in growing children. These latter irregularities are usually symmetrical.

CONGENITAL INSENSITIVITY TO PAIN

In this rare congenital abnormality, pain and, to some extent, temperature sensation are absent, though the ability to detect other sensory stimuli is preserved. The cause of the condition is unknown. The nervous system is otherwise normal on clinical examination and the sensory end organs in the skin are histologically normal on biopsy. The abnormality is familial and presents in early childhood with a liability to burns, dental sepsis, corneal injuries and bone lesions. The latter resemble the neuropathic 'Charcot' joints of adults. They result from fractures which unite poorly and also from epiphyseal separations, both of which lead to deformity. There may also be widening of the epiphyseal plate, an appearance which can resemble rickets. There is also progressive destruction of the articular surface of affected

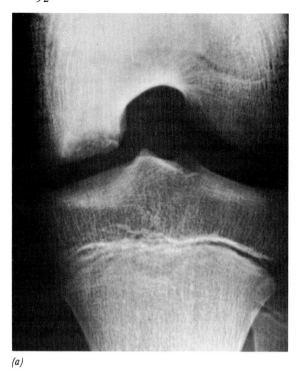

(a)

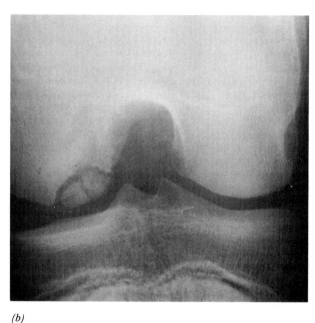

(b)

Figure 3.34. Osteochondritis Dissecans: (a) Right knee. A defect is present in the lateral femoral condyle due to the separation of two bony fragments which lie within it. (b) Left knee of another case examined at a later stage. The defect in this child lies in the medial femoral condyle and the bony fragments have become broken up and partly resorbed. Such defects are best seen in projections taken to show the intercondylar fossa owing to their situation on the curved surface of the femoral condyle

joints with fragmentation of bone at the attachments of the periosteum to the metaphyses and with the production of osteophytic outgrowths of bone. The ankle is the commonest joint to be affected, but the hips, knees and elbows may also be involved (*Figure 3.36*). The effects of the abnormality tend to lessen as the child grows older but they are not confined to lesions arising from trauma. Areas of chronic osteomyelitis are not uncommon; they arise from a combination of injury, infected burns and neglected lesions. The phalanges in particular may show progressive destruction of both bone and soft tissue. Areas of aseptic necrosis of bone can occur at sites adjacent to weight-bearing joints, especially in the tarsus and in the hips. This diagnosis should be considered in any case of 'osteochondritis' arising in an uncommon site or in which there is unusually extensive fragmentation. In infancy, cortical thickening due to organizing subperiosteal haematoma can lead to the suspicion that the patient may be a 'battered baby'. The presence of ordinary fractures of the skull and long bones may occur in a third of the cases of congenital insensitivity to pain (Siegelman et al., 1966). These fractures may suggest osteogenesis imperfecta or some other cause of pathological fracture, but the structure and form of the bones appear normal except in the region around the affected joints in congenital insensitivity to pain.

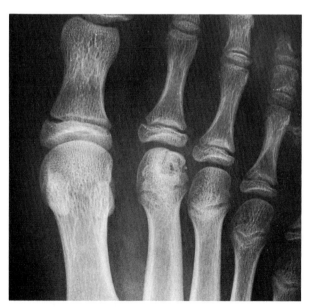

Figure 3.35. Freiberg's Disease: A portion of the head of the second metatarsal has become separated from the rest of the head. The separated fragment is liable to undergo necrosis and subsequent resorption leaving a defect in the metatarsal head which can persist for up to a year

MISCELLANEOUS BONE LESIONS

PERTHES' DISEASE

This is a condition which affects the epiphysis of the head of the femur; the cause of the lesion is either trauma and ischaemia, or both, but there is doubt as to the extent to which these two factors are involved. The usual view is that ischaemia due to a deficient blood supply is the basic cause. It has been suggested that the condition is primarily due to a direct injury of the epiphyseal ossification centre by compression against the roof of the acetabulum (Caffey, 1968). Histological evidence is hard to obtain because of the essentially benign nature of the condition. Most of the theories as to its aetiology have been based on the study of its radiological features. Any such theory as to the cause of Perthes' disease has to explain the following facts: (1) it has a characteristic but restricted age range, the peak incidence being between 3 and 8 years; (2) it is four or five times commoner in males; (3) it is more frequent in certain races than in others; and (4) it is occasionally familial.

A constant sequence of radiological changes occurs over a period of about 4 years from onset to healing. These changes have been ascribed to the effect of the presence of a fragment of dead bone in the epiphysis on the living bone surrounding it, and to the processes by which the dead bone is gradually broken up and absorbed. Only after this process has been completed can the affected epiphysis begin to reform. There is no doubt that Perthes' disease differs from avascular necrosis of the head of the femur (*see* page 95). It is important to diagnose the condition as early as possible because, if treatment is instituted soon enough, the full natural course of the disease may be curtailed and the residual deformity minimized. The earliest radiological sign of the condition is lateral displacement of the head of the femur relative to the medial wall of the acetabulum (Kemp and Boldero, 1966). This may only amount to a few millimetres in the early stages and it is difficult to assess. It requires radiographs accurately centred, without pelvic tilt or rotation, and also relies on comparison of the suspect hip with the normal hip on the opposite side. It is therefore less useful in bilateral cases, which comprise about 10–20 per cent of the total. Within a week or two an overall increase in the joint space of the affected hip occurs and it is caused not only by displacement of the head, but by a reduction in the size of the epiphyseal ossification centre which becomes flattened due to early compression and collapse (*Figure 3.37*). Both of these abnormalities are capable of complete resolution with rest, but whether this will occur or not depends on how far the cartilage surrounding the ossified part of the epiphysis has been deformed which cannot be judged from the radiological appearances at this stage of the disease. A small V-shaped area of osteolysis on the lateral aspect of the affected epiphysis ('Gage's sign') may afford evidence that the femoral head is liable to be deformed permanently. An increase or persistence of the lateral displacement of the femoral head may have the same significance, because it implies that the moulding influence of the acetabulum will not be applied to that part of the viable cartilage of the head lying outside the acetabulum.

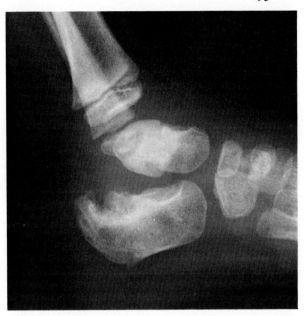

Figure 3.36. Congenital Insensitivity to Pain: Destructive lesions are present in the adjacent surfaces of the talus and calcaneum in a child aged 3½ years with absence of pain sensation since birth

The later features of Perthes' disease are fragmentation and increased density of the capital epiphysis. Changes may occur in the metaphysis at the same time and consist of areas of osteolysis and disturbance of the trabecular pattern (*Figure 3.38*).

The final outcome of the disease process is affected by the extent of the collapse and fragmentation of the head. It is therefore important to define the extent of these features. Cases in which only the anteromedial part of the femoral head is involved do better than those in which the lateral part is also involved, because the latter is predominantly subject to weight-bearing. In order to appreciate this feature, lateral views of the femoral head are essential and interpretation on the basis of an anteroposterior view alone can be highly misleading. The appearance of fragmentation is due to the break-up of the damaged epiphyseal bone which is removed by osteoclastic resorption. This may not infrequently be confused with the early stages of repair, because re-ossification begins from separate centres which subsequently coalesce.

A sign which may precede fragmentation of the epiphysis has recently been described (Jacobs, 1970). It may be due to gas within linear fissures in the ossific centre which form conspicuous dark lines lying inside the borders of the epiphysis. These must be distinguished from gas shadows within the synovial cavity produced by traction on the opposed surfaces. This is a normal phenomenon, but one which may provide evidence of the fact that the articular cartilage has not been damaged.

The process of healing can be followed radiologically by the progressive restoration of the epiphyseal bone to a normal texture and density. It is not possible to assess whether residual deformity of the femoral head will be permanent for at least 10–12 years after completion of

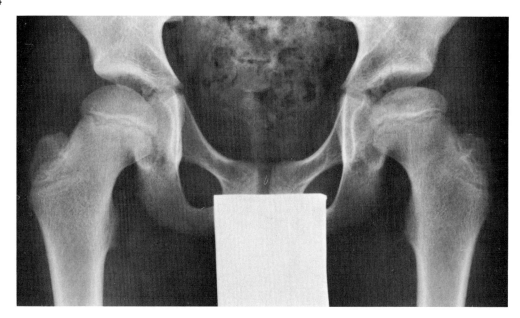

(a)

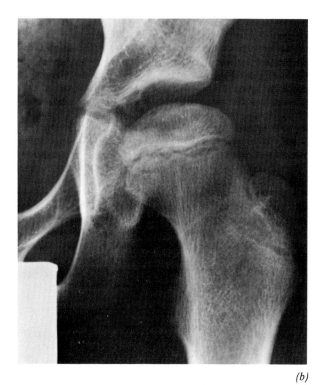

(b)

Figure 3.37. Perthes' Disease of the Left Hip Joint: A relatively early stage in the condition when the radiological features are confined to a widening of the joint space, a reduction in the height of the epiphysis, and minimal fragmentation of the articular surface of the left femoral head (a) Both hips. (b) Localized view of the left hip

treatment (Somerville, 1971). Restoration of the epiphysis to a completely normal appearance is not only possible but should be the ideal to which treatment is directed. This constitutes one of the chief differences between Perthes' disease and avascular necrosis. Various measurements of the femoral head and acetabulum have been devised to help in assessing residual deformity and these can assist in planning the duration of treatment. The reader is referred to the original paper of Heyman and Herndon (1950), where these are described in detail. If deformity of the cartilage as opposed to that of the bony ossific centre is severe, further treatment may be unrewarding. Arthrography can occasionally be helpful in showing the shape of the cartilaginous femoral head before re-ossification is complete.

Differential diagnosis

The only conditions likely to be confused with Perthes' disease radiologically are secondary avascular necrosis of the femoral head, the epiphyseal dysplasias or the epiphyseal dysgenesis which occurs in hypothyroidism. These latter conditions should be considered in any case with bilateral signs, but they do not show the characteristic sequence of changes seen in Perthes' disease.

SCHEUERMANN'S DISEASE

A large number of conditions of uncertain aetiology affecting various epiphyses and some of the carpal and tarsal bones, which have been thought to resemble Perthes' disease, have been grouped under various eponymous titles or under the general term of 'osteochondritis'. It is not proposed to deal with these conditions in detail. Most of them are benign, giving rise to few permanent sequelae, and some of them have little claim to be more than normal variations in epiphyseal ossification. Scheuermann's disease or juvenile kyphosis may, however, result in permanent spinal deformity and is therefore of some importance. Furthermore it is diagnosed, like Perthes' disease, largely on the basis of the characteristic pattern and sequence of the radiological changes it produces. Although the cause of this condition is still not determined, it is likely that ischaemia plays little part and that trauma, acting upon the end-plates of the affected vertebral bodies is the basic factor. There is a limited age incidence between 13 and 19 years and males are twice as often affected as females.

The earliest radiological feature is a loss of definition around the upper or lower anterior angles of the affected vertebral body. The disc spaces become progressively narrowed as the nucleus pulposus herniates through the damaged end-plate and separates the marginal epiphyses from the main part of the vertebral body (Williams and Pugh, 1963). These epiphyses are of the traction type (apophyses—*see* page 337) and play no part in growth. The epiphyses of the affected vertebral bodies tend to be smaller and more irregular and fragmented than the normal epiphyses. They frequently fail to fuse to the body and then persist as separate ossicles. The bony defects due to the nuclear herniation are characteristically situated in the anterior or middle third of the end-plates. They develop a reactive sclerosis around their edges, and persist as the familiar 'Schmorl's' nodes. The most commonly affected bodies are those between the 8th and 12th thoracic vertebrae (*Figure 3.39*). They become progressively deformed by failure of growth of the anterior half of the body in a craniocaudal direction. The bodies become wedge-shaped and this may lead to an increasing kyphosis. At the same time growth in an antero-posterior direction is stimulated, and results in an increase in the depth of the vertebral bodies. This latter feature serves to distinguish Scheuermann's disease from other causes of anterior wedging, such as crush fractures. It is common for cases to present with spinal deformity and back pains caused by the consequent strain on ligaments and muscles. In such cases the radiological appearances are those of the deformity and Schmorl's nodes. The early active stages of the disease are relatively rarely seen. Kyphosis may be quite severe and has occasionally led to cord compression; myelography may be desirable to localize its site and its degree.

AVASCULAR NECROSIS OF BONE

This condition in the hip differs from Perthes' disease, in the much more serious and permanent deformity which results. It may arise after fractures of the neck of the femur and may be a feature of sickle-cell disease. It may also occur in congenital dislocation of the hip, especially after unsuccessful reduction, or after septic arthritis of the hip in infancy. Avascular necrosis is commonest in the head of the femur, but it has also been described in the epiphyses of the distal phalanges following frostbite. Steroids and irradiation may also lead to bone necrosis.

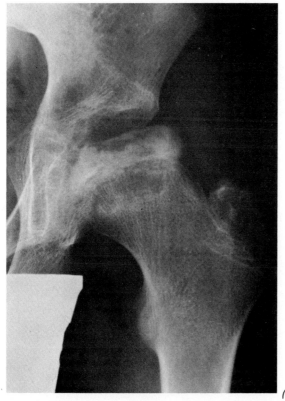

(a)

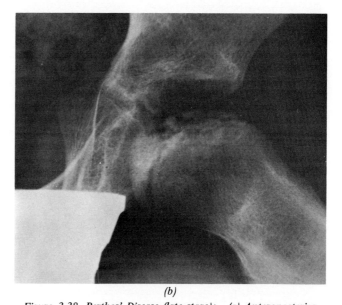

(b)

Figure 3.38. Perthes' Disease (late stage): (a) Anteroposterior view of same hip as in Figure 3.37 18 months later, showing a large defect in the femoral head which is more severely deformed. In addition, there are translucent areas present in the metaphysis. (b) Lateral view of the femoral head and neck showing that the defect lies anteriorly with the posterior third of the capital epiphysis remaining intact; several residual necrotic fragments are still present within the defect which have to be absorbed before healing will begin

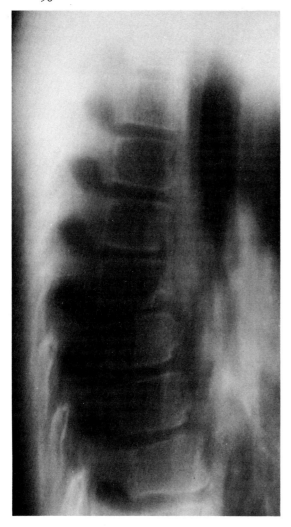

The radiological features are similar in all these instances. There is an increase in bone density, fragmentation, collapse and, in the most severe cases, complete destruction of the epiphysis. Permanent deformity almost always results and this can be aggravated by premature fusion of the epiphysis and arrest of normal growth.

ESSENTIAL OSTEOLYSIS

This is a condition of unknown aetiology. It is a rare but radiologically very striking condition, It has been referred to as the 'disappearing bone disease'. The affected bones, usually adjacent to a joint, show progressive destruction associated with tapering and thinning of the bones at a distance from the original focus. The wrists and ankles are the most frequent sites, but the hip and other joints can also be affected. Several varieties of the condition are described, some of which are inherited. In others there may be kidney lesions or associated abnormalities in the skin and central nervous system. In the type known as Gorham's massive osteolysis, biopsy of the affected areas of bone have revealed areas of fibrosis combined with vascular tissue resembling a haemangioma or lymphangioma.

Figure 3.39. Scheuermann's Disease: A tomogram showing multiple defects in the anteroinferior angles of the bodies of four of the lower thoracic vertebrae; the ring epiphyses are absent in the affected vertebrae, but can be seen in relation to the normal vertebra immediately below the abnormal ones. The disc spaces between the affected vertebrae are narrowed and a slight kyphosis has already developed

REFERENCES

INFLAMMATORY DISEASE OF BONES AND JOINTS

Alexander, C. J. (1970). 'The aetiology of juvenile spondylarthritis (Discitis).' *Clin. Radiol.* **21**, 178

Brass, A. and Bowdler, J.D. (1969). 'Non-specific spondylitis of childhood.' *Annls Radiol.* **12**, 343

Caffey, J. and Silverman, W. A. (1945). 'Infantile cortical hyperostoses—preliminary report on a new syndrome.' *Am. J. Roentgl.* **54**, 1

Cremin, B.J. and Fisher, R. M. (1970). 'The lesions of congenital syphilis.' *Br. J. Radiol.* **43**, 333

Eyre-Brook A. L. (1960). 'Septic arthritis of the hip and osteomyelitis of the upper end of the femur in infants.' *J. Bone Jt Surg.* **42B**, 11

Levin, E. J. (1970). 'Healing in congenital osseous syphilis.' *Am. J. Roentgl.* **110**, 591

Martel, W., Holt J. F. and Cassidy, J. T. (1962). 'Roentgenological manifestations of juvenile rheumatoid arthritis.' *Am. J. Roentgl.* **88**, 400

Padfield, E., and Hicken, P. (1970). 'Cortical hyperostosis in infants—a radiological study of sixteen patients.' *Br. J. Radiol.* **43**, 231

Roberts, P. H. (1970). 'Disturbed epiphyseal growth at the knee after osteomyelitis in infancy.' *J. Bone Jt Surg.* **52B**, 692

Rosberg, G. and Laine, V. (1967). 'Natural history of radiological changes of knee joint in juvenile rheumatoid arthritis.' *Acta Paediat. Scand.* **56**, 671

BONE LESIONS IN BLOOD DISORDERS

Bohrer, S. P. (1970). 'Acute long bone diaphyseal infarcts in sickle-cell disease.' *Br. J. Radiol.* **43**, 685

Brenner, G. and Allen, R. P. (1963). 'Skeletal changes in erythroblastosis foetalis.' *Radiology* **80**, 427

Caffey, J. (1957). 'Cooley's anemia: a review of the roentgenographic findings in the skeleton.' *Am. J. Roentgl.* **78**, 381

Middlemiss, J. H. and Raper, A. B. (1966). 'Skeletal changes in the haemoglobinopathies.' *J. Bone Jt Surg.* **48B**, 693

Silverman, F. N. (1948). 'The skeletal lesions in leukemia.' *Am. J. Roentgl.* **59**, 819

Willson, J. K. V. (1959). 'The bone lesions of childhood leukaemia, a survey of 140 cases.' *Radiology* **72**, 672

METABOLIC BONE DISEASE

Currarina, J., Neuhauser, E. B. D., Reyersbach, G. C. and Sobel, E. H. (1957). 'Hypophosphatasia.' *Am. J. Roentgl.* **78**, 392

Dent, C. E. and Friedman, M. (1965). 'Idiopathic juvenile osteoporosis.' *Q. Jl Med. N.S.* **34**, 177

――and Watson, L. (1968). 'Hereditary pseudo-vitamin D deficiency rickets.' *J. Bone Jt Surg.* **50B**, 708

― Richens, A., Rowe, D. J. F. and Stamp, T. C. B. (1970). 'Osteomalacia with long-term anticonvulsant therapy in epilepsy.' *Br. med. J.* **4**, 69

Du Bois, R., Farriaux, J.P., Maillard, E. and Maillard J. P., (1969). 'Primary hyperparathyroidism in a newborn infant.' *Annls Radiol.* **12**, 407

Holt, J. P. and Allen, R. J. (1967). 'Radiologic signs in the primary aminoacidurias.' *Annls Radiol.* **10**, 317

James, W. and Moule, B. (1966). 'Hypophosphatasia.' *Clin. Radiol.* **17**, 368

Mindelzun, R., Elkin, M., Scheinberg, I. H. and Sternlieb, I. (1970). 'Skeletal changes in Wilson's disease, a radiological study.' *Radiology* **94**, 127

Morreels, C. L., Fletcher, B.D., Weilbaecher, R. G. and Dorst, J. P. (1968). 'The roentgenographic features of homocystinuria.' *Radiology* **90**, 1150

Rajasuriya, K., Peiris, O. A., Ratnaike, V. T. and de Foneska, C. P. (1964). 'Parathyroid adenomas in childhood.' *Am. J. Dis. Child.* **107**, 442

Reilly, B. J., Leeming, J. M. and Fraser, D. (1964). 'Craniosynostosis in the rachitic spectrum.' *J. Pediat.* **64**, 396

Rose, G. A. (1964). The radiological diagnosis of osteoporosis, osteomalacia and hyperparathyroidism.' *Clin. Radiol.* **15**, 75

Steinbach, H. L. and Noetzli, M. (1964). 'Roentgen appearance of the skeleton in osteomalacia and rickets.' *Am. J. Roentgl.* **91**, 955

― and Young, D. A. (1966). 'The roentgen appearance of pseudohypoparathyroidism (PH) and pseudo-pseudohypoparathyroidism (PPH), differentiation from other syndromes associated with short metacarpals, metatarsals and phalanges.' *Am. J. Roentgl.* **97**, 49

TRAUMATIC BONE DISEASE

Caffey, J. (1946). 'Multiple fractures in the long bones of infants suffering from chronic subdural haematoma.' *Am. J. Roentgl.* **56**, 163

― (1957). 'Some traumatic lesions in growing bones other than fractures and dislocations: clinical and radiological features.' *Br. J. Radiol.* **30**, 225

― J. (1970). 'Traumatic cupping of the metaphyses of growing bones.' *Am. J. Roentgl.* **108**, 451

Gornall, P., Ahmed, S., Jolleys, A. and Cohen, S. J. (1972). 'Intra-abdominal injuries in the battered baby syndrome.' *Archs. Dis. Childh.* **47**, 211

Kempe, C. H. (1971). 'Paediatric implications of the battered baby syndrome.' *Archs Dis. Childh.* **46**, 28

Morscher, E. (1967). 'Growth cartilage and puberty.' *Annls Radiol.* **11**, 351

Salter R. B. and Harris, W. R. (1963). 'Injuries involving the epiphyseal plate.' *J. Bone Jt Surg.*, **45A**, 587

Siegelman, S. S., Heiman, W. G. and Manin, M. C. (1966). 'Congenital indifference to pain.' *Am. J. Roentgl.* **97**, 242

Silverman, F. N. (1953). 'The Roentgen manifestation of unrecognised skeletal trauma in infants.' *Am. J. Roentgl.* **69**, 413

MISCELLANEOUS BONE LESIONS

Caffey, J. (1968). 'The early roentgenographic changes in essential coxa plana. Their significance in pathogenesis.' *Am. J. Roentgl.* **103**, 620

Heyman, C. H. and Herndon, C. H. (1950). 'Legg-Perthes' disease—a method for the measurement of the roentgenographic result.' *J. Bone Jt Surg.* **32A**, 767

Jacobs, P. (1970). 'Intra-epiphyseal gas in osteochondritis.' *Clin. Radiol.* **21**, 318

Kemp, H. S. and Boldero, L. (1966). 'Radiological changes in Perthes' disease.' *Br. J. Radiol.* **39**, 744

Somerville, E. W. (1971) 'Perthes' disease of the hip.' *J. Bone Jt Surg.* **53B**, 639

Williams, H. J. and Pugh, D. G. (1963). 'Vertebral epiphysitis; a comparison of the clinical and roentgenological findings.' *Am. J. Roentgl.* **90**, 1236

4 CARDIOVASCULAR SYSTEM

INTRODUCTION

The quality and diversity of treatment in modern medicine and surgery is such that it is essential to have as comprehensive a diagnosis of the condition present as is possible. To obtain the precision of diagnosis thus required demands a multidisciplinary approach and in no field of medicine is this truer than in cardiological diagnosis. Radiology has a large part to play in making a final definitive diagnosis, in conjunction with the clinical history, physical signs, electrocardiograph, phonocardiograph and haemodynamic studies. When provided with information from all these sources, the clinician is in the best position to correlate them and confirm the final diagnosis.

It should be borne in mind that the only radiological examinations that do not endanger the patient are plain radiography, fluoroscopy and ultrasound. Cardiac catheterization and angiocardiography, which in most cases will be required to define the diagnosis accurately, carry a small risk for the patient. Full weight must be given to these facts when planning cardiological investigations and angiocardiography and catheterization should not be performed unless the results are likely to influence the management of the patient. The use of ultrasound in the diagnosis of cardiological conditions is now an established fact and the value of its application in paediatric cardiology is being more widely appreciated especially in congenital heart disease.

METHODS OF RADIOLOGICAL EXAMINATION

PLAIN RADIOGRAPHY

It is important to obtain a straight view of the chest in full inspiration. In older children this presents no problem as the child is co-operative, but in young infants and older children who are ill this method may not be possible. Several special frames have been devised to hold an infant upright in front of the x-ray cassette and these can give very satisfactory results. It is more usual to examine the infant lying supine on the cassette with his arms held above his head. At least two views should be taken, the postero-anterior view (or anteroposterior if the patient is supine) and the left lateral view.

Recently there has been a tendency not to take the left and right anterior oblique views used so frequently in former years, an omission that detracts from the information available from this part of the radiological examination. The postero-anterior view should show the condition of the lungs, the size and shape of the heart and mediastinal outline, the calibre of the pulmonary arteries and the size and position of the aortic arch as well as any bony abnormality in the thorax that might effect the shape and position of the heart. The lateral view is taken to locate lung pathology, to show abnormalities of the spine and sternum and the presence of a thymic shadow. It will also demonstrate the front and back of the heart outline and so aids determination of individual chamber enlargement. These views may be combined with a barium swallow to outline the oesophagus.

FLUOROSCOPY

It is an odd fact of life that, while most x-ray departments are now equipped with image-intensifiers and television chains, so that it is easy to examine a patient fluoroscopically as no dark adaptation is necessary, these facilities are used much less frequently for radiological diagnosis than in previous years. It must be recognized that, even with the most experienced radiographers in paediatric work, it is not infrequent

98

for the anteroposterior radiograph to be taken on partial or almost complete expiration. This results in a wholly false apparent enlargement of the heart being portrayed on the radiograph and an erroneous impression is given of the vascularity of the lungs. It is not uncommon for such patients to be sent for cardiac catheterization to elucidate the cardiac enlargement, a referral that could be avoided by a few seconds' fluoroscopy which would show that the heart is not in fact enlarged. The true size and shape of the heart and mediastinum are revealed while the patient takes a full inspiration, as he must during crying, and these can be recorded on film or video-tape.

Fluoroscopy also shows the pulsations of the heart and pulmonary arteries, the position of the aorta and the size of the individual chambers, especially when the oesophagus is outlined by barium. Impressions on the oesophagus produced by anomalies of the aortic arch and the arteries arising from it can readily be appreciated. Sometimes abnormal positioning of the main pulmonary artery can show in this way. In the adult, fluoroscopy is valuable for detecting intracardiac calcification but this is rarely seen in childhood.

CARDIAC CATHETERIZATION

An end-hole, smooth, radio-opaque catheter is inserted into an arm or saphenous vein towards the heart and directed under the fluoroscopic control of an image-intensifier and television. It should pass through the right atrium, right ventricle, main pulmonary artery and its branches, out into the lung fields until it wedges in a small peripheral pulmonary artery. The catheter may cross into the left side of the heart through a defect in the atrial or interventricular septum. In any position, blood aspirated and pressure recordings made from the catheter will indicate the oxygen saturation and pressure respectively of the blood in the anatomical structure in which the tip of the catheter is located. Thus cardiac catheterization is a combined haemo-dynamic and radiological study and the role of radiology is (1) to help in directing the catheter through the heart chambers and great vessels; (2) to locate the optimum anatomical sites from which blood sampling should be taken and determine whether this objective has been achieved; and (3) to recognize and record when the catheter takes an abnormal course (e.g. from the pulmonary artery through a patent ductus arteriosus to the descending aorta).

ANGIOCARDIOGRAPHY

Angiocardiography is serial radiography of the heart and great vessels after the blood within them has been rendered radio-opaque following the injection of a contrast medium. It is an unpleasant examination for the patient because the contrast medium as it passes through the heart and great vessels produces an intense feeling of warmth. The contrast medium entering the pulmonary arteries acts as an irritant and may produce coughing. For these reasons, in younger children it is performed under a general anaesthetic, though for older children sedation only is required.

The contrast medium used is one of the iodine-containing water-soluble contrast media such as Conray 420. It is injected through an NIH (National Institute of Health, USA) radio-opaque catheter whose end is sealed but which has six side-holes grouped within a centimetre of the tip. A side-hole catheter is less likely to produce damage to the heart muscle or endocardium than is one with an end-hole because the force of the injection is spread over a wider area. The success of the examination depends on getting as high a concentration of contrast medium in the blood at the end of the catheter as possible, thus producing the greatest opacification of the heart chambers on the radiographs. This can be achieved only by using a mechanical injector of some kind. The passage of the contrast medium through the heart chambers is recorded on a rapid series of radiographs or by cineradiography over a period of about 9 seconds. The radiographs are taken simultaneously in pairs at right angles to each other, one from the front being anteroposterior and the other from the side being a lateral radiograph; this method is known as biplane angiocardiography. Cineradiography can be performed single-plane or biplane. For the latter, pulsed exposures are necessary and electronic devices have to be introduced to ensure that the very short x-ray exposures are made only at the times the camera shutter is open. Speeds of up to 200 exposures per second are now obtainable by this means.

Undoubtedly the quantity and type of apparatus available at any centre will be limited by the money that is provided and will vary considerably from centre to centre. There is, however, no place for the occasional angiocardiograph. All angiocardiography must be done in centres which are adequately, if not ideally, equipped, and in which the staff have considerable experience in the examination and interpretation of the results.

Angiocardiography is classified according to the site in which the injection of contrast medium is made and it may be: (1) venous; (2) selective: (a) right-sided; (b) left-sided.

Venous angiography

The injection is made into a vein, which may be an antecubital vein or one of the more central veins. This method is seldom used now

Selective angiocardiography

RIGHT-SIDED

The injection is made usually into the right ventricle but occasionally into the right atrium. If, on right-sided catheterization the catheter tip is located in the pulmonary artery, pulmonary arteriography may be performed by injecting contrast medium.

LEFT-SIDED

The injection is made most frequently into the left ventricle but sometimes into the left atrium. The catheter may be placed in the left side of the heart either through a foramen ovale or atrial septal defect from the right atrium or, after percutaneous catheterization of the femoral artery, through the aorta into the left ventricle. If the foramen ovale is closed a trans-septal approach to the left atrium and left ventricle using a Brockenbrough or Ross needle to perforate the interatrial septum from the right side has been introduced recently. In the latter two cases catheters with an end-hole as well as side holes have to be used. If the catheter tip is located in the aorta, thoracic aortography can be performed. Very occasionally in children it may be desirable to place the catheter tip into the mouth of one of the coronary arteries and perform selective coronary arteriography.

It is also desirable to take a film of the abdomen at the conclusion of the procedure. This will demonstrate the urinary tract by virtue of the contrast medium excreted by the kidneys and may reveal any associated congenital anomalies that may be present (*see* Chapter 7, page 262 and *Figure 4.1*).

ULTRASOUND EXAMINATION OF THE HEART

In recent years ultrasound examination of the heart has become established as a reliable and valuable method of examination in adults which can give information about the heart not available otherwise. It is a non-invasive technique which causes the patient no discomfort. It gives information about the movement of the mitral (*Figure 4.2*), aortic and tricuspid valves and the size and function of the ventricles, and it is a sensitive method for detecting pericardial effusion and atrial myxoma. In recent years it has been applied in children and it has been shown that ultrasoundcardiography has considerable potential in the diagnosis of congenital heart disease (Godman and Kidd, 1974; Goldberg *et al.*, 1975).

RADIOLOGICAL FEATURES OF THE NORMAL HEART

PLAIN FILMS INCLUDING BARIUM SWALLOW

The postero-anterior view

The right border of the cardiovascular shadow is made up of two distinct portions with a well-marked notch intervening between them. The upper portion is straight and it is produced by the border of the superior vena cava. The lower portion is convex to the right and is

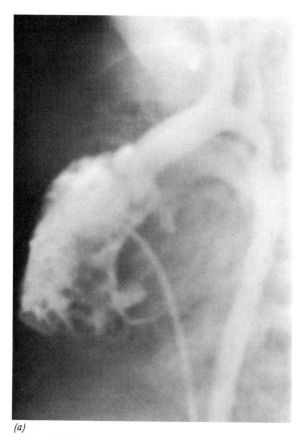
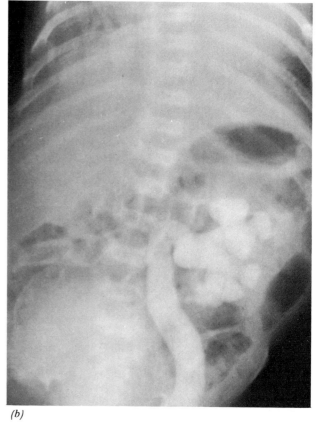

(a)   *(b)*

Figure 4.1. Urinary Tract Abnormality Associated with Congenital Heart Disease: (a) Angiocardiogram in lateral projection; injection of contrast medium into the right ventricle demonstrating transposition of the great arteries. (b) Film of the abdomen taken several hours later. A left hydronephrosis and hydro-ureter are shown due to a congenital obstructive lesion of the lower urinary tract. Such an association of cardiac and urinary anomalies is sufficiently common to make such a film a valuable procedure (see Chapter 7, page 262)

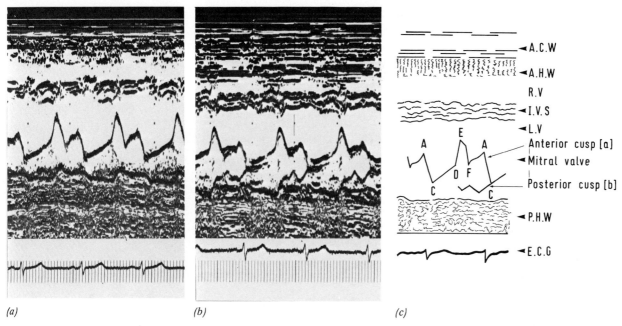

Figure 4.2. Normal Ultrasoundcardiogram with Reference Electrocardiogram: (a) and (b) same patient: (c) line drawing. Upward deflection of the trace is produced by movement of the anterior cusp of the mitral valve towards the anterior chest wall, therefore indicating opening of the valve; downward deflection of the trace indicates closing of the valve [(a) and (c)]. The valve opens on atrial contraction (A), then closes when the left ventricle contracts. (C) The mitral valve ring is drawn forwards during ventricular systole at the end of which (D) the valve opens (E). During early diastole the valve partially closes (F), a rapid movement which often takes place in two stages. It then remains partially open until the next atrial contraction. The posterior mitral valve cusp (b) moves in the opposite direction to the anterior cusp (a). ACW—anterior chest wall; AHW—anterior heart wall; RV—right ventricle; LV—left ventricle; PHW—posterior heart wall; IVS—interventricular septum

produced by the border of the right atrium. In most children the angle between the right atrium and diaphragm is clear-cut and acute, but in older children it may be filled in by the inferior vena cava or a pad of fat if the patient is obese. The outline of the left side of the cardiovascular shadow is produced from above down by: (1) the aortic knuckle which is formed by the aortic arch; (2) the short segment bulge of the main pulmonary artery; (3) a short bulge due to the left atrial appendage; (4) by the left ventricle which sweeps slowly down to the diaphragm (see Figures 4.3 and 4.6a).

The right pulmonary artery is seen as a comma-shaped opacity extending out from the side of the cardiovascular shadow at the level of the notch between the superior vena cava and the right atrium; the left pulmonary artery is seen on the left side of the cardiovascular shadow at a slightly higher level. Both pulmonary arteries branch dichotomously, gradually becoming smaller as they pass out towards the periphery of the lung fields, the larger branches extending down towards the lower lobes. The pulmonary veins are difficult to detect in childhood but may be seen in older children as almost vertical Y-shaped linear opacities extending down from the medial parts of the upper zones of the lung fields and crossing the hilar shadows to enter the left atrium. They may be seen also in the right lower zone where they pass transversely towards the left atrium. The azygos vein may be identified (Figure 4.4).

In some important details the radiograph of the infant differs from that of the older child or adult. In infancy the diaphragm is relatively high; as a result

the heart is more transverse in type than in older children and it appears larger (Figure 4.5). Also in infancy the aortic knuckle is not visible because the arch of the aorta is more in the sagittal plane than in later years. However, in a properly centred radiograph the trachea deviates slightly to the right in the mediastinum and this deviation is produced by the aortic arch on the left side. Thus the side of the aortic arch may be determined. In the infant also, the mediastinum may be obscured by the prominent shadow of the thymus which can be identified by its anterior position and a well-marked notch (sail shadow) on the mediastinal border usually on the right side (see Figure 5.3a). As the child gets older so the heart shadow resembles more closely the adult outline. This may be achieved by about the age of 8 years if the child has a long, narrow type of chest, but probably not till after age 10 years if his chest is short and broad (see Chapter 9, page 361).

The lateral view

The anterior and posterior borders of the heart are well seen, but in infants the superior part of the anterior aspect of the heart and the retrosternal space may be obscured by the shadow of the thymus. Posteriorly there is a clear space between the border of the heart and the spine known as the retrocardiac space. The anterior border is formed in its lower two-thirds by the anterior wall of the right ventricle and it is smoothly

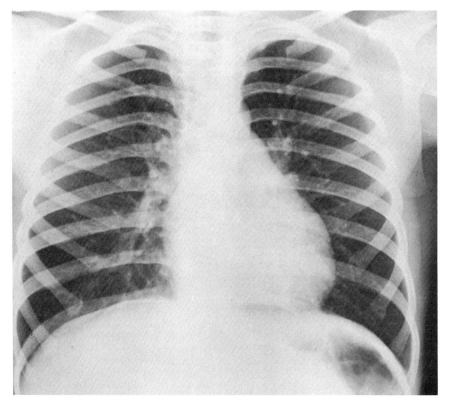

(a)

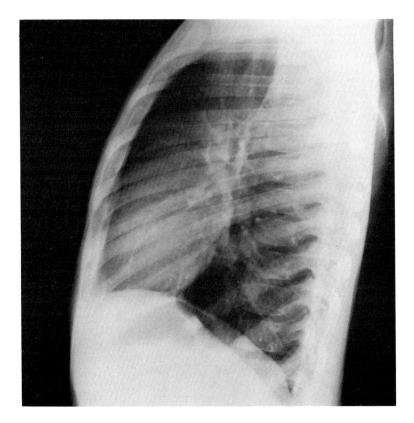

(b)

Figure 4.3. Normal Heart in a Child aged 7 years: (a) Postero-anterior projection.
(b) Lateral projection

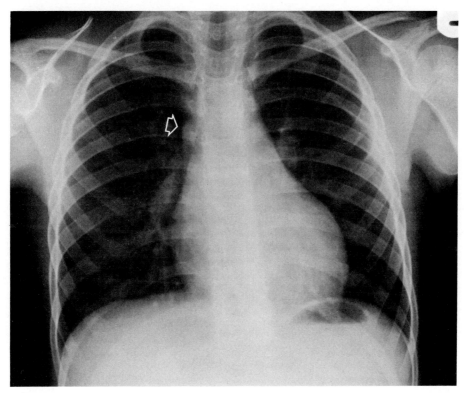

Figure 4.4. Normal Azygos Vein: The azygos vein may cause a localized projection on the upper part of the right mediastinal border (arrowed)

convex forwards (*Figures 4.3.* and *4.5*). In the majority of children just over a half of this part of the anterior border is in contact with the sternum but the amount of contact will vary with the degree of obliquity of the heart. The greater the obliquity, the less of the border that is in contact with the sternum and vice versa. Above the portion occupied by the right ventricle is a short segment formed by the appendage of the right atrium which overlaps the base of the ascending aorta. Above it is the ascending aorta which continues into the arch but this vascular pedicle is usually only poorly seen in early childhood. The posterior border of the heart is smoothly convex posteriorly and it is formed in nearly equal parts by the left ventricle inferiorly and the left atrium superiorly. The inferior vena cava passes up through the diaphragm to enter the right atrium and its posterior border is seen as a vertical linear shadow superimposed on the heart shadow just in front of the convexity of the posterior border of the left ventricle. About level with the upper border of the left atrium, the right pulmonary artery with its branches is seen end-on as an oval or rounded density and the left branch of the pulmonary artery is seen passing backwards and downwards and dividing into its smaller branches. In older children, the descending aorta may be seen passing downwards as a linear opacity with its anterior border just in front of the thoracic vertebral bodies (*Figures. 4.3b* and *4.6b*).

Oblique views

To obtain good oblique views of the heart the child must be rotated sufficiently so that a clear space is obtained between the heart and spine. The side of the oblique view depends on which of the patient's shoulders is in contact with the film. These anterior oblique views can be obtained only in children who can stand upright; for young infants and children the views have to be taken with the patient lying supine. In this case the x-ray tube must be in front of the patient and the cassette behind, the views being designated posterior oblique views, the side again referring to which shoulder is in contact with the cassette. The same radiological projections of the heart are obtained in the right anterior oblique and left posterior oblique views and also in the left anterior oblique and right posterior oblique views.

The right anterior oblique view is mainly useful for demonstration of the size of the left atrium, which forms the upper half of the posterior surface; the lower half of this surface is formed by the right atrium and inferior vena cava (*Figure 4.6c*).

The chief value of the left anterior oblique view is that the two ventricles are shown to the best advantage; the right ventricle forms the smooth slight convexity of the anterior surface of the heart and the left ventricle the lower half of the posterior surface, the two being separated inferiorly by the interventricular groove. The arch of the aorta and descending aorta may also be clearly shown in this view in older children (*Figure 4.6d*).

FLUOROSCOPY

The oesophagus

Much information about pathological states of the

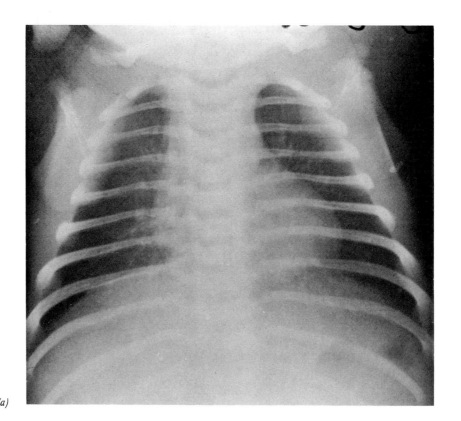

(a)

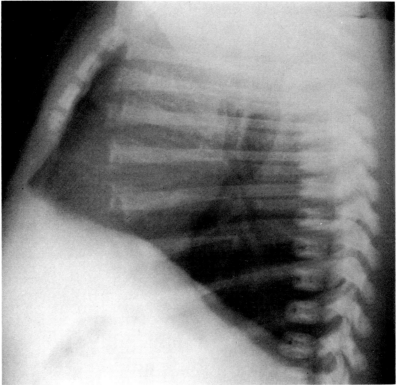

(b)

Figure 4.5. Normal Heart in an Infant aged 2 weeks: (a) Anteroposterior projection.
(b) Lateral projection

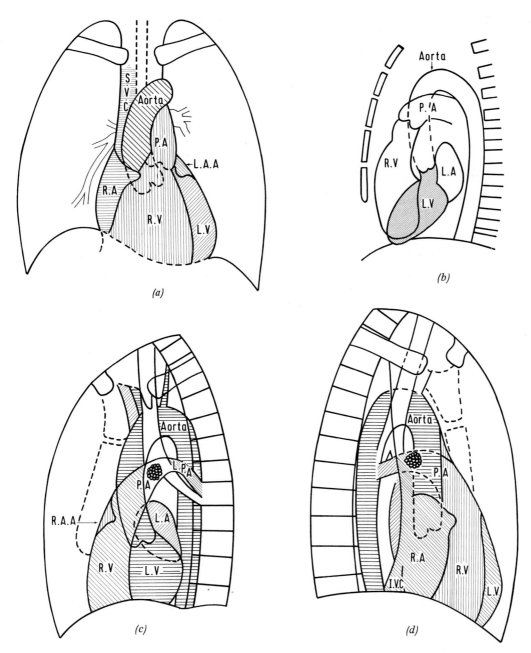

Figure 4.6. Diagram Illustrating the Relationship of the Cardiac Chambers to the Heart Outline: (a) Postero-anterior projection. (b) Lateral projection. (c) Left anterior oblique projection. (d) Right anterior oblique projection. IVC—inferior vena cava; LAA—left atrial appendage; LV—left ventricle; RA—right atrium; RV—right ventricle; LA—left atrium; LPA—left pulmonary artery; PA—main pulmonary artery; RAA—right atrial appendage; SVC—superior vena cava

heart and especially the great vessels can be obtained from study of the barium-outlined oesophagus. The oesophagus lies in close relationship to the right and posterior aspects of the arch of the aorta and then to the right side of the left main bronchus which separates it from the left pulmonary artery. Below this it lies posterior to the left atrium, and above the diaphragm it crosses over and in front of the lower part of the descending aorta. These structures may all produce impressions on the oesophagus, the degree of impression varying with the exact anatomical relationship, the age

of the patient and respiratory phase in which the radiograph has been taken. The older the patient the more marked are these impressions. The impressions from the aortic arch and left main bronchus are concave to the left, the aortic arch impression being the more prominent, but in young children these two impressions merge into a single, long segment concavity. These impressions are best seen in the postero-anterior and right anterior oblique views. In infancy and early childhood the left atrium produces a well-marked impression on the oesophagus below the level of those described above

106

and it is seen in the right anterior oblique and left lateral views as an anterior concavity. It deepens on expiration and it becomes less marked as the patient gets older. In childhood the descending aorta seldom makes an analysable impression on the lower end of the oesophagus.

Cardiovascular pulsations

Analysis of cardiac pulsations on fluoroscopy, recorded if required by cineradiography or preferably by videotape, can give very helpful information in certain circumstances. Pulsations of the left and posterior borders of the heart are deeper and more vigorous than those of the right and anterior borders; they are most marked on the lower left border. At this site in ventricular systole the heart border moves upwards and to the right though in diastole it moves in the opposite direction. Also during systole the bulge of the left border of the main pulmonary artery moves further to the left, returning to its former position in diastole. Pulsations in the aorta are seldom seen in the normal child because the aorta is poorly visualized, but they can be inferred by observations of the pulsations transmitted to the barium-filled oesophagus. As the left ventricle contracts in systole the lower part of the posterior heart border (in the lateral or left anterior oblique positions) moves forwards while the left atrial border moves backwards; in ventricular diastole the movements are in the reverse direction. Thus half-way up the posterior heart border a point of opposite pulsations is discernible and alterations in its position can have diagnostic significance. A similar point of opposite pulsations exists on the left heart border between the outlines of the main pulmonary artery and the left ventricle. The atrioventricular groove can be seen on fluoroscopy as a thin radiolucent line running obliquely down from the region of the pulmonary artery above to the right side of the lower border of the heart inferiorly. It moves downwards, forwards and to the left in ventricular systole and is best seen in the postero-anterior and right anterior oblique projections.

NORMAL APPEARANCES OF THE CARDIAC CHAMBERS AND GREAT VESSELS ON ANGIO-CARDIOGRAPHY

The right atrium is a crescentic chamber on the postero-anterior view. It is convex to the right where it forms the right heart border and concave to the left. The appendage is the upper medial cone-shaped part of the chamber which overlies the spine but it may extend across to the left to overlap the pulmonary artery or outflow tract of the right ventricle. The superior and inferior venae cavae enter the posterior part of the atrium. On the lateral view the atrium lies across the heart shadow and its posterior border is straight and directed diagonally upwards and forwards. Inferiorly its posterior edge is easily recognized if contrast medium refluxes back into the inferior vena cava.

The right ventricle is a cone-shaped chamber with its apex extending upwards and to the left towards the pulmonary artery (*Figure 4.7*). It covers most of the front of the heart from the spine to the left side. It consists

of the body, which is the inflow part of the ventricle, and the infundibulum, which is the smooth outflow tract from the body to the pulmonary valve. The crista supraventricularis is a muscle ridge posteriorly which separates these two parts of the ventricle. The body has muscular bundles in its wall and these give it a notched outline. It varies considerably in size from systole to diastole.

The main pulmonary artery is best seen on the lateral view extending upwards and backwards from the pulmonary valve. On the anteroposterior view the right pulmonary artery crosses the spine horizontally to divide into its branches on the right side (*Figure 4.7*). Frequently the right upper lobe branch is given off over the spine. The left branch is almost in direct continuity with the main pulmonary artery and as it passes almost straight backwards, it is best seen as the highest branch on the lateral view. The branches of the pulmonary artery can be traced into the periphery of the lung fields and they are larger and more numerous in the lower lobes.

The pulmonary valve is seen tangentially on the lateral view, in which it is best demonstrated (*Figure 4.7*). Two of the cusps show as thin curvilinear translucencies in the contrast medium, convex towards the ventricle in diastole and extending from the front to the back of the contrast shadow. Just above them there are small bulges, one forwards, one backwards, in the outline of the pulmonary artery; these are the valve sinuses. On ventricular systole the cusps open and they may be seen as translucent lines almost flush with the pulmonary artery walls. Two cusps may be similarly visible on the anteroposterior view. The pulmonary valve lies anterosuperiorly and to the left side of the aortic valve.

The left atrium. The pulmonary veins, three from each lung, drain into the posteriorly positioned left atrium which overlies the spine on the anteroposterior view. The left atrium is rounded in outline in this projection but it is oval on the lateral view (*Figure 4.7*). The appendage projects from the upper angle and is superimposed on the termination of the upper lobe veins on the anteroposterior view. On the lateral view the appendage extends forwards and upwards.

The left ventricle is acorn-shaped in both the anteroposterior and lateral views (*Figure 4.7*). Its apex points downwards and to the left and also anteriorly. Its walls are smooth and its outflow tract, which passes upwards and to the right towards the aortic valve, is short. It contracts vigorously, emptying itself almost completely on systole. The mitral valve is visible as a crescentic line across the outflow tract in the anteroposterior view. This appearance is due to the line of attachment of the posterior cusp and the translucency above it is produced by non-opaque blood entering from the left atrium. On the lateral view the two cusps of the mitral valve may be seen on the posterior borders of the ventricle. The left ventricular cavity usually overlaps the right ventricular cavity so the interventricular septum is not directly visualized. However, occasionally it may be seen as a vertical radiotranslucent stripe between the two ventricles in the lateral view when they happen to be orientated one in front of the other.

The aorta arises from the left ventricle above the aortic valve (*Figure 4.7*). Two valve cusps are seen as thin curvilinear translucent lines, convex towards the ventricle

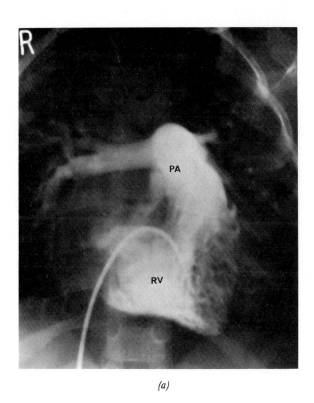

(a)

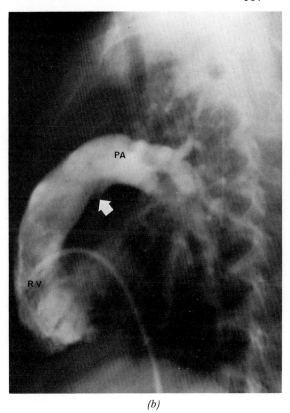

(b)

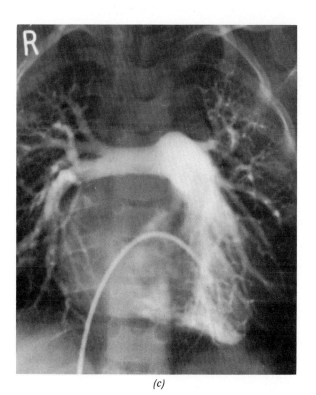

(c)

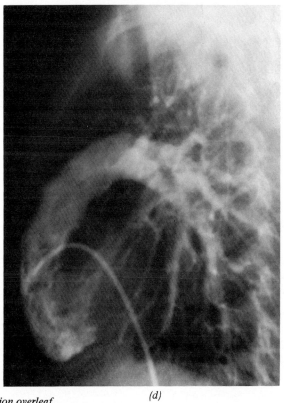

(d)

Figure 4.7. See caption overleaf

108

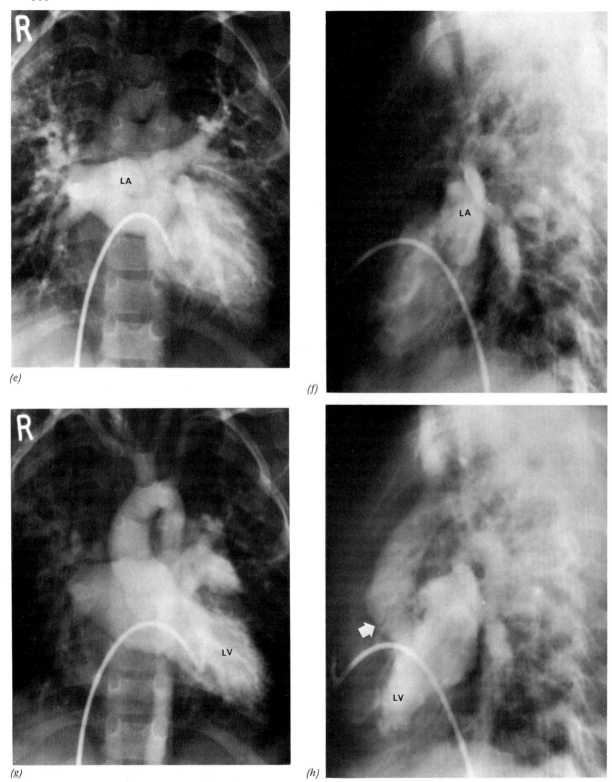

(e)

(f)

(g)

(h)

Figure 4.7. Normal Angiocardiogram: Contrast medium has been injected from a catheter in the right ventricle. (a) (see previous page) Anteroposterior and (b) lateral projections in which the contrast medium outlines the right ventricle (RV), the main pulmonary artery (PA) and its branches. The position of the pulmonary valve (arrowed) is shown in the lateral projection. (c) Anteroposterior and (d) lateral projections taken 2 seconds later. The contrast medium now lies in the branches of the pulmonary artery. (e) Anteroposterior and (f) lateral projections taken 6 seconds after the injection. The contrast medium fills the pulmonary veins and the left atrium (LA); the left ventricle is just beginning to fill. (g) Anteroposterior and (h) lateral projections taken 1 second later. The contrast medium fills the left atrium, left ventricle (LV) and aorta; the position of the aortic valve (arrowed) is shown in the lateral projection

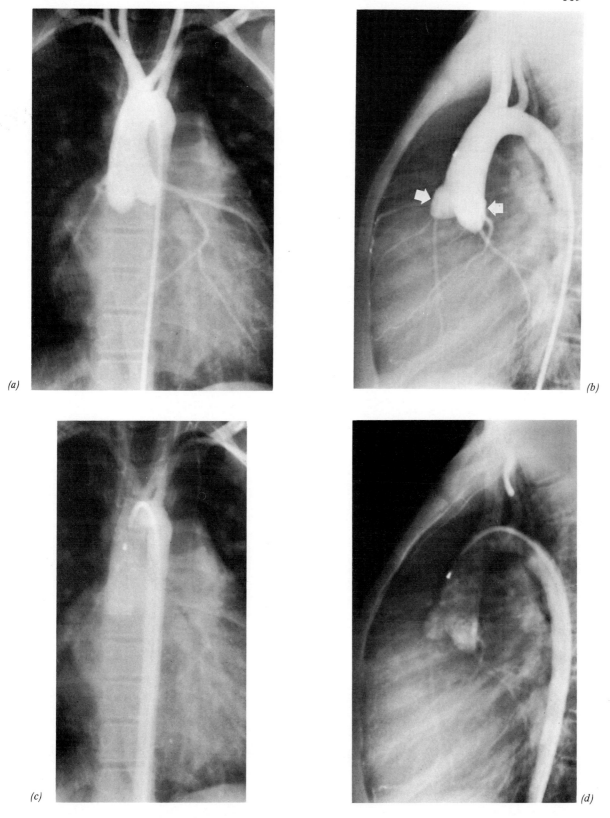

(a)

(b)

(c)

(d)

Figure 4.8. Normal Thoracic Aortogram: Contrast medium injected from a catheter in the ascending aorta. (a) Anteroposterior projection. The aortic valves, the ascending aorta and the aortic arch with its main branches are shown. (b) Lateral projection showing the coronary sinuses (arrowed) and the coronary arteries. (c) Anteroposterior projection and (d) lateral projection at a later stage when contrast medium fills the descending aorta

during ventricular diastole. They flatten against the aortic walls on ventricular systole. The three aortic sinuses are small projections from the aortic wall above the valve cusps. The two coronary arteries arise from the sinuses. In children the ascending aorta passes upwards and arches backwards in the sagittal plane to pass down in front of the spine as the descending aorta (*Figure 4.8*).

THE RADIOLOGICAL DIAGNOSIS OF ABNORMALITIES INVOLVING THE HEART

GENERAL

The heart is a relatively globular muscular organ attached to and suspended by the great vessels within the mediastinum. It is surrounded by the pericardium, pleura and lungs and rests inferiorly on the mobile muscular diaphragm, all these structures being enclosed within the rigid bony thorax. Thus alterations in the size, shape and orientation of the heart can be brought about not only by intrinsic abnormalities of the heart itself but also by volumetric changes in the lungs, differing heights of the diaphragm, by rotation or abnormalities of the bony thoracic cage. The position of the heart may be grossly influenced by lesions of the lungs, mediastinum, diaphragm and thoracic cage. Also in children orientation of the heart on its vertical axis varies from child to child, some having the heart rotated to the right, others to the left. All these factors have to be taken into account when assessing radiological cardiac abnormality. Study of the bony thorax, diaphragm level and lung fields can be very rewarding and may avoid some errors in diagnosis.

A further complication in assessing cardiac abnormality in childhood is the fact that in some children with congenital heart disease the heart does not have four chambers in the accepted anatomical positions. Criteria devised for assessment of individual chamber enlargement in these cases cannot be applied because the chambers are not occupying their normal part of the cardiac contour or they may be completely absent. However, in such patients fairly characteristic shapes of the cardiovascular shadow can be recognized even if individual chamber size assessment is not possible. These usually occur in patients with very severe abnormality of the heart who are deeply cyanosed.

Assessment of individual chamber size is most easily accomplished and is likely to be most accurate when only one chamber is involved; but children, in common with adults, frequently have more than one chamber enlarged. This introduces complications which certainly reduce the accuracy of radiological evaluation of the pathological lesions present. Nevertheless, in full realization that there are limitations to the value of the radiological signs described, every effort should be made to determine which chambers are enlarged and also the state of the aorta and pulmonary arteries. This information will be of great help in reaching a final diagnosis in any patient.

ENLARGEMENT OF INDIVIDUAL CARDIAC CHAMBERS

Enlargement of the right atrium

Gross degrees of enlargement of the right atrium may be recognized with relative ease but less marked degrees may be difficult to detect. When the right atrium is considerably enlarged the heart shadow projects more than usual to the right of the spine. The convexity of the right heart border increases in degree and the length of the convex segment extends so that the notch between it and the vertical superior vena caval shadow is at a higher level (*Figure 4.10*). In addition a shelf-like edge is formed just below this notch and this is well seen on the postero-anterior view. It is also evident projecting from the upper part of the anterior border of the heart in the left anterior oblique view. When the right atrium enlarges, the bulging of the right heart border extends right down to the level of the diaphragm on the postero-anterior view and the cardiophrenic angle becomes less acute than normal. In the right anterior oblique view, the right atrial enlargement will encroach on the lower part of the retrocardiac space narrowing this clear space inferiorly. In the lateral view, enlargement of the right atrial appendage causes a forward bulge of the upper part of the anterior heart border, filling in the lower part of the retrosternal space.

Enlargement of right ventricle

As the right ventricle enlarges the heart rotates in an anticlockwise direction, as viewed from above. This produces elevation of the apex away from the diaphragm, rounding of the upper part of the right heart border (*Figure 4.37a*) and accentuation of the main pulmonary artery segment above it. In many conditions, the main pulmonary artery will also be enlarged. All these features can be seen on the postero-anterior view, together with some increase in the transverse diameter of the heart. In the lateral view there is increased convexity of the lower two-thirds of the anterior surface of the heart and narrowing of the retrosternal space. In the left anterior oblique view the increased convexity of the anterior surface is better shown than in the lateral view, and the degree of obliquity of the patient required to show it is best determined on fluoroscopy. This view is particularly useful for demonstrating the backward and upward displacement of the left heart chambers produced by the enlargement of the right ventricle (*Figure 4.37b*). This is shown by elevation of the apex of the heart posteriorly, producing a convexity high on the posterior border and backward displacement of the interventricular groove, the impression being given that there is increased bulk of the anterior part of the heart. The depth of the heart is increased and the inferior vena cava is displaced back equally with the posterior border of the heart. The posterior part of the inferior border may appear to be rather flat. When the changes in the heart outline are present as described above, but the heart is not increased in size, then a diagnosis of right ventricular hypertrophy is justified.

Enlargement of the left atrium

On the postero-anterior view, enlargement of the left atrium may first show as widening of the upper part of the cardiac shadow due to some localized prominence of the left atrial appendage on the left heart border just below the pulmonary artery segment. If the append-age is considerably enlarged on actual shelf-like pro-jection may be produced at this site. The atrium also enlarges to the right and shows as an area of increased density to the right of the spine overlying the upper part of the right atrial shadow. This area of increased density is wider above than below. It has a sharply defined right border which is inclined slightly downwards and is convex laterally. If the left atrium is greatly enlarged its right border may extend superiorly beyond that of the right atrium, which is also displaced to the right, and the left atrial border may reach nearly to the right costal margin. The two atrial borders can be distinguished because the angle at which their right border meets the diaphragm is different, being about a right angle for the right atrium and an acute angle for the left atrium. Occasionally in childhood the left atrium will become so large that it elevates and splays the angle of bifurcation of the trachea; the right and left bronchi will then be more horizontal than normal and in particular the left main bronchus may be narrowed. This may produce collapse in the left lower lobe.

Smaller degrees of left atrial enlargement are best assessed in the right anterior oblique and left lateral views with the oesophagus outlined by barium (*Figure 4.13b*). As the left atrium enlarges it presses on the oesophagus in the segment below the left main bronchus. The oesophagus here is narrowed and displaced backwards with a concave impression on its anterior aspect. This impression is longer than the normal supero-inferior height of the atrium, i.e. greater than half the length of the posterior border of the heart. The length of this impression is important because on it depends the distinction between a left atrium which is normal in size and of normal prominence, i.e. a long segment of a short radius are as seen in a normal infant, and one which is pathologically enlarged which is a short segment of a long radius arc.

Enlargement of the left ventricle

When the left ventricle enlarges the heart rotates in a clockwise direction. On the postero-anterior view the apex of the heart is displaced outwards and downwards, increasing the transverse diameter of the heart and elongating the left border which also becomes more convex than normal (*Figure 4.19a*). The rotation accentu-ates the aortic knucle but the pulmonary artery seg-ment becomes less convex. The apex of the heart is also displaced backwards and the depth of the heart increased. In the left anterior oblique view the lower posterior border of the heart is seen to bulge posteriorly and inferiorly and a greater degree of rotation than normal is necessary for the heart to clear the spine. The distance between the posterior border and the border of the inferior vena cava is greater than normal. Prominence of the ascending aorta is frequently present in conditions that cause left ventricular enlargement and it should therefore be carefully sought as corroborative evidence of left ventricular enlargement. When the contour abnormalities described are present without increase of the transverse diameter of the heart then it is reasonable to infer ventricular hypertrophy.

Biventricular enlargement

Even in the presence of enlargement of both ventricles, careful analysis of the heart outline will reveal the true state of affairs in most patients. Features of both right and left ventricular enlargement will be noted and the observer should thus be alerted. In association with right ventricular enlargement which has produced most of the recognized features of this condition, one sign that does not receive sufficient attention as an indicator of the presence of co-existent significant left ventricular enlargement is the observation that the apex of the heart is not elevated and may in fact be displaced downwards. The apex is kept down by the counter-rotationary effect of left ventricular enlargement and, in the authors' experience, this can be a very useful and reliable sign.

DISPLACEMENT AND ROTATION OF THE HEART

The heart is relatively more mobile in the child than the adult. It is capable of displacement to either side or backwards and it may rotate towards the right or left side. Rotation to the right is limited by the anchoring effect of the superior and inferior venae cavae. Physio-logical rotation occurs throughout the cardiac cycle in response to diaphragmatic movement during respira-tion, and also in the presence of ventricular enlarge-ment. The aorta is capable of some displacement in response to physiological conditions and pathological states. Cardiac rotation in these circumstances must be allowed for when assessing individual chamber size.

Displacement of the cardiovascular shadow may also occur as a result of: (1) abnormalities of the bony thorax; (2) alterations in the diaphragmatic level; (3) pathological states of the lungs and mediastinum.

Abnormalities of the bony thorax

SCOLIOSIS CONVEX TO THE RIGHT

Even in small degrees of scoliosis the heart and aorta are displaced and rotated to the left into the concavity of the spine. In older children the aorta and main pulmonary artery may appear to be more prominent. In severe degrees, the left hemidiaphragm is elevated and the apex of the heart may be difficult to define because of it.

SCOLIOSIS CONVEX TO THE LEFT

This deformity is relatively rare. The heart is displaced and rotated to the right so that it lies more in the midline than normal, and there may be some widening of the vascular pedicle. If the scoliosis is severe the displacement of the heart may be such that most of it lies to the right of the spine. This may suggest dextrocardia, but with scoliosis the trachea also is displaced to the right.

KYPHOSIS

In uncomplicated kyphosis, the heart shadow remains central in position but it becomes more horizontal in direction owing to the vertical shortening of the spine and the relatively high diaphragm. This causes the heart shadow to be foreshortened on the postero-anterior view and more globular in outline. Kyphosis is frequently associated with scoliosis, and in these cases additional cardiac displacement is likely to be present.

STERNAL DEPRESSION

Depression of the lower third of the sternum is a common abnormality which most frequently exists without any associated congenital anomaly of the heart. All grades of depression are encountered from the very slight to the very severe; in childhood even minor degrees of depression of the sternum, which may not have been clinically recognized, can cause alteration in the x-ray outline of the heart (*see Figure 5.9* and page 178). Depression of the lower third of the sternum displaces the lower part of the heart backwards, flattens it from before backwards and displaces it to the left side. On the lateral radiograph the marked backward angulation of the lower end of the sternum is seen. On the postero-anterior view the ribs posteriorly are more horizontal than normal and may slope upwards and outwards in their posterior parts. Anteriorly the rib ends slope markedly downwards and medially and the transverse diameter of the thoracic cage appears to be wide. In the medial part of the right lower zone an ill-defined opacity is frequently seen. It is due to the soft tissues of the sloping edge of the funnel depression being projected partly edge-on. If the depression is of small degree, the heart shadow on the postero-anterior view may show some straightening of the left heart border with prominence of the main pulmonary artery segment. The apex is usually elevated. With severe degrees the heart is displaced to the left, the apex elevated and the transverse diameter increased. The lower part of the heart shadow is more radiotranslucent than the upper part. In the oblique views, the heart is displaced backwards and a greater degree of rotation is necessary for the posterior aspect of the heart to clear the spine. The flattening of the front of the heart is frequently very well seen in the left anterior oblique view.

Alterations in diaphragmatic level

The radiological interpretation of heart abnormalities depends largely on assessment of the cardiac contour and the appearances of the pulmonary arteries. Both of these features are profoundly sensitive to alterations of diaphragmatic level. This factor is particularly important in children in whom it is most difficult to control respiration. A standard appearance has to be agreed to allow for recognition of abnormalities. The accepted position of the diaphragm is that attained on deep inspiration; the right hemidiaphragm is then slightly higher than the left. With increasing elevation of the diaphragm, the transverse diameter of the heart enlarges and the heart becomes more transverse in type. The vascular pedicle widens, and there is a greater prominence of the superior vena cava. Of particular importance from the diagnostic point of view is the fact that as the diaphragm rises, the main pulmonary artery segment becomes more prominent. The pulmonary artery branches at the hila are elevated and more conspicuous. The peripheral pulmonary arteries widen and become crowded together throughout the lung fields. The high position of the diaphragm should make the observer suspect that the abnormalities may be more apparent than real and suggest examination of the child under fluoroscopy. Localized elevation or paralysis of the diaphragm and diaphragmatic herniae will displace the heart in a contralateral direction and are described in Chapter 6.

Depression of the diaphragm decreases the radiological size of the heart on the postero-anterior view. It becomes more vertical than in the normal individual. The vascular pedicle is elongated and its borders are well defined. The pulmonary arteries centrally and peripherally tend to be small, but if the depression is due to increased lung volume the central pulmonary arteries may be large.

Pathological states of the lungs and mediastinum

Pressure or traction on the heart caused by diseases of the lung, pleura or mediastinum may alter the position of the heart and of the great vessels and distort their outline. These conditions are dealt with in Chapter 5. Small areas of pulmonary fibrosis may alter the cardiovascular outline. Examples of this are the elevation of the pulmonary artery forming the hilum produced by fibrosis of the upper lobe and localized tenting of the cardiac outline resulting from a pleuropericardial adhesion.

The pulmonary lesion that seems to cause most difficulty in diagnosis is collapse (or agenesis) of the left lower lobe which is often present in patients with congenital heart disease. Collapse of the left lower lobe causes depression of the left pulmonary artery, which is therefore not so well seen, and compensatory emphysema of the left upper lobe. As a result of this, the peripheral pulmonary arteries are smaller and more spread out than normal in the left upper zone. The heart is displaced and rotated to the left, producing prominence of the main pulmonary artery segment. The opacity of the collapsed lower lobe will be visible through the heart shadow.

BRONCHIAL ARTERIES AND PULMONARY LYMPHATICS

The normal appearances of the lungs, pulmonary arteries and veins have already been described. In order to explain some of the radiological appearances that may result from heart disease further descriptions must be given of two structures which are not normally visible on the plain radiograph. These are the bronchial arteries and the pulmonary lymphatics.

The bronchial arteries arise from the descending aorta, enter at the hila and spread outwards with the bronchi into the peripheral interstitial tissue of the lungs.

The pulmonary lymphatics consist of two groups. The first group comprise the subpleural lymphatics, which form a network over the lung in the subpleural tissues. The second group consists of the deeper lymphatics, which accompany the bronchi, pulmonary arteries and veins. The subpleural lymphatics drain into the deep lymphatics and through them into the hilar glands. The superficial lymphatics are very fine and normally not visible. When they become overdistended they may contribute to the shadows cast by the inter-lobular septa of the lungs, as in left heart failure. In these circumstances the septa become oedematous and thickened and so they cast linear shadows on the radiograph. There are two types of these linear shadows. These are described by Kerley (1933) as 'B' lines, which are horizontal and best seen in the costophrenic angles, and 'A' lines, which are the deeper intrapulmonary septa. The latter are seen as thin straight lines extending from the periphery towards the hila and crossing normal vascular pathways (*see* page 115).

PULMONARY HYPERTENSION

Aetiology

The principal factors which control pulmonary blood pressure are (Steiner, 1972):
(1) Right ventricular output.
(2) Pulmonary capillary resistance.
(3) Elasticity of the lung.
(4) Degree of lung inflation.
(5) Pulmonary venous or left atrial pressure.

The normal pulmonary artery pressure is 30/12 mmHg measured at the sternal angle, with a mean of 22 mmHg. The normal pulmonary venous pressure is 6 mmHg. Arterial oxygen saturation is usually over 95 per cent; below 90 per cent desaturation and cyanosis occur.

Pulmonary hypertension may be arterial or venous (Steiner, 1972) (Table 1).

PULMONARY ARTERIAL HYPERTENSION

The pulmonary artery pressure is elevated but the pulmonary venous or capillary pressure may be normal.

PULMONARY VENOUS HYPERTENSION

The pulmonary venous and capillary pressures are raised but the pulmonary artery pressure can be normal or only slightly above normal values.

The radiological appearances of these two conditions differ mainly in respect of the presence of pulmonary oedema. It is very important when describing pulmonary

hypertension to determine whether it is arterial or venous in type, or, as is frequently the case, a combination of the two.

Table 1
CLASSIFICATION OF PULMONARY HYPERTENSION
(based on Steiner, 1972)
Pulmonary arterial or pre-capillary hypertension

(1) Hyperdynamic or hyperkinetic, due to increased pulmonary blood flow
  (i) Congenital heart disease
    (a) Ventricular septal defect including the Gerbode type
    (b) Atrial septal defect
    (c) Patent ductus arteriosus or any other left-to-right shunt

  (ii) Hyperdynamic circulation
    (a) Anaemia
    (b) Beriberi

(2) Vasoconstrictive hypertension
  (i) Arteriolar vasoconstriction
    (a) Increased pulmonary blood flow (congenital heart disease with right-to-left shunt)
    (b) Hypoxia
    (c) Response to drugs, i.e. acetylcholine
    (d) Secondary to pulmonary venous hypertension
  (ii) Obliterative pulmonary hypertension (obstructive)
    (a) Vasoconstrictive hypertension in congenital heart disease (Eisenmenger reaction)
    (b) Primary vasoconstrictive in children with congenital heart disease, i.e. persistent fetal pulmonary circulation
    (c) Thrombo-emboli
    (d) Tumour emboli
    (e) Bilharzia
    (f) Pulmonary arteritis
    (g) Diffuse interstitial pulmonary fibrosis
    (h) Idiopathic pulmonary hypertension

Pulmonary venous or postcapillary hypertension

  (i) Obstruction at mitral valve
    (a) Mitral valve disease
    (b) Cor triatrum
    (c) Left atrial tumour
  (ii) Left ventricular failure
  (iii) Pulmonary capillary or venous disease
  (iv) Constrictive pericarditis

In vasoconstrictive pulmonary hypertension the pulmonary vascular resistance can be increased in two ways. When the pulmonary venous pressure reaches the critical 25 mmHg plasma osmotic pressure level pulmonary oedema will follow. If it is held at this level chronically, pulmonary vascular contraction occurs, elevating pulmonary artery pressure further; this then may lead to organic vaso-occlusion, elevating the pulmonary artery

114

pressure still further. Alternatively, primary vascular disease in the pulmonary artery bed may cause the pulmonary vascular resistance; this may be seen with congenital heart disease.

At birth and shortly afterwards the pulmonary artery and aortic pressures are equal and the ductus arteriosus is patent. When the lungs expand, the pulmonary artery pressure is reduced over a few days while the pulmonary vascular resistance regresses to normal values. As these changes are occurring the pulmonary artery involutes to adult type and the pulmonary artery pressure becomes normal. If involution does not take place and congenital heart disease is not present, primary pulmonary hypertension is established. In some patients with left-to-right shunts, such as a ventricular septal defect, involution does not take place and pulmonary hypertension becomes established early. Medial hypertrophy with intimal proliferation may progress rapidly and this will lead to progressive pulmonary arterial hypertension; the pulmonary artery and aortic pressures may become equalized or even reversed (Eisenmenger reaction). In this situation acyanotic patients become cyanotic.

Radiological appearances

HYPERDYNAMIC OR HYPERKINETIC PULMONARY HYPERTENSION

On the postero-anterior chest film dilatation of the main pulmonary artery, the right and left branches and the branches throughout the lungs can be seen. The main pulmonary artery and the right and left branches at the hila are seen to pulsate vigorously on screening, especially if a left-to-right shunt is present. The degree of dilatation is proportional to the size of the shunt: the smaller the shunt the less the dilatation and vice versa. The heart will be enlarged if the shunt is great; the chambers which are enlarged are on the right side unless the primary lesion is a patent ductus arteriosus. In patients with only small left-to-right shunts, the heart size, shape and the appearances of the pulmonary arteries may be normal.

VASOCONSTRICTIVE HYPERTENSION

Patients with large left-to-right shunts may eventually develop vasoconstrictive pulmonary hypertension. This is due to persistent fetal-type vasculature or to secondary changes of medial and intimal thickening. The high peripheral vascular resistance is visible on the postero-anterior view of the chest. The pulmonary arteries are dilated centrally but the peripheral pulmonary arteries are either normal in size or contracted throughout the lung fields. There is thus a discrepancy in size between the central and peripheral pulmonary arteries, an appearance described by some as 'pruning' of the peripheral arteries (*Figure 4.9*). Affected patients are likely to have reversed shunts and to be cyanosed. These changes are most frequently seen with ventricular septal defects; they are also fairly frequent in patent ductus arteriosus but are infrequent in patients with atrial septal defects. The changes are well shown on pulmonary arteriography (*Figure 4.9b*) but it must be appreciated that such patients are poor risks for angiocardiography.

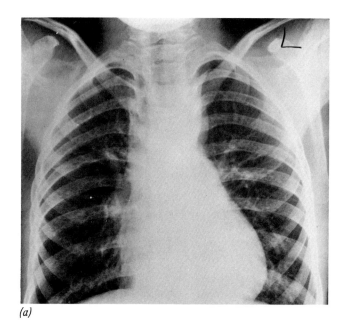

(a)

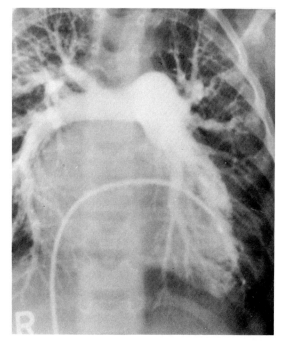

(b)

Figure 4.9. Pulmonary Arterial Hypertension: (c) Plain film in which the peripheral branches of the pulmonary arteries are disproportionately narrowed compared with the central branches. (b) Angiocardiogram in a similar case demonstrating the narrowing of the peripheral branches of the pulmonary artery compared with the widened central branches

PULMONARY HYPERTENSION IN ACQUIRED HEART
DISEASE

Pulmonary arterial hypertension

With left heart failure or mitral valve disease pulmonary
arterial hypertension develops as a result of pulmonary
venous hypertension. The pulmonary arterial hypertension is vasoconstrictive in type. At first, the constriction
is due to arteriolar spasm but organic occlusive changes
occur later in the pulmonary arterioles.

As the pressure begins to rise, the main pulmonary
artery and its central branches dilate but the peripheral
pulmonary arteries remain of normal calibre. When the
pulmonary artery pressure, in response to the raised
venous pressure, rises further there is constriction of the
peripheral pulmonary arteries in the dependent part of
the lungs. If the patient is old enough and well enough
to stand up these constrictive changes occur in the
lower zones and are usually easily visible. If the patient,
such as a young child, remains supine the constriction is
posterior and is not seen on the supine anteroposterior
film.

Pulmonary venous hypertension

Slight elevation of the pulmonary venous pressure causes
no radiological changes in the lung fields but as the
pressure rises the veins dilate. The degree of dilatation
correlates with the degree of elevation of the pulmonary
venous pressure. The dilatation is most marked in the
upper and middle zones, the lower lobe veins remaining
normal. If the patient is supine this differential is not
seen.

The appearances in the lung parenchyma are those of
pulmonary oedema. This leads to excess fluid in the
lymphatics and interstitial spaces and the passage of
fluid into the alveoli. As the venous pressure rises, fluid
accumulating in the extravascular tissues is first taken
up by the lymphatics. If they are overloaded the fluid
passes into the supporting tissues and intra-alveolar
spaces. When the pulmonary venous pressure is
chronically raised interstitial pulmonary oedema is
commoner than intra-alveolar oedema. In patients with
acute heart failure, intra-alveolar pulmonary oedema is
commoner than interstitial oedema because the pulmonary lymphatics and interstitial tissues become over-
whelmed with fluid.

The radiological changes of interstitial pulmonary
oedema are:

(1) Kerley's 'B' lines: These are linear shadows, up
to two centimetres long, seen at the edges of the lung
perpendicular to and continuous with the pleural surface.
They are due to oedematous interlobular septa and
dilated lymphatics within the septa.

(2) Kerley's 'A' lines: These are long septal lines
extending from the periphery towards the hila. They are
thin straight lines and are due to distended septa and
deep-draining lymphatics. They are usually visible in the
lower and mid zones.

(3) Perihilar haze, due to fluid in the interstitial
spaces around the hila, and in the peribronchial and
perivascular spaces extends out from the the hila towards
the periphery of the lung.

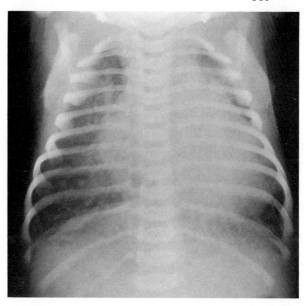

*Figure 4.10. Left Heart Failure and Pulmonary Venous Hyper-
tension: Anteroposterior chest film taken supine showing
cardiac enlargement involving predominantly the right atrium
and right ventricle. The pulmonary veins are dilated and there
are ill-defined shadows in the perihilar part of the lung fields,
due to intra-alveolar pulmonary oedema. The periphery of the
lung fields remains translucent*

(4) Peribronchial and perivascular cuffing; due to
oedema in the soft tissues around the bronchi and
pulmonary vessels. This produces thickening of their
walls and their radiological outline becomes blurred.

Intra-alveolar pulmonary oedema appears as confluent shadows in the lungs, of no characteristic distribution, more or less uniform in density and with ill-
defined edges. It is variable in extent and may resolve
irregularly. Intra-alveolar oedema may be central in
situation, extending out from the hila but sparing the
periphery of the lungs. It is usually bilateral but it
can be unilateral and may even be segmental or lobar in
distribution (*Figure 4.10*). The oedema is gravity-
dependent, being more marked on the side on which
the patient is lying and can appear and disappear very
rapidly.

Pleural effusions may also develop in patients with
left-sided heart failure. They may be bilateral or unilateral and if unilateral they are more frequent on the
right side than the left.

Pulmonary hypertension resulting from diseases of the lungs

In pulmonary heart disease there are two main causes
for the development of pulmonary hypertension.

(1) Hypoxia leading to vasoconstriction of the small
arteries.

(2) Pulmonary disease obliterating the pulmonary
vascular bed.

On the plain chest film, in the presence of extensive
inflammatory changes in the lung, the vascular pattern
may be overshadowed by the lesion in the lung. The

signs of the raised pulmonary artery pressure are dilatation of the main pulmonary artery and its central branches. The peripheral pulmonary arteries are usually normal in calibre but they may be small. After the lesion in the lungs has resolved the vascular changes will regress. Associated with the signs of pulmonary hypertension there may be enlargement of the right ventricle; also the right atrium, the superior vena cava and azygos vein may be prominent, suggesting right heart failure.

Primary pulmonary hypertension

This disease is most common in young women over the age of 20 years but it has been described in children and very rarely in infants during the first year of life. The postero-anterior view of the chest may show some enlargement of the heart. There is hypertrophy of the right ventricle and dilatation of the main pulmonary artery and its branches at the hila. The peripheral pulmonary arteries throughout the lung are normal or small in size.

CONGENITAL HEART DISEASE

INTRODUCTION

The plain film in congenital heart disease is of great importance but, on the whole, it is of less value than in patients in whom the heart disease is acquired. It is also fair to say that the older the child, the more information that is likely to be obtained from the plain radiograph. This information can be enhanced by a knowledge of the clinical features of the patient, and of course, of the haemodynamic data. Undoubtedly there are some conditions in which the diagnosis can be made with considerable certainty from the plain radiograph, such as in pulmonary valvular stenosis in older children. In many cases however the diagnosis can only be placed within a group of pathological states, the final diagnosis being made by more complicated radiology and/or haemodynamic studies. In interpreting the radiological appearances in any individual patient with heart disease it is essential to know whether the patient is in clinical heart failure, has the clinical signs of pulmonary hypertension, is cyanosed or has had previous cardiac surgery. All these conditions may alter the radiological appearances of the underlying congenital heart abnormality.

Classification of congenital heart disease has proved to be very difficult as the number of differing classifications indicates. Radiology is concerned with the identification and description of abnormal anatomy and the classification used here is based on that of Strickland (1972). It must be borne in mind that a congenital abnormality may be single or complicated by the presence of one or more additional abnormalities, which may or may not be essential for survival of the child. The conditions will be described singly, but also where two different conditions commonly co-exist (such as tricuspid atresia and atrial septal defect) they will be described as a combined entity.

COMMUNICATIONS BETWEEN SYSTEMIC AND PULMONARY CIRCULATION

Patent foramen ovale

In about 80 per cent of infants the foramen ovale closes in early life (the first few weeks or months) but in some it remains patent (Kaplan, 1968). In this state, however, no shunt occurs because the valve has a flap on the left atrial side and the higher pressure in the left atrium compared with the right atrium keeps the valve closed. If the right atrial pressure rises above that of the left atrium, as may occur in pulmonary valvular stenosis or ventricular septal defects, the valve may open and allow a right-to-left shunt through the foramen ovale with the development of cyanosis. In this case the radiological appearances are those of the primary condition. The patent foramen ovale may, however, allow the catheter to pass from right to left atrium during cardiac catheterization even though no shunt is demonstrable.

Atrial septal defect

Atrial septal defects may be of two types. (1) Ostium secundum (including the sinus venosus type). (2) Endocardial cushion defects (including the ostium primum defect and common atrioventricular canal).

OSTIUM SECUNDUM TYPE

The defect is an abnormal opening in the atrial septum in the region of the fossa ovalis (Jordan and Scott, 1973). It varies in size from a few millimetres to more than two centimetres in diameter. More than one defect may be present. The defect may extend inferiorly to involve the mouth of the inferior vena cava or superiorly to the superior vena cava or even posteriorly. The defect is usually an isolated abnormality; associated lesions occur in less than 10 per cent of cases and these include anomalous pulmonary venous drainage and pulmonary stenosis. In uncomplicated atrial septal defect, the primary shunt is from the left to the right atrium because the right atrium is more distensible and the right ventricle is less resistant to filling than the left ventricle (Bahnson and Williams, 1957). In small shunts the heart chambers are normal in size; in large shunts the right atrium and right ventricle are dilated, together with the main pulmonary artery and its branches. The left atrium and ventricle are usually normal in size but the aorta is small. The development of pulmonary hypertension is rare in children with atrial septal defect (Besterman, 1961).

Plain film

The heart is usually increased in its transverse diameter. Enlargement of the right atrium and the right ventricle and dilatation of the pulmonary arteries can be identified (*Figure 4.11*). On screening a typical 'hilar' dance can be shown. The diagnosis can usually be made on clinical grounds with plain radiography, but before surgery is performed it should be confirmed by cardiac catheterization.

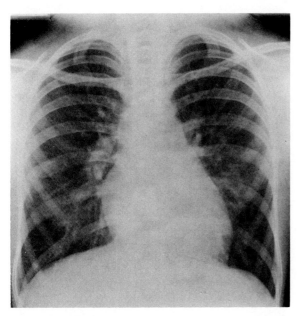

Figure 4.11. Atrial Septal Defect–Secundum Type: Plain film of the chest showing a heart with a normal transverse diameter. However, both lateral borders are convex due to enlargement of the right atrium and right ventricle. The central pulmonary arteries are enlarged but the aorta is relatively small

Cardiac catheterization

High oxygen saturation is obtained on sampling the blood from the right atrium. In addition the catheter may pass through the defect in the atrial septum and enter the left atrium, the pulmonary veins and the left ventricle.

Angiocardiography

Angiocardiography is usually unnecessary but an injection of contrast medium into the left atrium shows a shunt from left to right into the right atrium. An injection of contrast medium into the left ventricle shows that is outline is normal and thus excludes a primum type of atrial septal defect.

SINUS VENOSUS TYPE

In this condition the atrial septal defect is high in the septum, near the junction of the superior vena cava and right atrium, and in addition the right upper and middle lobe pulmonary veins (and sometimes all the veins from the right lung) drain into the superior vena cava above the defect. The superior vena cava in some patients overrides the defect so that some superior vena caval blood flows directly into the left atrium. (Gasul *et al.*, 1966).

Plain film

The radiological appearances are similar to those described under the secundum type of atrial septal defect, but the dilatation of the main pulmonary artery and its branches is usually less. In addition the upper part of the superior vena caval shadow may be absent or inconspicuous and a localized bulge may be seen at its lower end into which the pulmonary veins drain. There may also be recognizable increase in the vascularity of the upper zone of the right lung due to the anomalous veins crossing the pulmonary arteries to reach the lower part of the superior vena cava. Tomography may show the azygos vein in a higher position than normal and the anomalous veins entering the lower part of the superior vena cava.

Cardiac catheterization

Sampling in the lower part of the superior vena cava and in the right atrium will show increase in the oxygen saturation above that in the innominate veins or upper part of the superior vena cava. The catheter may pass from the superior vena cava into the right upper lobe veins (*see Figure 4.12b*).

Angiocardiography

Angiocardiography is usually unnecessary. However, an injection of contrast medium made into the lower part of the superior vena cava may fill the anomalous pulmonary veins retrogradely and prove their entry into the superior vena cava.

ENDOCARDIAL CUSHION DEFECTS

These are a spectrum of conditions which consist of a defect of the atrial septum associated with abnormal development of one or both atrioventricular valves. The commonest of these conditions is the primum type of atrial septal defect and the severest is a common atrioventricular canal in which there is complete failure of development of the endocardial cushions.

Ostium primum type

In this condition the defect is in .the lower part of the interatrial septum and it may extend down to involve the mitral and tricuspid valves. The anterior leaflet of the mitral valve is cleft to a varying extent. The tricuspid valve is usually normal but its septal cusp may be thickened and cleft. The interventricular septum is usually functionally intact, but its proximal part is always deficient. (Al Omeri *et al.*, 1965). As a result of the abnormalities of the valves there may be additional mitral and tricuspid regurgitation of varying degree in addition to the left-to-right interatrial shunt. Heart block may also occur.

Plain film

If heart block is absent and valve regurgitation minimal the plain film appearances are essentially the same as in the secundum type of atrial septal defect but the heart may be larger. If valve regurgitation is present, the

118

appearances depend on the valve involved and the severity of the regurgitation. Tricuspid regurgitation will lead to further increase in the size of the right atrium and right ventricle and mitral regurgitation to enlargement of the left ventricle; there is seldom much left atrial enlargement because the regurgitated blood rapidly shunts into the right atrium. Later pulmonary hypertension may develop and also left heart failure.

Angiocardiography

Angiocardiography performed with the catheter tip in the left ventricle will reveal the mitral regurgitation and the appearances of the outflow tract, described below. If the injection of contrast medium is made into the right ventricle, tricuspid regurgitation will be shown if it is present.

Common atrioventricular canal

This abnormality consists of an atrial septal defect, a ventricular septal defect and a complex common atrioventricular valve; there is communication between all four chambers with a predominant left-to-right shunt at atrial and ventricular levels. The common atrioventricular valve consists of anterior and posterior cusps at each ventricular end. Several associated valve deformities may be present. The anterior cusp is usually cleft to a varying extent; the lateral parts of this cusp are attached by chordae tendineae to an anterior papillary muscle in

each ventricle. The medial parts are attached by chordae to the adjacent interventricular septum or more commonly to the right side of the septum. This results in elongation and narrowing of the outflow tract of the left ventricle and produces a 'goose-neck' deformity of this region in the left ventricular angiocardiogram. The posterior cusp is irregular with thickened edges and is attached by normal chordae tendineae to the posterior papillary muscle of the left ventricle. On the right side it is attached either to the right side of the interventricular septum or to papillary muscles in the right ventricle. Interventricular communication occurs between the two cusps and between the chordal attachments to the septum. There are several variants of the above malformation (Rastelli *et al.*, 1966), and it may also be associated with additional deformities such as patent ductus arteriosus or pulmonary stenosis. The abnormality leads to left-to-right interatrial and interventricular shunting of blood, and also to regurgitation through the atrioventricular valve from the ventricles into the atria, especially into the right atrium. Pulmonary hypertension is frequent and is due to high pulmonary vascular resistance.

Plain film

The plain x-ray film appearances are similar to those of the primum type of atrial septal defect, with considerable cardiomegaly and dilated pulmonary arteries. The definitive diagnosis is made by left ventricular angiocardiography.

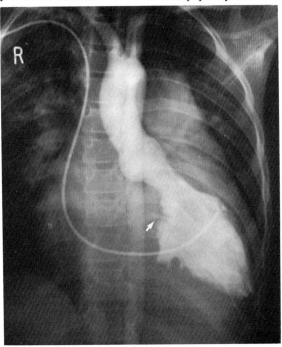

(a)

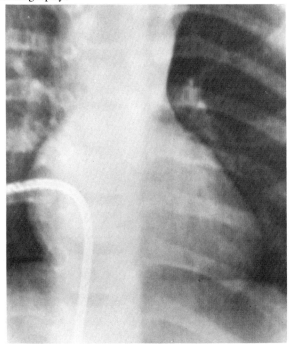

(b)

Figure 4.12. Atrial Septal Defect—Primum type: (a) Angiocardiogram in which contrast medium has been injected into the left ventricle. The outflow tract of this ventricle is elongated and concave inferiorly. This constitutes the 'goose-neck' deformity and is due to the abnormally low position of the mitral valve. The right border of the ventricle is serrated and a small jet of contrast medium (arrowed) demonstrates regurgitation into the left atrium through a cleft in the anterior cusp. (b) Film taken during cardiac catheterization. The catheter has entered an abnormal pulmonary vein draining into the superior vena cava

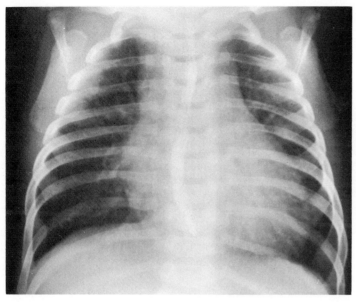

(a)

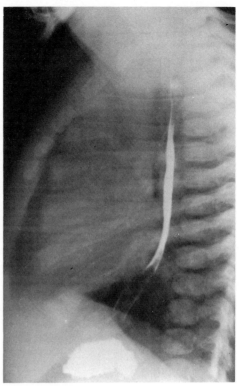

(b)

Figure 4.13. Ventricular Septal Defect: Plain films of the chest showing enlargement of both ventricles. Left atrial enlargement is demonstrated by the displacement of the barium-filled oesophagus to the right and backwards. The central branches of the pulmonary artery are increased in size due to pulmonary plethora. (a) Anteroposterior projection. (b) Lateral projection

Left ventricular angiocardiography The abnormality of the anterior cusp of the mitral valve causes a characteristic deformity of the outflow tract of the left ventricle. The right border of the outflow tract and the region of the upper part of the septum are serrated in outline with a linear defect near the middle of this serrated edge (*Figure 4.12*). The upper portion of this border bulges into the outflow tract and it produces an elongated narrowed channel, more horizontal than normal, an appearance described as a goose-neck deformity (Baron *et al.*, 1964). Mitral regurgitation through the defect in the anterior cusp may be shown as a jet of contrast medium from the region of the linear defect on the right border of the ventricle. In the lateral projection, irregularity of the upper part of the anterior border of the left ventricle and shunting of contrast medium forwards into the right ventricle may be seen. Contrast medium may also pass back into the left atrium.

Ventricular septal defect

Isolated ventricular septal defect is probably the most common congenital heart abnormality, being present in about 20 per cent of patients with congenital heart disease (Keith *et al.*, 1967). The defect occurs most frequently in the membranous septum. On the left ventricular side this is in the subaortic valvular region and on the right ventricular side, just below the crista supraventricularis. The remaining defects are seen either above the crista supraventricularis or in the muscular septum. The defect is usually single but there may be multiple defects. The defect may be small, about 3 to 5 millimetres in diameter, or so large that there is almost complete absence of the interventricular septum. The shunt in uncomplicated cases is from left to right; its degree depends on the size of the defect and the resistance of the pulmonary circulation. When pulmonary hypertension develops the shunt may reverse, leading to cyanosis. Small defects are considered to be those less than 0.5 centimetre in diameter and large defects those over 1.0 centimetre in diameter.

Plain film

The radiological appearances depend on the size of the defect and on the pulmonary resistance. A small defect causes no alteration in the appearances of the normal cardiovascular shadow. In large defects there is enlargement of the left ventricle, right ventricle, pulmonary arteries and left atrium and the aorta is small (*Figure 4.13*). When the pulmonary resistance is elevated, there is further dilatation of the central pulmonary arteries and the peripheral pulmonary arteries may be contracted in all zones of the lungs (*see page 114*).

Cardiac catheterization

The catheter will take the normal course from right atrium to pulmonary artery but occasionally it will cross through the ventricular septal defect from right-to-left ventricle. On blood sampling the left-to-right shunt will be identified entering the right ventricle.

Angiocardiography

In cases of ventricular septal defect coming to cardiac catheterization right ventricular angiocardiography

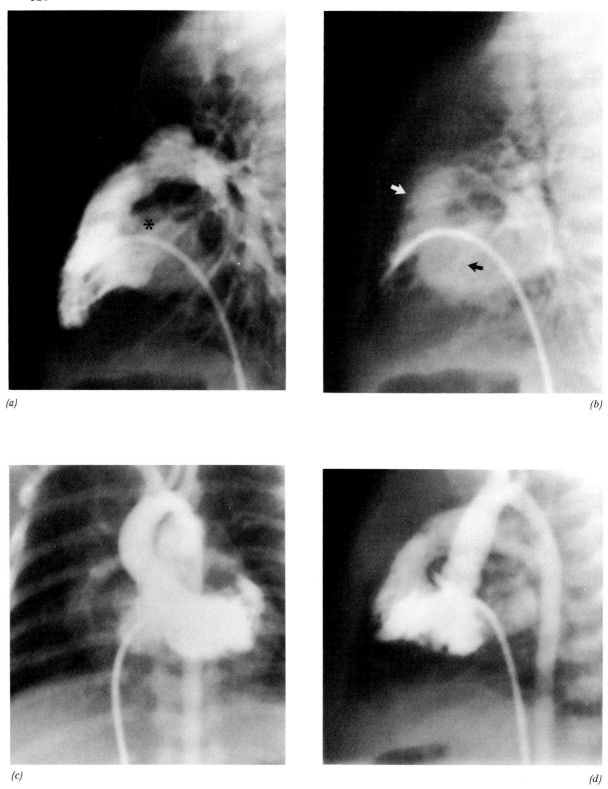

Figure 4.14. Ventricular Septal Defect: (a) Right ventricular angiocardiogram in the lateral projection taken 1 second after injection. Contrast medium has passed backwards through the ventricular septal defect into the left ventricle (*). (b) Film of the same case taken 1 second later. The outflow tract of the right ventricle (white arrow) has refilled with contrast medium passing through the septal defect from the left ventricle (black arrow). (c) Left ventricular angiocardiogram in the anteroposterior projection. Contrast medium has passed from the left ventricle both into the ascending aorta and through the septal defect into the right ventricle and pulmonary artery. (d) Lateral projection of the same case

should be performed in order to confirm the diagnosis, and particularly to exclude corrected transposition of the great arteries, double outlet right ventricle or single ventricle. It is most important to exclude the presence of any of these possible alternative diagnoses if surgery is contemplated. Right ventricular angiocardiography will show several features: enlargement of the right ventricle and normal origin of the pulmonary artery and aorta; large pulmonary arteries centrally and peripherally in the lungs; momentary shunting of contrast medium from the right ventricle through the defect into the left ventricle during an extrasystole and also a large left atrium and left ventricle (*Figure 4.14a* and *d*). Early in the examination, there may be dilution of the contrast medium in the outflow tract of the right ventricle, produced by non-opaque blood entering through the ventricular septal defect from the left ventricle. In the latter stages of the examination, contrast medium from the left ventricle will pass forwards through the ventricular septal defect into the outflow tract of the right ventricle and pulmonary artery, producing refilling of these regions (*Figure 4.14b*). If pulmonary hypertension with reversal of the shunt has developed, right ventricular angiocardiography will show filling of the left ventricle and aorta through the defect in the interventricular septum. If the catheter passes through the foramen ovale into the left atrium and left ventricle, left ventricular angiocardiography may be performed. This will show rapid shunting of the contrast medium forwards from the left ventricle to the right ventricle, through the ventricular septal defect (*Figure 4.14c* and *d*).

Rarely the ventricular septal defect is so large that the interventricular septum is absent or nearly completely absent so that effectively a single or undivided ventricle is present. This condition is frequently associated with transposition of the great arteries on angiocardiography, injection of the contrast medium into the expected site of the right ventricle will show a single rather rounded ventricle and no evidence of an interventricular septum. If the great arteries arising from the ventricle are transposed, this will also be demonstrated (*Figure 4.15*).

VENTRICULAR SEPTAL DEFECT WITH AORTIC REGURGITATION

Rarely a ventricular septal defect is associated with prolapse of one of the aortic valve cusps, usually the right coronary cusp, which superimposes aortic regurgitation onto the left-to-right shunt through the ventricular septal defect. If the aortic regurgitation is small, the radiological appearances of the heart are those of uncomplicated ventricular septal defect. If the regurgitation is marked, there is disproportionate enlargement of the left ventricle. The aortic regurgitation can be shown by retrograde aortography.

VENTRICULAR SEPTAL DEFECT–GERBODE TYPE

In this condition the abnormality is a defect in the membranous interventricular septum posterior to and

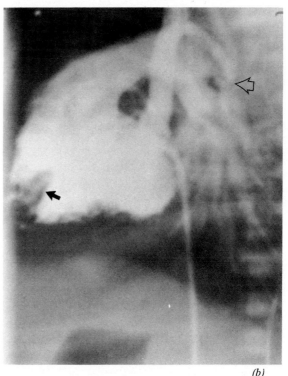

(a)

(b)

Figure 4.15. Single Ventricle: Angiocardiogram with the contrast medium injected from the expected site of the right ventricle. The large common ventricle is opacified and from this the contrast medium passes to normally sited pulmonary artery and aorta. Only a small interventricular septum is present (black arrow). There is also a coarctation of the aorta (white arrow). (a) Anteroposterior projection. (b) Lateral projection

above the attachment of the septal cusp of the tricuspid valve, or the defect may involve the tricuspid valve and adjacent part of the muscular septum. The typical shunt is from left ventricle to right atrium (Gerbode *et al.*, 1958) but there may also be a shunt from left to right ventricle.

Plain film

On the postero-anterior view, enlargement of the right atrium is usually visible as increased rounding of the right heart border. There will also be enlargement of the right ventricle, left atrium and pulmonary arteries. The aorta is small.

Cardiac catheterization

High oxygenated blood is obtained from the right atrium. The catheter does not usually pass across the defect.

Angiocardiography

The injection of contrast medium must be made into the left ventricle. This will show enlargement of the left ventricle and a normal origin of the aorta. Very rapid and intense filling of the enlarged right atrium occurs. There will also be some filling of the right ventricle through the defect in the upper part of the interventricular septum (*Figure 4.16*).

PATENT DUCTUS ARTERIOSUS

This is a common condition. The ductus arteriosus arises in the region of the origin of the left pulmonary artery and it passes to the inferior aspect of the aorta just distal to the origin of the left subclavian artery. At the site of entry of the ductus the aorta frequently shows a localized bulge on its inferior border and it may also be kinked forwards at this level. The ductus may be funnel shaped, being wider at the aortic end. It varies in width from 2 centimetres to a few millimetres. The ductus may be a centimetre or so in length or it may be so short that the pulmonary artery opens directly into the descending part of the arch of the aorta. If the aorta is right-sided the ductus may enter the right pulmonary artery or pass from the left subclavian artery to the left pulmonary artery. The ductus normally is functionally closed about 20 hours after birth (Moss *et al.*, 1963), and it is permanently occluded in 4 weeks' time in most infants (Mitchell, 1957). It may persist in patients with low oxygen tension and in the children of mothers who have

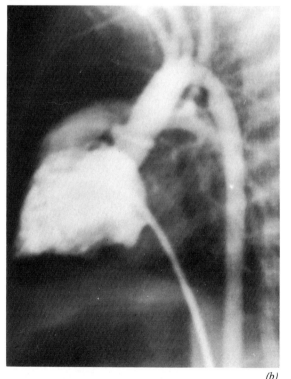

(a)

(b)

Figure 4.16. Ventricular Septal Defect—Gerbode type: Left ventricular angiocardiogram. Contrast medium passes into the ascending aorta and into the right atrium (arrowed), the right ventricle (*) and pulmonary artery; the left ventricle is enlarged. (a) Anteroposterior projection. (b) Lateral projection

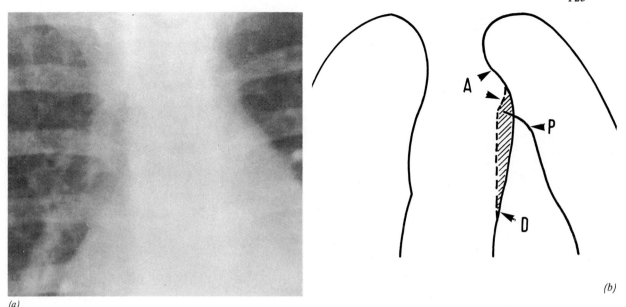

(a)

(b)

Figure 4.17. Patent Ductus Arteriosus (Jönsson's sign): (a) Plain film. (b) Line diagram. The outline of the left border of the aorta, from the aortic arch (A) to the descending aorta (D), forms a continuous convex line. The normal concavity differentiating the aortic 'knuckle' from the descending aorta is obliterated by the infundibulum of the ductus arteriosus. The latter is overlapped by the enlarged pulmonary artery (P)

had German measles in the first trimester of pregnancy (Pitt, 1957), or for no known reason.

If the ductus arteriosus remains open, blood will be shunted from aorta to pulmonary artery because after birth the pressure in the pulmonary artery is lower than that in the aorta. If large enough, this shunt will cause hyperkinetic pulmonary hypertension in the presence of normal peripheral pulmonary resistance. The pulmonary arteries, the left atrium, left ventricle and the ascending aorta and arch of the aorta have to cope with the additional flow. In less than 10 per cent of patients (Cleland et al., 1969) the peripheral resistance will remain significantly elevated after birth and this will lead to the production of pulmonary hypertension. In a very small number (2 per cent, Wood, 1956) the peripheral resistance is very high and the pulmonary artery pressure then may equal that in the aorta (Eisenmenger syndrome). Intermittent reversal of the shunt will, therefore, occur. Obviously the size of the ductus is important in determining the degree of shunting of blood: a small ductus produces little shunting and therefore these patients are unlikely to develop pulmonary hypertension. If the ductus is large it may produce a torrential shunt which can overload the pulmonary circulation and lead to death of the patient with heart failure and pulmonary oedema. More commonly the peripheral pulmonary resistance increases rapidly due to medial hypertrophy of the small arteries and this protects the lungs from oedema but leads to established pulmonary hypertension. Apart from pulmonary hypertension with reversal of the shunt and heart failure, various complications may supervene such as bacterial endocarditis, calcification and aneurysm formation. Finally, patent ductus arteriosus may occur in combination with other congenital heart lesions, for example, with ventricular septal defect; in some of these conditions its presence may be essential to the preservation of life, such as in aortic atresia.

Plain film

The radiological features of patent ductus arteriosus depend on the size of the shunt between aorta and pulmonary circulation, the degree of pulmonary hypertension, the age of the patient and the presence of any concomitant congenital heart lesions. If the shunt is small the appearances on the radiograph will be normal. If the shunt is large there will be enlargement of the left ventricle with increased rounding of the left heart border, downward displacement of the apex of the heart and increase in the transverse diameter of the heart (*Figure 4.18a*). The left atrium is enlarged and produces backward displacement of the oesophagus on barium swallow. The main pulmonary artery and its branches at the hila are dilated and pulsatile and the lungs are pleonaemic. The right ventricle will be enlarged if pulmonary hypertension is present.

The striking feature of a patent ductus arteriosus in older children is the enlargement of the aorta, particularly the arch; it is best seen on the postero-anterior film as enlargement of the aortic knuckle and is well shown on fluoroscopy with barium swallow. In a young infant enlargement of the aorta may not have developed or it may be difficult to recognize since it lies deep in the normally rather wide mediastinum.

In older children and adults a sign described by Jönsson and Saltzman (1952) may be seen. This consists of a bulge, due to the infundibulum of the ductus, shown on the left border of the aorta on the postero-anterior view and the bulge is overlapped by the dilated main pulmonary artery (*Figure 4.17*). This sign when present is reliable as evidence of the presence of patent ductus arteriosus. If pulmonary hypertension develops early in life, the aorta may remain small. In the presence of pulmonary hypertension, the peripheral pulmonary arteries will be narrowed in calibre and the central pulmonary arteries dilated. If a patent ductus is present

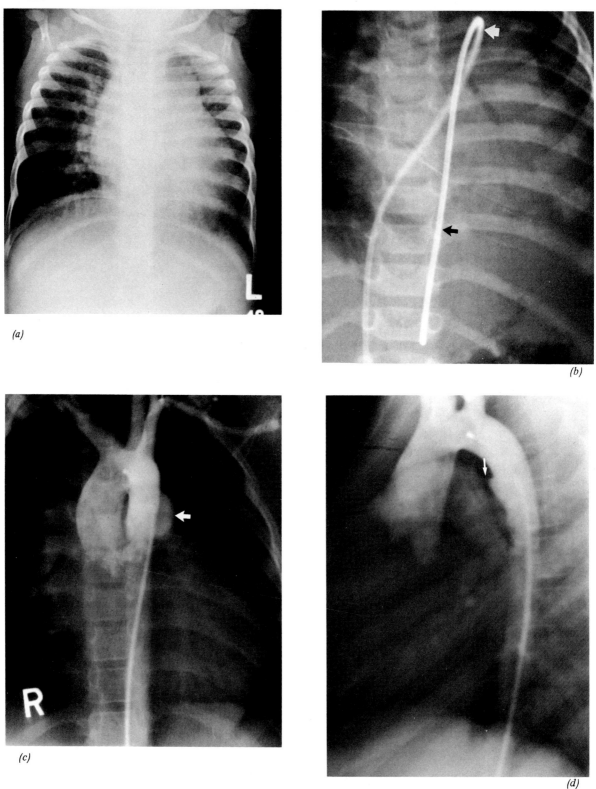

(a)

(b)

(c)

(d)

Figure 4.18 Patent Ductus Arteriosus: (a) Plain film showing an enlarged heart and dilated pulmonary arteries. The left ventricle and aorta are also increased in size. (b) A cardiac catheter is shown passing medially and backwards from the pulmonary artery through the patent ductus arteriosus (white arrow) into the descending aorta (black arrow). (c) Thoracic aortogram in the anteroposterior projection. Contrast medium is shown passing from the aorta to the pulmonary artery (arrowed). (d) Lateral projection of the same case; the contrast medium outlines the patent ductus arteriosus (arrowed)

in association with another congenital heart lesion, the radiological features will depend on the relative haemodynamic importance of the two lesions, e.g. a small patent ductus in association with a large ventricular septal defect will cause no alteration in the appearances on the radiography due to the ventricular septal defect but a large patent ductus with a small ventricular septal defect will increase the size of the shunt and therefore the size of the pulmonary arteries, left side of the heart, and the aorta compared with those expected from the ventricular septal defect alone.

Cardiac catheterization

On right heart catheterization, the aorto-pulmonary artery shunt will be identified by increased oxygen saturation in the pulmonary artery. The catheter may pass through the patent ductus arteriosus into the descending aorta (*Figure 4.18*), and its tip pass below the level of the diaphragm. Sometimes the catheter will pass upwards from the patent ductus into the aortic arch instead of going downwards. Once the catheter has passed into the ductus a small hand-injection of contrast medium will confirm the presence of the ductus by showing contrast medium passing down the aorta.

Right ventricular angiocardiography

On right ventricular angiocardiography, if the aorto-pulmonary shunt is from left to right there will be dilution of the contrast medium in the main pulmonary artery on diastole due to the non-opaque blood entering the pulmonary artery from the patent ductus arteriosus.

On aortography, with the catheter tip in the descending part of the aortic arch, the patent ductus arteriosus will be outlined precisely as the contrast medium enters the pulmonary artery (*Figure 4.18*). A closed ductus arteriosus is sometimes shown as a small diverticulum from the upper surface of the left pulmonary artery (*Figure 4.18*).

If the shunt is reversed from right to left there will be filling of the ductus arteriosus and descending aorta from the pulmonary artery on right ventricular angiocardiography.

Aorto-pulmonary septal defect

In this condition, which is rare, there is a communication between the ascending aorta just above the aortic valve and the main pulmonary artery through which a left-to-right shunt occurs (Neufeld *et al.*, 1962). The degree of shunting will depend on the size of the defect and the peripheral pulmonary resistance. The shunt is usually large.

Plain film

The plain film radiological appearances are similar to those of patent ductus arteriosus. However, the main pulmonary artery may be disproportionately large (*Figure 4.19a*). Also the ascending aorta may be larger than expected for the size of the arch.

Cardiac catheterization

On cardiac catheterization a shunt into the main pulmonary artery will be shown and the catheter will pass

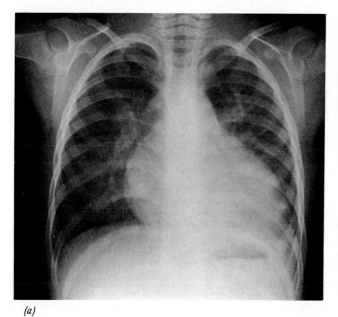

(a)

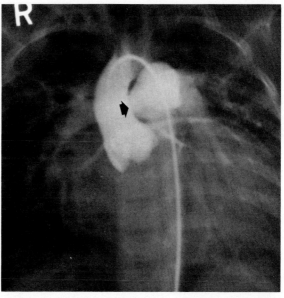

(b)

Figure 4.19. Aorto-pulmonary Septal Defect: (a) Plain film showing enlargement of the heart, mainly involving the left ventricle. There is also enlargement of the pulmonary artery and aorta with plethora of the lung fields. (b) A thoracic aortogram in which contrast medium injected into the ascending aorta passes directly through the aorto-pulmonary septal defect (arrowed) into the main pulmonary artery

anteriorly from the main pulmonary artery to the ascending aorta and thence posteriorly around the arch.

Retrograde aortography

Retrograde aortography with the catheter tip just above the aortic valve will show the shunt from the ascending aorta to the main pulmonary artery (*Figure 4.19b*). Right and left ventricular angiocardiography will show that the aorta and pulmonary artery arise normally from their respective ventricles.

Truncus arteriosus

In this condition the primitive truncus arteriosus fails to differentiate into aorta and pulmonary artery. A single large artery, the truncus arteriosus, over-rides the interventricular septum (Collett and Edwards, 1949; Bruins and Dekker, 1968), and arises from a large single valve which represents the combined aortic and pulmonary valves. The number of cusps lining this valve varies between two and six. Truncus arteriosus is usually associated with a ventricular septal defect or sometimes a single ventricle, and it carries all the blood leaving the heart. The truncus arteriosus supplies the systemic

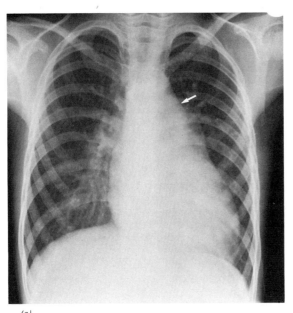

(a)

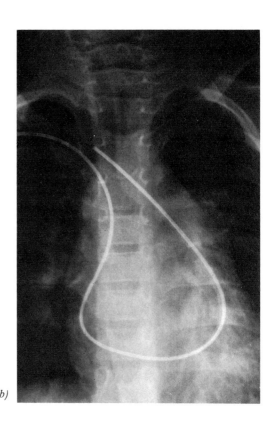

(b)

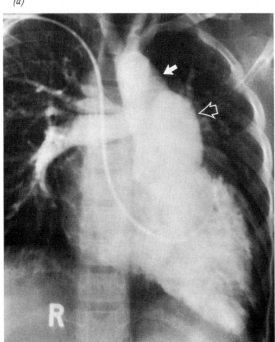

(c)

Figure 4.20. Truncus Arteriosus: (a) Plain film showing biventricular enlargement and a large left-sided 'aorta' (arrowed) due to the truncus which projects over the pulmonary artery whose main branches are both at the same level. (b) A film taken during cardiac catheterization. The catheter has been introduced into the right atrium and right ventricle whence it passes into the truncus arteriosus and innominate artery. (c) Angiocardiogram in the anteroposterior projection. Contrast medium has been injected into the right ventricle and the truncus arteriosus (solid arrow) is opacified. The pulmonary arteries (outline arrow) are shown to arise from the truncus by a common trunk. There is a stenosis of the artery supplying the right upper lobe (cont. on next page).

arteries, the pulmonary arteries and the coronary arteries. There are various forms of the malformation. Both pulmonary arteries may arise from the common trunk, either separately or through a main pulmonary arterial trunk communicating with the base of the truncus just above the valve. In other cases, no pulmonary arteries arise from the common trunk, the lungs being supplied by bronchial arteries.

Plain film

On the plain radiograph both ventricles are shown to be enlarged and the heart apex is usually elevated. As there is no main pulmonary artery at its normal site, the pulmonary artery segment frequently tends to be concave, giving a 'sitting-duck' appearance to the heart on the postero-anterior view. This appearance is commoner in younger patients. The truncus arteriosus appears as a large aorta and it is right-sided in 25 per cent of cases. The appearances of the hila and pulmonary arteries depend on the type and size of pulmonary arteries present (*Figure 4.20a*). The lungs may be normal in appearance or they may be pleonaemic or oligaemic. If they are oligaemic, they may have a spotted appearance due to bronchial artery supply, but they are most frequently pleonaemic. The left pulmonary artery may be seen at a level higher than normal and curves upwards and outwards into the lung field even as far up as the aortic arch.

Cardiac catheterization

The catheter will fail to pass from the right ventricle into the pulmonary artery. It will, however, enter the aorta easily from the right ventricle. Blood samples from the right ventricle will show increased oxygenation.

Right ventricular angiocardiography and retrograde aortography

Both of these examinations should be performed. Right ventricular angiocardiography will show the right and left ventricles communicating through a ventricular septal defect and the large truncus arteriosus arising by a single valve from both ventricles over the ventricular septal defect (*Figure 4.20*). If the lungs are supplied by bronchial arteries the condition cannot be distinguished from pseudotruncus (pulmonary atresia). When pulmonary arteries are present they will fill simultaneously with the aorta. Retrograde aortography, with the catheter tip just above the valve will show either the pulmonary arteries arising through a common trunk (*Figure 4.20*) or arising separately from the truncus. If a common pulmonary trunk is present the absence of a separate pulmonary valve distinguishes the condition from aorto-pulmonary septal defect.

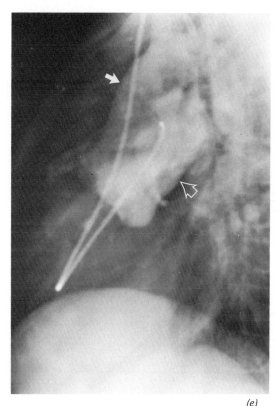

(d)   *(e)*

Figure 4.20 (cont.) (d) Lateral projection of the same case. The origin of the aorta (solid arrow) and pulmonary arteries (outline arrow) from the truncus arteriosus is again shown. The origin of the truncus lies over a defect in the upper part of the interventricular septum through which contrast medium fills part of the left ventricle. (e) Lateral projection in which the contrast medium has been injected from a catheter with its tip in the truncus arteriosus near the origin of the common pulmonary trunk. The aorta (solid arrow) and the pulmonary arteries (outline arrow) are both opacified but no separate pulmonary valve is shown

128

Ruptured sinus of Valsalva

Rupture of a sinus of Valsalva of the aorta is a very rare anomaly, seldom encountered in children. The affected sinus may be anaeurysmal and the rupture occurs sometime after birth into the right atrium, right ventricle or pulmonary artery. The anterior (right coronary) sinus is most frequently involved (Sakakibara and Konno, 1962). Aneurysms of the sinus of Valsalva may be acquired as a result of bacterial endocarditis. If the defect is small it will have few haemodynamic consequences. If the rupture of the anaeurysm is sudden, heart failure and death may rapidly ensue. If the patient survives, cardiac catheterization will detect the shunt into the right side of the heart and retrograde aortography, with the catheter tip just above the aortic valve, will show the shunt and site of rupture.

Coronary artery fistula

Fistulous communications between the coronary arteries and the right heart are very rare (Gasul, 1966). They may occur between the right coronary artery and the right ventricle (most common), left coronary artery and right ventricle, left coronary artery and coronary sinus and also between a single coronary artery and the right ventricle. Fistulas into the left atrium and left ventricle have been reported.

Plain film

On plain radiography the heart is usually normal in size and shape and the pulmonary vessels are normal. If the shunt is large the heart may be increased in size and the pulmonary arteries dilated.

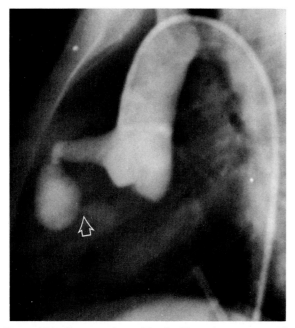

Figure 4.21. Coronary Artery Fistula: Thoracic aortogram. The origin of the right coronary artery is dilated and its distal portion is aneurysmal. There is a small fistula (arrow) between this latter part and the right ventricle

Cardiac catheterization

Cardiac catheterization shows the shunt into the right side of the heart.

Angiocardiography

Right ventricular angiocardiography excludes a ventricular septal defect. This is important in differential diagnosis. Thoracic aortography and coronary arteriography will show the dilated and tortuous coronary artery communicating with the right atrium, right ventricle or coronary sinus (*Figure 4.21*).

Anomalous origin of the left coronary artery from the pulmonary artery

Anomalous origin of the right coronary artery from the pulmonary artery is usually an incidental finding and not clinically significant. Anomalous origin of both coronary arteries from the pulmonary artery leads to death in a few weeks. These two conditions will not be discussed further.

Anomalous origin of the left coronary artery from the pulmonary artery is uncommon but clinically significant. The right coronary artery arises normally from the aorta but the left coronary artery arises from the pulmonary artery, the two being connected by intercoronary anastomoses. After birth the pressure in the main pulmonary artery falls and blood then flows from the right coronary artery through the intercoronary anastomoses to the left coronary artery and thence into the pulmonary artery, the adequacy of the circulation to the left ventricle depending on the size of the intercoronary anastomoses. The blood flow is retrograde down the left coronary artery (Sabiston *et al.*, 1960).

Plain film

The heart is usually grossly enlarged, the left ventricle and left atrium being particularly affected (*Figure 4.22*). On screening, the left ventricle may lack pulsations and it may alter its shape excessively with respiration. Signs of left heart failure may be present with dilated pulmonary arteries and Kerley's 'B' lines (*see* page 115 and *Figure 4.10*).

Cardiac catheterization

Cardiac catheterization should be conducted with caution as these patients are very liable to develop ventricular fibrillation. The shunt into the pulmonary artery may be detected. Pulmonary hypertension is seldom encountered.

Thoracic aortography

Thoracic aortography is the method of choice for

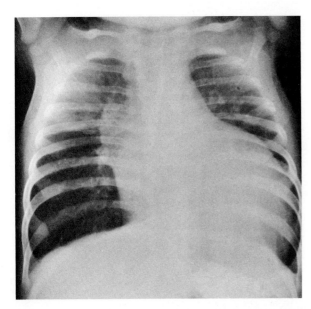

Figure 4.22. *Anomalous Origin of the Left Coronary Artery from the Pulmonary Artery: Plain film showing marked enlargement of the left ventricle consequent upon the myocardial ischaemia. Both lower lobes are hyperinflated*

demonstrating the abnormality by contrast medium injection. The catheter tip is placed just above the aortic valve. This examination will show the dilated right coronary artery filling early. There is absence of immediate filling of the left coronary artery but in the late stages the left coronary artery will fill retrogradely and contrast medium will pass through it to enter the main pulmonary artery.

OBSTRUCTION AND REGURGITATION

Aortic stenosis

Obstruction to the outlet from the left ventricle may occur at valvular level, supravalvular level or subvalvular level, the first being the most common. The last may be due to a diaphragm crossing the subvalvular region or to thickening of the wall of the outflow tract, as seen in hypertrophic obstructive cardiomyopathy.

AORTIC VALVULAR STENOSIS

The basic abnormality is a bicuspid valve with thickening of the valve tissue and varying degrees of commissural fusion (Braunwald *et al.*, 1963) (*Figure 4.23*). In infants and young children the valve ring may be underdeveloped. Calcification may occur in later life. If the obstruction is significant, hypertrophy of the left ventricle occurs and there is dilatation of the ascending aorta above the valve (post-stenotic dilatation).

Plain film

The heart size is usually normal. If left ventricular hypertrophy is present there may be rounding of the lower

part of the left heart border, together with downward and backward displacement of the apex. The ascending aorta may be dilated. Cardiac pulsations are usually normal. Left heart failure may supervene.

Cardiac catheterization

Right-sided catheterization excludes associated anomalies such as ventricular septal defect and patent ductus arteriosus.

On left-sided catheterization through the femoral artery, if the catheter will pass across the aortic valve, a pressure gradient across the valve between the left ventricle and aorta will be shown. If the catheter will not pass across the aortic valve, the trans-septal route may be used, in order to pass another catheter through the left atrium and mitral valve to record the pressure in the left ventricle.

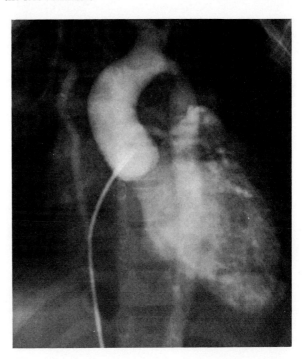

Figure 4.23. *Bicuspid Aortic Valve: The aortic valve is shown to be bicuspid. There is also a coarctation of the aorta*

Left ventricular angiocardiography

If the catheter will cross the aortic valve from the ascending aorta, left ventricular angiocardiography can be performed. If it fails to cross the valve a trans-septal approach to the left ventricle can be used for this purpose. The valve cusps may be normal in thickness or thickened (*Figure 4.24*) and the valve will be dome-shaped or restricted in movement, with a central or eccentric jet of contrast medium passing from the valve orifice into the ascending aorta, which is dilated. The left ventricular wall is thickened and the valve ring may be small. However, if the catheter should fail to enter the left ventricle, retrograde aortography, with the contrast medium injected just above the valve, will outline the aortic surface of the valve and demonstrate any regurgitation through it.

130

SUBVALVULAR AORTIC STENOSIS

This abnormality is less common than valvular stenosis. The condition consists of a membranous diaphragm or fibrous ridge encircling the outflow tract of the left ventricle about 1.0 centimetre proximal to the valve, the latter being normal.

Plain film

The plain film appearances are the same as for valvular stenosis with the important exception that post-stenotic dilatation of the aorta is infrequent (Champsaur *et al.*, 1973).

Cardiac catheterization

A catheter inserted from the aorta into the left ventricle shows a pressure gradient below the aortic valve across the outflow tract.

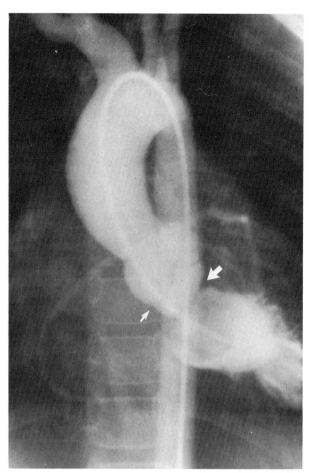

Figure 4.25. Subvalvular Aortic Stenosis: Left ventricular angiocardiogram. The left ventricle is hypertrophied. There is a short-segment eccentric narrowing (large arrow) of the outflow tract about 1 cm below the normal aortic valve (small arrow); the ascending aorta is dilated

Left ventricular angiocardiography

Left ventricular angiocardiography may show a thin linear translucency in the contrast medium in the outflow tract produced by the diaphragm or fibrous ridge (*Figure 4.25*). This encircles the outflow tract wholly or in part about 1 centimetre proximal to the normal aortic valve. It is, however, possible for the diaphragm to be so orientated that it is never parallel to the central x-ray beam and therefore it will not be shown in either plane. Cineradiography performed after localized injection of contrast medium into the left ventricular outflow tract will almost invariably show the lesion.

IDIOPATHIC HYPERTROPHIC SUB-AORTIC STENOSIS (HYPERTROPHIC OBSTRUCTIVE CARDIOMYOPATHY)

In this condition there is marked hypertrophy of the wall of the left ventricle and especially the interventricular septal part of the left ventricular outflow tract (Goodwin *et al.*, 1960). The hypertrophy is usually asymmetric but it may be diffuse and it causes

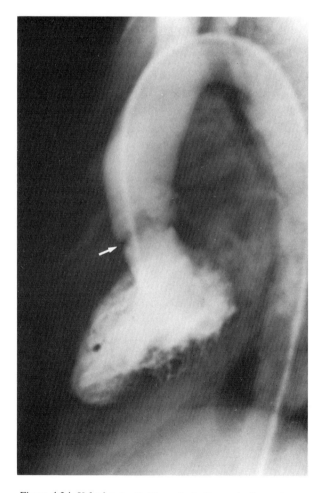

Figure 4.24. Valvular Aortic Stenosis: Left ventricular angiogram in lateral projection. The thickened, irregular and rigid aortic valve (arrowed) is clearly shown

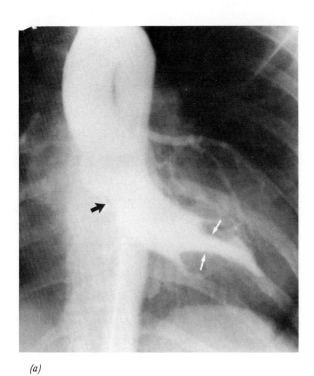
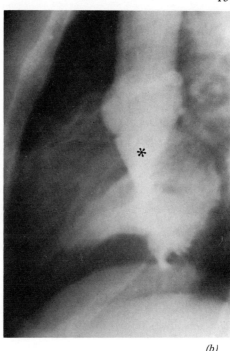

(a)

(b)

Figure 4.26. Obstructive Hypertrophic Cardiomyopathy: Contrast medium has been injected into the left ventricle from a catheter which has been passed retrogradely through the aortic valve. (a) Anteroposterior projection showing narrowing of the cavity of the left ventricle by muscle bundles (white arrows) projecting into it below the level of the aortic valve (black arrow). (b) Lateral projection in which the cone-shaped outflow tract of the left ventricle (*) is shown

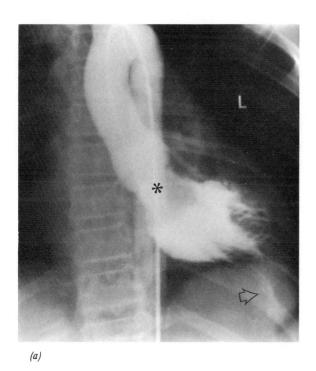
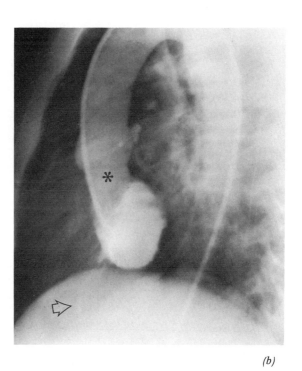

(a)

(b)

Figure 4.27. Non-obstructive Hypertrophic Cardiomyopathy: Left ventricular angiocardiogram: films taken in systole, showing the distal part of the left ventricular cavity (arrowed) almost completely obliterated by the hypertrophic muscle. In this type however the outflow tract (*) remains widely open. (a) Anteroposterior projection (b) Lateral projection

concentric narrowing of the outflow tract. The obstruction is due to protrusion of a nodular mass of hypertrophied septum into the outflow tract during systole. This part of the septum may bulge into and narrow the right ventricular outflow tract. The left ventricular papillary muscles are also hypertrophied. They may contract early in systole, drawing the mitral valve cusps forward and causing mitral regurgitation (Goodwin and Oakley, 1972).

Plain film

The appearances are the same as those of aortic valvular stenosis except that there is no dilatation of the ascending aorta. Some patients also show right ventricular enlargement.

Cardiac catheterization

On left heart catheterization a pressure gradient is shown across the subvalvular region of the left ventricle and during the examination the magnitude of the gradient may vary considerably. It may be intensified by administration of isoprenaline.

Left ventricular angiocardiography

The wall of the left ventricle is usually thickened and the ventricular cavity is irregularly narrowed and reduced in capacity. There are filling defects in its margin produced by the irregular muscle bundles (*Figure 4.26*). These appearances are especially marked in systole. The outflow tract is narrowed by a mass of hypertrophied muscle in the upper part of the interventricular septum, which produces an anterior filling defect below the aortic valve on the lateral view. In addition the anterior cusp of the mitral valve is drawn forward during early systole, and this leads to additional narrowing of the outflow tract from the posterior aspect; on the lateral view the anterior and posterior defects give a cone-shaped appearance, apex downwards, to the outflow tract (*Figure 4.26*). Mitral regurgitation may also occur. The aortic valve and aorta are normal. Occasionally hypertrophic obstructive cardiomyopathy may be associated with a membranous diaphragm across the outflow tract.

In other patients there may be no obstruction in the outflow tract (*Figure 4.27*).

Right ventricular angiocardiography

Right ventricular angiocardiography may show narrowing of the outflow tract of the right ventricle in an antero-posterior plane due to hypertrophy of the interventricular septum.

SUPRAVALVULAR AORTIC STENOSIS

Supravalvular aortic stenosis is a localized or diffuse concentric narrowing of the aorta just above the sinuses and the coronary arteries. Three types have been described (Perou, 1961).

(1). Hourglass type. This is the commonest type. It consists of considerable thickening of the media of the aorta which leads to a constricting annular ridge at the superior margin of the sinuses of Valsalva.
(2) Membranous type. This is produced by a diaphragm with a central hole in it.
(3) Hypoplastic type. In this type there is uniform hypoplasia of the ascending aorta, the whole ascending aorta being small in calibre.

The coronary arteries are proximal to all these narrowings; they are therefore subjected to high pressure and become tortuous and dilated. Supravalvular aortic stenosis may occur in association with idiopathic infantile hypercalcaemia. Congenital supravalvular aortic stenosis and peripheral pulmonary artery stenosis may also occur in sporadic and familial forms not associated with other abnormalities (*see* page 136).

Cardiac catheterization

On left heart catheterization a pressure gradient is shown above the aortic valve.

Thoracic aortography

This examination shows a constriction of the ascending aorta above the level of the aortic sinuses and also shows widened coronary arteries (*Figure 4.28*). Narrow segments in the aorta may also be seen distal to the ascending aorta.

Pulmonary arteriography

This investigation may show localized stenoses in the pulmonary artery and its branches.

Aortic regurgitation

Congenital aortic regurgitation may occur as an isolated lesion and it is uncommon. It may also co-exist with another congenital abnormality such as high ventricular septal defect, aortic stenosis or aneurysm of the sinus of Valsalva. It may result from superimposition of bacterial endocarditis on an existing congenital abnormality, particularly a bicuspid aortic valve.

Plain film

If the degree of regurgitation is marked the heart may be enlarged and there will be evidence of left ventricular enlargement.

Thoracic aortography

Thoracic aortography is the examination of choice. Contrast medium injected into the root of the aorta will regurgitate into the left ventricular cavity (*Figure 4.29*).

Hypoplastic left heart syndrome

The severest form of this complex is atresia of the mitral valve, slit-like left ventricular cavity, very small ascending aorta, aortic atresia and patent ductus arteriosus which supplies blood retrogradely through the hypoplastic aorta to the coronary arteries. In milder cases the mitral valve may be hypoplastic rather than atretic, the left ventricular cavity may be nearer normal in size and the aortic valve is atretic or hypoplastic. The width of the ascending aorta may be up to 50 per cent of normal size, (Lev, 1952; Noonan and Nadas, 1958).

The foramen ovale is usually patent. The right atrium is dilated and hypertrophied and the tricuspid valve is normal. The right ventricle is markedly dilated and hypertrophied and the pulmonary artery arises normally from it. The ductus arteriosus is large and forms a direct communication to the descending aorta which is of normal calibre. The pulmonary veins drain into the left atrium which is most frequently normal or small in size, but occasionally may be large. The mitral valve is stenotic or hypoplastic in 75 per cent of cases and atretic in the rest (Noonan and Nadas, 1958). The left ventricular cavity is small or cannot be identified. The aortic valve is atretic or hypoplastic. The ascending aorta is very narrow and the coronary arteries originate at its base. The great arteries arise from the small aortic arch.

Plain film

Usually the heart is enlarged with obvious right atrial and right ventricular enlargement. The pulmonary arteries are dilated secondary to venous obstruction. The apex is elevated.

Cardiac catheterization

Cardiac catheterization shows raised right ventricular and pulmonary artery pressures, and oxygen desaturation may be present in these regions. The catheter may pass through the patent ductus arteriosus into the descending aorta.

Thoracic aortography

The best way of demonstrating the lesion is to make a hand injection of contrast medium with the tip of the catheter in the aorta just distal to the patent ductus arteriosus, the patient being in the anteroposterior position. The injection of contrast medium is repeated with the patient in the lateral position. The procedure is recorded on cineradiography. This is usually all that is necessary to show the lesion in a desperately ill neonate. Right ventricular angiocardiography may also show the lesion (*Figures 4.30* and *4.31*).

MITRAL LESIONS

Congenital mitral stenosis

In about 50 per cent of cases congenital mitral stenosis occurs as an isolated lesion. In the remainder it is associated either with the left heart syndrome or with

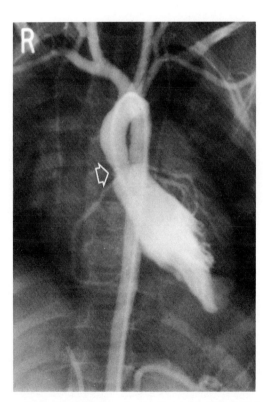

Figure 4.28. Supravalvular Aortic Stenosis: Left ventricular angiocardiogram in which the contrast medium has been injected from a catheter passed through the aortic valve from the thoracic aorta. The ascending aorta is narrowed (arrowed) above the aortic sinuses; the coronary arteries are well shown and are widened

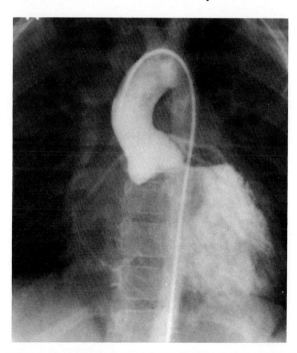

Figure 4.29. Congenital Aortic Regurgitation: A thoracic aortogram in the anteroposterior projection. The contrast medium is shown to be regurgitating through the region of the left cusp of the aortic valve into the left ventricle

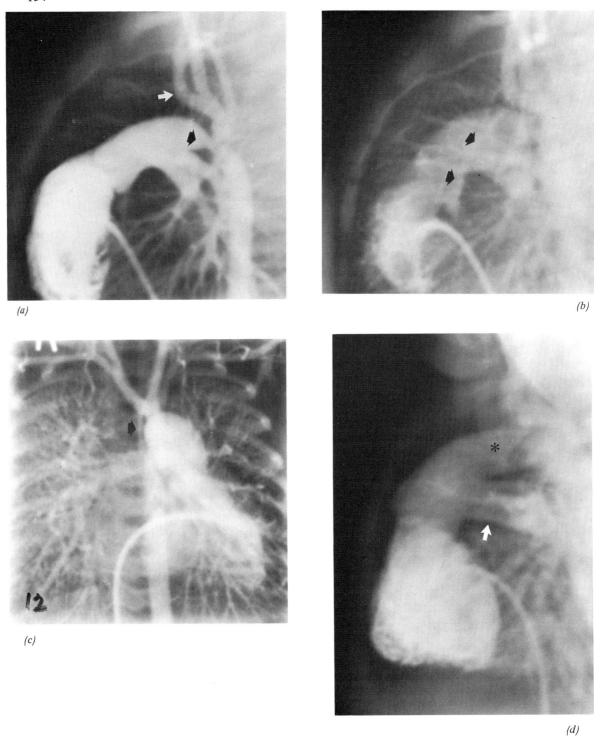

Figure 4.30. *Hypoplastic Left Heart Syndrome. Aortic Atresia: Right ventricular angiocardiogram. (a) Lateral projection. A film taken early in the series showing filling of the dilated pulmonary artery. Contrast medium passes through the large patent ductus arteriosus (black arrow) to fill the descending aorta. The aortic arch and its branches fill retrogradely and there is a coarctation of the aorta at the level of the ductus. Note the forward convexity (white arrow) transcribed by the junction between the arch of the aorta and the innominate artery. (b) Later film in the series showing retrograde filling of the hypoplastic ascending aorta (arrowed) back as far as the coronary arteries. (c) Anteroposterior projection taken at the same time as (b), again showing retrograde filling of the hypoplastic ascending aorta. (d) Right ventricular angiocardiogram of another case in lateral projection. This shows that in this condition the patent ductus arteriosus (*) may be as large as the pulmonary artery (arrowed)*

patent ductus arteriosus, aortic stenosis or coarctation of the aorta (Kaplan, 1968). The valve may be markedly thickened and narrowed and it may encroach on the outflow tract of the left ventricle, partially obstructing it. The left ventricle may be small, normal or dilated. The left atrium will be hypertrophied and dilated and there will be dilatation of the right ventricle and right atrium. Changes in the pulmonary artery and veins such as have already been described will develop in the presence of pulmonary venous and arterial hypertension. A supravalvular stenosing ring may sometimes be present above a normal mitral valve.

Plain films

The heart is usually enlarged with evidence of left atrial and right ventricular enlargement. On the lateral view the oesophagus is displaced backwards by the enlarged left atrium. The changes of pulmonary venous and arterial hypertension may be present and they have already been described in detail (*see* page 115).

Cardiac catheterization

This will show pulmonary hypertension and raised pulmonary capillary (wedge) pressure.

Right ventricular angiocardiography and pulmonary arteriography

These examinations may show enlargement of the left atrium with delayed emptying.

MITRAL REGURGITATION

Isolated congenital mitral incompetence is rare. It may be due to abnormal insertion of chordae tendineae into the valve cusps or there may be clefts in the cusps (Talner *et al.*, 1961). The lesion is most frequently associated with other conditions such as ventricular septal defect or cardiomyopathy.

The plain film findings are the same as those found with congenital mitral stenosis. The diagnosis is made by selective left ventricular angiocardiography, when the left atrium is shown to fill during systole from the left ventricle (*Figure 4.32*).

Cor triatrium

In this condition the pulmonary veins drain into an accessory left atrial chamber (or dilated common pulmonary vein) proximal to the true left atrium. The accessory chamber communicates with the true left atrium by an orifice which is small in size. The mitral valve is normal. The accessory chamber is most frequently larger than the true left atrium. Obstruction to the venous return is usual and leads to pulmonary hypertension with arteriolar changes, dilatation of the main pulmonary artery and right ventricle. The lesion may be accompanied by an atrial septal defect which can be small or large. If the septum between the two left atria is not perforated two co-existent atrial septal defects must be present. Oxygenated blood then passes

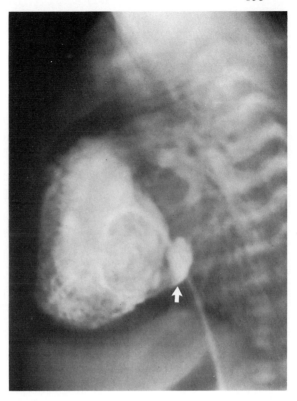

Figure 4.31. Hypoplastic Left Heart Syndrome with Both Mitral and Aortic Atresia: Right ventricular angiocardiogram in lateral projection. Film taken early in the series showing filling of a minute left ventricle (arrowed) through a ventricular septal defect

into the right atrium and the condition is similar to anomalous pulmonary venous drainage.

Cardiac catheterization

Cardiac catheterization shows the degree of pulmonary hypertension and elevated pulmonary wedge pressures. In some patients the catheter also enters the lower left atrial chamber and shows normal pressures which contrast with the raised pulmonary wedge pressure. A shunt into the right atrium may also be shown.

Right ventricular angiocardiography or Pulmonary arteriography

In the later stages of either of these examinations the two left atrial chambers may be shown. If the catheter tip is manipulated into the lower chamber and a contrast medium injection made, it will show that the chamber is small in size and has a normal left atrial appendage (Somerville, 1966).

Pulmonary stenosis

Pulmonary stenosis may occur alone (isolated) or in association with many other congenital heart lesions. Pulmonary stenosis may occur at valve level (valvular), proximal to the valve (infundibular) or distal to the valve.

In valvular stenosis the valve cusps are fused to form a diaphragm which has a central or eccentric hole in it.

136

The diaphragm may be thin and mobile or thick and rigid. Infundibular stenosis consists of a ring of fibromuscular tissue which encircles the outflow tract of the right ventricle. It may be high and just under the valve, low in position at the junction of the body and infundibulum of the right ventricle or in a middle position. The two types of stenosis may occur separately or in combination.

In all types of stenosis the right ventricle hypertrophies. In infundibular stenosis the hypertrophy is confined to the body, whereas in valvular stenosis it extends to involve the outflow tract as well. When the outflow tract is involved, the thickened hypertrophied muscle causes the walls of the outflow tract to approach each other closely in late systole so that an additional secondary stenosis may be produced. This secondary systolic stenosis may be severe but it is intermittent in the cardiac cycle; this feature distinguishes it from organic infundibular stenosis, which is constant and varies its degree only slightly throughout the cardiac cycle.

The third type of pulmonary stenosis consists of localized narrowing of the main pulmonary artery or its branches and is known as pulmonary artery stenosis (*Figure 4.33*). It may also lead to right ventricular hypertrophy.

ISOLATED PULMONARY STENOSIS

When this is at valvular level, it is one of the commonest organic infundibular stenosis, which is constant and to severe, depending on the size of the central hole in the stenotic valve. The valve ring may also be smaller than normal. Valvular stenosis is much commoner than infundibular stenosis. In valvular stenosis, and occasionally in high infundibular stenosis, poststenotic dilatation of the main pulmonary artery is seen and this may be very marked. When the poststenotic dilatation is well developed it frequently extends into the left branch of the pulmonary artery, presumably because the central jet tends to pass into the left branch which is continuous with the main artery. The pressure in the right ventricle may become very high (200 mmHg or higher) and hypertrophy of the right atrium occurs as a result.

Plain film

The appearances depend on the severity of the stenosis and its site. If the stenosis is valvular the poststenotic dilatation of the main pulmonary artery is visible as a localized bulge of the left heart border at pulmonary artery level. This dilatation shows evident pulsation on screening, and it extends into the left pulmonary artery, so that the left pulmonary artery is large and pulsatile and the right pulmonary artery is small. The dilatation extends into the first and second order branches, but the peripheral pulmonary arteries are smaller than normal, i.e. the periphery of the lungs is oligaemic (*Figure 4.34a*).

If the stenosis is infundibular in type, the pulmonary artery segment is usually concave, because the main pulmonary artery is not dilated. The branches at the hila are equally small. If the stenosis is severe the peripheral pulmonary arteries are small and the lungs are oligaemic. In the presence of severe stenosis a bronchial artery circulation may be recognized. The bronchial arteries enlarge and enter the lungs at the hila where they

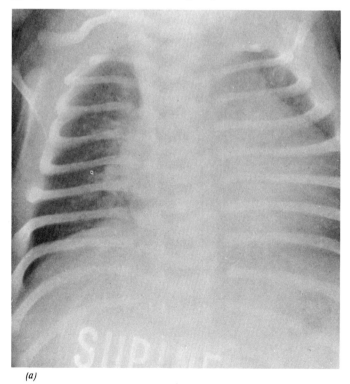 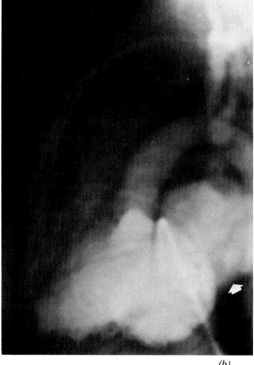

(a) *(b)*

Figure 4.32. Congenital Mitral Regurgitation: (a) Plain film showing enlargement of the right ventricle and of the pulmonary veins in the region of the right hilum. (b) Left ventricular angiocardiogram showing regurgitation of contrast medium into the enlarged left atrium (arrowed)

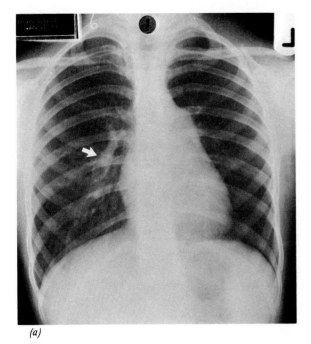

(a)

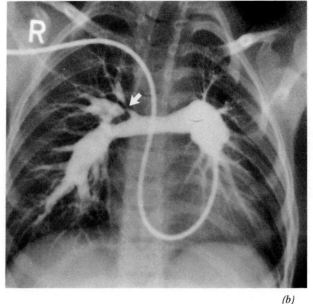

(b)

Figure. 4.33. Peripheral Pulmonary Artery Stenosis: (a) Plain film of chest showing a normal sized heart with a prominence of the upper part of the left cardiac border due to the enlarged main pulmonary artery. The peripheral arteries are diminished in calibre except for the right lower lobe artery which is dilated (arrowed). (b) Pulmonary arteriogram performed with the catheter tip in the main pulmonary artery. There are narrowed segments (arrowed) with post-stenotic dilatations distal to them in the branches of the right pulmonary artery. The dilatation of the lower lobe pulmonary artery is confirmed and it is due to post-stenotic dilatation. The narrowed segment is however not shown on this film

anastomose with the branches of the pulmonary artery. They are seen as small opacities, giving a spotty appearance to the hila and perihilar regions. When the stenosis is marked, right ventricular hypertrophy may be recognized by increased rounding of the left heart border, elevation of the apex and increased forward convexity of the anterior surface of the heart, the latter features being best seen in the left anterior oblique and lateral views. Right atrial hypertrophy may also be shown by increased rounding of the lower part of the right heart border. The aortic arch is usually small and insignificant on the postero-anterior view and this is due in part to the low cardiac output and in part to the rotation that occurs due to the right ventricular hypertrophy, so that the arch lies more in the sagittal plane than normally. It is surprising how little the transverse diameter of the heart increases in isolated pulmonary stenosis. If the heart is much enlarged then an associated abnormality should be suspected.

Cardiac catheterization

The catheter will follow the normal course. It will record raised pressure in the body of the right ventricle and low pressure in the pulmonary artery. On withdrawal from the pulmonary artery a rapid rise in pressure will occur at valve level if valvular stenosis is present but in the infundibulum if infundibular stenosis is present, or there will be an intermediate pressure in the outflow tract when both valvular and infundibular stenoses occur together. If the stenosis is in the main pulmonary artery or in a major branch a pressure gradient will be shown at its site.

Angiocardiography

Right ventricular angiocardiography will show the site and type of pulmonary stenosis present and the degree of associated right ventricular hypertrophy.

In valvular stenosis the stenotic valve is shown as a translucency in the contrast medium, usually domed so that it is convex to the pulmonary artery in systole. If the valve is thin it collapses irregularly in diastole (*Figure 4.34d*). If the valve is rigid a transverse translucent line is seen at the site of the valve which moves little throughout the cardiac cycle (*Figure 4.35*). Contrast medium will form a jet issuing from the valve into the dilated main pulmonary artery, the width of the jet depending on the size of the central hole (*Figure 4.34c*). The hypertrophy of the ventricle is shown by the presence of rounded filling defects in the ventricular outline due to thick muscle bundles in the body of the ventricle and tubular narrowing of the outflow tract in late systole due to hypertrophy of the outflow tract (*Figure 4.34e*). In diastole the outflow tract will dilate widely.

If the stenosis is infundibular there will usually be concentric narrowing over a limited area just proximal to the valve cusps or in the region of the junction of body and infundibulum (*Figure 4.36*) or between these two points. The degree of narrowing will remain fairly constant, but it will vary to some extent during the different phases of the cardiac cycle. Sometimes the narrowing is most marked from side to side but in others it is most marked from before backwards. The plane of the narrowed segment is sometimes oblique.

If the stenosis is in the pulmonary artery, localized narrowing may be seen in the main pulmonary artery

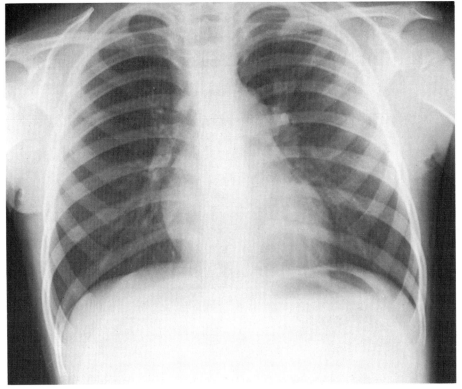

(a)

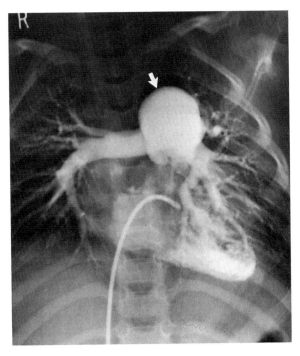

(b)

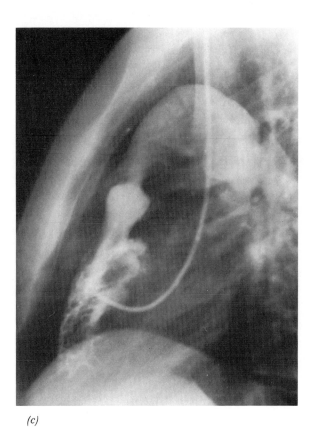

(c)

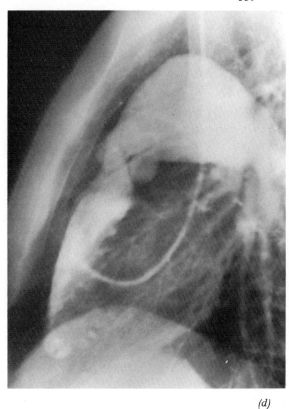

(d)

Figure 4.34. Pulmonary Valvular Stenosis: (a) Plain film showing a normal sized heart and oligaemic lungs. The main pulmonary artery is enlarged due to post-stenotic dilatation. (b) Right ventricular angiocardiogram. The main pulmonary artery distal to the stenosed pulmonary valve is markedly enlarged (arrowed) ('post-stenotic dilatation'). The peripheral branches of the pulmonary arteries are narrowed. (c) Lateral angiocardiogram showing the contrast medium passing through the stenosed pulmonary valve. (d) Lateral angiocardiogram with the contrast medium filling the greatly dilated main pulmonary artery and outlining the valve cusps on either side of the stenosed orifice. (e) Lateral angiocardiogram showing upward ballooning of the pulmonary valve cusps below the greatly dilated main pulmonary artery

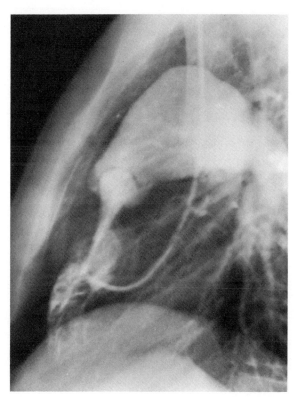

(e)

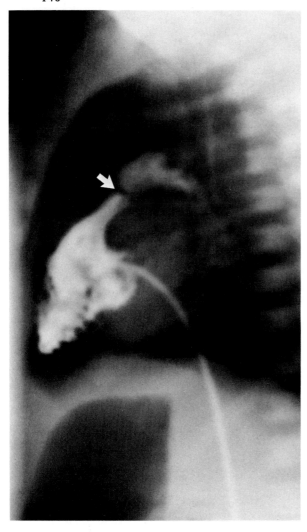

Figure 4.35. Pulmonary Valvular Stenosis in the Neonate: Right ventricular angiocardiogram in the lateral projection. The stenosed pulmonary valve is rigid and is shown as a transverse linear defect (arrowed) in the column of contrast medium

itself, at the bifurcation of the main pulmonary artery involving the origin of one or both branches, or in one of the branches. If the stenosis is in a branch there is usually dilatation (post-stenotic) of a length of the artery distal to the stenosis; in the lung fields this dilatation may be easier to recognize than is the stenosis on the angiocardiogram (*Figure 4.33*).

Pulmonary stenosis and ventricular septal defect (Fallot's tetralogy)

The site of the pulmonary stenosis may be valvular or infundibular or both. The ventricular septal defect may be small or large. Fallot described the condition that bears his name as consisting of pulmonary stenosis, ventricular septal defect, right ventricular hypertrophy and over-riding aorta. The hypertrophy of the right ventricle arises in response to the obstruction to the

outflow from the ventricle; the over-riding aorta comes about because the interventricular septum is displaced backwards by the right ventricular hypertrophy so that the aorta is directly over the septum. Thus the aorta is situated partly over the outlet from each ventricle. There is a spectrum of cases of increasing severity. At one extreme is the acyanotic patient with mild pulmonary valvular stenosis, a small ventricular septal defect, a normally situated aorta and a shunt from left to right (acyanotic Fallot). At the other extreme is the patient with severe pulmonary valvular and infundibular stenosis with a high resistance at the outlet from the right ventricle, a large ventricular septal defect with equalized right and left ventricular pressures, considerable right to left shunt, over-riding aorta and marked cyanosis. In Fallot's tetralogy the ventricular septal defect is large and it is usually infracristal in position. In about half the cases the stenosis is entirely infundibular, in 10 per cent the stenosis is valvular and in 20 per cent it is combined valvular and infundibular (Keith *et al.*, 1967). In the remaining 20 per cent pulmonary atresia is present, i.e. pseudotruncus (*see* page 141). If infundibular stenosis is present the outflow tract of the right ventricle distal to it and the main pulmonary artery are frequently small in calibre or hypoplastic. The degree of right ventricular hypertrophy is proportional to the degree of stenosis. In 25 per cent of cases the aorta is right-sided and about one-fifth of cases are associated with a persistent left superior vena cava. If the resistance of the outflow tract of the right ventricle is greater than that of the systemic circulation, the blood flows directly from the right ventricle into the aorta and the patient is cyanosed. This condition occurs in the majority of patients with Fallot's tetralogy and about 10 per cent also have an atrial septal defect (Pentalogy of Fallot). If the pulmonary stenosis is severe, then a bronchial artery circulation may develop to supplement the poor perfusion of the pulmonary arteries; even arteries from the neck and mediastinum may take part in these anastomoses.

Plain film

The heart is not usually enlarged. The right ventricle is hypertrophied, producing rounding of the lower part of the left heart border and elevation of the apex on the postero-anterior view. In the left anterior oblique view and left lateral view there is increased convexity of the anterior surface of the heart and the apex of the heart is small and elevated posteriorly (*Figure 4.37*). On the postero-anterior view the right heart border is usually normal.

In those cases with infundibular stenosis the main pulmonary artery is small and therefore the pulmonary artery segment is concave in most patients (*Figure 4.37*). If valvular stenosis alone is present the pulmonary artery segment may be bulging. The pulmonary arteries and the hila are small and the peripheral pulmonary arteries are also small. The aorta is usually large; this may be obvious on the postero-anterior view but is probably best recognized on the left anterior oblique view. The arch may be left- or right-sided, with the descending aorta on the corresponding side. The position of the arch can usually be seen on the postero-anterior view in older patients by

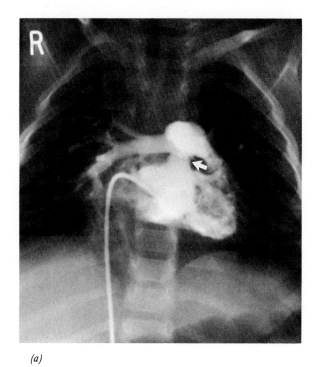

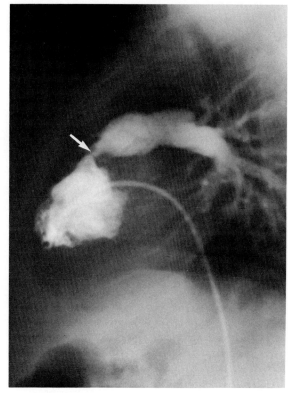

(a)

(b)

Figure 4.36. Infundibular Pulmonary Stenosis: (a) Right ventricular angiocardiogram in the anteroposterior projection. The outflow tract of the right ventricle is narrowed (arrowed) and there is a moderate degree of post-stenotic dilatation of the main pulmonary artery. (b) Lateral projection showing the narrowed infundibulum (arrowed) below the pulmonary valve

recognizing the position of the aortic knuckle. In younger patients the aortic knuckle may not be seen but its position can be inferred because the trachea is deviated to the side opposite the arch (*Figure 4.37c*) and on barium swallow the indentation produced on the oesophagus is on the same side as the arch. Should these features not be clear on the plain film they should be clarified on screening. The combination of a large aorta, concave pulmonary artery segment, rounded left heart border and elevated apex gives the heart a 'coeur-en-sabot' or 'sitting duck' appearance which, in a cyanotic patient, should strongly suggest Fallot's tetralogy (*Figure 4.37*).

Cardiac catheterization

The catheter· may pass from right ventricle into the pulmonary artery and in this position the pressure will be low. On withdrawal, a step-up in pressure will occur at the pulmonary valve and also at the infundibular stenosis. Pressure in the right ventricle will be elevated up to systemic level. The catheter may pass from the right ventricle through the ventricular septal defect into the ascending aorta, where desaturated blood will be sampled.

Right ventricular angiocardiography

Right ventricular angiocardiography is the examination of choice. It should show the size of the right ventricle,

the position of the ventricular septal defect; the type, site and severity of the pulmonary valvular and infundibular stenosis; the size of the outflow tract of the right ventricle; the pulmonary valve ring and the pulmonary arteries; the presence of peripheral pulmonary stenosis; and the size and position of the aorta (*Figure 4.38*). The pulmonary artery usually fills just before the aorta but occasionally they fill simultaneously.

Pulmonary atresia

Pulmonary atresia may occur either with a ventricular septal defect or with an intact interventricular septum.

PULMONARY ATRESIA WITH VENTRICULAR SEPTAL DEFECT

In this condition, which is known as extreme Fallot's tetralogy or pseudotruncus, the cardiac malformation is the same as in Fallot's tetralogy except that the pulmonary valve is atretic. There is no communication between the right ventricle and the pulmonary arteries. A fine membrane may replace the normal pulmonary valve and distal to it is a well-formed main pulmonary artery. In other cases the atretic valve may consist of thickened tissue or the main pulmonary artery may be absent, only its branches being present. The pulmonary arteries are supplied by a large patent ductus arteriosus

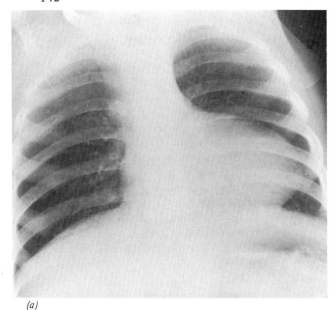

(a)

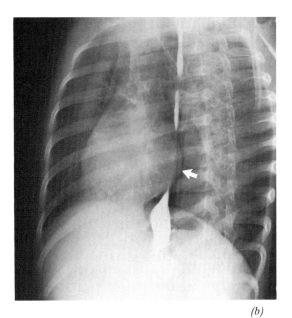

(b)

Figure 4.37. Tetralogy of Fallot: (a) Plain film showing elevation of the cardiac apex and convexity of the lower part of the left heart border due to the large right ventricle. The upper part is concave due to the small main pulmonary artery ('coeur en sabot'). (b) Left anterior oblique projection of the chest showing increased convexity of the anterior border of the heart due to the large right ventricle; the apex of the heart is elevated posteriorly (arrowed) but the heart is not generally enlarged. (c) Postero-anterior projection showing a heart of normal size and shape but with deficient peripheral pulmonary vessel shadows. The aortic arch is right sided (arrowed) and indents and displaces the trachea to the left

(c)

and/or bronchial arteries. It is important in such cases to demonstrate whether a main pulmonary artery is present or not, because remedial surgery may be possible.

Plain film

The plain film appearances are similar to those of severe Fallot's tetralogy, but in addition the heart may be enlarged. The aorta is usually very large and easily recognized (*Figure 4.39a*).

Cardiac catheterization

The findings are the same as in Fallot's tetralogy except that the catheter does not enter the pulmonary artery. It will enter the aorta with ease.

Right ventricular angiocardiography

The findings are similar to those of Fallot's tetralogy, with a large aorta receiving blood from both ventricles.

If the outflow tract of the right ventricle fills it does not communicate with the main pulmonary artery (*Figure 4.39*). After the aorta has been outlined the pulmonary arteries are filled through a patent ductus arteriosus or by bronchial or other arteries (*Figure 4.40*). The main pulmonary artery may fill retrogradely from its branches. Every attempt should be made to get the catheter to enter the aorta and to bring the tip to the descending part of the arch. Here injection of contrast medium will demonstrate the blood supply to the pulmonary arteries and show whether a main pulmonary artery is present. If it is not possible to get the catheter into the aorta through the right ventricle then retrograde aortography should be performed (*Figure 4.39b*).

PULMONARY ATRESIA WITH INTACT VENTRICULAR SEPTUM

This abnormality may take two forms and in both

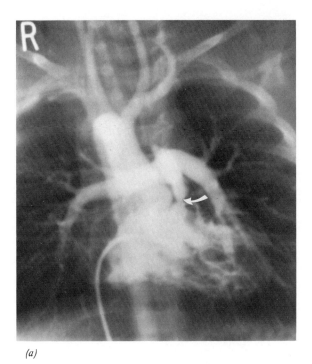

(a)

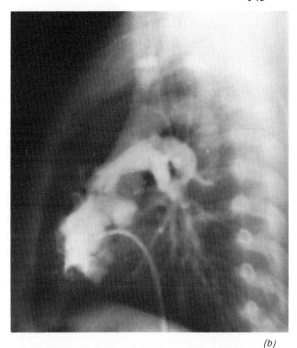

(b)

Figure 4.38. Tetralogy of Fallot: (a) Anteroposterior angio-cardiogram injected from the right ventricle. The pulmonary valve is stenosed (arrowed) and the calibre of the pulmonary artery and its main branches reduced. The dextroposed ascending aorta is filled at the same time. There is a right-sided aortic arch and descending aorta. (b) Lateral projection showing the pulmonary stenosis with the ascending aorta displaced forwards as well as to the right and superimposed on the pulmonary artery. (c) Right ventricular angiocardiogram of another case in which a Blalock's operation has been carried out. The aorta and pulmonary artery are both opacified. The latter receives contrast medium both through the stenosed pulmonary valve and through the right subclavian artery (arrowed) which has been anastomosed to the right pulmonary artery

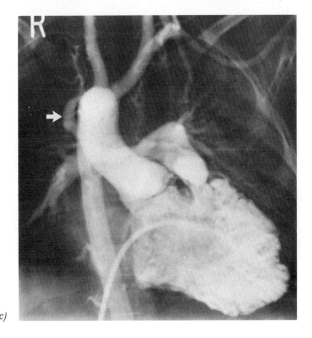

(c)

types the obstruction is at valvular level (Greenwold *et al.*, 1956). In each type a communication across the atrial septum is essential. This is usually through the foramen ovale but there may be a secundum type atrial septal defect. In addition a patent ductus arteriosus is essential to support a pulmonary artery supply. A main pulmonary artery is frequently present in addition to the branches to both lungs. The circulation is from right atrium through the foramen ovale into the left atrium to the left ventricle and aorta and then through the ductus to the pulmonary arteries and then back to the left atrium, the systemic blood flow returning to the right atrium through the vena cava.

Type 1

This condition is the commoner type. The cavity of the right ventricle is small and narrow. It is surrounded by a large mass of muscle. The tricuspid valve has a small ring. It is relatively normal in structure and only moderately incompetent. Myocardial sinusoids in the ventricular wall frequently communicate with the coronary arteries. The right atrium is usually small.

Type 2

In this condition the right ventricular cavity is either

144

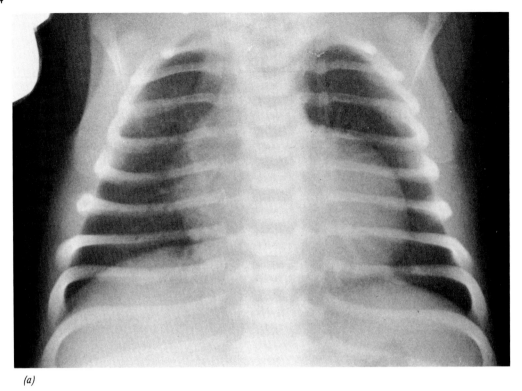

(a)

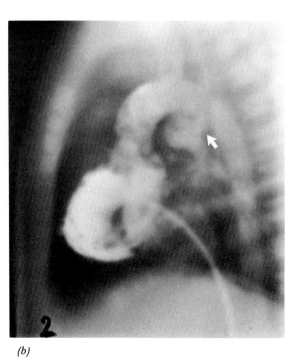

(b)

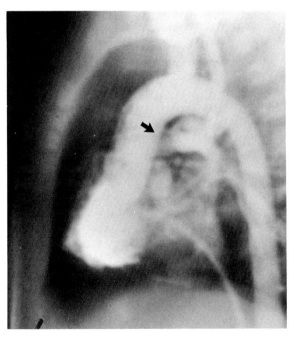

(c)

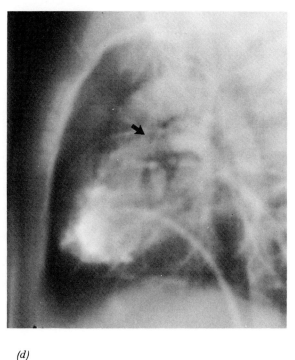

(d)

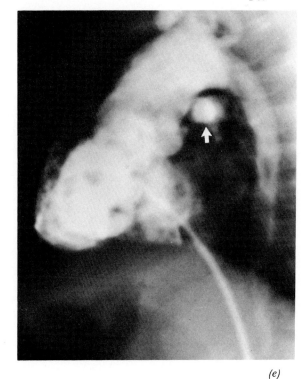

(e)

Figure 4.39. Pulmonary Atresia with Ventricular Septal Defect:
(a) Plain film showing an enlarged right ventricle and right
atrium and markedly oligaemic lung fields. (b) Right ventricular angiocardiogram in the lateral projection. Film taken
early in the series showing filling of the aorta which overrides
the defect in the ventricular septum. Filling of the pulmonary
arteries through a patent ductus arteriosus (arrowed) has
occurred but the main pulmonary artery has not yet been opacified. (c) and (d) Later films from the same examination showing
filling of the main pulmonary artery (arrowed) retrogradely
from its branches. Some opacification of the left ventricle
has occurred through the septal defect. (e) Right ventricular
angiocardiogram of another case in the lateral projection. Filling
of the small pulmonary artery branches (arrowed) has occurred
through a patent ductus arteriosus and contrast medium has
passed through a septal defect into the left ventricle. (f) Thoracic
aortogram of the same case in the lateral projection showing
the branches of the pulmonary artery unobscured by the contrast medium in the heart and ascending aorta. The main pulmonary artery is absent

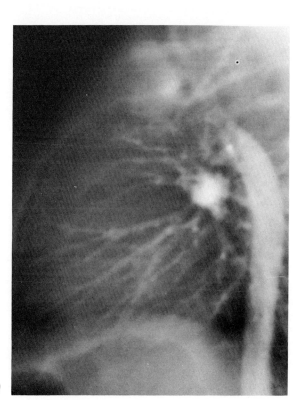

(f)

normal in size or dilated. The tricuspid valve is usually incompetent. The right atrium is large.

Plain film

Though exceptions occur, those patients with small ventricles tend to have normal sized or only slightly enlarged hearts. Those patients with normal or large ventricles have larger and sometimes enormous hearts If the patient survives, the heart tends to increase rapidly in size. In most patients the pulmonary artery segment is concave. The lungs are usually oligaemic but if the ductus arteriosus is large the pulmonary arteries may be nearly normal in size.

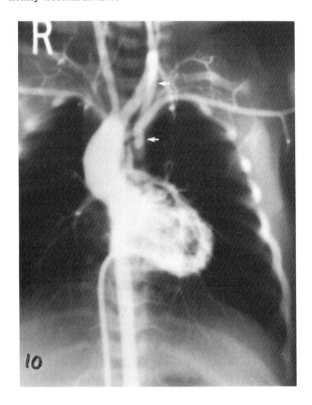

Figure 4.40. Pulmonary Atresia: Right ventricular angiocardiogram in the anteroposterior projection. Contrast medium has filled the right-sided aorta and its branches. Some contrast medium has also reached the pulmonary arteries through a branch of the left common cartoid artery (arrowed)

Cardiac catheterization

This examination should be done as soon as possible after birth. In Type 1 ventricles it may not be possible to enter the right ventricle with the catheter. The findings are similar to those of tricuspid atresia from which they can be distinguished by a left ventricular angiocardiograph which in pulmonary atresia fails to show a ventricular septal defect. The pressure in the right ventricle is high but the catheter will not pass into the pulmonary artery. It will go from the right atrium into the left atrium and left ventricle where desaturated blood is obtained.

Right ventricular angiocardiography

Every effort must be made to get the catheter to enter the right ventricle and to make the injection into this chamber. In Type 1 a small, smooth-walled, flask-shaped ventricle will be shown and there will be no filling of the pulmonary artery from it (*Figure 4.41*). Contrast medium refluxes into the right atrium and thence through the foramen ovale into the left atrium, left ventricle and aorta from which the pulmonary arteries fill through a patent ductus arteriosus. Frequently, small linear sinusoids fill from the ventricular cavity and outline the coronary arteries and coronary sinus.

The Type 2 the large ventricular cavity is shown and tricuspid regurgitation is marked. As these patients may benefit considerably from surgery if the atretic valve is a diaphragm and the main pulmonary artery is present, it is important to perform an aortogram to try to fill the pulmonary artery through the patent ductus arteriosus.

Pulmonary regurgitation

Pulmonary regurgitation may occur in patients with pulmonary hypertension or after pulmonary valvotomy, but it may also occur as a separate entity. It is not clinically important but radiologically the pulmonary artery may be dilated and pulsatile.

Tricuspid atresia

In this condition the tricuspid valve and inflow part of the right ventricle are absent. If the patient is to survive an interatrial communication is essential, either through the foramen ovale or an atrial septal defect. The left atrium and left ventricle are large and hypertrophied. The aorta is increased in calibre. The right ventricular chamber is small and consists mostly of the infundibulum up to the pulmonary valve. This diminutive remnant of the right ventricle communicates with the left ventricle through a small ventricular septal defect which is usually in the muscular septum. About 30 per cent of cases of tricuspid atresia are associated with transposition of the great arteries according to Keith *et al.* (1967). These authors have classified tricuspid atresia with and without transposition of the great arteries into six types in all.

Plain film

The heart size is usually normal and the lungs are oligaemic. On the postero-anterior view the right heart border tends to be straight. The left heart border is rounded with a shelf below the pulmonary artery segment, the latter being deeply concave; this gives a square shape to the left heart border (*Figure 4.42a*). In the right anterior oblique position, left atrial enlargement may be recognized. In the left anterior oblique view the lower half of the anterior border is flattened and its upper part convex forwards. The enlargement of the left side of the heart can be recognized in this view.

Unfortunately the radiological appearances in this condition vary considerably and it may be impossible to

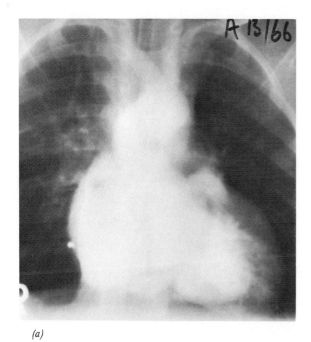

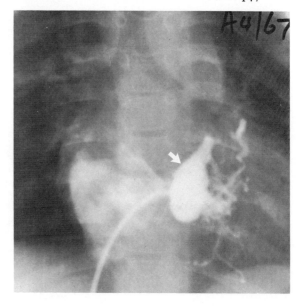

(a)

(b)

Figure 4.41. Pulmonary Atresia with Hypoplastic Right Ventricle and Intact Interventricular Septum: (a) Angiocardiogram in the anteroposterior projection with the contrast medium injected into the right atrium. This shows the typical circulation of tricuspid atresia. (b) At a subsequent catheterization the catheter passed directly into the right ventricle (arrowed) and the injection was made from there. The right ventricle is hypoplastic and the pulmonary valve is atretic. Contrast medium regurgitates through the tricuspid valve into the right atrium and has filled the coronary vessels through myocardial sinusoids

recognize tricuspid atresia from the plain film alone. In the cases where there is a large ventricular septal defect and the outflow tract of the right ventricle is well developed, the pulmonary artery segment will not be concave and it may even be bulging. The lungs then may be pleonaemic. In the left anterior oblique view, the front of the heart is more convex than in those cases in which the outflow tract is small.

Cardiac catheterization

The catheter does not enter the right ventricle. It passes from the right atrium through the interatrial septum into the left atrium and left ventricle where desaturated blood is obtained on sampling. The pressures in the right atrium and left atrium are usually elevated.

Angiocardiography

The diagnosis may be reached on angiocardiography by making the first injection into the right atrium (*Figure 4.42*) and a supplementary injection into the left ventricle. The right atrium may be large. Contrast medium passes across the atrial septum into the left atrium and thence into the left ventricle. From the left ventricle it enters the aorta if the great vessels are in normal relationship and passes through the ventricle septal defect into the remnant of the right ventricular and the small pulmonary artery. A characteristic feature derives from the absence of the inflow part of the right ventricle. This is shown as an inverted V-shaped area between the contrast medium in the right atrium and the left ventricle on the postero-anterior view which is devoid

of contrast medium, i.e. at the expected site of the inflow tract of the right ventricle. If the great arteries are transposed this will be shown after the contrast medium has reached the left ventricle, but in much more detail after the injection has been made into the left ventricle. Left ventricular angiocardiography also shows the ventricular septal defect well and the anatomy of the outflow part of the right ventricle, the position and size of the great arteries and the presence of a patent ductus arteriosus.

Ebstein syndrome

This condition is rare. The tricuspid valve leaflets are abnormal and attached partly to the valve ring and partly to the wall of the right ventricle. The valve, which is usually funnel-shaped, stenotic and incompetent, is displaced into the right ventricle. The valve displacement produces a large proximal chamber which consists of the right atrium and the atrialized part of the right ventricle (Edwards, 1953), together with a small right ventricular cavity. A defect is present in the interatrial septum in 42 per cent of cases, a patent foramen ovale being more common than an atrial septal defect, (Watson, 1974).

Plain film

The pulmonary artery segment will be concave or straight, and the aorta and pulmonary arteries small. Pulsations of the right heart border are reduced. The appearances vary with the severity of the lesion from

148

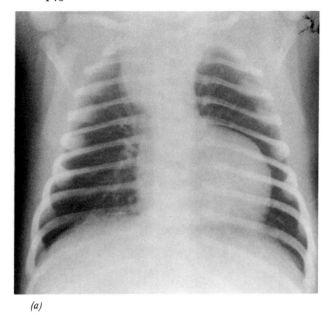

(a)

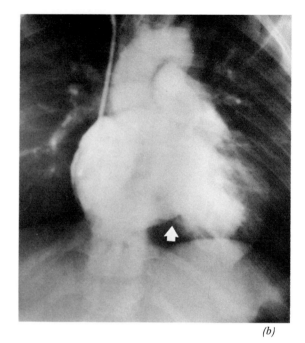

(b)

Figure 4.42. Tricuspid Atresia. (a) Plain film showing a square heart outline with a straight right border and a shelf-like projection of the left heart border below the concave pulmonary artery segment. The lung fields are oligaemic and the aorta is right sided. (b) Right atrial angiocardiogram in the antero-posterior projection. The right atrium is large and the contrast medium passes from it into the left atrium, left ventricle and through a ventricular septal defect into the outflow tract of the right ventricle and pulmonary artery. The characteristic notch (arrowed) in the inferior border of the heart due to the absence of the inflow tract of the right ventricle is well shown. (c) Lateral projection of the same case. The small outflow tract of the right ventricle (arrowed) is shown filled through the ventricular septal defect

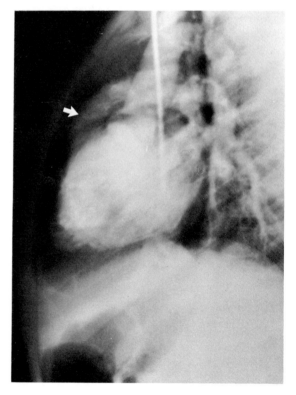

(c)

a normal heart outline to one with huge enlargement of the right atrium. This shows as increased convexity of the right heart border on the postero-anterior view and of the front of the heart in the left anterior oblique view.

Cardiac catheterization

These patients are prone to develop arrhythmias with catheterization, which may therefore be hazardous.

The catheter tip will take the normal course but curls up into the right atrium and so reveals its large size.

Right atrial angiocardiography

If the injection of contrast medium is made into the right atrium, the huge size of this chamber will be shown as well as the displacement of the tricuspid valve to the left side. The right atrium takes a long time to empty and this causes poor demonstration of the right ventricle and pulmonary artery. On the antero-posterior view two notches may be seen on the inferior border of this chamber. The right one is due to the normal atrio-ventricular groove and the left one to the displaced tricuspid valve. The part of the chamber between the notches is the atrialised portion of the right ventricle and cineradiography may show asynchronous contraction of the two parts of the right atrium.

If the injection is made into the right ventricle the incompetence of the tricuspid valve will be shown by the contrast medium regurgitating into the large right atrium. After this has occurred, similar appearances to those described above will be shown.

MALPOSITION OF THE HEART

Dextrocardia

This condition is a congenital anomaly in which the position of the cardiac chambers and great vessels is reversed from side to side but normal from before backwards. The heart and great vessels are thus a mirror image of the normal and this is accompanied by transposition of the viscera (Van Praagh *et al.*, 1964). About a fifth of these cases also have bronchiectasis (Kartagener's syndrome) (*see* page 189). There is seldom any intracardiac abnormality in adolescent and adult patients who have dextrocardia associated with transposition of the viscera (situs inversus) but this is not the case in infants and young children in whom ventricular or atrial septal defects, transposition of the great arteries and pulmonary stenosis frequently coexist with dextrocardia. The right atrium and inferior vena cava are always on the opposite side to the stomach; i.e. if the gastric air bubble is under the right hemidiaphragm, the left side of the heart shadow will be formed by the right atrium and inferior vena cava. Dextrocardia should be distinguished from *dextroversion or dextrorotation* in which the cardiac chambers and great vessels are rotated to the right but not inverted in position. The viscera are normal in site (situs solitus), the gastric air bubble is under the left hemidiaphragm and the cardiac apex is directed to the right side (*Figure 4.43*). Patients with dextrorotation usually also have severe intracardiac abnormalities. Occasionally there may be inversion of the ventricles or more rarely inversion of the atria and this may be accompanied by asplenia or polysplenia. The latter occurs as part of the *asplenia complex*. It may be inferred radiologically when the liver shadow is shown to be in the midline and when there is evidence of a diaphragmatic hernia accompanied by a malrotation of the intestine on the barium meal (Campbell and Deuchar, 1967). The occurrence of Howell–Jolly bodies in the red blood cells in the presence of cyanotic congenital heart disease is said to be pathognomonic of this syndrome (Moller *et al.*, 1971). If transposition of the viscera (situs inversus) coexists with a heart that is normally positioned then isolated laevocardia is said to be present. There are always intracardiac abnormalities in such cases.

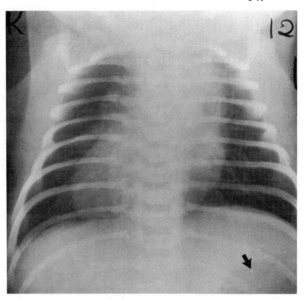

Figure 4.43. Dextrorotation: The cardiac apex is directed to the right although the gastric air bubble (arrowed) is shown to lie in its normal position on the left side. Such a combination indicates that other severe intracardiac anomalies are likely to be present

LESIONS OF THE GREAT VESSELS

Transposition of the great arteries

Advances in palliative and corrective surgery in the last two decades have included the treatment of transposition of the great arteries (Bonham-Carter, 1973) and this has led to a great interest in these malformations. There have been many classifications of these lesions recently which have shown the very complex nature of the abnormalities. Only the more common and simpler abnormalities will be dealt with here and the interested reader is referred to more detailed works for further reading (Van Praagh *et al.*, 1964).

The term 'transposition of the great arteries' is taken to mean that the origins of the aorta and pulmonary artery are reversed from before backwards so that the aorta arises in front from the anterior ventricle and the pulmonary artery arises behind from the posterior ventricle. The term 'inversion' implies that the relationship of the great arteries or ventricles is reversed from side to side, i.e. the aorta arises to the left of the pulmonary artery. It is important to know that transposition may be present either with or without inversion of the great arteries, ventricles or atria. If the aortic valve is to the right of the pulmonary valve D-transposition is said to be present. If the aortic valve is to the left of the pulmonary valve then L-transposition is present.

D-loop and L-loop can be defined as follows. When the morphologically right ventricle is to the right side of the morphological left ventricle a D-loop is present and when the morphologically right ventricle is to the left of the morphological left ventricle L-loop is present.

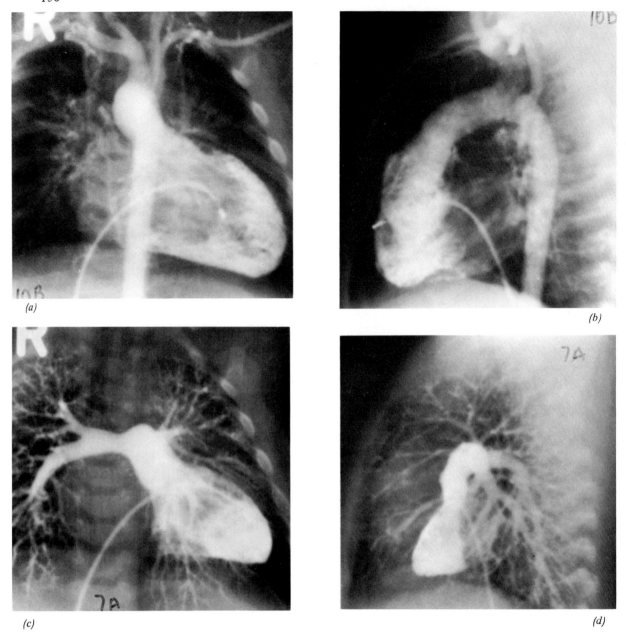

(a)

(b)

(c)

(d)

Figure 4.44. Transposition of the Great Arteries–D-loop: (a) Right ventricular angiocardiogram in the anteroposterior projection. Direct filling of the aorta is shown. The ascending aorta is displaced upwards and to the left. Filling of the pulmonary arteries has occurred through a patent ductus arteriosus. (b) Lateral projection of the same case. The forward displacement of the ascending aorta, the widened sweep of the aortic arch and the patent ductus arteriosus are well shown. (c) and (d) Left ventricular angiocardiogram in the same child. The pulmonary artery which is displaced posteriorly and centrally is shown to arise from the outflow tract of the left ventricle (c) Anteroposterior projection (d) Lateral projection

A simple classification of transposition of the great arteries is given by Paul *et al.* (1968).

    (1) Transposition with two ventricles and spleen present
        (a) Complete
        (b) Corrected
        (c) Double outlet right ventricle
    (2) Transposition with single ventricle and spleen present
    (3) Transposition with asplenia

COMPLETE (D-LOOP) TRANSPOSITION OF THE GREAT ARTERIES

This is the commonest type of transposition of the great arteries and is a frequent cause of cyanosis and heart failure in the newborn. The venous drainage to the atria is normal. The course of the blood flow is: (1) from the right atrium to the right ventricle, thence to the aorta returning via systemic veins to the right atrium; and (2) from the left atrium to the left ventricle, thence to the pulmonary artery and the pulmonary veins returning to the left atrium. There are therefore two separate circulations. Communication between them must exist either through an atrial septal defect, a ventricular septal defect or through a patent ductus arteriosus or combinations of these. The larger or the more numerous the communications, the better is the outlook.

Plain film

The heart may be normal in size at birth but it will progressively enlarge. The lungs are pleonaemic. The appearances of the heart will vary considerably. It is difficult to identify the individual chambers but the heart has a globular outline or, more characteristically, an outline resembling the shape of an egg set obliquely across the chest, the blunt end to the right of the spine. The vascular pedicle is narrow and the pulmonary artery segment concave in spite of the pleonaemia of the lungs. If, however, associated pulmonary stenosis is present the heart may not be enlarged and the lungs may show normal vascularity or be oligaemic (*Figure 4.46*).

Cardiac catheterization

The catheter in most cases will pass from the right atrium into the right ventricle and thence into the ascending aorta. It will also pass from the right atrium through a foramen ovale or atrial septal defect into the left atrium and left ventricle.

Angiocardiography

Right ventricular angiocardiography shows immediate and dense filling of the aorta which arises anteriorly in continuity with the outflow tract of the right ventricle. The aortic valve is high and anterior in position and it is to the right of the pulmonary artery. On the lateral view, the aorta forms a wide arch and the ascending aorta is further forwards than normal (*Figure 4.44*). The venous return from the head and arms is to the right atrium. If a patent ductus arteriosus is present it will be shown at the same time as the descending part of the arch of the aorta through it (*Figure 4.45*). If a ventricular septal defect is present contrast medium will pass backwards into the left ventricle and the pulmonary artery will fill.

Left ventricular angiocardiography will show the large pulmonary artery arising in continuity with the outflow tract of the left ventricle. The pulmonary artery is more central in position on the anteroposterior view than is normal but it is posterior on the lateral view, i.e. it is behind and to the left of the aorta. The pulmonary valve is therefore posterior and inferior in position. Contrast medium will return from the pulmonary circulation to the left atrium and refill the left ventricle and pulmonary artery. If an atrial septal defect

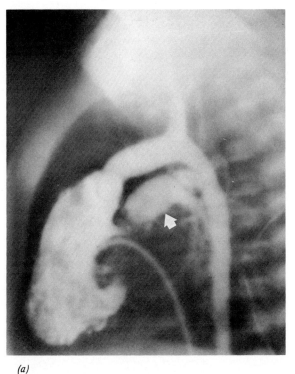

(a)

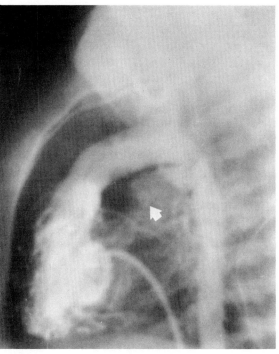

(b)

Figure 4.45. Transposition of the Great Arteries: (a) Right ventricular angiocardiogram in the lateral projection. The aorta arises entering from the right ventricle. Filling of the main pulmonary artery (arrowed) posteriorly and its branches has occurred through a patent ductus arteriosus. (b) Film taken 1/16th second later in systole, showing the contrast medium washed out of the pulmonary artery (arrowed) by non-opaque blood which must have entered it from the left ventricle

is present contrast medium will pass from the left atrium to the right atrium. If pulmonary stenosis is an associated lesion, it will be shown to be valvular or subvalvular in site.

CORRECTED (L-LOOP) TRANSPOSITION OF THE GREAT ARTERIES

In this condition most commonly the aorta arises from an anterior left-sided ventricle which is morphologically a right ventricle (i.e. it has the shape and structure of a right ventricle) and the pulmonary artery arises posteriorly and to the right of the aorta from a right-sided ventricle which is morphologically a left ventricle. Right atrial blood goes to the posterior ventricle and into the pulmonary artery and left atrial blood goes to the anterior ventricle and aorta. The circulation is thus normal unless there are associated abnormalities; these are frequent, the commonest being ventricular septal defect.

Plain film

The appearances will vary with the associated abnormalities, but so far as the transposition is concerned the heart size and shape may be normal. Instead of the pulmonary artery segment being concave, there is a long-segment, smooth, shallow convexity to the left of the upper part of the cardiovascular border due to the abnormal position of the aorta (*Figure 4.47a*). The

aorta may very occasionally be in this position in association with complete transposition of the great arteries.

Cardiac catheterization

The findings are normal in the absence of a ventricular septal defect.

Angiocardiography

The catheter will enter the posterior venous ventricle from the right atrium. Injection of contrast medium into this chamber will show that it is acorn shaped and like a left ventricle with short outflow tract and smooth walls; from it the pulmonary artery arises centrally and posteriorly. Contrast medium will return to the left atrium and pass to the arterial ventricle, which is anterior and shaped like a right ventricle with a long outflow tract and trabeculation of its walls. The ascending aorta is anterior and on the left side and runs parallel to the pulmonary artery (*Figure 4.47b* and *c*).

Atrial septostomy

Marked clinical improvement can be obtained in infants with transposition of the great arteries by the creation or enlargement of an atrial septal defect by balloon catheter (Rashkind and Miller, 1965, 1966).

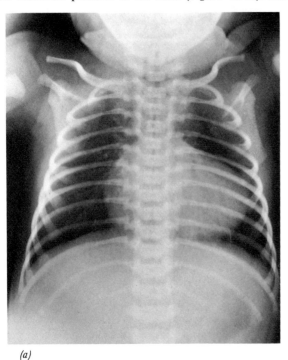

(a)

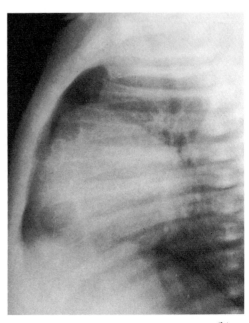

(b)

Figure 4.46. Transposition of the Great Arteries Associated with Pulmonary Stenosis: Plain films showing the heart lying transversely with an elevated apex, convexity of the anterior and posterior borders and oligaemic lung fields. (a) Anteroposterior projection. (b) Lateral projection

DOUBLE OUTLET RIGHT VENTRICLE

In this condition the pulmonary artery arises normally from the right ventricle. The aorta takes origin entirely from the right ventricle and its site of origin is on the posterior wall above the tricuspid valve and to the right of the pulmonary artery. The aortic valve is therefore high and on the same horizontal level as the pulmonary valve but these two valves are side by side in the coronal plane. A ventricular septal defect is almost always present and it is usually infracristal in position (Neufeld *et al.*, 1961). Many associated abnormalities have been reported, the most frequent of which are coarctation of the aorta and pulmonary stenosis. The condition is important in that if it is mistaken for simple ventricular septal defect this may be closed surgically with fatal results.

Plain film

The appearances are similar to those of ventricular septal defect.

Cardiac catheterization

The catheter may pass out of the right ventricle into either or both of the great arteries. As the blood from the ventricular septal defect may stream almost entirely into the aorta, the oxygen saturations may be normal. Right ventricular pressure is always at systemic level.

Right ventricular angiocardiography

This is the only examination by which the diagnosis can be made. As the origin of the pulmonary artery from the right ventricle is normal, the diagnostic features must rely on the position of the aorta (*Figure 4.48*). The aortic valve lies in front of the plane of the interventricular septum and the ascending aorta is directed forwards instead of downwards and backwards. The aorta is not so far forward as in complete transposition of the great arteries but the aortic and pulmonary valves are on the same level. On the anteroposterior view, the outflow tract may be seen to split, the right limb going into the aorta and the left one to the pulmonary artery. On the lateral view the aorta and pulmonary artery are in the same anteroposterior plane and there is discontinuity between the aortic valve and the mitral valve. In the later stages of the angiocardiograph the normal left ventricle fills from the left atrium and it is shown to be posterior to the right ventricle. The high position of the aortic valve as the aorta fills from the left ventricle through the ventricular septal defect is again evident. Ultrasound examination will demonstrate the discontinuity between the posterior wall of the aorta and the anterior cusp of the mitral valve.

SINGLE VENTRICLE WITH OUTLET CHAMBER AND TRANSPOSITION OF THE GREAT VESSELS

This is the commonest type of single ventricle and accounts for 79 per cent of all cases of single ventricle. Transposition of the great arteries occurs in 84 per cent of these cases (Van Praagh *et al.*, 1964, 1965). The most common type consists of a single left ventricle with an outlet chamber which is the outflow tract of the right ventricle. Associated stenosis of the pulmonary or aortic valve or coarctation of the aorta may occur. Other types of single ventricle are described. These comprise single right ventricle and undivided ventricles (absence of interventricular septum).

Plain film

The heart is usually normal in size or slightly enlarged if there is obstruction to the pulmonary blood flow, moderately enlarged if there is aortic flow obstruction and greatly enlarged when there is excessive pulmonary blood flow. The vascular pedicle may be narrow in the anteroposterior view but wide on the lateral view. If the aorta is transposed into the L-position there may be a smooth convexity of the upper part of the left heart border.

Cardiac catheterization

The catheter findings are similar to those of ventricular septal defect but the catheter may pass out of the ventricle into the pulmonary artery which is medially placed and this should suggest the possible diagnosis.

Angiocardiography

Injection of the contrast medium into the ventricle shows the pulmonary artery to arise centrally from the ventricle. The small outlet chamber fills by a ventricular septal defect and is shown as an anvil-shaped chamber on the left and anterior apsect of the heart from which the aorta arises anterior to the pulmonary artery. The outlet chamber may be anterior to the pulmonary artery and the great arteries will therefore be superimposed on the anteroposterior view.

Coarctation of the aorta

Coarctation of the aorta is a congenital narrowing of the aortic arch or descending aorta. It is most frequently situated in the descending part of the arch just distal to the origin of the left subclavian artery. It may coexist with other congenital abnormalities, particularly with patent ductus arteriosus. Its incidence is 1 in 16,000 children.

It may be classified into: (1) pre-ductal and (2) post-ductal, the type depending on the relationship of the coarctation to the entrance of the ductus arteriosus into the aorta. The pre-ductal type is sometimes known as the infantile type. If this condition is severe, the descending aorta gets its blood supply from the pulmonary artery through a large patent ductus arteriosus. In the post-ductal or adult type the descending aorta is supplied from the aortic arch. The aorta may be narrowed over a short or long segment and in infants the arch may be hypoplastic as well. Frequently the aortic valve is bicuspid in type. A patent ductus arteriosus is also a common accompaniment; it is usually small but may be very large and then is the dominant lesion. Many associated intracardiac conditions have been described, such as ventricular septal defect; they are usually present with the pre-ductal type of coarctation, but are rare in the adult or post-ductal type. Very rarely the coarctation of the aorta may be sited in the lower thoracic or abdominal aorta. About 25 per cent of patients with Turner's syndrome have a coarctation of the aorta.

It is helpful to describe the radiological appearances in older children on the one hand and infants on the other. The features are related to the age of the patient and the severity of the coarctation.

COARCTATION IN OLDER CHILDREN

In most of these patients the narrowing involves only a short segment but in about 10 per cent of patients it may be more extensive. If the obstruction is severe there may be dilatation of the ascending aorta which continues into the innominate and left subclavian arteries. Just distal to the coarctation the descending aorta is locally dilated (post-stenotic dilatation). The left ventricle is hypertrophied and sometimes also the left atrium. To circumvent the constriction a collateral circulation develops chiefly through the internal mammary and thyrocervical and intercostal arteries, the blood flowing retrogradely in the intercostal arteries to supply the descending aorta. The intercostal arteries become tortuous and their upward convexities erode the inferior surface of the ribs producing notching in their middle and posterior parts (*Figure 4.49a*). This rib notching usually occurs on both sides but it may be confined to one side. If it is on the right side only the

coarctation may be proximal to or at the origin of the left subclavian artery or in the artery itself, so that no collateral circulation develops on the left side. If an aberrant right subclavian artery is present arising distal to the left subclavian artery and the coarctation is between the origins of these arteries then rib notching will occur only on the left side. This is because the aberrant right subclavian artery will carry the collateral circulation by retrograde flow into the descending aorta. Absence of rib notching does not exclude a coarctation, and its frequency diminishes with decreasing age, being uncommon below the age of 8 years.

On the postero-anterior view the heart may be normal in size or slightly enlarged with rounded lower left heart border and depression of the apex due to the left ventricular hypertrophy. The ascending aorta may be prominent. In the upper part of the left mediastinal border there will be two bulges, the upper one due to the dilated left subclavian artery and the lower to the post-stenotic dilatation of the descending aorta (*Figure 4.49b*). The power part of the descending aorta may be prominent too because of displacement to the left side. Rib notching may be seen on the under-surface of the rib in their posterior parts and it occurs most frequently from the fourth to the tenth ribs. It must be remembered that an appearance of notching on the under-surface of ribs is a normal anatomical feature on the medial 1—1½ inches of the ribs; pathological notching therefore must be lateral to this. An anteroposterior film, especially with the tube angled upwards a few degrees, may show the rib notching better than a postero-anterior film. On barium swallow the oesophagus will

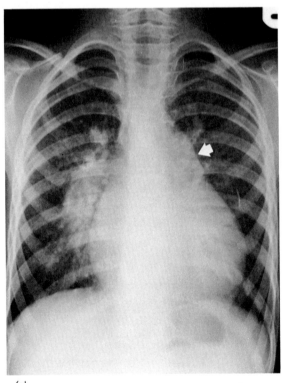

(a)

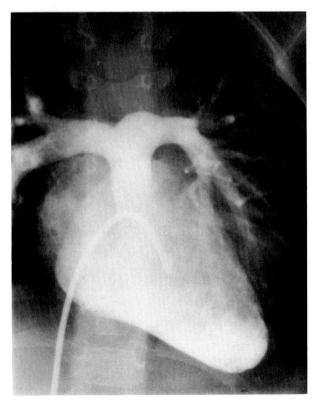

(b)

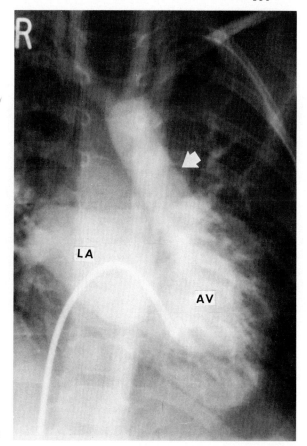

(c)

Figure 4.47. Corrected (L-loop) Transposition of the Great Arteries. (a) Plain chest film showing cardiac enlargement and a smooth convexity of the upper part of the left heart border due to the abnormally placed ascending aorta (arrowed). The pulmonary arteries are dilated because of shunting through a ventricular septal defect. (b) Angiocardiogram of another case. Contrast medium injected through a catheter placed in the venous ventricle. This resembles a left ventricle with smooth walls and an acorn shape. Filling of the centrally placed pulmonary artery occurs from it. (c) Later stage of the same angiocardiogram as in (b). The contrast medium has outlined the left atrium (LA) and arterial ventricle (AV) from which the ascending aorta (arrowed) arises on the left side. The descending aorta lies to the left of the spine

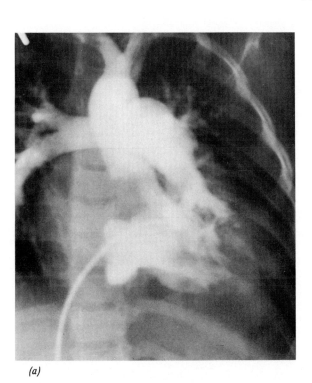

(a)

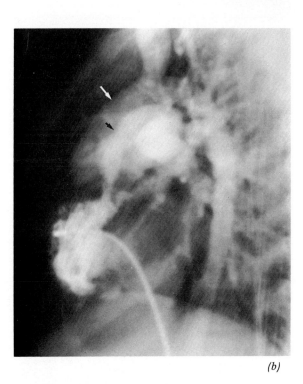

(b)

Figure 4.48. Double Outlet Right Ventricle: Right ventricular angiocardiogram showing the aorta and pulmonary artery arising from the right ventricle. The aorta (white arrow) lies anterior to the pulmonary artery (black arrow). (a) Anteroposterior projection. (b) Lateral projection

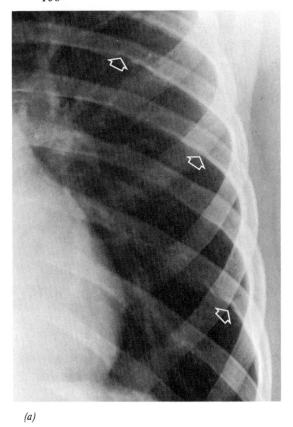

(a)

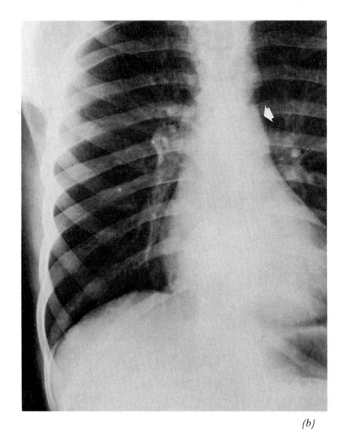

(b)

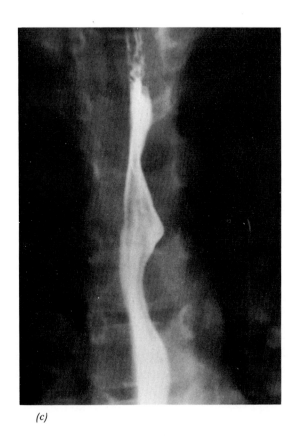

(c)

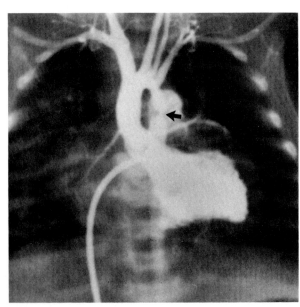

(d)

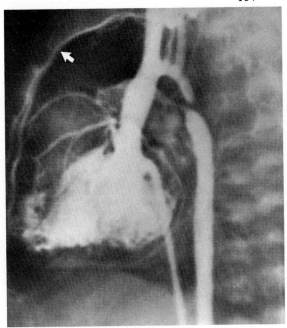

Figure 4.49. Coarctation of the Aorta: (a) 'Rib notching' on the underside of several ribs (arrowed) in a case of coarctation of the aorta. (b) Postero-anterior view of the chest showing a normal sized heart with a rounded lower left heart border. There is a convexity of the left border of the descending aorta below the prominent aortic 'knuckle', due to the post-stenotic dilatation (arrowed). Rib notching is present but is not very marked. (c) A barium swallow in the same case as in (b) showing a well marked 'reversed three' impression on the left border of the oesophagus due to the aortic arch above and the post-stenotic dilatation below the site of the coarctation. (d) Left ventricular angiocardiogram in the anteroposterior projection. The site of the coarctation is well shown (arrowed). The aortic arch proximal to it is narrowed and an anomalous left carotid artery arises from it. (e) Lateral projection of the same case. The collateral circulation through the internal mammary arteries (arrowed) is well shown

be displaced to the right and forwards just below arch level by the post-stenotic dilatation (*Figure 4.49c*). In the left anterior oblique position the left ventricular hypertrophy will be well shown. Rib notching is not a specific sign of coarctation of the aorta. It may be seen in generalized neurofibromatosis, pulseless disease, angiomatous malformations of the chest wall, pulmonary atresia, subclavian artery obstruction, after Blalock—Taussig operations for Fallot's tetralogy and sometimes after thoracotomy.

Cardiac catheterization

Normal pressures are shown on the right side of the heart. Elevated systolic pressures will be shown in the left ventricle and ascending aorta.

Thoracic aortography

In most patients it is not necessary to perform contrast medium examinations to diagnose coarctation of the aorta, but a good demonstration of the exact anatomy can be of great assistance to the surgeon.

COARCTATION IN INFANTS AND YOUNG CHILDREN

In the authors' experience the adult type of coarctation is seen most commonly in young children and its angiographic features are similar to those already described. If the coarctation lies proximal to the ductus, it may be short segment in type; or it may be long segment, extending up as far as the left subclavian artery or sometimes as far as the innominate artery. Often the two types are combined with a hypoplastic arch and a short segment coarctation at its distal end. In extreme cases the aortic lumen may be completely occluded. In this case the distal part of the aorta is supplied by the right ventricle through a large patent ductus arteriosus. Infants with coarctation frequently present with large hearts and signs of left heart failure.

Plain film

There are usually no specific radiological features of coarctation in infancy, the radiograph showing a large heart with dilated pulmonary arteries and enlargement of the left atrium and left ventricle.

Cardiac catheterization

The catheter takes the normal course through the right heart and the right ventricular pulmonary artery and pulmonary wedge pressures are elevated.

Angiocardiography

In young infants it is adequate to perform biplane right ventricular angiocardiography or pulmonary arteriography, prolonging the examination long enough to show the aorta. No further descriptions of the signs of coarctation of the aorta are necessary (*see above*). Occasionally the arch is hypoplastic but no localized coarctation is present (*Figure 4.50*).

Interruption of the aortic arch

This condition consists of absence or atresia of the aortic arch occurring at one of several locations and they have been classified by Abbott (1936) and Celoria and Patton (1959). The interruption may occur either beyond the left subclavian artery, beyond the

158

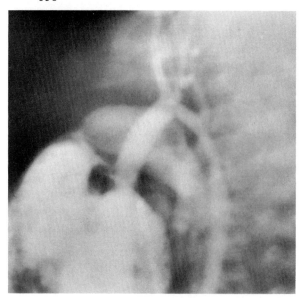

Figure 4.50. Hypoplastic Aortic Arch: Angiocardiogram in the lateral projection. The whole of the aortic arch is narrowed but no localized stenosis is present

left common carotid artery or beyond the innominate artery, the distal part being supplied by a small or large patent ductus arteriosus. Any of these types may have an associated aberrant right subclavian artery and additional congenital heart lesions are common (Roberts *et al.*, 1962) such as transposition of the great arteries, aortic stenosis, ventricular septal defect, etc.

Though interruption of the aortic arch would seem to have an obvious relationship to coarctation of the aorta, its behaviour is quite different and most patients die within a month. There are no specific radiological appearances on the plain film, only cardiac enlargement and dilated pulmonary arteries. Right heart catheterization is necessary to identify any associated cardiac abnormalities. Though aortography is the examination of choice to demonstrate the lesion, it can usually be shown well by right ventricular angiocardiography or pulmonary arteriography. The appearances of the aortic arch will vary according to the site of the interruption as described above. The defect in the aortic arch is best shown on the lateral view.

Congenital anomalies of the aortic arch and its branches

Congenital anomalies of the aortic arch and its branches are many and varied and they cannot be dealt with fully here. A recent very full description of them has been given by Kerley and Pattinson (1972), to which the reader is referred. The majority of these anomalies are asymptomatic and incidental findings on routine chest radiographs but, because of their importance in differential diagnosis, they deserve description. Others are associated with congenital heart disease, particularly cyanotic heart disease. A small proportion cause symptoms of tracheo-oesophageal compression by the production of a vascular ring around the oesophagus and trachea. The ring is composed of differing elements

which are combinations of the aorta, one of its branches, the ligamentum arteriosum or patent ductus arteriosus, or the pulmonary artery. Symptoms arising from the vascular ring, particularly stridor, usually occur in infancy.

DOUBLE AORTIC ARCH

Two main groups of double aortic arch are described. In each the ascending aorta is normal above the valve but superiorly it divides into two branches, a right and a left, which pass on their respective sides of the trachea and oesophagus to unite behind to form the descending aorta. Thus a ring is formed around the trachea and oesophagus. These rings may be divided into two groups (Kerley and Pattinson, 1972).

In group I, which accounts for 65 per cent of cases the descending aorta is left-sided and the ductus arteriosus is also left-sided. In group II the descending aorta is right-sided and the ductus arteriosus is left-sided. In either group, the components of the double aortic arch on the left and right side may be equal in size or one may be smaller. In addition part of one arch may be absent or represented by a fibrous band. Usually each arch gives origin to the common carotid and sub-clavian arteries of its own side.

Plain film

There are no specific plain film features in childhood. On barium swallow the appearances differ according to the type of abnormality present, the size of each arch and the severity of the constriction. The two arches produce smooth short segment indentations on the walls of the oesophagus, usually at slightly different levels, the right one most frequently being slightly higher. The oesophagus is thus narrowed. The part of the arch behind the oesophagus causes a deep impression and displaces the oesophagus forwards. Sometimes the posterior impression may be oblique. The anterior surface of the oesophagus may be impressed by the trachea. The trachea will also be indented at the same level in front and on each side and this is best shown by tracheography after the instillation of contrast medium such as propyliodone (*Figure 4.51*).

Thoracic aortography or right ventricular angiocardiography

Thoracic aortography or right ventricular angiocardiography will show the anatomical type of double aortic arch present, the former giving the best demonstration and the latter being easier to perform.

RIGHT-SIDED AORTIC ARCH

Right-sided aortic arch can be classified into two groups. In group 1 the descending aorta is on the right of the spine and in group 2 it is on the left of the spine. Each group is divided into subgroups according to the origin of the branches and the origin and course of the ligamentum arteriosum or patent ductus arteriosus. (Klinkhammer, 1969). Certain types may produce

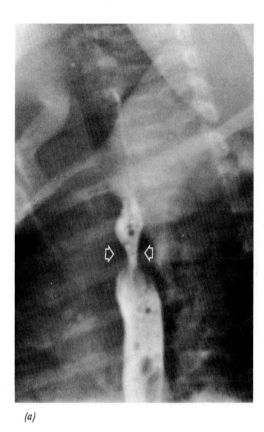

(a)

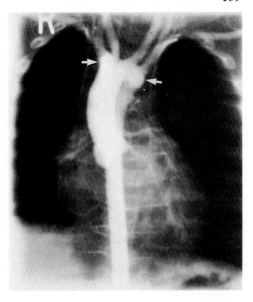

(b)

Figure 4.51. Double Aortic Arch: (a) Barium swallow in the left anterior oblique projection showing anterior and posterior indentations on the oesophagus due to the two aortic arches which form a vascular ring around it (arrowed). (b) Aorto-cardiogram of another case in the anteroposterior projection showing the ascending aorta dividing into right and left branches (arrowed) which unite posteriorly to form the descending aorta

tracheo-oesophageal compression by forming a ring through the ligamentum arteriosum or left subclavian artery and therefore cause symptoms. The radiological appearances have already been described (*see* page 158). In children the arch does not usually indent the trachea but displaces it to the left. It will indent the oesophagus and this will be seen on barium swallow. If one type of deformity (Type IA3) is present and is associated with a left-sided ligamentum arteriosum the trachea may be indented on the right side; a deep short segment impression may also be produced on its left border and on the left and posterior aspect of the oesophagus by the ligamentum arteriosum.

In association with another type of right-sided aortic arch (Type 2B) the left subclavian artery is the last branch to arise from the arch; it passes upwards from left to right behind the oesophagus producing an oblique impression on it as well as a posterior indentation.

ANOMALOUS ORIGINS OF THE BRANCHES OF THE AORTIC ARCH

Many variations of the origins of the branches of the aorta have been described. Most of them will be encountered as incidental findings on angiocardiography and aortography and they are usually symptomless. Every artery can be involved. They may, however, be of importance when catheterization of the arch is being undertaken. It is impossible to describe all of them here but a few will be selected.

Anomalous right innominate artery

The innominate artery arises more distally than normal and therefore passes upwards and to the right in front of the trachea, producing an indentation on its anterior surface at about aortic arch level. The indentation is best seen on tracheography.

Anomalous left common carotid artery

The left common carotid artery may arise more proximally than normal. It passes upwards from right to left indenting the front of the trachea.

Anomalous right subclavian artery

This is the anomaly most frequently seen radiologically. The artery arises as the last branch from a left-sided aortic arch distal to the origin of the left subclavian artery. The artery passes upward and to the right to reach the anterior surface of the first right rib: 80 per cent pass behind the oesophagus, 15 per cent between the trachea and oesophagus and 5 per cent in front of the trachea. Anomalous right subclavian artery may coexist with various other conditions and it is particularly frequent with Fallot's tetralogy. It also occurs occasionally with coarctation of the aorta and with oesophageal atresia.

160

Radiological appearances

There are no characteristic plain film appearances. On barium swallow an oblique indentation is visible at or below aortic arch level, running upwards from left to right. If the origin of the artery is dilated, there may be an indentation of the left side as well. In the oblique and lateral views the impression is seen to be posterior in position and the oesophagus is displaced anteriorly. If the artery passes in front of the oesophagus, a similar impression may be produced with an anterior indentation. The artery will be readily recognized at aortography or angiocardiography.

Anomalous pulmonary venous drainage

Anomalous pulmonary venous drainage comprises a group of conditions in which there are defects in the normal connection of the pulmonary veins into the left atrium. The anomalous veins either drain directly into the right atrium or into the systemic veins. If all the pulmonary veins are involved the condition is referred to as total anomalous pulmonary venous drainage. If only one or some pulmonary veins are involved the condition is referred to as partial anomalous pulmonary venous drainage. If all the veins of one lung are involved the condition is known as hemi-anomalous pulmonary venous drainage. If total anomalous pulmonary venous drainage is present, all the systemic and pulmonary venous blood mixes completely in the right atrium and a communication between the right and left heart is essential. This communication is usually at atrial level. If the pulmonary venous drainage is partial, an atrial septal defect is not essential but is frequently present.

TOTAL ANOMALOUS PULMONARY VENOUS DRAINAGE

This may be at either supracardiac, cardiac or infracardiac levels but mixed types occur (Darling *et al.*, 1957). In the supracardiac type all the right pulmonary veins drain into a common trunk which passes behind the left atrium. It is joined by the veins from the left lung and it drains on the left side of the mediastinum into a persistent left cardinal vein which enters the left innominate vein. From thence, the blood passes down the right superior vena cava into the right atrium, part going through the atrial septal defect into the left atrium and part into the right atrium and right ventricle to the lungs. The greater part goes into the right side of the heart because of the relatively low peripheral resistance of the lungs. In the cardiac type all the veins usually drain into the coronary sinus and thence into the right atrium or directly into the right atrium. In the infracardiac type the usual drainage is by a common trunk into the portal vein but it may be into the inferior vena cava (*Figure 4.53*) and in the mixed types a combination of these three anomalies exists.

Plain film

In the supracardiac type, the dilated venae cavae produce widening of the mediastinum which is usually symmetrical. This gives the cardiovascular shadow a 'figure-of-eight' or 'cottage loaf' appearance on the postero-anterior view (*Figure 4.52a*). The heart is enlarged and has an outline similar to that of an atrial septal defect. The pulmonary arteries are dilated and on the lateral view the dilated superior venae cavae are seen as an opacity in the middle mediastinum.

In total anomalous pulmonary venous drainage into the portal vein the appearances are different. There is obstruction to the venous return and the heart is not enlarged. The pulmonary vascular markings are prominent and they have a spotty or mottled appearance; in addition the translucency of the lung may be impaired by oedema.

Cardiac catheterization

The catheter may pass from the right atrium up the right superior vena cava into the left innominate vein and then down the left superior vena cava and into the right common venous trunk. From this oxygenated blood is aspirated; the saturation of the blood in the right atrium is higher than normal. The catheter may pass across the atrial septal defect into the left atrium.

Right ventricular angiocardiography

The right ventricular angiocardiograph will outline the bilateral venous drainage into the common trunk. The contrast medium continues up the left superior vena cava and down the right superior vena cava in the later stages of the examination (*Figure 4.52b* and *c*). If the drainage occurs into the portal vein a common trunk is formed by the right and left pulmonary veins and this passes through the diaphragm to fill the portal vein.

PARTIAL ANOMALOUS PULMONARY VENOUS DRAINAGE

This is more common from the right than the left lung and it usually occurs in conjunction with an atrial septal defect.

The anomalous vein may drain into the right atrium, superior vena cava or inferior vena cava. If the veins drain into the superior vena cava they do so from the upper and middle lobes. If they drain into the inferior vena cava most of the right lung veins converge into a single vein which enters the inferior vena cava. Sometimes the right lung is hypoplastic and the heart is displaced to the right. This is known as the scimitar syndrome (*Figure 4.5a*) and is associated with anomalous arterial supply from the aorta to the lower part of the lung (Neill, 1956). When the partial anomalous venous drainage occurs on the left side the draining vein usually passes up to the left innominate vein (*Figure 4.54b*).

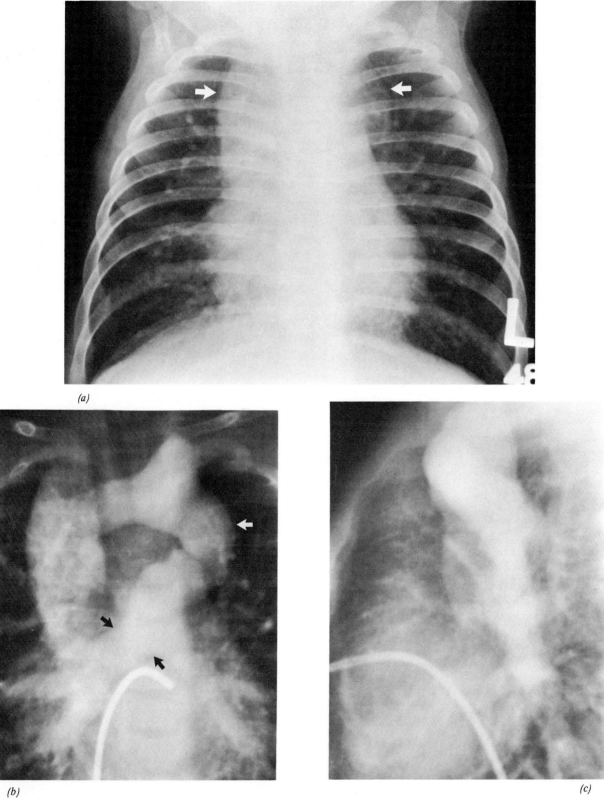

(a)

(b)   (c)

Figure 4.52. Total Anomalous Pulmonary Venous Drainage Supracardiac Type: (a) Plain film showing convex widening of the upper mediastinal borders on both sides due to the right and left superior venae cavae (arrowed) which carry the blood return from the lungs through the anomalous pulmonary veins. This appearance constitutes the 'cottage loaf' heart. (b) Angiocardiogram in the antero-posterior projection. The pulmonary veins are shown uniting to form a common pulmonary trunk (black arrows), whence the contrast medium passes through the left superior vena cava (white arrow), innominate vein and right superior vena cava to enter the right atrium (c) Lateral projection of the same case

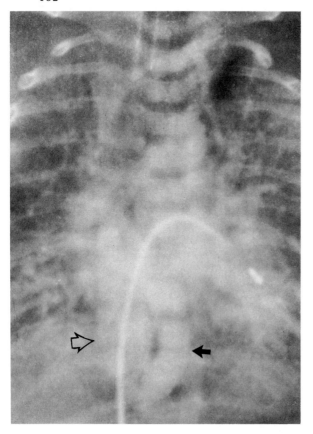

Figure 4.53. Total Anomalous Pulmonary Venous Drainage Infracardiac Type.: Right ventricular angiocardiogram in another case in which the common pulmonary vein (black arrow) is shown to pass downwards through the diaphragm to enter the inferior vena cava (white arrow)

ACQUIRED HEART DISEASE

Endocardial fibro-elastosis

This is the commonest form of endomyocardial disease in children and it particularly affects infants. Some of the patients rapidly go into heart failure and may die quickly, but most survive with treatment and outgrow it.

The left side of the heart is usually involved. It occurs either as an isolated disease or, more commonly, superimposed on congenital heart lesions such as aortic stenosis, aortic atresia and coarctation of the aorta. It must be distinguished from the form of endomyocardial fibrosis described by Davies (1948) which occurs in Africans and in which characteristically fibrosis of the endocardium of the outflow tracts of both ventricles develops.

Endocardial fibro-elastosis is considered to be fairly common and its pathogenesis is unknown. The condition leads to hyperplasia of the endocardium with surface deposits of fibrin. It affects the left ventricle and atrium, occasionally the right side also and it involves the aortic and mitral valves. It produces a smooth glistening appearance in the lining of the chambers which are described as being like porcelain, (Hudson, 1965). The valves become regurgitant or stenotic. In the majority of patients the left ventricle is dilated but there is a contracted type in which the ventricle is normal or small in size (Edwards, 1960).

Plain film

There is marked general cardiac enlargement, the enlargement predominantly affecting the left ventricle and left atrium. The pulmonary arteries may be normal, but if left heart failure has developed the pulmonary arteries are dilated. On screening the heart pulsations are considerably reduced.

Angiocardigraphy

In the dilated type, the left ventricle is large with thickened walls and there is little change in the size of the ventricle between systole and diastole. The left atrium is also enlarged and may contract vigorously, but contrast medium lingers for a long time in the left ventricle. The other cardiac chambers may be normal in size.

In the contracted type the left ventricle is small or normal in size and it contracts poorly. The left atrium, however, is enlarged and the pulmonary arteries may be dilated.

Myocarditis (excluding rheumatic fever and tropical disease)

Myocarditis may be due to specific causes such as known infectious diseases (bacterial, viral, rickettsial, fungal or protozoan) or there may be no identifiable cause.

Plain film

Often the abnormal draining veins can be seen on the plain radiograph and by their direction the abnormal connections can be inferred (*Figure 4.54a*). They are better shown by tomography.

Cardiac catheterization

The catheter tip may well enter the anomalous vein from which highly saturated blood is aspirated and the shunt into the superior vena cava or inferior vena cava will be identified.

Anomalous connection of inferior vena cava to the left atrium

This anomaly occasionally occurs and it is usually associated with complicated intracardiac lesions. It can be shown by injecting contrast medium into the inferior vena cava through the cardiac catheter.

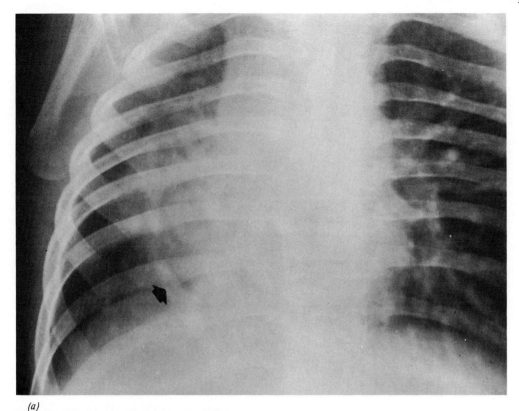

(a)

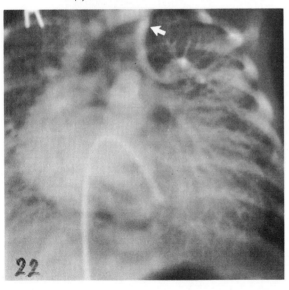

(b)

Figure 4.54. Partial Anomalous Pulmonary Venous Drainage: (a) Plain film of the chest in which the heart is displaced to the right and there is a curvilinear opacity (arrowed) due to an anomalous vein draining blood from the right lung into the inferior vena cava ('scimitar syndrome'). The vessels of the left lung are increased in calibre due to the left-to-right shunt and consequent pleonaemia (b) Angiocardiogram of another case in which an anomalous pulmonary vein (arrowed) drains the blood from the left upper lobe into the innominate vein

Plain film

The heart is usually generally enlarged and the enlargement increases as the disease progresses. On recovery the heart will decrease in size and may assume normal appearances. If left heart failure is present the pulmonary arteries will be dilated. The heart outline may be sharply defined because of the lack of contractility and this is particularly evident on screening. The myocarditis may be complicated by a pericardial effusion and there may also be pleural effusions.

Cardiac catheterization and angiocardiography are not usually performed in patients with myocarditis.

Glycogen storage disease of the heart

In glycogen storage disease of the heart there is diffuse myocardial hypertrophy produced by deficiency in the activity of a single enzyme. The glycogen content of the heart muscle is greatly increased as is that in other organs, such as the liver, and the muscles. The hypertrophy involves the whole of the ventricular muscle but it is most marked in the left ventricle and the interventricular septum is frequently very thick.

Plain film

There is a generalized cardiomegaly, usually to a considerable degree. Both ventricles are enlarged and the cardiac apex points downwards to the left. The atria are enlarged and the pulmonary arteries dilated if left heart failure is present.

Angiocardiography

There are few reports of angiocardiography in these patients and no useful description can be given here.

Cardiomyopathy associated with muscular and neuromuscular dystrophy

In Friedreich's ataxia the heart may be enlarged with hypertrophy of both ventricles and mural thrombi. In progressive muscular dystrophy severe degenerative changes occur in the cardiac muscle as well as in the skeletal muscle. The muscles are fatty and fibrous. In both these conditions there may be cardiac enlargement and dilated pulmonary arteries from left heart failure.

RHEUMATIC FEVER AND RHEUMATIC HEART DISEASE

In the Western world rheumatic fever is now less common than it was before the Second World War, but in some other parts of the world this falling trend has not been evident. The age range for first attacks is commonly 5 and 15 years of age. Detectable carditis in first attacks of rheumatic fever occurs in 45–55 per cent of patients (Keith *et al.*, 1967). Involvement of the myocardium may lead to dilatation of the mitral and aortic valve rings and valvular regurgitation. If the myocardial changes are extensive congestive heart failure may develop. On the other hand the myocarditis may be mild and go undiagnosed. Endocarditis may lead to acute valvulitis with diffuse involvement of the valve leading to small discrete nodules which develop along the line of impact of the valve cusps. These changes lead to valvular regurgitation and in association with the myocardial changes, ventricular dilatation. Pericarditis also occurs and it is always accompanied by some underlying myocarditis. Detectable pericardial effusion may develop. Chorea now only occurs in about 15 per cent of patients with rheumatic fever.

Plain film

In the acute stages of rheumatic fever, radiological examination is seldom undertaken and contributes little. The heart may be generally enlarged due to myocarditis. The enlargement is generalized, some of which may be due to pericardial effusion. At this stage the heart outline may be globular in shape. If screening is done pulsations of the heart borders will be noticed to be diminished and in these patients the heart appears to be flabby, altering its shape more than normal with respiration. If heart failure is present, the pulmonary arteries will be dilated. Opacities in the mid and lower zones of the lungs may be due to rheumatic pneumonia. It is usually some years before radiological signs of chronic rheumatic heart disease are established, if at all.

Chronic mitral valve lesions

When the mitral valve is involved, the left atrium enlarges producing widening of the waist of the heart and a bulge on the left heart border just below the main pulmonary artery segment due to enlargement of the atrial appendage. On the right side overlying the upper part of the right atrial shadow a double density may be identified due to the left atrial enlargement. In the lateral and right anterior oblique views, backward displacement of the oesophagus due to the enlargement of the left atrium will be seen. The left atrium seldom enlarges in childhood sufficiently to compress the left main bronchus. Calcification in the mitral valve is also most unlikely to develop in childhood. As the obstruction to the left side increases pulmonary venous and arterial hypertension will develop and the radiological signs of these states have already been described (*see* page 115). If significant mitral regurgitation is present, the left ventricle will be enlarged with elongation of the left heart border and depression of the apex.

Aortic valve lesions

In aortic valve lesions the left ventricle will be enlarged and the ascending aorta may be prominent and pulsatile.

In the authors' experience it has not proved necessary to perform angiocardiography on these patients in childhood in view of the reluctance of surgeons to operate in this age group.

PERICARDIAL DISEASE

Pericardial effusion

Pericardial effusion may be either acute, subacute or chronic. If the fluid develops rapidly it will embarrass the heart function with the development of tamponade. On the other hand, if the fluid develops slowly large quantities can collect before cardiac embarrassment is caused.

Pericardial effusion may be due to septic infections, viral infections, trauma, including surgery, rheumatic fever, tuberculosis, myxoedema and hypoproteinaemia.

With small effusions the heart outline and size may not be altered from normal. In adults 300–400 ml must accumulate before radiological detection is possible. When a pericardial effusion first develops the fluid will gravitate to the most dependent part of the pericardial sac, which is postero-inferior in the erect position. Accumulation at this site will cause obliteration of the

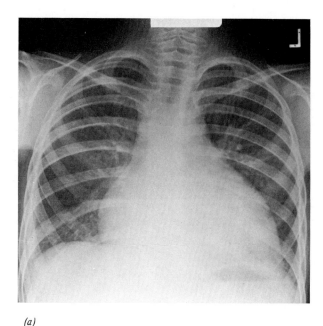

(a)

Figure 4.55. Pericardial Effusion: (a) Plain chest film taken erect. The heart outline is enlarged with convex lateral borders but with an acute right cardiophrenic angle. The pulmonary arteries are of normal size and the aorta is small and does not project to form a knuckle. (b) Right ventricular angiogram showing considerable elevation of the right ventricular lumen (arrowed) by the pericardial fluid beneath it

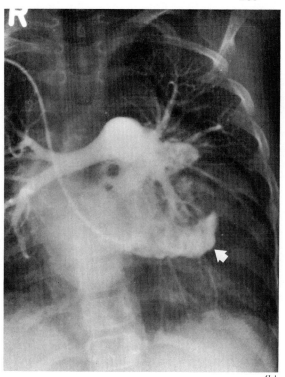

(b)

inferior vena caval shadow on the lateral view and posterior bulging of the inferior heart outline. As further fluid collects, it extends up laterally, flattening the borders and increasing the size of the heart shadow (*Figure 4.55a*). If at this stage the patient is x-rayed lying down, the heart outline will change to a globular shape as the fluid runs up towards the great vessels. As further fluid collects, the heart outline will increase in size and its lateral walls will be convex. The cardiophrenic angles remain acute. On screening, the cardiac pulsations will be very poor or absent and, because of this lack of pulsation, the heart shadow on the radiograph will appear to be unusually sharp. The pulmonary arteries are normal in size and not dilated. On barium swallow the oesophagus is displaced backwards and to the right over the full length of the heart shadow. The aortic knuckle is small. Rarely the effusion on resolution may become encysted by pericardial adhesions. This usually happens on the right side where a localized broad-based bulge, inseparable from the heart outline, is shown against the right atrial border.

Cardiac catheterization and angiocardiography

If a catheter is passed into the right atrium its tip will be held up before it reaches the lateral edge of the right atrial shadow. The normal right atrial wall radiographically is thin and measures between 1 and 2 millimetres in thickness. Similarly, if contrast medium is injected down the catheter, or run in through the superior vena cava, the space between the right limiting edge of the contrast medium and the radiological soft-tissue shadow of the right heart wall will be wider than normal. This is due to the fluid separating the right edge

of the pericardium from the lateral wall of the right atrium. Right or left ventricular angiocardiography will show the ventricle raised from the inferior surface of the heart by the pericardial effusion (*Figure 4.55b*). In addition, ultrasound cardiography is an excellent non-invasive technique for detecting pericardial effusion (Feigenbaum *et al.*, 1965).

Chronic constrictive pericarditis

Chronic constrictive pericarditis is rare in the first decade but increases in frequency in the second decade. Roshe and Shumaker (1959) collected 68 cases from the literature in which pericardectomy had been performed before the age of 15 years, 65 for constrictive pericarditis.

In this condition the pericardium is thickened and two layers adhere together. It leads to interference with myocardial function. Its aetiology is varied and includes tuberculosis, coxsackie virus infection and trauma though in many cases no cause can be found.

Plain film

The heart may be enlarged but frequently is not. The borders of the heart are straightened. The notch between the superior vena cava and the right atrium and also the indentation between the main pulmonary artery and the left heart border disappear, giving the heart a triangular or globular outline. The constriction may extrude the left atrium posteriorly and this will show by backward deflection of the oesophagus on barium swallow. Pericardial calcification is rare in children. Pulsations are seen to be reduced on all heart borders on screening.

Congenital defects of the pericardium

Congenital defects in the pericardium are not common. The pericardium may be completely absent or the defect may be localized. Chang and Leigh (1961) collected 108 cases from the literature, 67 per cent of which were on the left side, the lesion being three times more common in males than in females.

Plain film

The main pulmonary artery and its left branch may be herniated through the defect producing a very prominent pulmonary artery segment. Sometimes the left atrial appendage herniates through a defect and it then becomes very prominent as a bulge below the main pulmonary artery segment. Occasionally the whole heart may be shifted to the left without tracheal displacement but with exaggeration of the aortic knuckle, pulmonary artery and left heart border and a deep notch between pulmonary artery and aorta.

If a pneumothorax is produced artificially or pathologically, air will pass through a pericardial defect and produce a pneumopericardium.

Right ventricular angiocardiography

Right ventricular angiocardiography will show the abnormal positions of the pulmonary artery and left atrium and will also exclude other causes for the abnormal cardiac outline.

Congenital pericardial cysts and diverticula

Congenital pericardial cysts are benign. They are usually smooth in outline and are most frequently related to the lower right heart border. They may not communicate with the pericardial sac. These lesions will form a bulge on the right heart border.

CARDIAC TUMOURS

Cardiac tumours are rare but are now being diagnosed more frequently. They may be histologically benign or malignant and the malignant ones may be primary or secondary, the latter being more common. In children secondary tumours are most frequently due to leukaemia or lymphoma and the pericardium is usually involved.

The benign tumours seen in children are rhabdomyoma, fibroma, myxoma and teratoma.

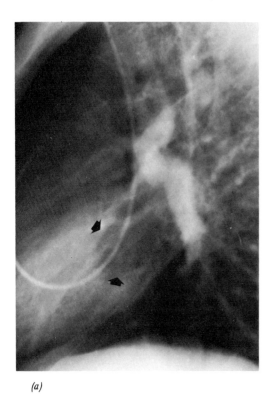
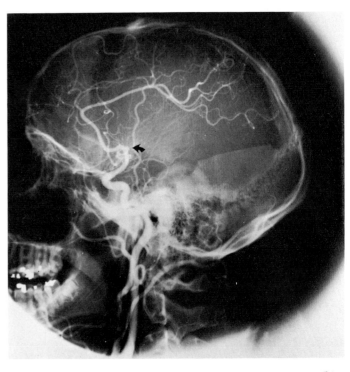

(a) *(b)*

Figure 4.56. Left Atrial Myxoma: (a) Angiocardiogram in which contrast medium injected from the pulmonary artery fills the left atrium. The tumour is shown as a translucency (arrowed) projecting through the mitral valve. (b) Carotid arteriogram in the same case showing complete occlusion of the middle cerebral artery by a fragment of tumour which has broken off, forming an embolus (arrowed)

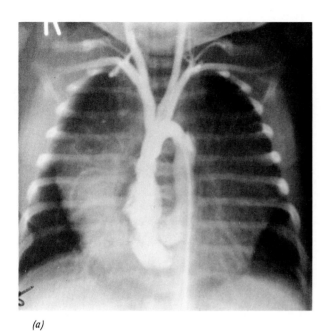

(a)

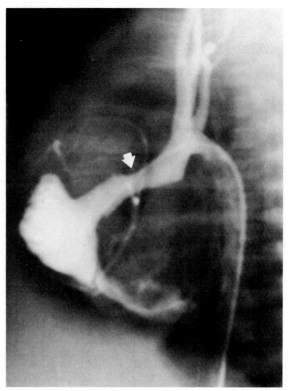

(b)

Figure 4.57. Malignant Tumour of the Heart: Left ventricular angiocardiogram showing narrowing of the cavity of the ventricle by a large filling defect. The outline of the heart by contrast is markedly increased in size. The ascending aorta (arrowed) is narrowed and displaced forwards together with the left ventricle. (a) Anteroposterior projection. (b) Lateral projection

Rhabdomyoma

Rhabdomyoma of the heart is a very rare tumour. In more than half the cases the tumour is associated with tuberose sclerosis and this association is almost the rule in older children. On plain films the heart is usually enlarged. On angiocardiography there will be a constant filling defect in one of the cardiac chambers, if the tumour is large enough to encroach upon the cavity of the chamber.

Fibroma

Most cardiac fibromas have been reported in children. The plain film may show either diffuse cardiomegaly or left ventricular enlargement.

Myxoma

Myxoma is the commonest primary cardiac tumour in adults but it is rare in childhood (McWhirter and Tetteh-Lartey, 1974). Three quarters occur in the left atrium (Pritchard, 1951) and the rest in the right atrium. The tumour is a gelatinuous, friable mass arising from the interatrial septum which may produce intermittent obstruction of the atrioventricular valves, particularly the mitral valve. It produces arterial emboli (Figure 4.56b), intermittent cardiac murmurs and systemic reactions such as fever, raised sedimentation rate, leucocytosis and increase in the plasma globulins.

Plain film

Plain films may show some enlargement of the left atrium or right atrium according to the site of the tumour in the respective atria. Multiple echoes behind the anterior cusp of the mitral valve and interference with the valve cusp movement will reveal the presence of a left atrial myxoma on ultrasoundcardiography (Rees et al., 1973).

Angiocardiography and pulmonary arteriography

If the tumour is in the right atrium, angiocardiography with injection of the contrast medium into the right atrium or one of the venae cavae will show a filling defect in the atrium produced by the tumour, and it may herniate into the right ventricle during atrial systole.

If the tumour is in the left atrium, pulmonary arteriography, continued until the left side of the heart is filled, will show a filling defect in the left atrium (Figure 4.56a). This may herniate into the mitral valve orifice on atrial systole and return to the left atrium on ventricular systole.

Malignant tumours

Primary malignant cardiac tumours are very rare in childhood. They are most frequently sarcomatous but malignant teratomas and primary mesotheliomas have been reported. The neoplasm may be extracardiac, intracardiac or both (*Figure 4.57*). They lead to the development of pericardial effusion and heart failure.

Secondary malignant tumours usually present with pericardial effusion.

HEART DISEASE IN COLLAGEN DISEASES

In recent years there have been considerable advances in the understanding of the so-called collagen diseases. There may be involvement of the heart and this is manifested most often as endocarditis, myocarditis or pericardial effusion. These cardiac lesions are seen in rheumatoid arthritis, systemic lupus erythematosus, dermatomyositis, periarteritis nodosa and diffuse scleroderma, all of which may occur in children though most of them are relatively rare (Walker, 1968).

REFERENCES

Abbott, M. E. S. (1936). *Atlas of Congenital Cardiac Disease*. New York; *American Heart Association*

Al Omeri, M., Bishop, M., Oakley, C., Bentall, H. H. and Cleland, W. P. (1965). 'The mitral valve in endocardial cushion defects.' *Br. Heart J.* **27**, 161

Bahnson, H. T. and Williams, G. R. (1957). 'Physiologic considerations of intracardiac pressures following closure of atrial septal defects.' *J. thorac. Surg.* **34**, 685

Baron, M. G., Wolf, B. S., Steinfeld, L. and Van Mierop, L. H. S. (1964). 'Endocardial cushion defects. Specific diagnosis by Angiocardiography.' *Am. J. Cardiol.* **13**, 162

Besterman, E. (1961). 'Atrial septal defect with pulmonary hypertension.' *Br. Heart J.* **23**, 587

Bonham-Carter, R. E. (1973). 'Progress in the treatment of transposition of the great arteries.' *Br. Heart J.* **35**, 573

Braunwald, E., Goldblatt, A., Aygen, M. M. Rockoff, S. D. and Morrow, A. G. (1963). 'Congenital aortic stenosis. I. Clinical and haemodynamic findings – 100 patients. II. Surgical treatment and the results of operation.' *Circulation* **27**, 426

Bruins, C. and Dekker, A. (1968). In *Paediatric Cardiology*, p. 649. Ed. by Hamish Watson. London; Lloyd Luke

Campbell, M. and Deuchar, D. C. (1967). 'Absent inferior vena cava, symmetrical liver, splenic agenesis and situs inversus and their embryology.' *Br. Heart J.* **29**, 268

Celoria, G. C. and Patton, R. B. (1959). 'Congenital absence of the aortic arch.' *Am. Heart J.* **58**, 407

Champsaur, G., Trusler, G. A. and Mustard, W. T. (1973). 'Congenital discrete subvalvar aortic stenosis. Surgical experience and long-term follow-up in 20 paediatric patients.' *Br. Heart J.* **35**, 443

Chang, C. H. and Leigh, T. F. (1961). 'Congenital partial defect of the pericardium associated with herniation of the left atrial appendage.' *Am. J. Roentgl.* **86**, 517

Cleland, W., Goodwin, J., McDonald, L. and Ross, D. (1969). *Medical and Surgical Cardiology*, p. 585. Oxford and Edinburgh; Blackwell Scientific Publications

Collett, R. W. and Edwards, J. E. (1949). 'Persistent truncus arteriosus: a classification according to anatomic types.' *Surg. Clins N. Am.* **29**, 1245

Darling, R. C., Rothney, W. B. and Craig, J. M. (1957). 'Total pulmonary venous drainage into the right side of the heart: Report of 17 autopsied cases not associated with other major cardiovascular anomalies.' *Lab. Invest.* **6**, 44

Davies, J. N. P. (1948). 'Endocardial fibrosis in Africans.' *E. Afr. med. J.* **25**, 10

Edwards, J. E. (1953). 'Pathological features of Ebstein's malformation of the tricuspid valve.' *Proc. Mayo Clin.* **28**, 89

– (1960). 'Congenital malformations: E. Malformations of endocardium and pericardium. In *Pathology of the Heart* (2nd edn), p. 417. Ed. by S. E. Gould. Springfield; Thomas Thomas

Feigenbaum, H., Waldhausen, J. A. and Hyde, L. P. (1965). 'Ultrasound diagnosis of pericardial effusion.' *J. Am. med. Ass.* **191**, 711

Gasul, B. M. (1966). In *Heart Disease in Children*, p. 1. Ed. by Gasul, B. M., Arcilla, R. A. and Lev, M. J. B. Philadelphia; Lippincott

– Arcilla, R. A. and Lev, M. J. B. (1966). *Heart Disease in Children*. Philadelphia; Lippincott

Gerbode, F., Hultgren, H., Melrose, D. and Osborn, J. (1958). 'Syndrome of left ventricular–right atrial shunt: successful surgical repair of defect in five cases with observation of bradycardia on closure.' *Ann. Surg.* **148**, 433

Godman, M. J. and Kidd, B. S. L. (1974). 'Echocardiography in the evaluation of the newborn infant with cyanotic congenital heart disease.' *Br. Heart J.* **36**, 396

Goldberg, S. J., Allen, H. D. and Sahn, D. J. (1975). *Pediatric and Adolescent Echocardiography–A Handbook*. Chicago; Year Book Medical Publishers

Goodwin, J. F., Hollman, A., Cleland, W. P. and Teare, D. (1960). 'Obstructive cardiomyopathy simulating aortic stenosis.' *Br. Heart J.* **22**, 403

– and Oakley, C. M. (1972). 'The cardiomyopathies.' *Br. Heart J.* **34**, 545

Greenwold, W. E., DuShane, J. W., Burchell, H. B., Bruwer, A. and Edwards J. E. (1956). 'Congenital pulmonary atresia with ventricular septum; two anatomic types.' (Abstr.) *Circulation* **14**, 945

Hudson, R. E. B. (1965). *Cardiovascular Pathology*. Baltimore; Williams & Wilkins

Jönsson, G. and Saltzman, G. F. (1952). 'Infundibulum of patent ductus arteriosus–a diagnostic sign in conventional roentgenograms.' *Acta Radiol.* **38**, 8

Jordan, S. C. and Scott, O. (1973). *Heart Disease in Paediatrics*, p. 76. London; Butterworths

Kaplan. S. (1968). In *Pediatric Cardiology*. Ed. by Hamish Watson. London; Lloyd Luke

Keith, J. D., Rowe, R. D. and Vlad, P. (1967). *Heart Disease in Infancy and Childhood* (2nd ed). New York; Macmillan

Kerley, P. (1933). 'Radiology in heart disease.' *Br. med. J.* **2**, 594

Kerley, P. and Pattinson, N. (1972). In *A Textbook of X-Ray Diagnosis*, Ed. by Shanks, S. C. and Kerley, P. Vol. II pp. 358–421. Philadelphia; Saunders

Klinkhamer, A. C. (1969). *Esophagography in Anomalies of the Aortic Arch System*. Amsterdam; Excerpta Medica

Lev, M. (1952). Pathologic anatomy and interrelationship of hypoplasia of the aortic tract complexes.' *Lab. Invest.* **1**, 61

McWhirter, W. R. and Tetteh-Lartey, E. V. (1974). 'A case of atrial myxoma.' *Br. Heart J.* **36**, 839

Mitchell, S. C. (1957). 'The ductus arteriosus in the neonatal period.' *J. Pediat.* **51**, 12

Moller, J. H., Amplatz, K. and Wolfson, J. (1971). 'Malrotation of the bowel in patients with congenital heart disease associated with splenic anomalies.' *Radiology* **99**, 393

Moss. A. J., Emmanouilides, G. and Duffie, E. R., Jr. (1963). 'Closure of the ductus arteriosus in the newborn infant.' *Pediatrics, Springfield* **32**, 25

Neill, C. A. (1956). 'Development of the pulmonary veins with reference to the embryology of anomalies of pulmonary venous return.' *Pediatrics, Springfield* **18**, 880

Neufeld, H. N., Du Shane, J. W., Wood, E. H., Kirklin, J. W. and Edwards, J. E. (1961). 'Origin of both great vessels from the right ventricle. I. without pulmonary stenosis.' *Circulation* **23**, 399

— Lester, R. G., Adams, P., Anderson, R. C., Lillehei, C. W. and Edwards, J. E. (1962). 'Aorticopulmonary septal defect.' *Am. J. Cardiol.* **9,** 12

Noonan, J. A. and Nadas, A. S. (1958). 'The hypoplastic left heart syndrome: an analysis of 101 cases.' *Pediat. Clin. N. Am.* **5,** 1029

Paul, M. H., van Praagh, S. and van Praagh, R. (1968). In *Pediatric Cardiology*, 576. Ed. by Hamish Watson London; Lloyd Luke

Perou, M. L. (1961). 'Congenital supravalvular aortic stenosis. A morphological study with attempt at classification.' *Archs Path.* **71,** 453

Pitt, D. B. (1957). 'Congenital malformations and maternal rubella.' *Med. J. Aust.* **1,** 233

Prichard, R. W. (1951). 'Tumours of the heart; review of the subject and report of one hundred and fifty cases.' *Archs Path.* **51,** 98

Rashkind, W. J. and Miller, W. W. (1965). 'Creation of an atrial septal defect without thoracotomy: a palliative approach to complete transposition of the great vessels.' (Abstract, Oct., 1965). Section on cardiology, American Academy of Pediatrics

— (1966) 'Creation of an atrial septal defect without thoracotomy. A palliative approach to complete transposition of the great arteries.' *J. Am. med. Ass.* **196,** 991

Rastelli, G-C., Kirlin, J. W. and Titus, J. L. (1966). 'Anatomic observations on complete form of persistent common atrioventricular canal with special reference to atrioventricular valves.' *Mayo Clin. Proc.* **41,** 296

Rees, J. Russell, Ross. F. G. M. and Keen, G. (1973). 'Lentiginosis and left atrial myxoma.' *Br. Heart J.* **5,** 874

Roberts, W. C., Morrow, A. G. and Braunwald, E. (1962). 'Complete interruption of the aortic arch circulation.' *Circulation* **26,** 39

Roshe, J. and Shumacker, H. B. Jr. (1959). 'Pericardiectomy for chronic cardiac tamponade in children.' *Surgery* **46,** 1152

Sabiston, D. C., Jr., Neill, C. A. and Taussig, H. B. (1960). 'The direction of blood flow in anomalous left coronary artery arising from the pulmonary artery.' *Circulation* **22,** 591

Sakakibara, S. and Konno, S. (1962). 'Congenital aneurysm of sinus of Valsalva: anatomy and classification. *Am. Heart J.* **63,** 405

Somerville, J. (1966). 'Masked cor triatriatum.' *Br. Heart J.* **28,** 55

Steiner, R. E. (1972). In *A Textbook of X-Ray Diagnosis,* Vol. II, p. 107. Ed. by Shanks, S. C. and Kerley, P. London; H. K. Lewis

Strickland, B. A. (1972). In *A Textbook of X-ray Diagnosis*, Vol. II, p. 215. Ed. by Shanks, S. C. and Kerley, P. London; H. K. Lewis

Talner, N. S., Stern, A. M. and Sloan, H. E., Jr. (1961). 'Congenital mitral insufficiency.' *Circulation* **23,** 339

Van Praagh, R., Ongley, P. A. and Swan, H. J. C. (1964). 'Anatomic types of single or common ventricle in man. Morphologic and geometric aspects of 60 necropsied cases.' *Am. J. Cardiol.* **13,** 367

— van Praagh, S., Vlad, P. and Keith, J. D. (1965). 'Diagnosis of the anatomic types of single or common ventricle.' *Am. J. Cardiol.* **15,** 345

Walker, C. H. M. (1968). In *Pediatric Cardiology,* p. 824–825. Ed. by Hamish Watson. London; Lloyd Luke.

Watson, Hamish (1974). 'Natural history of Ebstein's anomaly of tricuspid valve in childhood and adolescence. An international co-operative study of 505 cases.' *Br. Heart J.* **36,** 417

Wood, P. H. (1956). *Disease of the Heart and Circulation* (2nd edn), p. 380. London; Eyre & Spottiswoode

5 RESPIRATORY SYSTEM

METHODS

GENERAL CONSIDERATIONS

The radiological examination of the lungs in the older child presents no special problems and the methods used are the same as in adults. In infants and children up to the age of 5 or 6 years, however, difficulties may arise owing to the child's inability to co-operate fully with the radiographer, especially as regards arrest of respiration and timing of the radiographic exposure in relation to respiratory phase. These disadvantages may be to some extent offset by the use of modern apparatus which is capable of accurately timed and very short exposures, and full advantage should be taken of such facilities in the diagnosis of respiratory disease in the newborn or very young infant. The practice of examining these infants with mobile apparatus in the wards on the grounds that they are too ill to be moved to the radiological department is to be discouraged. Although modern mobile units are capable of very much better performance than was the case 10 or 20 years ago, they still fall short of that which can be achieved by the larger fixed units. The fact that ill babies can be moved with little distress in a modern incubator is also a strong argument in favour of this policy, because the disturbance to the infant by the examination will be no greater, perhaps less, than would be the case if a mobile unit were used.

RADIOGRAPHIC TECHNIQUE

The positioning of infants for radiography of the chest should be such as to ensure the minimum disturbance and, for this reason, the present authors prefer to take films in an anteroposterior projection with the child supine, except when it is important to show air—fluid levels. It is considered that the greater ease and rapidity of the procedure and the avoidance of crying and movement offset the loss of the advantages obtained by the use of the erect position. However, in cases in whom the erect position is considered essential, the use of an efficient device for immobilizing and maintaining the infant in the desired position may be a great help. Faulty positioning, particularly rotation, may make interpretation difficult. The presence or absence of rotation may be easily assessed by noting the position of the clavicles or of the anterior ends of the ribs relative to the spine. While it is desirable to obtain chest films that are exposed in full inspiration, it is often difficult to ensure this in all cases (see Figure 5.1). It may be better to expose the film during quiet respiration, in order to avoid making an exposure during forced expiration. This latter event is very liable to happen if the infant is crying because during crying short inspiratory gasps are separated by relatively long periods of expiration against an almost closed glottis. Recently it has become possible to trigger a radiographic exposure at the height of inspiration by the use of a thermocouple which is sensitive to changes of temperature caused by the flow of air in and out of the mouth during respiration. In our experience, however, the increase in the accuracy of timing has been insufficient to compensate for the disturbance to the child and the prolonged time needed for the examination, which is inevitable when using such a device. In spite of the small increase in radiation involved, it has been our practice in neonates to obtain two anteroposterior films, with a slight difference in penetration, and a lateral film in most cases. This routine very often makes assessment of minimal changes easier because the chances of a well-timed film are increased, and, although a lateral film in many cases may contribute little, it may be of value in conditions such as pneumomediastinum and when the thymus is prominent.

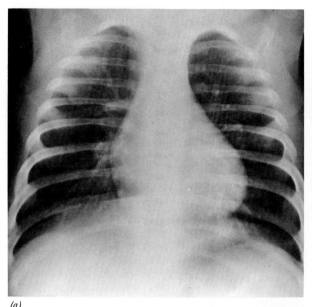

(a)

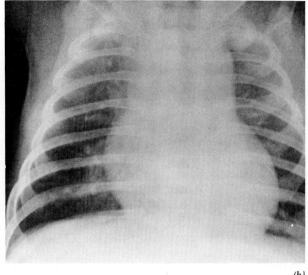

(b)

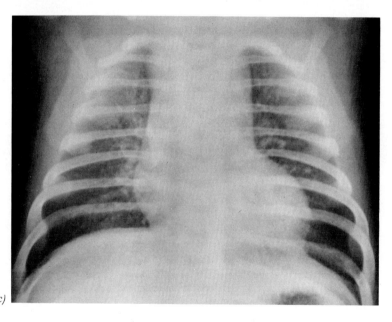

(c)

Figure 5.1. Effect of Respiratory Phase on the Appearances of the Lungs, Heart and Mediastinum of the Normal Infant: (a) Film taken in full inspiration. The mediastinum is relatively narrow and the diaphragm low in position. The lungs occupy a large proportion of the thorax. (b) Anteroposterior chest film of a normal infant taken during the expiratory phase of the respiratory cycle. The shadow of the heart and upper mediastinum are wide and the lung fields appear disproportionately small with a prominent vascular pattern. (c) Film taken in a neutral phase. The lung mediastinum is still wide, due in part to the thymus, and the vascular pattern of the lungs is still prominent

FLUOROSCOPY

Fluoroscopic examination is seldom required. However, it may be very useful, if not essential, in certain situations. For example in some cases of airway obstruction, it may be uncertain whether a difference in translucency between the two lung fields indicates obstructive emphysema on one side or collapse on the other. In such cases, observation of mediastinal movement on respiration may provide the clue as to which is the diseased side since the inspiratory shift is always towards this side.

Combined with a barium swallow, screening may help in the detection of vascular rings or other causes of compression of the trachea or pharynx and, in cases of recurrent pneumonia, may indicate the presence of a hiatus hernia or other predisposing cause of inhalational pneumonitis.

In any case in which the possibility of obstruction of the upper respiratory tract is present, a lateral and sometimes an anteroposterior radiograph of the neck, taken to show the details of the soft tissues, is an essential part of the examination (*see Figure 5.34a*). This technique will often enable a diagnosis to be made without the need for more complex investigations. The use of contrast media may be dangerous in such cases and should be used, if at all, with discretion.

MAGNIFICATION TECHNIQUE

The difficulty in resolving small structures such as the finer vascular branches or thickened interlobular septa and distinguishing these from miliary or lobular areas of consolidation or collapse has prompted the use of a magnification technique. However, this method cannot be carried out unless an x-ray tube with a suitably small focal spot is available.

TOMOGRAPHY

As in adults, tomography may, in certain limited situations, be a useful adjunct to plain radiography. Its main disadvantage in the young child is that adequate blurring of unwanted shadows outside the plane under investigation necessarily demands a relatively long exposure time. However, with sedation when necessary, useful results may almost always be obtained, particularly in localizing mediastinal opacities and in separating structures within the lungs from one another.

BRONCHOGRAPHY

Although bronchography has been employed less frequently in children during the last few years, coincident with the decline in the frequency of bronchiectasis, it is still an examination which is required in a diminishing number of conditions. It is very important to ensure that an adequate period of postural drainage and percussion therapy is arranged before the investigation in order to empty the bronchial tree of retained secretions as far as is possible. If this is not done, inadequate filling of the bronchial tree results, and the investigation may need to be repeated.

It is our practice to carry out bronchography under a general anaesthetic, because it is considered to be safer, more convenient and less frightening for the child than the use of local anaesthesia as in adults. The nature of the anaesthetic used is a matter for the anaesthetist to decide, but the safety and variety of modern anaesthetic agents makes the use of inflammable gases such as ether an unjustifiable risk. Some controversy exists over whether muscle relaxants should be used to arrest respiration during the injection of the contrast medium. The present authors incline to the view that the negative pressure produced during inspiration constitutes the most effective force in securing filling of the more peripheral parts of the bronchial tree. Gravity, as employed in posturing the patient at the time of injection, is mainly of use in transporting the contrast medium to the orifice of the main segmental bronchi and is thus an important means of ensuring that each segment is properly filled. Squeezing the bag to apply positive pressure to the gas within the airway in order to blow the contrast medium into the smaller bronchi is often ineffective as may be observed on fluoroscopy. It results mainly in a to and fro oscillation of the contrast medium and if this is the only force applied, filling of the bronchi will be patchy.

Dionosil Aqueous is the type of contrast medium preferred. With the use of general anaesthesia, its mildly irritating effect on the upper respiratory tract is not an important disadvantage. In our experience its viscosity is higher than is desirable, but this can be improved by storing it in a refrigerator prior to the examination. For each lung $1-1.5$ ml per year of age is used and normally both lungs are examined one after the other on the same occasion, thus avoiding two general anaesthetics.

The two posterior oblique projections are the most useful for delineating the whole of the bronchial tree, supplemented by an anteroposterior and occasionally by a lateral view as needed (*Figure 5.2*). Selective catheterization of particular segmental bronchi is not essential. We have no experience of the use of transcricoid catheterization of the trachea by the Seldinger technique as described by Sargent and Turner (1968), but it would seem likely that such a method would have advantages over transglottic catheterization, if for any reason general anaesthesia was inadvisable or unavailable.

LUNG SCANNING

Scintiscanning of the lungs is now a well established technique. It involves the use of a radioactive isotope of iodine incorporated in a macro-aggregated albumen the molecular size of which enables it to be arrested temporarily in the pulmonary capillaries. This is basically a test of pulmonary perfusion and has attained a place in the investigation of such conditions as pulmonary infarction in adults. Its application in children has not, as yet, become widespread. Its use in such conditions as hypoplasia of the lungs or pulmonary artery, and in long-standing chronic infections has been suggested (Pendarvis and Swischuk, 1969). The presence of persistent perfusion defects which are unsuspected on plain radiographs may be disclosed. However, the authors feel that an increase in the scope of this investigation in children may have to wait until isotopes with a shorter half life than iodine 131, such as indium 113, and more rapid scanning devices, such as the gamma camera are more widely available. Even so, it is likely to be more useful as a correlative study than as a primary diagnostic procedure though in certain cases it could replace bronchography or arteriography.

THE THYMUS

The presence of the normal thymus as a visible opacity in the mediastinum of infants during the first year of life may be a source of difficulty in interpretation. This is mainly because of its variable size, not only in different children, but from time to time in the same child. In addition, the size, shape and visibility may vary. Classically the thymus is shown as a triangular opacity in the upper mediastinum, and its basal angle projects laterally over the lung field to give the well recognized 'sail shadow (*Figures 5.3a* and *9.34*). However, it may also present a lateral convexity, merging into the lower mediastinal border with no 'angle' at all, or it may merely lead to a general widening of the mediastinum. A lateral view is very useful in confirming that the upper part of the retrosternal space is occupied by the thymus. Its lower border is usually clearly identified. The presence of the thymus and the necessity for its positive identification constitutes one of the arguments in favour of 'routine' lateral views in all small infants.

The frequency with which the thymus is visible radiologically in the neonate has been stated to be 50 per cent on the basis of a survey of over 1000 chest films (Tausend and Stern, 1965). It was unilateral in two-thirds of the cases, and it occurred more commonly on the right side than on the left (4:1). There is no doubt

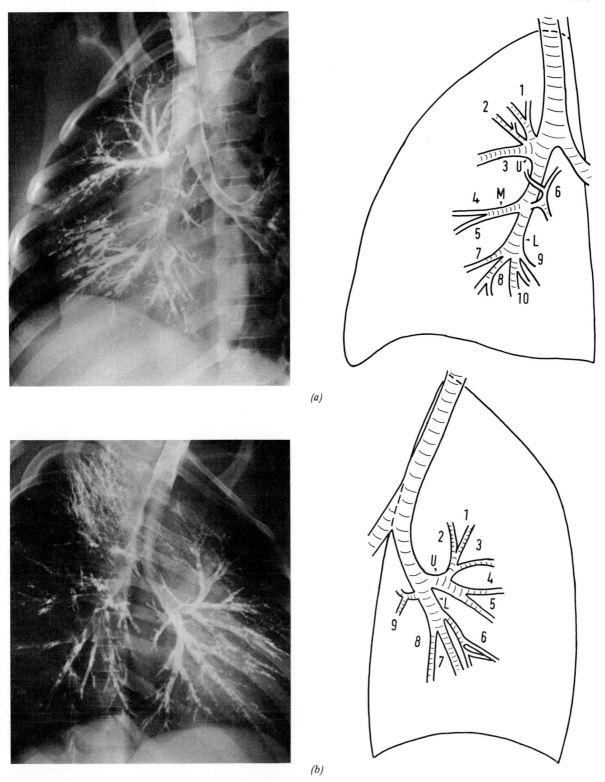

(a)

(b)

Figure 5.2. Normal Bronchograms: (a) Right posterior oblique projection showing the bronchial tree of the right lung. Main lobar bronchi: U–upper lobe, M–middle lobe, L–lower lobe. Segmental bronchi: 1–posterior, 2–apical, 3–anterior (upper lobe); 4–lateral, 5–medial (middle lobe); 6–apical, 7–anterior basal, 8–middle basal, 9–posterior basal, 10–medial basal or cardiac (lower lobe). (b) Left posterior oblique view showing the bronchial tree of the left lung. Main lobar bronchi: U–upper lobe, L–lower lobe. Segmental bronchi: 1–apical, 2–posterior 3–anterior 4–superior lingular, 5–inferior lingular (upper lobe); 6–anterior basal, 7–middle basal, 8–posterior basal, 9–apical (lower lobe). The smooth regular tapering of the segmental bronchi and their branches from their origin to the periphery of the lung is an important sign that they are free from disease (either stenosis or bronchiectasis)

174

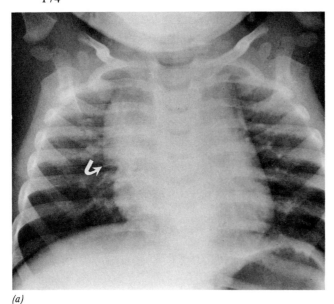
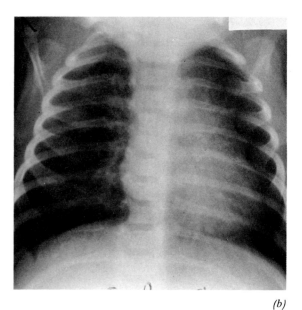

(a)   *(b)*

Figure 5.3. Thymus: (a) An anteroposterior view of a normal infant's chest. The thymus projects over the medial part of the right lung field, where its inferolateral angle is well defined (arrowed) and constitutes the 'sail shadow'. (b) The thymus projecting over the left lung field has a scalloped outline due to indentation by the costochondral junctions

that the sail sign is of great help in identifying an opacity as thymus, though it is only present in a minority of cases. A scalloped outline of the lateral border of the thymus may also be a helpful sign in identification. It is due to indentation by the costochondral junctions (*Figure 5.3b*) and this feature thus confirms that the opacity lies in the anterior mediastinum. The thymus may also be outlined by air in the mediastinum, either as a result of spontaneous pneumomediastinum in airway obstruction, or when introduced deliberately by injection from the neck to produce a mediastinogram. In such cases, the thymic lobes may be displaced laterally and upwards over the upper zones of the lungs, resulting in a striking exaggeration of the sail shadow which has been graphically described as the 'spinnaker sign'(*see Figure 5.32c*).

In many cases, doubt may arise as to whether an opacity projecting from the upper mediastinum is due to a normal thymus or to disease. The chief conditions to be differentiated from a thymic shadow are segmental consolidation of the upper lobes, loculated effusions, cysts and tumours of the mediastinum, distension of the superior vena cava on one or both sides as is found in some cases of total anomalous pulmonary venous drainage, and the presence of aberrant thyroid tissue in the retrosternal space. In such cases, tomography may be of help in differentiating these lesions. A careful search for other confirmatory abnormalities, such as splaying or erosion of ribs or enlargement of intervertebral foramina, may sometimes point to the diagnosis. If the case is still obscure, it has been suggested that the administration of steroids should be considered (Caffey and Silbey, 1960). This will have the effect of causing a temporary reduction in the size of the thymus and allow any other opacity to be shown unobscured. They suggest 10 mg of prednisolone or 8 mg of triamcinolone daily for 7—14 days for this purpose. The maximum effect is produced in about 7 days and a return to normal in the size of the thymus will occur in from 7 to 14 days after

stopping the steroids. Care should obviously be taken that this method is not used in any case in whom the use of steroids is undesirable on other grounds.

Mediastinography by the injection of air into the neck has been advocated for the elucidation of mediastinal tumours in general and could presumably be of use in outlining the thymus also. The radiological appearances in cases of thymic tumours are discussed elsewhere (*see* page 202).

CONGENITAL ABNORMALITIES

PULMONARY AGENESIS AND HYPOPLASIA

These conditions are not common, but they are important to recognize, because unilateral agenesis may render a child liable to serious respiratory embarrassment if a foreign body is aspirated into the bronchial tree or if a pleural effusion or pneumothorax develops (Davidson, 1956). Hypoplasia of the lung, while not potentially so dangerous a condition, may result in arterial unsaturation owing to perfusion of underventilated areas of lung.

Diagnosis of agenesis is not usually difficult because the whole hemithorax is opaque apart from a tendency for the normal lung to herniate across the midline. In the earliest stages the thorax is symmetrical with equal movement of the two sides, but there is progressive flattening of the abnormal hemithorax and narrowing of its rib spaces. The extent of the agenesis may vary from complete absence of both lung and bronchi to an abnormal bronchial tree with some non-functioning lung tissue. Bronchography may demonstrate the extent and calibre of any bronchi that are present, but it is not without danger to the patient, and therefore, it should only be embarked upon if the information likely to be obtained is essential for the management of the child. Hypoplasia of one or both lungs will result in a reduction in volume and diminished aeration of the abnormal areas, again without any concomitant asymmetry of the thorax in the initial stages. In the course of time a hypoplastic lung may become emphysematous and will then appear on the radiograph to be of normal volume but it will be hypertranslucent. Hypoplasia should be suspected in cases in which there is mediastinal displacement with no apparent cause to account for it (*Figure 5.4a*). Bronchography and pulmonary arteriography will demonstrate accurately the extent of the condition (*Figure 5.4b*) and the latter examination is in some respects a safer procedure.

Associated congenital abnormalities are common and may be of assistance in suggesting the diagnosis. Such abnormalities are hemivertebrae, rib anomalies and the absent radius syndrome, usually on the ipsilateral side. Diaphragmatic hernia or eventration is also commonly associated with some degree of hypoplasia of the lungs, usually on the side of the hernia, but occasionally on the contralateral side. This may lead to a very confusing radiological appearance, and there may be difficulty in localizing the defect in the diaphragm. Atresias and malrotation of the intestinal tract, genito-urinary and cardiac anomalies, especially patent ductus arteriosus or a septal defect, may also be present.

ABNORMALITIES OF SEGMENTATION OF THE LUNG; SEQUESTRATED LOBE

Abnormal pleural fissures are common and usually of little significance. An azygos lobe, in which a medial portion of the apical segment of the right upper lobe is separated by the displaced azygos vein from the rest of the right upper lobe, may occasionally present a bizarre radiological appearance, especially when the lobe is consolidated or an effusion within the abnormal fissure is present.

In the case of a sequestrated lobe or segment, in addition to the abnormal segmentation of the lung, the blood supply to it is abnormal, arising from a systemic artery, usually the aorta or one of its branches. These sequestrated segments can be intralobar, when they lie within the visceral pleura, or extralobar when they are situated outside the pleura or even below the diaphragm (Kohler, 1969).

The sequestrated lung segment presents radiologically as a well defined opacity which may be rounded or lobulated in outline and which is frequently cystic. It is characteristically in a lower zone and is most common on the left side (*Figures 5.5* and *5.6*). Extrathoracic lesions may present as a paraspinal mass below the diaphragm. Although tomography will often help to delineate the mass and reveal an air-containing cavity within an apparently solid lesion, aortography is the method of choice because it will establish the diagnosis unequivocally by direct demonstration of the abnormal blood supply. This information is not just of academic interest; it is essential in order to provide exact knowledge of the anatomy of the arterial connections which will help in planning the operative approach (*Figure 5.7*). Thoracic aortography is preferable to angiocardiography, because the filling of the pulmonary arteries and veins produced in the latter examination may obscure the arteries supplying the sequestrated segment. Differentiation from arteriovenous malformations will also be possible by either investigation. Bronchography will not demonstrate the abnormal segment directly but may sometimes be of use in revealing bronchiectasis of adjacent lung segments which may be present as a hitherto unrecognized complication.

ARTERIOVENOUS FISTULA AND OTHER VASCULAR ABNORMALITIES

Arteriovenous fistulae are of two types: communications between branches of the pulmonary arteries and the pulmonary veins, and communications between systemic arteries and pulmonary veins. The former result in a

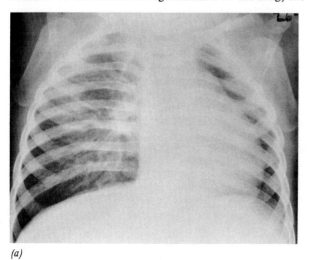

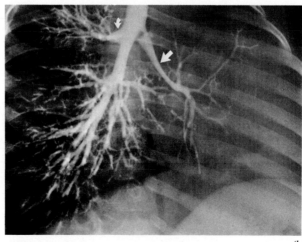

(a)   *(b)*

Figure 5.4. Pulmonary Agenesis and Hypoplasia: (a) Anteroposterior film of chest showing displacement of the heart to the left and a reduction in the size of the left lung. (b) Bronchogram showing hypoplasia of the left lower lobe bronchus (straight arrow) and of its peripheral branches which are much reduced in calibre and in number. The left upper lobe bronchus is absent. The bronchial tree on the right side is normal except for the upper lobe bronchus (curved arrow) which originates abnormally close to the carina and supplies a smaller area of lung than usual

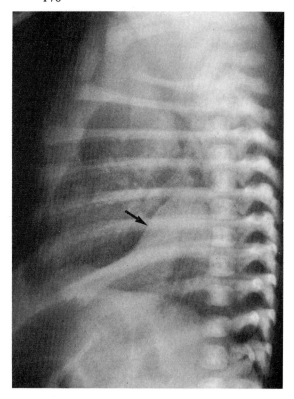

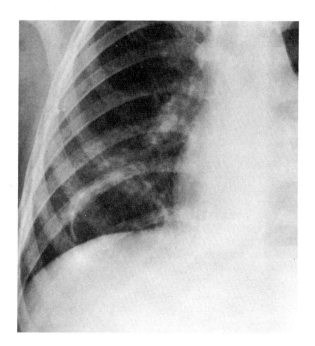

Figure 5.6. Sequestrated Segment of Lung (cystic type): A thin-walled 'cyst' in the right lower zone constitutes the sequestrated segment

Figure 5.5. Sequestrated Segment of Lung (solid type): This appears as a uniform triangular opacity overlying part of the lower lobe, with a well-defined anterior border (arrowed)

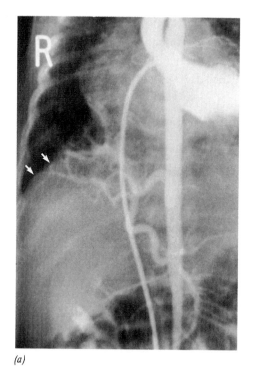

(a)

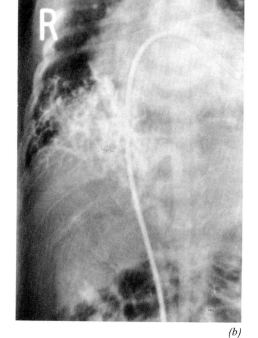

(b)

Figure 5.7. Sequestrated Segment of Lung: Left ventricular angiocardiogram showing a segment at the base of the right lung supplied by two arteries arising from the aorta, one of which traverses the diaphragm (arrowed). (a) Early film. (b) Later film in which the smaller vessels within the abnormal segment are opacified

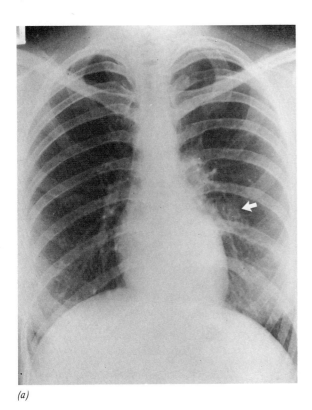

(a)

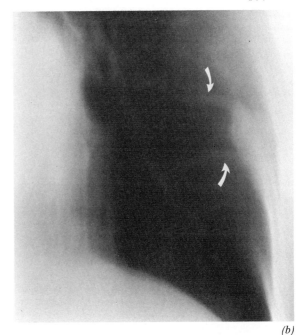

(b)

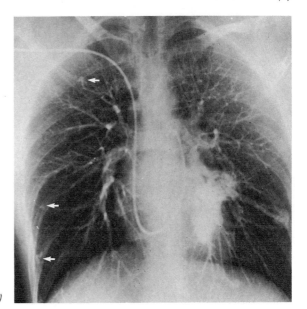

(c)

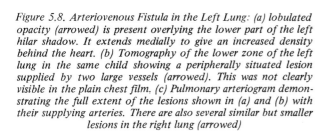

Figure 5.8. Arteriovenous Fistula in the Left Lung: (a) lobulated opacity (arrowed) is present overlying the lower part of the left hilar shadow. It extends medially to give an increased density behind the heart. (b) Tomography of the lower zone of the left lung in the same child showing a peripherally situated lesion supplied by two large vessels (arrowed). This was not clearly visible in the plain chest film. (c) Pulmonary arteriogram demonstrating the full extent of the lesions shown in (a) and (b) with their supplying arteries. There are also several similar but smaller lesions in the right lung (arrowed)

right-to-left shunt, and there may be cyanosis and poly-cythaemia, the latter in a left-to-right shunt with no serious symptoms. Multiple arteriovenous fistulae are common, occurring in over a third of all cases (Good, 1961). There is an association with similar lesions elsewhere in the body. These may occur locally in the nasal cavity, in the alimentary tract or all over the body as in the rare condition of hereditary haemorrhagic telangiectasia (Osler—Weber disease).

A rounded or lobulated opacity is present on the plain chest film in almost all cases but the chest radiograph may be normal if the fistula is small. Often there are linear shadows connecting the opacity with the hilum and left atrium; these represent the arterial supply and venous drainage. Pulsation may be detected on

fluoroscopy and rib notching may be present if the fistula occurs between the intercostal arteries and pulmonary veins. The heart may be enlarged when the volume of the shunt is very great. Tomography will often give a clearer picture of the vessels supplying and draining the lesion and it will help in differentiating arteriovenous fistulae from anomalous pulmonary veins because with the latter there will be no arterial element. Pulmonary arteriography, angiocardiography or thoracic arteriography will demonstrate the lesions and their blood supply directly, according to their site, and pulmonary arteriography is especially important in revealing multiple lesions which may be unsuspected from the plain film (*Figure 5.8*).

Radiographic examination of the chest in relatives of

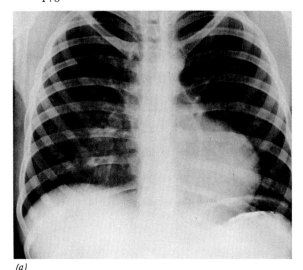

(a)

Figure 5.9. Sternal Depression: (a) Postero-anterior view of chest in a child with sternal depression. The heart is displaced to the left with elevation of its apex and there is a relative loss of translucency in the medial part of the right lower zone due to the obliquity of the chest wall caused by the inward displacement of the lower end of the sternum. The anterior ends of the ribs slope more steeply downwards than usual. (b) Lateral view of the sternum showing its abnormal position. The distance between it and the spine is reduced, leading to the lateral displacement of the heart

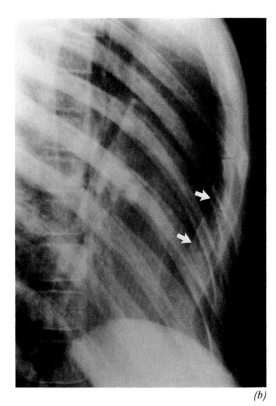

(b)

cases of Osler–Weber disease is valuable because this condition is inherited as an autosomal dominant and unrecognized fistulae may be revealed (Jeresaty *et al.*, 1966).

STERNAL DEPRESSION

Sternal depression, a permanent deformity of the thorax in which the lower part of the sternum is displaced backwards relative to the rest of the anterior chest wall, may be a source of disability serious enough to warrant surgical intervention. More often it will present as an incidental finding in an individual whose chest is being x-rayed for some other condition. The radiological features will vary with the severity of the depression. It may flatten the heart and displace it to the left. It may also produce an opacity in the medial part of the right lower zone which may be misinterpreted as evidence of pleural or pulmonary disease. Lateral or oblique views will readily reveal the true nature of the condition. It should be appreciated that in small infants with airway obstruction, a very considerable degree of sternal recession may occur, and what may appear on a lateral chest film to be a severe deformity may rapidly revert to normal following relief of the pulmonary condition.

RESPIRATORY DISTRESS IN THE NEWBORN INFANT

Respiratory distress in the neonatal period may result from many different causes, some of which may give rise to characteristic radiological appearances. The response to treatment or the natural evolution of these conditions

may be followed with accuracy by serial examinations. However, the two most important functions of radiology in neonatal respiratory distress are: first, to differentiate intrathoracic disease from intracranial damage which may produce similar clinical effects due to interference with the function of the respiratory centres; and second, to demonstrate the presence of pneumothorax or pneumomediastinum because in such cases the use of artificial ventilation may be dangerous (Steiner, 1954).

HYALINE MEMBRANE DISEASE

Although it is true that a similar clinical picture can result from many causes, there is no doubt that there exists a specific entity with characteristic clinical, radiological and pathological features which has been designated as the respiratory distress syndrome or hyaline membrane disease. This condition is related to prematurity and to anoxia in the perinatal period. Other factors concerned in its development are maternal diabetes or delivery by Caesarean section.

The pathological changes found in the lungs of these infants are patchy alveolar collapse with dilatation of the respiratory bronchioles and alveolar ducts, combined with the presence of hyaline membrane, which lines the walls of the alveoli and is predominantly composed of fibrin. It has been suggested that this material originates from the pulmonary capillaries which become abnormally permeable as a result of intra-uterine anoxia. Pulmonary immaturity has also been postulated as a factor in the origin of this condition because expansion of the alveolar spaces during the initiation of respiration at birth is more difficult in premature infants than in normal infants owing to lack of surfactant, a substance

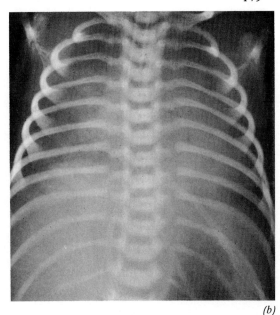

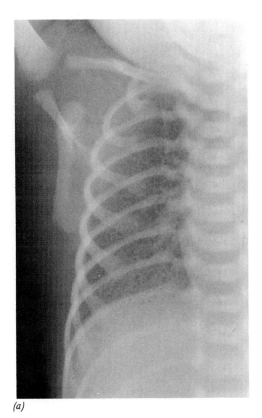

(a)

(b)

Figure 5.10. Hyaline Membrane Disease: (a) early stage. There is a generalized diminution in translucency and the vascular markings are obscured by a diffuse slightly granular pattern throughout the right lung. (b) The lung fields are diffusely opaque with loss of the vascular pattern and of the outlines of the heart and diaphragm due to almost complete de-aeration

which normally reduces surface tension in the smaller airways.

Radiological features

The appearances produced in this condition are often easy to recognize. Even in cases where the initial film fails to demonstrate a diagnostic picture, this will eventually be disclosed in subsequent films if they are taken over the next few hours or days. The most typical picture is a combination of fine granular or miliary opacities which are sometimes uniformly distributed over both lung fields, but are usually most marked in the lower zones. A branching pattern of linear translucencies radiating from the hila is also present. The latter represent air in the normal bronchial tree which has been made visible by a reduction in the air content of the surrounding lung tissue. This appearance is known as an air bronchogram and is not in any way specific to the respiratory distress syndrome because it can be seen in any condition in which the contrast between the lung parenchyma and the air-filled bronchi is increased in this way. The heart is often significantly enlarged (*Figure 5.10*). As the condition becomes more widespread and severe, the heart borders are less well defined and may be rendered invisible as the result of a progressive loss of contrast between the lung tissue and the soft-tissue density of the heart. There is a notable absence of over-inflation or of significant reduction in lung volume, and

in consequence mediastinal displacement does not occur. There is a characteristic evolution of these radiological features. They usually appear within a few hours of birth and are always present in the first 12 hours; however, a negative or atypical film in the first 4 hours of life does not exclude the diagnosis. In a proportion of cases subsequent films will show progressive clearing of the lung fields. In others the 'reticulogranular' pattern and the air bronchogram become gradually more extensive until there is total de-aeration of the lungs (*Figure 5.10b*). The lung fields are then opaque and there is complete loss of the heart outline. This development may occur very rapidly but more usually it occurs over the course of a few days; it is indicative of a bad prognosis. In other cases there is the development of coarser, more blotchy opacities representing extensive areas of collapse, or of interstitial emphysema. This is manifested by areas of linear translucency which do not have the regular branching pattern of the air bronchogram but are scattered more haphazardly over the lungs especially in the peripheral zones. In a few cases this may progress to the development of a pneumomediastinum.

Some infants who undoubtedly suffer from hyaline membrane disease have localized and not diffuse changes in the lungs. In these cases the reticulogranular pattern affects only one lung or one lobe; such a distribution may indicate pulmonary haemorrhage or pneumonia superimposed upon the underlying condition.

It should also be noted that the appearances described above are not entirely specific, because they may occur

180

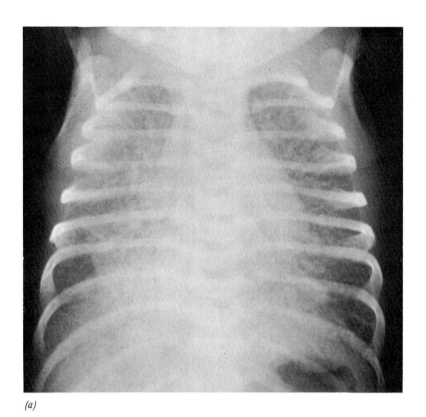

(a)

Figure 5.11. Hyaline Membrane Disease: (a) Plain film of a preterm infant with a diffuse loss of translucency over both lung fields, an air bronchogram and loss of part of the outline of both heart borders. (b) Right ventricular angiocardiogram in the antero-posterior projection. This was carried out because the clinical impression was that the child suffered from a congenital heart lesion. No such abnormality was shown except for a patent ductus arteriosus which had not yet closed. The right-to-left shunt through it allowed filling of the descending aorta from the pulmonary artery. Contrast medium was shown to pass abnormally slowly through the pulmonary circulation and the peripheral pulmonary arteries were small. (c) Lateral projection of the same case. Contrast medium fills the ductus arteriosus (arrowed) and the descending aorta

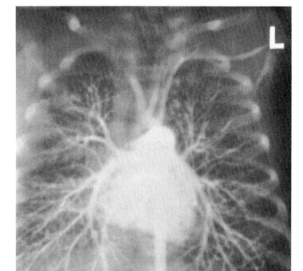

(b)

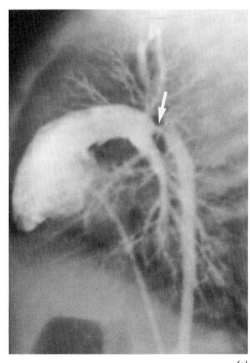

(c)

in infants subsequently shown at autopsy to have other conditions. There may be a proportion as high as 30 per cent who have conditions such as pulmonary haemorrhage, atelectasis, pneumonia or simple immaturity on histological examination (Finnegan *et al.,* 1970). Conversely, as already stated, the appearance found in infants with hyaline membrane disease may depend very much on the stage at which the chest radiograph is obtained and a single film may in consequence be misleading.

Appearances in premature infants

The interpretation of the changes occurring in hyaline membrane disease presupposes a knowledge of the normal appearances in the lungs of premature and full-term infants at the time of birth and in the few hours following birth. In full-term normal infants, complete uniform expansion of the lungs should occur within a few minutes of the first inspiration, the lower zones aerating most rapidly owing to the greater effectiveness of the diaphragm in favouring expansion. In premature infants, however, expansion may occur more slowly and in a less uniform manner. Residual areas of atelectasis may be present, especially in the lower lobes and on the left side after birth but in the absence of any complicating factors, these should expand within 8 hours (Fawcitt, 1956) (*Figure 5.12*).

Another factor which has been discussed recently is the process of removal of the amniotic fluid which normally fills the alveolar spaces during intra-uterine life and which is displaced by air during the onset of extra-uterine respiration. This process usually occurs rapidly and leads to no detectable effects on the radiological appearances, but in some cases it may be delayed. It is

likely that the normal compression of the thorax during vaginal delivery may be largely responsible for the removal of the amniotic fluid from the lungs. Delayed removal has been reported to occur more frequently in infants born by Caesarean section. This is discussed further elsewhere (*see* page 182).

OTHER CAUSES OF RESPIRATORY DISTRESS

A number of other conditions which may lead to respiratory distress in the newborn infant may be recognized by the radiological appearances they produce. Some of these are discussed elsewhere and they will only be listed here.

Congenital heart lesions of various types may lead to heart failure in the first weeks of life; among these, coarction of the aorta, hypoplastic left heart syndrome, transposition of the great arteries and total anomalous pulmonary venous drainage, especially when engorgement of the lungs due to obstruction to the venous return is present, may give rise to difficulty in diagnosis from hyaline membrane disease (*see* Chapter 4).

Pulmonary agenesis or hypoplasia (see page 174).
Congenital lobar emphysema (see page 193).
Diaphragmatic hernia (see page 216).
Tracheo-oesophageal fistula (see page 210).
Pneumothorax (see page 193).
Pneumonia (see page 184).

Primary atelectasis, in which the lung either does not expand normally at birth or expands irregularly and subsequently collapses, is particularly frequent in premature infants who have relatively immature lungs. Radiologically there may be uniform opacity of the lungs with an air bronchogram and loss of the heart

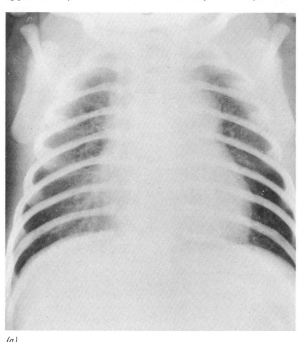

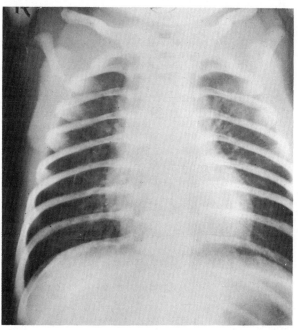

(a)   (b)

Figure 5.12. The Expansion of the Lungs in the Premature Infant: Films of the chest of a preterm infant (birth weight 2.54 kg). (a) At 45 minutes after birth showing some failure of expansion in the lower zone of the right lung. (b) At 24 hours when the lungs are both completely expanded

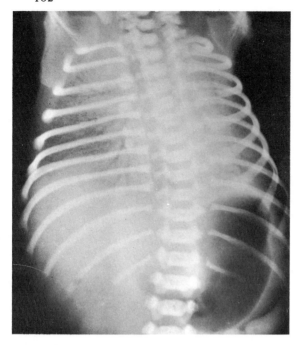

Figure 5.13. The Lungs in Extreme Immaturity: A chest film of an infant born at 30 weeks' gestation who survived only 4 hours. The lungs have failed to expand to any extent and are diffusely opaque except for an extensive air bronchogram. The appearances are very similar to those in the late stages of hyaline membrane disease

borders, an appearance which may resemble the most severe grade of hyaline membrane disease (*Figure 5.13*). The opacity is denser than in the latter condition and it usually only involves the whole or part of one lung and the mediastinum is also displaced. Moreover, the characteristic evolution of hyaline membrane disease does not occur.

The *aspiration syndrome,* in which amniotic fluid has been inhaled during delivery may, in some respects, be contrasted with hyaline membrane disease. It is a condition which is found predominantly in postmature, and not premature infants and there is a history of meconium-staining of the liquor. The radiological appearances resemble those of an inhalational pneumonitis of postnatal origin (*see Figure 5.14*) The opacities are coarser, irregularly distributed and of uneven size. They may be associated with areas of focal collapse, emphysema and generalized hyperinflation of the lungs. An air bronchogram and pneumomediastinum are not seen, but pneumothorax and pleural effusion are common (20—25 per cent of cases). Rapid clearing of the opacities may occur or on the other hand, the condition may deteriorate with the development of confluent areas of bronchopneumonia.

Bronchopulmonary dysplasia is a condition which has been recently described in infants treated with 80—100 per cent oxygen or who have undergone endotracheal intubation and been artificially ventilated on a respirator (Northway and Rosan, 1968). These infants show a radiological picture, very similar to hyaline membrane disease, which progresses from a reticulogranular pattern to complete opacity of the lungs and loss of heart outline, signs which may persist for periods

of up to 10 days. Following this stage small, cyst-like translucent areas develop due to focal emphysema and the heart borders again become invisible. Gradual weaning from the need for high oxygen concentrations may thus become possible. Finally, chronic lung changes may develop with streaky linear opacities, hyperinflation and cardiomegaly and in a proportion of cases, death from cor pulmonale may occur.

Pulmonary haemorrhage may occur in the neonatal period often in association with prenatal hypoxia or with haemorrhagic disease of the newborn. The radiological appearances may resemble those seen in the aspiration syndrome and there are patchy opacities scattered over the lung fields. On the other hand, a reticulogranular pattern may occur which may be indistinguishable from hyaline membrane disease although it is usually slightly coarser (Fawcitt, 1956).

Transient tachypnoea of the newborn (wet lung disease) is a mild form of respiratory distress in newborn infants which has recently been described (Avery *et al.,* 1966). Symptoms arise from 1 to 6 hours after birth. They reach a peak between 6 and 36 hours and usually subside within 96 hours of birth.

Radiological abnormalities in this condition consist of an increase in prominence of the vascular markings which at the same time lose their sharp outline. They become ill defined, thick and nodular, resembling the appearances in passive vascular engorgement. Mild hyperinflation and thickening of the interlobar and interlobular septa are also described. Small pleural effusions and a moderate cardiomegaly are present in a proportion of cases. These appearances may be related to an increase in fluid content of the lung, either interstitial, septal or

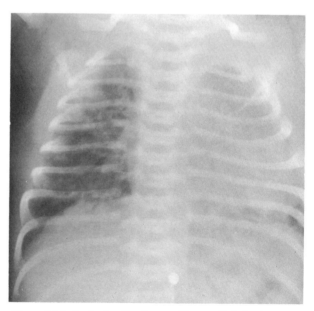

Figure 5.14. Aspiration Syndrome: Discrete ill-defined opacities are present in the right lung. The left border of the heart has been obscured due to the de-aeration of the adjacent lung tissue and there is an air bronchogram overlying the heart shadow. The appearances are those of an inhalational pneumonitis resulting from aspiration of amniotic fluid and the meconium contained within it due to prolongation of labour and premature attempts to breathe (by courtesy of Dr. G. R. Airth, Southmead Hospital)

pleural. It is postulated that the cause of the condition is a delay in the rate at which the amniotic fluid normally present in the lungs during intra-uterine life is absorbed. This is usually achieved within a few minutes of birth but may take longer, especially if there is a defect in the lymphatic drainage of the lung. The condition has also been noted to occur more commonly in infants born by Caesarean section and in such cases, an absence of the normal squeezing of the thorax during vaginal delivery may be a relevant factor.

The *Wilson–Mikity syndrome* was first described in 1960. It always affects premature infants and usually those born before 30 weeks or with an average birth weight of 1280 grams. There is a high mortality but those infants who survive tend ultimately to recover, though symptoms may persist for a number of years. The onset is relatively gradual and is not apparent until from 6 to 35 days after birth. Cough, cyanosis and dyspnoea are then progressive over a period of several weeks followed in favourable cases by a gradual improvement. When death occurs in fatal cases it is from cor pulmonale (Wilson and Mikity, 1960).

Radiological appearances are at some stage of the condition characteristic. There are bilaterally symmetrical, coarse, streaky opacities radiating from the hilar regions, interspersed with small circular translucent areas from 1 to 4 mm in diameter, giving a 'bubbly' appearance throughout both lungs. The cardiac outline remains well defined but is sometimes mildly enlarged. The peripheral pulmonary vessels are not increased in calibre but the main pulmonary artery may be enlarged. Moderate hyperinflation of the lungs is present and the coarse streaky opacities tend to persist after the translucent areas have disappeared (*Figure 5.15*). Resolution occurs only slowly over a number of years, the hyperinflation of the lungs being the last feature to disappear.

The nature of this condition remains obscure, but it may be regarded basically as a pulmonary dysmaturity, in which the lungs of severely premature infants are called upon to perform a respiratory function for which they are not yet ready. This results in a progressively abnormal air distribution within the lung and a disturbance in the relationship between air flow and vascular

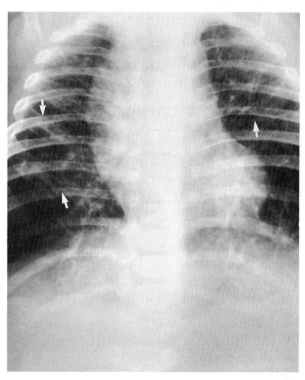

(a)

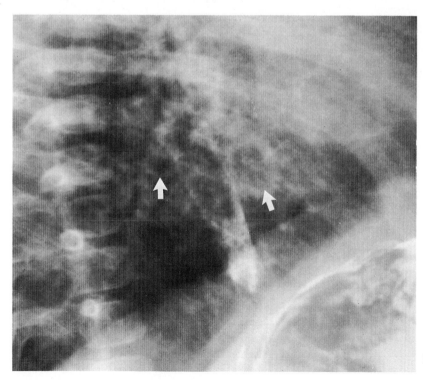

(b)

Figure 5.15. Wilson-Mikity Syndrome: Hyperinflation of the lungs with coarse linear opacities radiating from both hilar regions; a number of small circular translucent areas are present (arrowed). This infant was 5 months old and was dyspnoeic at rest with attacks of cyanosis, since a few weeks after birth. There was no history of prolonged oxygen administration. (a) Anteroposterior view. (b) Lateral view (barium is present in the oesophagus and stomach)

perfusion through a poorly developed capillary network (Hodgman *et al.*, 1969). It has also been suggested that this condition may represent a common response of immature lungs to a number of different factors. The resemblance of the radiological appearances to those seen in bronchopulmonary dysplasia (*see* page 182) tends to support this view.

INFLAMMATORY DISEASE

PNEUMONIA

Introduction

Pneumonic consolidation which results in loss of aeration due to inflammatory exudate in the alveoli may be easily recognized by the opacity which it produces on the radiograph. However, the pattern may be very variable. It depends on the size and situation of the areas of lung involved and the presence of associated airway obstruction which leads to superimposed collapse or local hyperinflation. There may also be pleural involvement which results in local pleural thickening or effusion. Such variations, however, are seldom sufficiently well correlated with the type of organism which causes the pneumonia to enable a positive opinion to be given as to the aetiology, purely on the basis of the radiological appearances. The site and distribution of the inflammatory infiltration may however be fairly accurately assessed and a given case may be classified as alveolar or interstitial. The former may be either lobar, segmental or lobular in distribution (*Figure 5.16*). However, mixed types frequently occur (*Figure 5.17*). The rate at which the pneumonic process extends or resolves may also be determined.

Interpretation of the radiological appearances is more difficult in young infants than it is in adults owing to the small size of the opacities in children. This is especially so because lobular or interstitial consolidations are the commonest type in this age group. Magnification techniques may prove helpful as stated on page 000' The obliteration of the normal vascular pattern of the lung field and the presence of an air bronchogram may be useful signs in the identification of alveolar consolidation. These signs are not specific evidence of pneumonia because other causes can result in de-aeration of the alveoli. Interstitial infiltration will result in linear or reticular opacities which are difficult to distinguish from widened pulmonary vessel shadows, the latter being due to congestion of pleonaemia. It may be possible, however, to identify opacities occurring in parallel lines with a line of translucency between them or running alongside the normal vessels. Alternatively, where a bronchus is seen end-on, a round translucency surrounded by a dense ring-like opacity may be present (*Figures 5.18* and *5.41b*). With such appearances the presence of peribronchial thickening may be inferred. This need not always be inflammatory in origin but the diagnosis of interstitial pneumonia may usually be made if the clinical picture is consistent or the presence of other radiological features, such as hilar lymphadenopathy or pleural involvement, are observed.

Confusion may sometimes be caused by the fact that when the chest is examined radiologically, the pneumonia has already begun to resolve and the resulting appearances may be interpreted as cavitation, obstructive hyperinflation or interstitial emphysema. Furthermore, in children, an element of collapse commonly accompanies

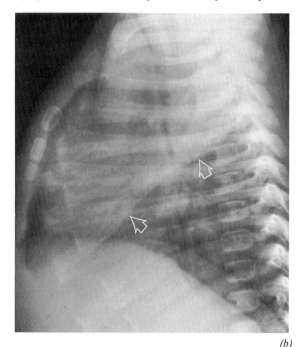

(a)   *(b)*

Figure 5.16. Lobar Pneumonia: Consolidation of the whole of the left upper lobe. (a) Anteroposterior view in which the greater part of the left heart border is obscured due to the lack of aeration of the portion of the left upper lobe which is in contact with it (mainly the lingular segment). This constitutes the 'outline or silhouette' sign which can be helpful in the detection and localization of limited areas of consolidation or collapse. (b) Lateral view in which the sharply defined lower border of the opacity due to the oblique interlobar fissure defines the extent of the consolidated area of lung (arrowed)

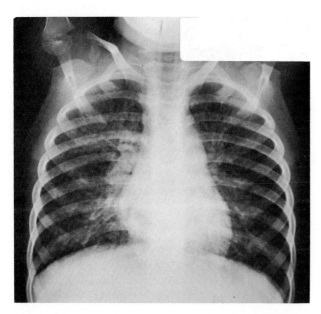

Figure 5.17. Bronchopneumonia: Small discrete opacities are present distributed diffusely throughout the lungs. These are due to consolidation which is limited to pulmonary lobules. They are accompanied by an increase in the width of the vascular shadows which are ill defined. In some areas there are linear translucencies representing air in the smaller bronchi outlined by inflammatory exudate

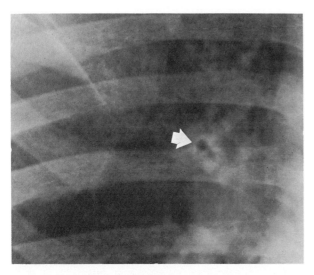

Figure 5.18. Peribronchial Thickening: In some types of inflammatory disease of the lungs, particularly those due to viruses, the exudate occurs mainly in the interstitial tissues as in this case. Ring-shaped shadows (arrowed) represent peribronchial and interstitial thickening due to such exudates

an inflammatory condition. The localization of segmental areas of pneumonia may be helped by observation of the silhouette sign, which is present when the cardiac, mediastinal or diaphragmatic borders of the lung become ill defined or disappear (*Figure 5.16*). This occurs when the contrast between the soft tissues and the air-containing lung adjacent to them is removed by the presence of

consolidation in a segment of the lung which borders on one of these structures. Such appearances may be particularly useful in making the diagnosis and localizing the lesion when a lateral view is not available.

Staphylococcal pneumonia

This is a disease which is relatively common in childhood, especially in the first year of life and one which is likely to produce recognizable radiological appearances. In the earliest stage of the disease, these appearances may not be specific and may resemble other segmental or lobular consolidations (*Figure 5.19a*). In the later stages, thin-walled air-containing lesions or pneumatoceles develop (*Figures 5.19b* and *c*). The inflammatory process frequently spreads to the pleural cavity with the production of an empyema of pyopneumothorax. These features may give a bizarre picture which is sufficiently distinctive to allow a full diagnosis to be made. Pneumatoceles usually appear about a week after the onset of the condition and they resolve after successful treatment leaving no visible residual opacities. On the radiograph a pneumatocele has a thin, regular, spherical wall in its fully developed state and it may contain an air–fluid level in an erect film (*Figure 5.19c*). However, in the earliest stages of development it appears within an area of consolidation as a small air space which subsequently enlarges. Its wall may be thick and nodular. Initially it is a peribronchial abscess arising from a small area of necrosis in the bronchial wall. With breakdown of the necrotic wall communication between the abscess and the lumen is established. This allows ingress of air on inspiration into the cavity but egress is obstructed. Air-trapping within the 'abscess' cavity converts it into a form of 'tension cyst'. Relief of the obstruction to the egress of air following treatment accounts for the rapid deflation and disappearance of the pneumatocele.

Pleural effusion or empyema developing in the course of pneumonia in an infant is almost diagnostic of a staphylococcal origin. These sequelae may, in some cases, be the presenting feature and there may be no apparent antecedent consolidation (*Figure 5.20*). Air within the pleural cavity may vary in amount from a small loculated collection resembling a pneumatocele to a large 'tension' pneumothorax. The appearances produced, especially in supine films, may be very bizarre; plaques or strands of fibrin may be present within the pleural cavity which may give rise to linear opacities crossing the hemithorax. An erect film will often clarify the picture by demonstrating an air–fluid level.

Differentiation of pneumatoceles arising in staphylococcal pneumonia from lung cysts, true abscesses or lobar hyperinflation may sometimes be difficult but the rapid variation in size and appearance of the pneumatoceles is a helpful feature. Pneumatoceles have, on occasions, been described in other types of pneumonia but in practice they are very rare except in staphylococcal pneumonia. The initial area of consolidation may extend rapidly and produce an increase in the volume of the affected lobe or segment. This may suggest the presence of a neoplasm or other expanding lesion and cases have been described in which a lobectomy has been performed as a result of these radiological appearances. The rarity of rapidly growing

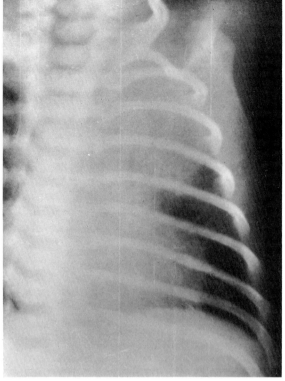

(a)

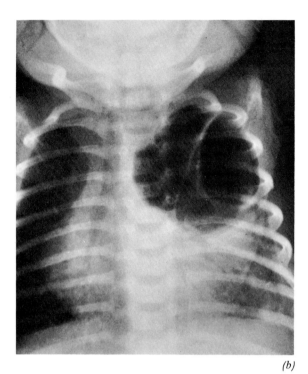

(b)

Figure. 5.19. Staphylococcal Pneumonia: (a) Segmental consolidation in part of the left upper lobe in the early stages of a staphylococcal pneumonia. (b) Later stage of the same case when a number of distended, thin-walled, air-containing cavities (pneumatoceles) have developed within the left upper lobe at the site of the previously consolidated segments. An air bronchogram is present in the lower part of the left lung and there is a small lamellar pleural effusion along the lateral chest wall. (c) An erect film showing two pneumatoceles (arrowed) in another case of staphylococcal infection. The upper one contains an air-fluid level and has a characteristically thin, smoothly rounded outline

children under 2 years of age. Pneumatoceles are not seen, however, in this type of pneumonia.

Viral pneumonia

In any given case, the differentiation of pneumonia due to viruses from other forms of infective agent may be impossible but certain features occur with sufficient frequency to give rise to a suggestive radiological picture.

(1)   An interstitial pneumonia in which the bronchial walls and interstitial spaces are infiltrated by cells or oedematous fluid, results in a reticular or linear pattern of opacities with parallel streaks outlining the air content of the larger bronchi. This may also result in ring shadows when the bronchi are seen end-on. Thickening of the interlobular septa may also contribute to this appearance. The changes are most commonly diffuse but may sometimes be confined to one part of the lung.

(2)   Perihilar opacities which resemble pulmonary oedema appear. They are rapidly progressive and may be accompanied by pleural effusion, as occurs for instance in influenzal pneumonia.

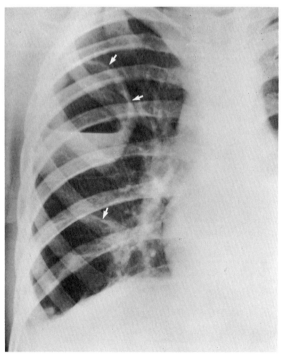

(c)

tumours in the lung at the age at which staphylococcal pneumonia is common should prevent this error. Pleural involvement may, of course, occur in any type of pneumonia, but in the young infant the only organisms commonly causing this are *staphylococci* and *Haemophilus influenzae,* the latter predominantly affecting

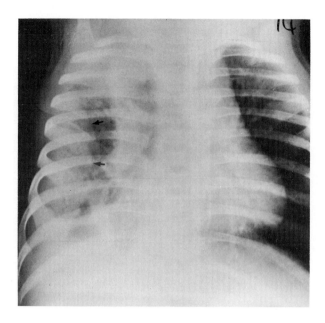

Figure 5.20 Staphylococcal Pneumonia–Empyema: Consolidation of part of the right lung with an empyema lying on the inner aspect of the right lateral chest wall (arrowed) in an infant with staphylococcal pneumonia

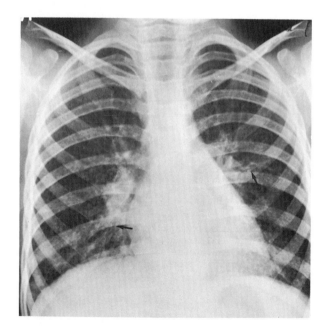

Figure 5.21. Viral Pneumonia: Chest film of a child with glandular fever. There are discrete opacities in both lower zones. Enlargement of the bronchopulmonary glands has produced a large right hilar shadow. Well marked 'tramline' shadows can be seen in the left hilar region and at the right base due to peribronchial thickening (arrowed)

(3)   A bronchopneumonic pattern of small, widely scattered, nodular or even miliary opacities extending symmetrically over both lung fields; an appearance especially characteristic of varicella pneumonia.

(4)   Hilar gland enlargement which is usually bilateral.

In infants, an interstitial type of pneumonia is described as occurring as a result of infections with respiratory syncitial virus, adenoviruses, measles and rubella and in primary atypical pneumonia. All these conditions resemble each other so far as the radiological appearances are concerned and cannot be differentiated from each other except on clinical grounds. Varicella pneumonia may cause a nodular or miliary pattern which though not in any way specific, is distinguishable from a secondary bacterial pneumonia complicating chicken pox by its symmetrical, widely diffused distribution and persistence. Furthermore, in surviving patients, the lesions tend to heal by calcification. Varicella is thought to be responsible for many of the cases in which scattered miliary calcifications occur in the lungs as an incidental radiological finding (Knyvett, 1966).

Pneumocystis carinii pneumonia

An interstitial pneumonia may also occur as a result of infection with *Pneumocystis carinii,* and it is particularly common among premature or debilitated infants in hospitals or nurseries. A combination of radiating perihilar opacities resembling pulmonary oedema with a fine reticulogranular pattern like that of hyaline membrane disease is described (*Figure 5.22*) (Feinberg *et al.*, 1961). However, differentiation from other types of pneumonia and from other conditions seen in premature infants, such as hyaline membrane disease, heart failure or the Hamman–Rich syndrome is certainly not easy. The symptoms and radiological signs are usually more extensive than would be expected from the physical signs, but pleural involvement and enlargement of the hilar glands are usually absent.

Inhalational pneumonia

Children, especially small infants and those with disorders of swallowing or gastro-oesophageal reflux are liable to develop pneumonia after inhaling foreign material into the lungs (*Figure 5.23*). This may be meconium in the newborn infant, or milk in the postnatal period. Foreign materials, especially paraffin or substances of similar chemical nature may cause pneumonia in the older child (*Figure 5.24*). The inhalation of solid objects may cause bronchial obstruction, to which pneumonia may be secondary, and these have therefore been considered elsewhere (*see* page 198). The direct effect on the lung of inhalation of paraffin or kerosene is favoured as the mechanism which gives rise to pneumonia. It is no longer thought to be due to re-excretion into the lungs after the paraffin has been absorbed into the blood-stream. A potentially very serious involvement of the lungs has been recently

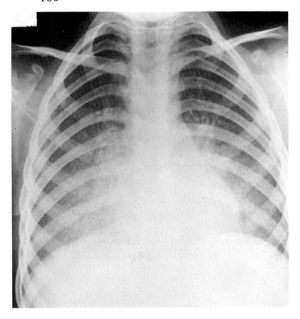

Figure 5.22. Pneumonia due to Pneumocystis Carinii: Chest film of a child with leukaemia treated by immunosuppressive drugs. The diffuse hazy opacity of both lungs fields was considered to be due to infection with Pneumocystis carinii and cleared up rapidly after treatment with pentamidine

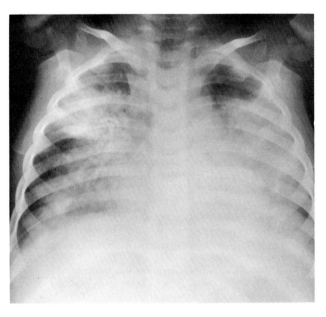

Figure 5.24. Paraffin Pneumonia: Extensive consolidation of both lungs after the ingestion and subsequent inhalation of paraffin. In spite of the area of lung involved, the child survived with complete resolution of the opacities in a few weeks

described following the ingestion of weedkillers containing the substance 'Paraquat'. In this case a progressive fibrosis of the lungs is produced with the subsequent development of cor pulmonale.

The radiological appearance of inhalational pneumonia is not particularly characteristic of the cause, but has a tendency to persist or recur in spite of treatment and this fact should lead to suspicion of an inhalational cause. The site of the lesions may vary but the lower lobes or perihilar regions are commonly affected in 'paraffin' pneumonia, and the right upper or middle lobes in the regurgitating infant.

TUBERCULOSIS

Infection by the tubercle bacillus has become much less common in recent years due to the spread of immunization and more efficient treatment of infectious individuals. Nevertheless, with the existence of relatively large numbers of Mantoux-negative children who have not received BCG, the possibility of contracting the disease in childhood is still by no means negligible. The detection of primary pulmonary lesions in these children is of great importance because early treatment will, in most cases, prevent the development of more serious forms of the disease and its complications.

Primary tuberculosis

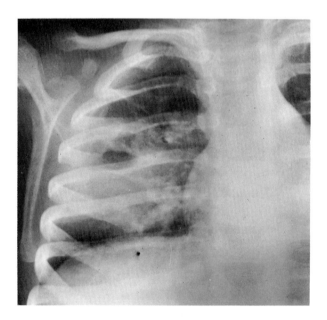

Figure 5.23. Inhalational Pneumonia: An area of consolidation in the right midzone in an infant with hiatus hernia. There is a translucency within the consolidated part of the lung representing an abscess cavity and pleural thickening or a localized effusion is present on its lateral surface. This pneumonia is due to inhalation of food regurgitated from the stomach during sleep

It has been pointed out that in 65 per cent of children, the primary lesions in the lung were detected, not as a result of symptoms, but as a result of routine surveys of schoolchildren or contracts. Such lesions were also found in the lungs of 25 per cent of children examined after a

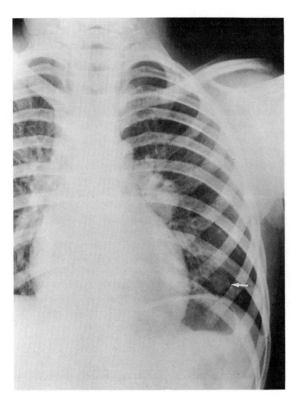

Figure 5.25. Primary Tuberculous Infection: A small, rounded primary focus (arrowed) is present at the left base with enlarged bronchopulmonary lymph glands at the left hilum

or environmental factors and the age of the child. Most of the cases occur under 3 years of age. Inadequate treatment may also be a contributory factor (Joffe, 1960).

Pneumatoceles may occur in association with primary tuberculous disease but they are rare. They may develop within a few weeks of the commencement of treatment with antituberculous drugs or steroids, but they resolve spontaneously.

Tuberculous bronchopneumonia and miliary tuberculosis

These conditions are rarely seen with efficient treatment of the primary infection but when the primary lesion has not been recognized, they may appear as evenly diffused opacities varying from 1.0 mm in miliary tuberculosis to 0.5 cm in bronchopneumonia (*Figure 5.26* and *5.27*).

SARCOIDOSIS

This is a rare disease in children and in them its radiological appearances differ to some extent from the pattern seen in adults.

Hilar gland enlargement with or without parenchymal lung lesions affords a non-specific radiological picture which is difficult to distinguish from other inflammatory diseases, particularly from viral pneumonia. The possibility that renal lesions may coexist should not be forgotten because nephrocalcinosis and renal failure are features which may have a serious outcome.

BRONCHIECTASIS

Once a relatively common disease of childhood, the incidence of bronchiectasis has fallen markedly over the past few years, associated with the use of broad-spectrum antibiotics in the treatment of pneumonia and other respiratory tract infections. The radiological demonstration of bronchiectasis is now less important than it used to be because surgical treatment is less commonly required and accurate localization of the disease is therefore not so vital. Nevertheless, in spite of the decline in infection as a factor in the causation of bronchiectasis and the more rapid recognition and treatment of inhaled foreign bodies, food or blood, there remain a small number of cases who suffer from hereditary or congenital types. The basis of these is a structural weakness in the bronchial wall or an immunological defect such as agammaglobulinaemia.

Bronchography, in addition to localizing the site of the diseased bronchi, may allow differentiation of tubular, saccular and fusiform types of bronchiectasis (*Figure 5.28*). The prognosis of these types varies and they occur at different stages of the disease. The tubular type is the earliest stage of the disease in children. It may develop into the saccular form, in which the terminal segment of the bronchus is predominantly affected and which is often irreversible. Alternatively, it may develop into the fusiform or irregularly dilated type, the prognosis of which is much better (Field, 1961).

Abnormalities of the bronchial anatomy may accompany bronchiectasis and they are easily detected by bronchography. An example is Kartagener's triad where

Mantoux conversion (Weber *et al.*, 1968). The recognition of primary lesions may not, however, be easy because the radiological appearances of the tuberculous lesions may resemble other types of inflammatory disease (*Figure 5.25*). The combination of a localized parenchymatous focus, enlarged bronchopulmonary or paratracheal glands and thickened lymphatic channels connecting the two, may be incomplete or obscured by segmental collapse or pleural effusion. The group of glands enlarged is related to the site of the primary parenchymatous lesion and this may occur in any part of the lung. It is important, however, to recognize that the paratracheal glands may be the only group to be involved and in such cases the enlarged glands may resemble a mediastinal mass. Tuberculous glands may compress a segmental bronchus and lead to collapse of the affected segment; this occurs in about a third of all cases. The right middle lobe bronchus is especially vulnerable to compression in this manner and re-expansion of the consequent collapse of the middle lobe may not occur for several months.

A well penetrated film may enable localized narrowing of the trachea or main bronchi to be detected, a finding which may point to the site of enlarged glands. The parenchymatous foci may involve a whole segment. They can be multiple and rarely they may break down to form a cavity. On the radiograph the cavity is shown as an irregular translucent area within the large opacity of the parenchymatous focus. The walls of the cavity are ill defined and fluid levels may not be seen. The factors predisposing to the formation of such a cavitating primary lesion are lack of resistance, poor nutritional

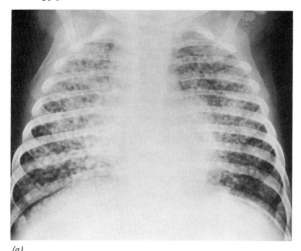

(a)

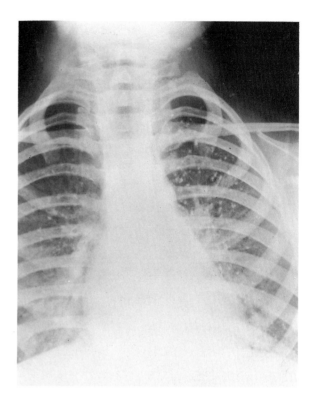

(b)

Figure 5.26. Miliary Tuberculosis: (a) Small discrete opacities evenly distributed over both lungs; both hilar shadows are increased in size due to enlargement of the bronchopulmonary glands and the upper part of the mediastinum is widened due to enlargement of the paratracheal glands. (b) Small calcified opacities in a child who had recovered from miliary tuberculosis several years previously. Calcified cervical lymph glands are present in the neck

bronchiectasis is present together with sinus infection or absence of the frontal sinuses and dextrocardia. The latter is part of a generalized situs inversus which includes a mirror image reversal of the bronchial anatomy, with a lingular segment on the right and a middle lobe on the left side. Defects in the cartilage of the bronchial wall may result in dilatation of the bronchi. On fluoroscopy or cineradiographic studies they may be seen to expand and collapse with respiratory movement.

IMMUNE DEFICIENCY DISEASES

A number of conditions in which widespread infections occur throughout the body due to a defect in the normal defence mechanism, have been described. This group of diseases will be briefly considered here because the most frequent radiological signs are related to the respiratory tract, although other systems are also involved. Most of these diseases are congenital in origin. They may be classified into two groups: (1) those in whom humoral immunity is defective and the level of serum gammaglobulin is low; (2) those in whom there is a defect in cellular immunity and the thymus is small or completely absent. In the former group, there is an increased liability to pyogenic infections and in the latter to viral, fungal or protozoan infections.

These conditions have certain radiological features in common. Recurrent attacks of pneumonia, in which the consolidation is usually lobular or interstitial in distribution, are liable to occur. *Pneumocystic carinii* is a frequent cause and it may produce symmetrical perihilar hazy opacities (*see* page 187). In the normal infant the posterior nasopharyngeal soft tissue opacity due to the adenoids is easily visible after the age of about

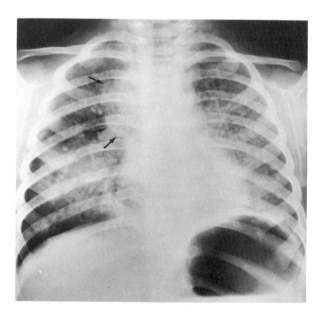

Figure 5.27. Tuberculous Bronchopneumonia: Discrete opacities in both lung fields which are rather larger and less evenly distributed than in miliary tuberculosis. An opacity in the right lower zone together with enlarged right paratracheal glands (arrowed) represents the 'primary complex'

12 months on the routine lateral radiograph of the sinuses. In the immune deficiency disease the lymphoid tissue around the pharynx is absent and this soft tissue opacity is not seen. This produces an 'empty' naso-pharynx resembling that seen after adenoidectomy. This is a sign which is only of value after the first year of life and in the absence of previous surgery. Bronchiectasis may also be a frequent complication.

The opacity in the upper part of the mediastinum normally caused by the infantile thymus is absent in the type of immune deficiency disease with thymic alymphoplasia. It must be pointed out that even with the aid of tomography or pneumomediastinum, it is easier to demonstrate the presence of a thymus of normal size than to determine whether it is absent or abnormally small. Radiological abnormalities due to involvement of other systems may be present, among which are included the irregular defects due to monilial oesophagitis and those in the small intestine and colon, due to lymphoid hyperplasia. A skeletal dysplasia closely resembling achondroplasia has also been described in association with thymic alymphoplasia. The most wide-spread and striking abnormalities occur in chronic granulomatous disease. This is a condition which results from inability of the phagocytes to kill bacteria which have been ingested. Radiologically demonstrable granulomatous lesions develop in the lungs, mediastinum, bones and genito-urinary tract (Sutcliffe and Chrispin, 1970). The pulmonary lesions comprise patchy areas of consolidation which tend to become confluent, often with perihilar hazy opacities and an air bronchogram. More massive opacities involving a lobe, or even the whole lung, are not uncommon, and these may break down to form lung abscesses. Enlarged hilar glands, pleural effusion and widening of the mediastinum with irregular ill-defined margins also occur. Round, well-defined opacities in the lungs produce a particularly charac-teristic appearance. This has been termed *encapsulating pneumonia*.

Features due to the effect of this disease on other organs are:

(1) Dilatation of the oesophagus which fails to contract normally.
(2) Calcified intra-abdominal abscesses.
(3) Hydronephrosis with a small contracted bladder.
(4) Osteomyelitis. Osteomyelitis especially involves the small bones of the hands and feet. Though the bone destruction may be extensive and unusually persistent, it will heal with an almost complete reconstruction of the bone architecture.

AIRWAY OBSTRUCTION

Obstruction to the air passages may produce effects which are easily detected on chest radiographs. These

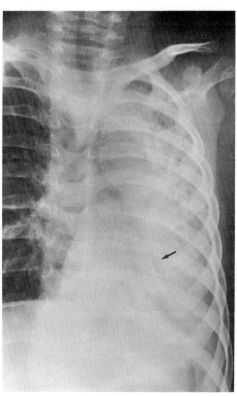

(a)

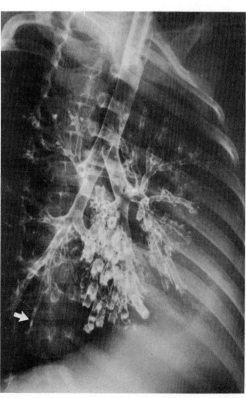

(b)

Figure 5.28. Bronchiectasis: (a) The left hemithorax is opaque except for a few linear translucent areas representing the dilated bronchi. The heart and the trachea are displaced to the left, indicating a considerable degree of collapse of the left lung. There is hyperinflation of the right lung. (b) Bronchography showing dilatation and lack of tapering of most of the bronchi of the left lung. This is in contrast to the bronchi of the right lung (arrowed) which taper in the normal manner

changes will not only indicate the presence of obstruction but by their site and distribution may give useful information as to the part of the bronchial tree involved.

COLLAPSE

This is the most obvious effect of obstruction of a bronchus and is due to absorption of the air within the alveoli and distal bronchioles of the affected segment. The air cannot be replenished on inspiration because the obstruction in the bronchus prevents this happening. A segmental or subsegmental opacity is produced on the radiograph. There is also displacement of interlobar fissures, diaphragm and mediastinal structures towards the opacity and crowding of the ribs on the same side which result from the loss of volume of the affected portion of lung. These changes need to be differentiated from inflammatory consolidation without collapse of similar areas of lung. This differentiation rests mainly on the evidence of loss of lung volume in the presence of collapse.

HYPERINFLATION

If the obstruction of the bronchus is less complete and is of such a type that air can pass peripherally on inspiration but cannot be expelled on expiration, the part of the lung distal to the site of the obstruction will become progressively over-distended. Its volume will increase, even at the expense of the unaffected parts of the same lung or of the opposite lung (*Figure 5.29*).

Such a condition is referred to as 'air trapping' or 'obstructive emphysema'. The latter term is inaccurate because there is no destruction of the alveolar walls as takes place in true emphysema and the condition is reversible. The increase in volume of the affected part of the lung may be so great and the unaffected parts so markedly compressed that a hyperinflated lobe may fill the whole hemithorax and even herniate across the midline. This may suggest that the whole lung is involved, especially on the left side, where the compressed lower lobe may be entirely hidden behind the heart. Depression and relative immobility of the diaphragm, mediastinal displacement, blunting of the costophrenic angle and bulging of the lung into the intercostal spaces are other indications of increased lung volume. The latter is particularly likely to be present when the more superficial parts of the lung are involved and this may occur if the obstruction is situated in the finer bronchioles. This is likely to be the case when there is inflammatory oedema or when the bronchioles contain mucous plugs as a result of bronchiolitis.

Hyperinflation may occur with airway obstruction at any age, but it is particularly common in the infant in whom the calibre of the bronchi is small and the variation in bronchial diameter on inspiration and expiration is marked. If the chest radiograph of a small child shows a difference in translucency between the two lung fields, it may be difficult to determine whether the side which is hyperlucent is the site of obstructive emphysema or whether there is collapse present on the more opaque side which has produced compensatory hyperinflation of the opposite lung. In such cases, fluoroscopic examination or films taken on inspiration and expiration may

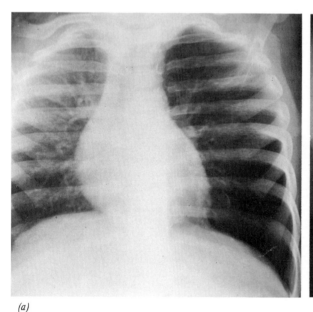
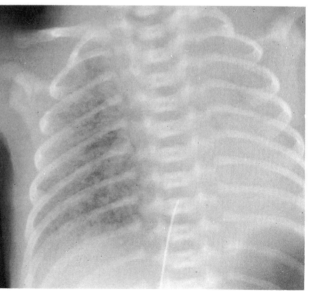

(a)   (b)

Figure 5.29. (a) Obstructive Hyperinflation: Chest film of a child following inhalation of a foreign body which lodged in the left main bronchus. The whole of the left lung is hypertranslucent with depression of the left hemidiaphragm, displacement of the heart and mediastinum to the right and widening of the rib spaces on the left side. (b) Interstitial Emphysema. An infant with extensive de-aeration of the lungs due to respiratory distress syndrome. An irregular pattern of translucencies is present throughout the right lung due to air in the interstitial spaces of the lung. There is also air along the mediastinal border of the lung. This condition is often followed by a pneumomediastinum (see Figure 5.32 page 195). An umbilical catheter has been passed through the ductus venosus and its tip lies in the right atrium. Radiological examination is very helpful in ensuring that such catheters are correctly placed

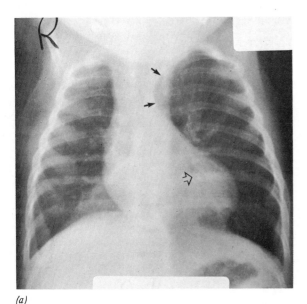

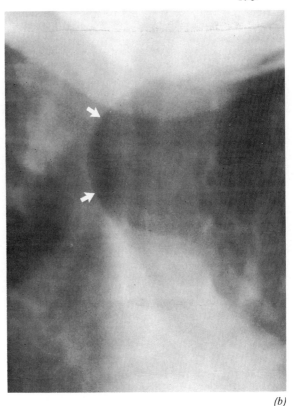

(a)

Figure 5.30. Congenital Lobar Emphysema: (a) Obstructive hyperinflation of the left upper lobe which has come to fill the whole of the left side of the thorax and is beginning to herniate across the midline (solid arrows). The left lower lobe is compressed medially and is not visible. The lingular bronchus is seen behind the heart (outline arrow) (b) Later stage of the same case showing an increase in the extent of the herniation of the mediastinum to the right (arrowed).

(b)

be useful, because if the mediastinum moves to one side or the other during respiration, it will move towards the side of the obstruction on inspiration (or on sniffing) and towards the normal side on expiration (or on coughing). This applies whether the obstruction has resulted in collapse or in hyperinflation. However, the mediastinum may be fixed on inspiration, especially when the obstruction is of long duration and, in such cases, this sign cannot be elicited. Barium should always be introduced into the oesophagus if fluoroscopy is performed, because occasionally this may disclose a cause for the obstruction such as mediastinal tumour or vascular impression due to an aberrant subclavian or pulmonary artery.

Bronchography is seldom necessary and may be dangerous, especially in newborn infants.

CONGENITAL LOBAR EMPHYSEMA

Progressive hyperinflation of a complete lobe may occur in infants within the first few weeks of life. The affected lobe may continue to expand resulting in compression of the other lobes and even of the opposite lung. Emergency lobectomy may then be required to prevent death from asphyxia. In over half such cases, no obstructive cause may be found. In the remainder, various potentially obstructive conditions may be present such as chondromalacia of the bronchial wall, redundant bronchial mucosa, congenital stenosis and extrinsic pressure from an aberrant left pulmonary artery arising as a branch of the right pulmonary artery. Both the upper lobes and the right middle lobe are predominantly affected. Recognition of this type of respiratory distress in the newborn

infant is important in view of the serious outcome in many cases if untreated.

The radiological features are usually similar to those described above and the hyperinflation may appear to involve the whole of one lung. The unaffected lobes, which are compressed against the heart or mediastinum, are difficult to detect. As the condition progresses the emphysematous lobe herniates across the midline (*Figure 5.30*). Following lobectomy, the compressed parts of the lung may re-expand readily, even if the condition has been present for some time. Occasionally this condition may occur before birth. In such cases the abnormal lobe will be opaque, because it is full of fluid. It occupies a larger volume than normal, with displacement of heart and trachea to the opposite side. Following aeration of the lungs, the radiological appearances gradually change to those of lobar hyperinflation. In the initial stages, there may be difficulty in diagnosis because there may be confusion with conditions such as empyema, chylothorax, right-sided diaphragmatic hernia with a solid viscus in the chest and intrathoracic tumours. In all these conditions as opacity within the chest is associated with an increase in the size of the hemithorax.

SPONTANEOUS PNEUMOTHORAX

This may occur as a complication of airway obstruction when this results in hyperinflation over a long period, and this may occur in asthma. The condition may, in such circumstances, be unsuspected clinically because the signs may be masked by those of the asthma. In the neonate, pneumothorax may result both from obstruction due to aspirated blood or amniotic fluid or from

194

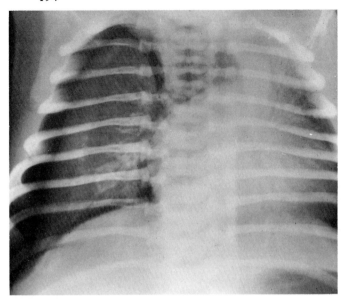

Figure 5.31. Pneumothorax: Right-sided pneumothorax in an infant. The right lung has not completely collapsed in spite of the rise in intrapleural pressure evident from the displacement of the heart to the left, and bulging of the mediastinum across the midline. The left upper lobe is collapsed

the use of artificial ventilation at too high a pressure. The diagnosis of a pneumothorax may depend therefore on radiological examination. It is very important to recognize the presence of a pneumothorax because it may require urgent treatment, particularly when a high intrapleural pressure has built up and led to mediastinal displacement with compression of the opposite lung. Radiography of the highest quality is necessary for the detection of a pneumothorax. Sometimes oblique views may be helpful in revealing the lung edge when this is not clearly shown in the anteroposterior view. The edge of the relaxed lung with air around it may be well shown on a radiograph taken on expiration and this view should be included when a pneumothorax is suspected. This of course may not be possible in small infants. Serial films may also be helpful in detecting a progressive increase in the amount of the intrapleural air. The lung beneath a pneumothorax in an infant may remain relatively expanded, and this may aggravate the displacement of the mediastinal structures and the compression of the unaffected lung. It has been suggested that this may be due to the presence of air in the interstitial and perivascular spaces (*Figure 5.31*). Abnormal pleural fissures or normal skin folds on the surface of the back or in the axilla may cause confusion by producing a curvilinear shadow which resembles a lung edge. Skin folds can usually be seen to extend outside the limits of the lung field. A pneumothorax may sometimes be loculated, especially just above the diaphragm and, in such cases it may be difficult to recognize.

PNEUMOMEDIASTINUM

Air may enter the mediastinal spaces outside the pleural cavities and from this site it may extend widely over the chest wall, into the neck and even over the scalp. The causes of this condition are similar to those of pneumothorax. It is likely that, in many cases, both conditions may arise at the same time by a similar mechanism. The alveoli rupture and this allows air to pass into the perivascular spaces from where it may track either subpleurally and result in a pneumothorax, or along the interstitial spaces towards the hila and thence into the mediastinum. Pneumomediastinum is a potentially dangerous condition especially in infancy, but it is usually not those cases in whom the clinical signs are most widespread and dramatic that have the most serious outcome. Fatal results are more likely to occur in the child in whom the mediastinal air is trapped within the thorax and in whom the inspiratory expansion of the lungs and the venous return of blood to the heart are impeded. For this reason, radiological diagnosis of the condition may be very important.

The radiological appearances are characteristic in a case in whom the air has spread widely, but they may be difficult to recognize when the air is limited to the intrathoracic structures. Linear air shadows outline the heart and the great vessels, and separate the anterior border of the heart from the sternum (*Figure 5.32*). They may also outline the thymus and give rise to an appearance described as the 'spinnaker' sign (*Figure 5.32c*) (*see* page 174). The smallest degree of separation of the thymus from the cardiac and other mediastinal tissues is significant and oblique projections are often helpful in detecting this sign of pneumomediastinum. Air may also collect between the pleura and the diaphragm in an extrapleural pneumothorax and produce a circumscribed translucent area which is difficult to distinguish from a loculated intrapleural pneumothorax.

The lung fields may show a streaky or coarsely granular pattern, not only as a result of the air in the extrapleural spaces but also due to air in the interstitial tissues of the lung itself. Pneumothorax and even pneumopericardium may coexist with air in the mediastinum, but distinction between them can usually be made from

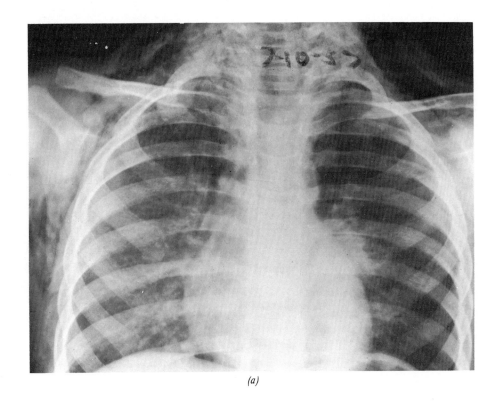

(a)

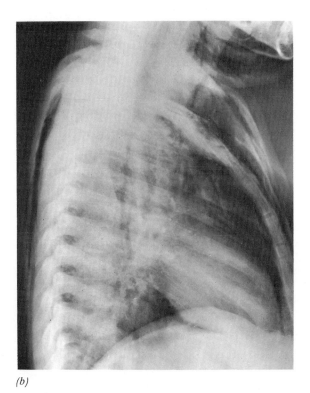

(b)

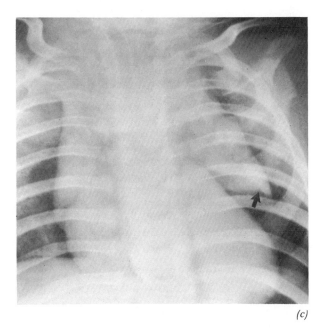

(c)

Figure 5.32. Pneumomediastinum: (a) Anteroposterior view of the chest showing extensive linear translucencies due to air tracking along the mediastinal borders and within the soft tissues of the neck and chest wall. These appearances followed obstruction of the left main bronchus due to inhalation of a foreign body. (b) Lateral view of the same case. (c) Another case in which the mediastinal air is much less extensive but has led to separation of the shadow of the thymus (arrowed) from the left heart border ('spinnaker sign')

196

the fact that mediastinal air is relativley immobile, whereas a change of position will cause a shift of air lying free in the pleural cavity or pericardium.

Newborn infants who have developed a spontaneous pneumomediastinum may present with an apparent dextrocardia. This is said to be due to the fact that the anterior mediastinum extends further to the left than to the right of the midline. As a result air accumulating in this space will tend to force the heart over to the right (Franken, 1970). It is often difficult to exclude an isolated dextrocardia in such cases, especially in view of the fact that the pneumomediastinum may lead to circulatory disturbances. Such a diagnosis should be regarded as unproven in any case in which mediastinal air is present, until the air has been absorbed. The condition is much less serious in older children than in the newborn period because in the former it appears to escape from the thorax much more readily and this is presumably due to the greater size of the thoracic inlet and to the greater ease of dissection of the tissue planes. In these circumstances it is rapidly absorbed and no particular treatment is normally required.

UPPER RESPIRATORY TRACT OBSTRUCTION

Apart from the radiological features common to most cases of obstructive disease of the respiratory tract which have been described above, radiology may often provide information as to the specific cause of the obstruction and to its site. Obstruction of the upper respiratory tract in infants commonly causes stridor in addition to other clinical signs. Radiological investigation of cases presenting in this way may be of considerable value (Scott Dunbar, 1970).

Choanal atresia is usually easy to diagnose clinically, but it may sometimes be confused with other conditions, especially when it is unilateral. The installation of iodized oil into the nostrils followed by lateral films in the supine position using a horizontal beam, will give an accurate outline of the atretic septum. These may be supplemented by anteroposterior or occipitomental views if required. The use of a few drops of 0.5 per cent ephedrine as a nasal decongestant will often be helpful. By shrinking the nasal mucosa it will ensure that contrast medium outlines the nasal cavity completely. If both sides are to be examined, the contrast medium in one side should be drained out before the other side is injected.

Cysts of the pharynx or larynx are often well demonstrated on plain soft tissue lateral films of the neck, preferably taken both in inspiration and expiration. Contrast medium is seldom required and may obscure the lesion, but occasionally midline tomograms may reveal the outline of the abnormal swelling more clearly. Thyroglossal cysts are recognized from their characteristic site at the base of the tongue. Laryngeal or aryepiglottic cysts enlarge and deform the outline of the epiglottis and vallecula and project upwards into the hypopharynx.

Tracheal stenosis has become well recognized recently as a complication of intubation or as a sequel to local

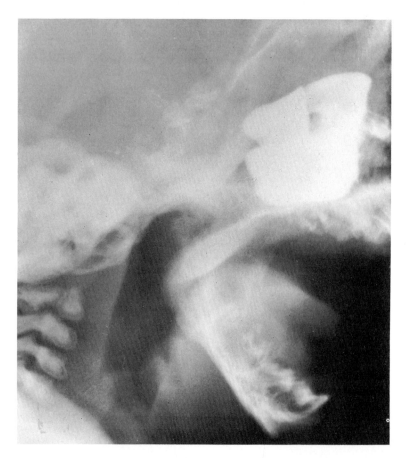

Figure 5.33. Choanal Atresia: Iodized oil has been instilled into both nostrils and a lateral film taken with the child supine. The obstruction between the nasal cavity and the nasopharynx is defined. A thin, bony septum is often present

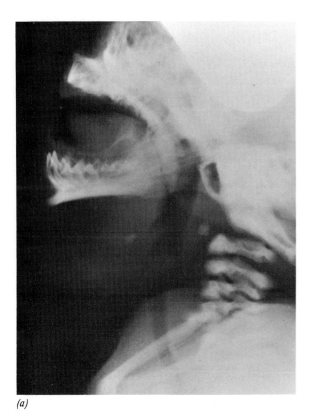

(a)

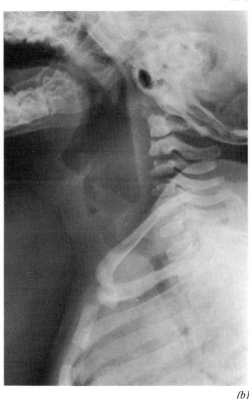

(b)

Figure 5.34. Normal Variations in the Calibre of the Pharynx and in the Course of the Trachea with Respiratory Phase: (a) Lateral film of the neck of an infant taken in relative inspiration, showing the pharynx, larynx and trachea outlined by the air within them; the trachea is straight and shows only minimal tapering from above downwards. (b) Lateral film of the neck of an infant taken in expiration. The pharynx appears distended and the trachea is buckled due to the elevation of the carina by the upward movement of the diaphragm

trauma. It may also occur as a primary condition and may, in such cases, be associated with premature calcification of the laryngeal and tracheal cartilages. It is necessary to avoid confusion with the normal variation in the calibre of the lumen of the trachea, which occurs on inspiration and expiration; this leads to a surprising degree of kinking or buckling in response to the upward movement of the diaphragm during forceful expiration or crying (*Figure 5.34*). With any type of laryngeal obstruction the trachea may collapse on inspiration, but in tracheal stenosis the trachea will not expand during expiration. A condition of 'idiopathic stridor' has recently been described in infants. They manifest an unusual degree of tracheal narrowing during respiratory activity. This either affects the upper part of the trachea on inspiration or involves the lower half on expiration, the latter being seen particularly in infants with 'peripheral' obstruction such as occurs in bronchiolitis or asthma (Wittenborg *et al.*, 1967). Cineradiography is usually required to demonstrate this phenomenon and this may also show the downward and forward movement of the aryepiglottic folds and epiglottis on inspiration when these are abnormally lax and mobile.

Inflammatory disease of the pharynx, larynx and epiglottis are common causes of upper respiratory obstruction and are potentially very serious. Radiological examination is seldom necessary to demonstrate these conditions directly but it may be required to exclude pulmonary disease. In this event a chest radiograph may show subglottic narrowing of the trachea due to inflammatory oedema and this sign may point to the presence of laryngotracheobronchitis. A soft tissue lateral film of the neck may reveal the extent of a *retropharyngeal abscess* (*Figure 5.35a*). Occasionally it may also demonstrate its source in those cases where it arises secondarily to tuberculous disease of the cervical spine. The film may also distinguish between this condition, subglottic oedema or stenosis and epiglottitis. In the latter, the larynx and trachea are shown to be normal and the epiglottis and aryepiglottic folds are enormously swollen (*Figure 5.35b*). However, when this condition is suspected it is essential to examine the patient erect, because lying the child down in a supine position can cause fatal asphyxia.

Vascular rings due to abnormal arteries arising from the aorta or pulmonary artery are well recognized as a cause of stridor and may be readily demonstrated by the impression which they produce on the oesophagus. They should be regarded seriously in any infant who has a combination of stridor and a right-sided aortic arch, because the latter may be associated with a complete vascular ring encircling both oesophagus and trachea, a condition readily relieved by surgical means. The trachea and oesophagus are usually displaced towards one another. In the case of an aberrant right pulmonary artery or of the rare type of aberrant right subclavian artery which passes between the trachea and oesophagus, they may be shown to be separated from each other.

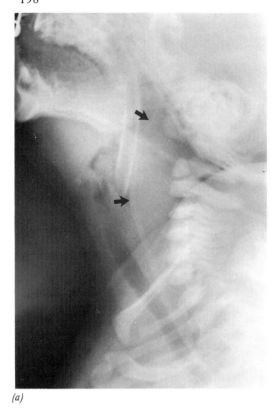

(a)

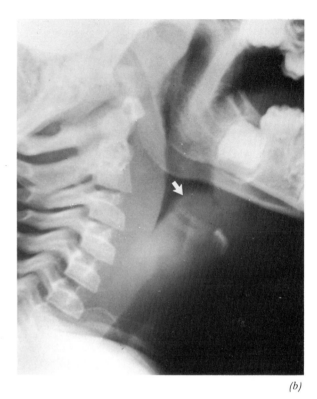

(b)

Figure 5.35. (a) Retropharyngeal Abscess: Anterior displacement of the pharynx, larynx and trachea by a large retropharyngeal abscess (arrowed). An intranasal tube has been inserted to prevent occlusion of the pharyngeal airway. (b) Epiglottitis: The epiglottis (arrowed) and the upper part of the larynx are swollen with considerable narrowing of the airway. There is also swelling of the posterior wall of the pharynx due to spread of the inflammatory process

INHALED FOREIGN BODIES

Children between the ages of 2 and 3 years are particularly liable to inhale foreign bodies but such an accident may happen at any age. A specific history that would suggest the presence of a foreign body may not be elicited. The condition presents as stridor, 'asthma' or a respiratory infection. Some foreign bodies, such as metallic or mineral objects or teeth, are radiopaque but a large proportion of those which are inhaled by children are not opaque (*Figure 5.36*). Their presence then may have to be inferred from the effects on the lungs of the obstruction which they produce. However, the routine use of over-penetrated anteroposterior and oblique films may allow a direct demonstration of non-opaque foreign bodies which may be shown as an interruption in the translucent air column in the trachea or main bronchi. Segmental collapse of the part of the lung supplied by the obstructed bronchus is the commonest radiological appearance, particularly in the case of vegetable matter, such as peanuts. These types of foreign body are a serious problem because of the severe inflammatory reaction which they provoke. If not removed within a short time there is a risk of permanent fibrosis and bronchiectasis developing in the collapsed segment. It is therefore important to examine any such case radiologically and to recognize the characteristic appearances as soon as possible. A proportion (possibly as much as a third) of inhaled foreign bodies produce a ball-valve type of obstruction which leads to distal hyperinflation

and even pneumomediastinum (*Figure 5.29* and *5.32*), but some, particularly the larger metallic objects, may cause no disturbance in aeration (Theander, 1970).

Localization of the foreign body is usually not difficult but it should be remembered that they move spontaneously. Rarely they may be coughed up, but more commonly they are displaced peripherally with an exacerbation of the obstructive effects. In difficult cases tomography may be helpful in showing the foreign body within the bronchus. Fluoroscopy may also assist by allowing observation of the inspiratory mediastinal shift in cases in whom the side affected is in doubt.

BRONCHIAL ASTHMA

Obstruction of the peripheral airways is common at all ages, being seen frequently in the infant with a descending infection, which readily causes sufficient oedema of the mucosa in the finer bronchioles to lead to air trapping. In the older child, asthma is a frequent cause for radiological examination of the chest. It may lead to gross deformity of the bony thorax and also to generalized hyperinflation of the lungs which results in flattening of the diaphragm, small heart shadow and increased vascular markings both at the hila and in the peripheral part of the lung fields. These changes were found to correlate well with the severity of the asthma as assessed on clinical grounds and by tests of pulmonary function (Gillam *et al.*, 1970). Areas of segmental collapse may also be present but are usually transient. Occasionally they are more permanent and are followed by bronchiectasis. In such cases associated infection or rarely mucus plugs are the significant causative factors (*Figure 5.37*). It is important to distinguish these transient areas of segmental collapse from the more serious segmental pneumonia which is found most commonly in the right middle lobe and lingular segments of the left upper lobe. Such episodes of pneumonia may resemble pure collapse closely because an element of atelectasis almost always accompanies the consolidation, but the clinical signs particularly pyrexia, raised sedimentation rate and leucocytosis should help to indicate the correct diagnosis.

Thickening of the bronchial walls or peribronchial tissues is also a sign of associated infection, and once established this tends to persist, but it does not necessarily imply the presence of bronchiectasis. Radiologically it is manifested by fine, gently tapering, parallel linear shadows in the line of the larger bronchi, or as a thick-walled circle, when a bronchus is seen end-on. Tomography may be of value for confirming the presence of such shadows. They may be localized or extend over most of both lung fields and, although they may be obscured during episodes of acute infection, they reappear once this subsides. Bronchography rarely demonstrates significant bronchiectasis but it may show narrowing at the point of origin of the segmental and subsegmental bronchi throughout the lungs (*Figure 5.37b*). Pneumothorax and pneumomediastinum are both found in association with asthma but the clinical signs they produce may be obscured by the hyperinflation present. It is therefore particularly important to examine the chest radiologically in cases of severe or prolonged attacks of asthma or following a sudden collapse in

asthmatic patients. Cardiomegaly is also an important feature to detect as it can be associated with sudden unexpected death. While it is obviously desirable to avoid unnecessarily frequent radiography in children who suffer from asthma, any child sufficiently ill to be admitted to hospital should certainly be examined in order to exclude possibly serious complications such as pneumothorax and also to assess the need for treatment of associated infection.

CYSTS AND TUMOURS OF THE LUNGS AND MEDIASTINUM

PULMONARY METASTASES

Tumours of the lung in children are either metastatic or arise from the local extension of tumours of adjacent structures such as ribs or lymph glands. Metastases are shown radiologically as multiple rounded opacities situated in any part of the lung field. The common sites for the primary tumour in such cases are the kidney (Wilm's tumour), bone (osteogenic sarcoma), suprarenal gland (neuroblastoma, carcinoma), the brain (medulloblastoma) and the blood (leukaemia). In children with such primary tumours a chest x-ray is essential before operative or other treatment is instituted. An association between pulmonary metastases and spontaneous pneumothorax has been reported in older children (Spittle *et al.*, 1968). This is particularly the case with metastases from osteogenic sarcoma and it is suggested that the mechanism

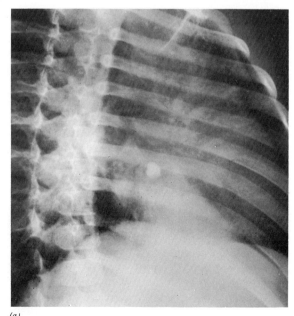

(a)

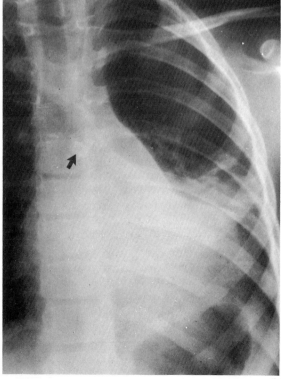

(b)

Figure 5.36. Inhaled Foreign Body: (a) A small pebble impacted in the anterior basal segmental bronchus of the left lower lobe. The collapsed segment distal to the foreign body can be clearly seen as a wedge-shaped opacity with its base on the diaphragm. (b) Collapse of the whole of the left lower lobe due to a tooth (arrowed) lodged in the left main bronchus

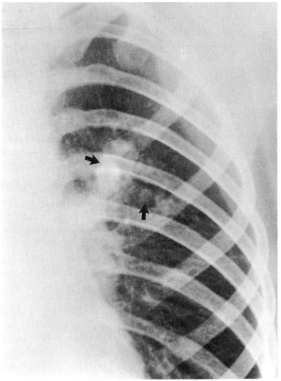

(a)

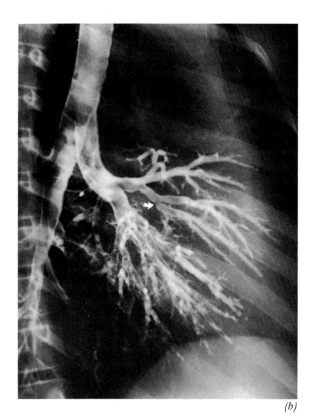

(b)

Figure 5.37. Bronchial Asthma–Mucous Plug: (a) Plain film showing a branched opacity (arrowed) due to a dilated bronchus filled with mucus. This opacity projects from the upper part of the hilum of the left lung. It subsequently disappeared spontaneously. The hilar shadows are prominent as is frequently seen in asthma. (b) Bronchogram of the same case showing occlusion of the apical and posterior segmental bronchi of the upper lobe. The lingular bronchi show a localized narrowing at their origins due to spasm (arrowed)

is probably necrosis of the metastatic deposit leading to a bronchopleural fistula.

CYSTS OF THE LUNG

Cystic lesions of the lungs are radiologically not uncommon but in the majority of such cases, the 'cysts' are probably acquired as the result of infection, ball valve obstruction of smaller bronchi and oedema of the bronchial walls blocking the pores of Kuhn. Pathological confirmation of those lesions which are 'true cysts' is made more difficult by the fact that bronchial epithelium may extend into, and line the walls of chronic abscess cavities once the infection has become quiescent.

True congenital cysts of the lung are often of the same nature as the bronchogenic cysts of the mediastinum. Rogers and Osmer (1964) reviewed a series of 46 cases of 'bronchogenic cysts' and found that 70 per cent were situated within the lungs. They postulate that, although both pulmonary and mediastinal cysts of bronchogenic origin arise from an abnormality in the budding of the developing tracheobronchial tree, the final site of the cyst depends on the time at which the anamoly develops. Radiologically the cyst is shown as a sharply defined round or oval opacity. It is either of uniform density if it contains fluid, or it contains an air–fluid level. It has a relatively thin wall (*Figure 5.38*). The latter feature is, however, not always helpful in the diagnosis between congenital cysts and acquired cavities.

Pneumothorax is a complication of lung cysts, and although it is relatively infrequent, it may make recognition difficult because it may obscure the primary lesion. Tomography is usually unnecessary, but it may in some cases help to distinguish a cyst from overlying structures. Bronchography is chiefly useful in demonstrating the presence of associated bronchiectasis but contrast medium will occasionally enter the cyst itself.

Cysts, or cystic cavities, are not infrequently present in association with sequestrated lobes or segments (*see* page 175), and arteriography either of the pulmonary arterial system or aortography may be helpful in demonstrating the abnormal blood supply.

Hydatid cysts are rarely seen in children in Britain but, in those parts of the world where the disease is common, the lungs are often affected. They most frequently occur in the upper lobes, unlike bronchogenic cysts which occur predominantly in the lower lobes.

CONGENITAL CYSTIC DISEASE OF THE LUNGS

Multiple lung cysts present a difficult problem especially in the differentiation of lesions of varied origin from one another. Pneumatoceles resulting especially from staphylococcal infections of the lungs may be particularly confusing and they may indeed be regarded as 'transient cysts'. However, there seems no doubt that multiple cystic cavities may occur as a congenital malformation and these have been referred to under such terms as congenital cystic adenomatous malformation or congenital cystic disease of the lung (Craig *et al.*, 1956). These may be regarded as different forms of the same basic anomaly, although with histological and radiological differences. The former may cause cyanosis and tachypnoea in newborn infants and it is associated with prematurity and maternal hydramnios. On radiological examination, translucent areas of variable size and shape are scattered through an area of opaque lung with well-defined margins. Mediastinal displacement is present owing to the fact that the abnormal portion of the lung fields tends to occupy a larger space than normal. In true congenital cystic disease, on the other hand, the heart and mediastinum are central and there is often no demonstrable local opacity surrounding the cysts.

An appearance suggestive of multiple cystic spaces in the lung may occur in relation to a large number of different conditions and has been referred to by the term 'honeycomb lung'. This seems to be a purely descriptive label and has no specific aetiological significance. Among the conditions which may give this radiological appearance are included histiocystosis X, tuberose sclerosis, congenital bronchiectasis of the saccular type, diffuse cystic lymphangiectasis, Wilson—Mikity syndrome and biliary cirrhosis, in which both lung cysts and renal tubular cysts may be associated features.

MEDIASTINAL TUMOURS

A considerable variety of tumours and cysts of the neck and mediastinum occur in children, the latter almost always of developmental origin in contrast to cysts of the lung. The tumours are either benign or malignant and may be classified according to their histological nature into neurogenic, teratomatous, lymphatic or vascular types. Their radiological appearance, however, tends to be similar whatever the histological type and the distinction between them has to be made on their situation and the effects they produce on adjacent structures such as the spine, ribs, oesophagus and trachea. The neurogenic tumours, ganglioneuromas and neuroblastomas are characteristically situated in the posterior mediastinum alongside the spine. Involvement of bone is not uncommon in the spine, where the intervertebral foramina may be widened, or the pedicles destroyed or thickened. This occurs especially in the case of tumours which have a portion extending into the spinal canal. In such cases myelography may help in defining the extent of such intraspinal prolongation. The trachea or oesophagus may be displaced or compressed. Calcification may occur in primary neuroblastoma (*Figure 5.39*) of the mediastinum and it takes the form of discrete punctate opacities best seen on tomograms. In the series reported from the Mayo Clinic, (Ellis and DuShane, 1956) neurogenic tumours were the commonest type, comprising a third of all mediastinal cysts and tumours. Teratomata and the related dermoid cysts on the other hand are situated in the anterior mediastinum and are also not uncommonly calcified. They are midline lesions and may grow to a large size before they are discovered; they often extend up into the neck (*Figure 5.40*).

Lymphatic tumours include both those arising from

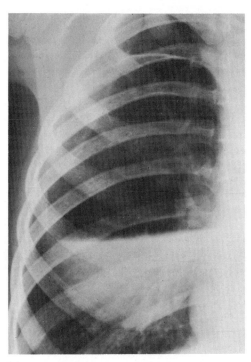 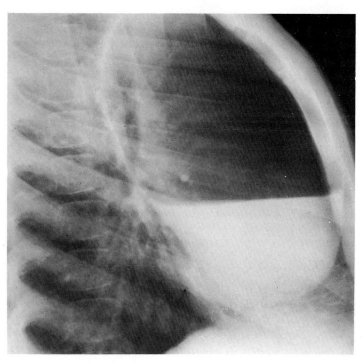

(a)   *(b)*

Figure 5.38 Lung Cyst: A cystic lesion in the anterior part of the right lung with a thin, smooth wall, containing an air—fluid level. This lesion was found to be lined by bronchial epithelium and was considered to be a bronchogenic cyst. (a) Anteroposterior view.
(b) Lateral view

202

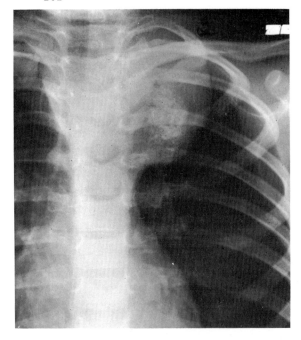

Figure 5.39. Neuroblastoma of Mediastinum: A smoothly rounded mass projects over the apex of the left lung. Fine calcification is present within the tumour and the posterior part of the interspace between the third and fourth ribs is widened

lymph glands such as lymphoma, lymphosarcoma and leukaemia and those arising in the thymus. The bilateral, hilar or paratracheal masses are not usually difficult to recognize but thymic tumours have to be differentiated from the normal thymus on the one hand and from dermoid cysts, teratomata and retrosternal goitres on the other. The normal thymus only presents a problem in the young infant. Vascular tumours occur mainly in the upper mediastinum and they may extend into the neck. Haemangiomata, though mostly benign, may occasionally be malignant. Lymphangiomata tend to be cystic, often of a multilocular type and they present in the first year of life. Such tumours may ramify extensively within the tissues and be difficult to excise. Nevertheless, injection of contrast medium into them is inadvisable.

MEDIASTINAL CYSTS

Congenital cysts of the neck and mediastinum which may be of varied origin and histological nature, resemble each other in their radiological appearances. The features are those of a soft tissue mass with rounded contours and, where these are visible on the radiograph, the margins are sharp and well defined. The group of mediastinal cysts referred to by the generic term of 'foregut cysts' originate from oesophageal, gastric or bronchial epithelium, often with a muscular wall. They present as a mass in the central part of the mediastinum which is often related to the bifurcation of the trachea, but sometimes it extends upwards into the thoracic inlet or neck. About a third of the bronchogenic cysts contain air and, in consequence, show an air—fluid level in an erect film. Those lying beneath the carina may move on

swallowing. All the cysts in this group are commonly associated with other anomalies, such as oesophageal atresia, malrotation of the gut and congenital heart disease. Some of the commonest and most characteristic of these associated lesions are those involving the cervicodorsal spine, either hemivertebrae, fusion of vertebrae or an anterior or posterior spina bifida. Anterior meningocele can very rarely be associated with them, and can also produce a mediastinal mass.

Cysts in the neck may lie in the midline as exemplified by thyroglossal cysts, or laterally as in the case of branchial or pre-auricular cysts. Many of these communicate with the skin through an external sinus or with the pharynx through an internal orifice. Occasionally fistulae from the cyst communicate both with the skin and the pharynx. Radiological demonstration of the extent and connections of such sinuses may be undertaken by injecting contrast medium into the external orifice. This may be of considerable help in localizing such structures before surgical treatment. Alternatively, the cysts which do not connect with a sinus may be aspirated by needle puncture and filled with contrast medium.

MISCELLANEOUS LUNG DISEASE

FIBROCYSTIC DISEASE (MUCOVISCIDOSIS)

The lungs are the site in which the most serious effects occur. Recent improvements in the outlook for children afflicted with fibrocystic disease have resulted very largely from more effective control of the obstructive and infective sequelae of such pulmonary lesions. Although radiological examination of the chest shows appearances which are relatively unspecific and the definitive diagnosis rests on the result of the chemical examination of body secretions, radiology is of value in controlling the efficacy of therapy and in alerting the paediatrician to the presence and extent of lung involvement at a stage before this has become irreversible and is no longer responsive to treatment. The basic abnormality in this condition is related to the physical properties of mucus. It is too viscid and therefore not only fails to perform its normal function, but it leads to obstruction of the narrower bronchi with consequent infection and damage to those parts of the lung distal to the site of blockage.

Hodson and France (1962) have correlated these basic pathological changes with the appearances on the radiograph. Obstructive airway disease results either in generalized hyperinflation or collapse of the affected segment or lobule, depending on the size of the bronchus involved and the degree of the obstruction. The appearances are in no way different from those seen in obstruction from any other cause, in particular bronchiolitis. The hyperinflation affects both lungs and it results in depression of both sides of the diaphragm and a relative reduction in the size of the heart. This picture may be regarded as the basic radiological feature upon which the other signs are superimposed. Areas of pneumonitis or small abscesses give rise to localized peripheral opacities which are often arranged in groups and they may resemble those seen in adult pulmonary tuberculosis (*Figure 5.41*). Such opacities are especially characteristic of the disease and they usually appear

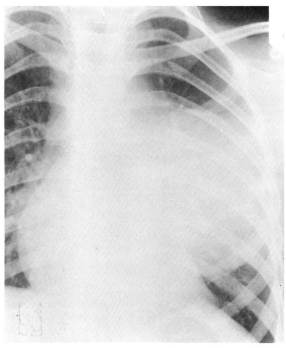

(a)

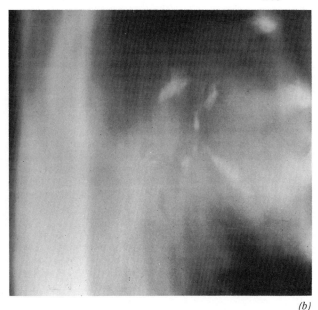

(b)

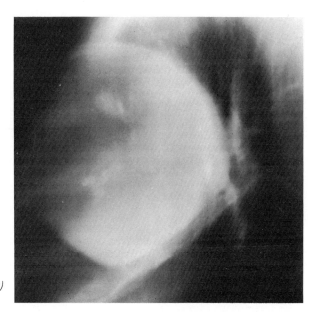

(c)

Figure 5.40. Mediastinal Teratoma: A large ill-defined opacity obscures the midzone of the left lung. (a) Anteroposterior view. (b) Tomogram in frontal plane showing discrete areas of dense calcification within the mass. (c) Tomogram in lateral plane showing the rounded outline of the tumour and compression of the lingular segments of the left upper lobe bounded below by the oblique fissure

during an acute febrile episode. These opacities may disappear in a few weeks or months but frequently recur and may be succeeded by abscess cavities or thin-walled cystic lesions similar to, but more persistent than, the pneumatoceles of staphylococcal pneumonia. These inflammatory foci may be difficult to distinguish from distended bronchi filled with mucopus. The latter however have a branched finger-like shape and radiate from the hilum. They also have a predilection for the upper lobes (*Figure 5.37*). Such 'mucous plugs' may be purely obstructive and therefore disappear when the obstruction is relieved. On the other hand, if they persist for longer than a month, they indicate the presence of permanent bronchiectasis. This condition also occurs in the form of multiple scattered cavities distributed irregularly over the whole of the lungs. Peribronchial

thickening is a very common feature which is recognizable on radiographs as parallel linear shadows or a circular ring shadow. This opacity is much thicker and more obvious than a normal bronchus seen end-on. Such features, when present in the periphery of the lung fields, are always pathological and once they appear usually remain as a permanent change. The hilar glands are very commonly enlarged in fibrocystic disease, especially during acute infective episodes and in advanced cases there may be pulmonary hypertension which leads to cardiomegaly and right-sided heart failure in due course.

A good correlation has been found between the radiological appearances and pulmonary ventilatory function. The signs most useful in the assessment of decreased pulmonary ventilation were air trapping and

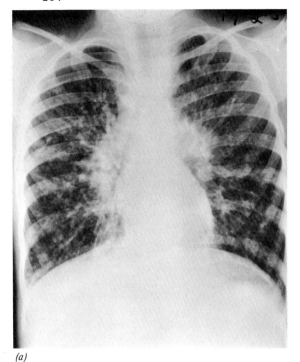
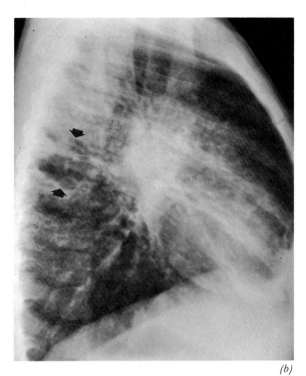

(a)   *(b)*

Figure 5.41. Fibrocystic Disease of the Lungs: (a) Anteroposterior view showing widely diffused opacities extending throughout both lungs. There are enlarged hilar glands and increased bronchovascular markings. The heart is relatively small due to the hyperinflation of the lungs. (b) Lateral view of the same child showing an oval cavity (arrowed) in the apex of the lower lobe due to an abscess. Peribronchial thickening is shown by a small round translucency outlined by a dense ring-like opacity

hyperinflation, peribronchial thickening and the presence of cavities due to abscesses and bronchiectasis (Reilly *et al.*, 1971).

PROGRESSIVE INTERSTITIAL FIBROSIS OF THE LUNGS (HAMMAN–RICH SYNDROME)

Fibrosis of the lungs may result from many causes, either inflammatory or obstructive in nature. It has been recognized that there exists a form of interstitial fibrosis which is progressive and is not due to any known primary cause. Such a condition was first described in adults by Hamman and Rich (1935). It is now known to affect children and to lead ultimately to death from respiratory or cardiac failure. This occurs after an average course of about 4 years (Livingstone *et al.*, 1964).

The radiological appearances of the Hamman–Rich syndrome comprise fine granular opacities diffusely distributed throughout the lung fields but they vary in size. They may be very small and then give rise to a uniform ground glass appearance (*Figure 5.42*). They may form areas of patchy consolidation alternating with small translucencies which, together with the opacities, may resemble the appearance described as 'honeycomb lung'. The hilar shadows are often large and this is due to engorgement of the hilar vessels and main pulmonary arteries, which is often accompanied by cardiomegaly. With such a relatively unspecific radiological picture, the diagnosis may be difficult. The constant or progressive

nature of the lesions may be suggestive of the Hamman–Rich syndrome. The conditions which are most likely to be confused with it are chronic pneumonia or bronchiectasis, particularly the interstitial pneumonias due to viral infections such as influenza, measles and chickenpox, pneumonia due to *Pneumocystis carinii*, idiopathic pulmonary haemosiderosis, idiopathic pulmonary hypertension, and some types of congenital heart disease with persistent heart failure and pulmonary oedema.

Two other conditions have recently been described in children which resemble the Hamman–Rich syndrome very closely.

Desquamative interstitial pneumonitis gives a radiological picture composed of patchy areas of interstitial infiltration on a uniform ground glass background symmetrically distributed on the two sides and indistinguishable from the Hamman–Rich syndrome (Rosenow *et al.*, 1970). However, the histological findings on lung biopsy are diagnostic. The prognosis is very much better and complete radiological clearing may occur on steroid therapy.

Pulmonary alveolar proteinosis has been described in children (Wilkinson *et al.*, 1968). It is a condition of unknown aetiology in which protein and lipoid material accumulate in the alveoli and result in an alveolar–capillary block. Radiography of the lungs shows a diffuse uniform opacity of both lung fields with perihilar shadowing and a well marked air bronchogram. The radiological signs are more extensive than would be expected from the clinical state of the patient, and they may occasionally improve following treatment with acetyl cysteine or proteolytic enzymes.

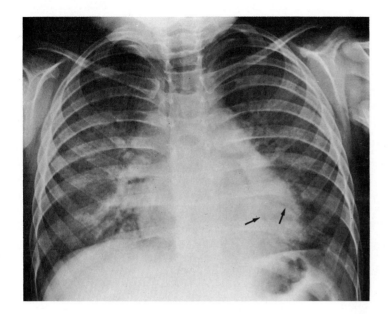

Figure 5.42. Progressive Interstitial Fibrosis of the Lungs: A diffuse haziness of both lung fields is present leading to an air bronchogram (arrowed), best seen in the lower zones, and a loss of definition of the heart borders

Figure 5.43. Pulmonary Haemosiderosis: The uniform hazy opacity of both perihilar regions is seen in the later stages of this condition and is due to a combination of oedema and fibrosis

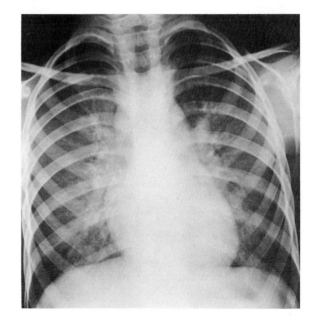

PULMONARY HAEMOSIDEROSIS

The deposition of iron in the lungs in the form of haemosiderin may occur in conditions in which long continued back pressure and venous congestion is present, such as mitral stenosis. In children, however, it may occur without a primary cause but in association with an iron deficiency anaemia. The disease pursues a remittent course over several years, ultimately resulting in death from cardiac or respiratory failure or widespread alveolar haemorrhage.

The radiological appearances are also variable and depend on the phase of the disease in which the examination is made. In the acute exacerbations, there are small discrete opacities from 1 to 3 mm in diameter throughout the lungs often with a clear space within them. These opacities resolve during the remissions, but the lung fields remain lacking in translucency. Sometimes a reticular or granular appearance, either due to alveolar oedema or the progressive interstitial fibrosis persists (*Figure 5.43*). How much of this opacity is due to the haemosiderin deposits is uncertain. The diagnosis may usually be made by examining the sputum or gastric washings for cells containing iron. The nodular opacities of the acute phase appear to represent small areas of haemorrhage into groups of alveoli surrounding a terminal bronchiole. The cause of the haemorrhage is unknown; it is most likely to be due to an abnormality of the pulmonary arterioles or capillaries.

INJURIES OF THE LUNG

The lungs may be involved in chest injuries, whether fractures of the ribs are present or not. In the former case the presence of associated haemothorax or pneumothorax may obscure the radiological signs cf damage to the lung itself. When present without signs of pleural or rib injury, haematomata are shown as ill-defined opacities of variable density and extent within the lung. These do not usually require any special treatment. They may predispose to infection and be persistent, in which case they may appear as coin lesions of indeterminate nature. This appearance may lead to difficulties in diagnosis and even, occasionally, to exploratory thoracotomy, if the true nature of the opacity is not recognized. Furthermore, the lesions may cavitate, often within a few days of the injury, and they may gradually resolve over several weeks. Air–fluid levels are not uncommon and the lesions may then resemble abscesses, cysts or pneumatoceles. The situation of the opacity need not bear any relation to the site or type of injury. The opacity may even occur on the opposite side to the injury. This type of lesion may result from non-penetrating chest injuries in children. They may arise from laceration of lung tissue due to sudden compression of an area of air-containing lung. Chest films in cases of trauma should therefore include a film taken with a horizontal beam if at all possible, even where the injury is extra-thoracic, in order to ensure the demonstration of air–fluid levels in cavitating lesions.

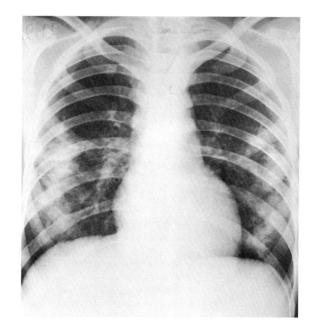

Figure 5.44. Wegener's Granulomatosis: Symmetrical fairly large opacities in the peripheral part of the middle and lower zones of both lungs in a child with periarteritis nodosa. At autopsy these proved to be due to multiple infarcts

EOSINOPHILIC LUNG

Lung lesions may occur in children in association with eosinophilia, for instance, in bronchial asthma, in which the association is by no means constant, and in two other less common conditions.

Loeffler's syndrome

Transient lobular infiltrations, resembling bronchopneumonia, but more widely scattered over the lung fields, may occur in children who are the hosts of a variety of parasites. In the United Kingdom, this association between lung opacities and eosinophilia due to parasites most commonly occurs in ascariasis but in other parts of the world it may occur in relation to other parasitic infestations. The condition is benign and usually clears up rapidly. It is commonly regarded as an allergic manifestation, but a connection with so-called 'larva migrans' has been postulated. In this state a direct irritative effect on the pulmonary tissues may be caused by the migration of the larval stages of certain parasites occurring during the processes of maturation of the adult organism.

Wegener's granulomatosis

Periarteritis nodosa, when it involves the respiratory tract, has different features from those seen in the more typical form of the disease. This has led to the adoption of the above eponymous nomenclature, but most authorities are agreed that the conditions do not differ in their basic pathology. Wegener's granulomatosis commonly presents with a respiratory illness which is often regarded as 'asthma', bronchitis or pneumonia. However, the blood eosinophilia, which is a frequent feature and the presence of eosinophils in the sputum may point to the diagnosis (Rose and Spencer, 1957).

The radiological appearances may be suggestive of the condition if the possibility of the diagnosis is kept in mind. Irregular, homogeneous opacities occur together with smaller miliary shadows, in all areas of the lung fields. These are never segmental in type but there is a tendency for them to be distributed around the perihilar regions, sparing the extreme periphery. This appearance has some resemblance to that of the 'batswing' opacities of pulmonary oedema, and this may suggest the likelihood of a 'vascular' aetiology (*Figure 5.44*). The individual lesions may clear and then reappear elsewhere or they may calcify. Histologically they have the characteristics of necrotizing granulomata and in some instances they appear to arise as areas of infarction related to the arterial lesions.

The diagnosis of this condition is difficult and the radiological appearances, though unusual, are not specific. The existence of systemic signs of periarteritis nodosa in other organs, manifested by bleeding from the alimentary tract, haematuria, hypertension and, in particular, of ulcerating lesions of the upper respiratory tract, paranasal sinuses and middle ear cleft, may be very helpful in making the diagnosis.

REFERENCES

METHODS

Pendarvis, B. C. and Swischuk, L. E. (1969). 'Lung scanning in the assessment of respiratory disease in children.' *Am. J. Roentgl.* **107**, 313

Sargent, E. N. and Turner, A. F. (1968). 'Percutaneous transcricothyroid membrane selective bronchography; a simple, safe technique for selective catheterisation and visualization of segmental and subsegmental bronchi.' *Am. J. Roentgl.* **104**, 792

THYMUS

Caffey, J. and Silbey, R. (1960). 'Regrowth and overgrowth of the thymus after atrophy induced by the oral administration of adrenocorticosteroids to human infants.' *Paediatrics* **26**, 762

Tausend, M. E. and Stern, W. Z. (1965). 'Thymic patterns in the newborn.' *Am. J. Roentgl.* **95**, 125

CONGENITAL ABNORMALITIES

Davidson, S. W. (1956). 'Some anomalies of the respiratory system.' *J. Fac. Radiol.* **8**, 1

Good, C. A. (1961). 'Certain vascular abnormalities of the lungs.' *Am. J. Roentgl.* **85**, 1009

Jeresaty, R. M., Knight, H. F. and Hart, W. E. (1966). 'Pulmonary arteriovenous fistulas in children.' *Am. J. Dis. Child.* **111**, 256

Köhler, R. (1969). 'Pulmonary sequestration.' *Acta Radiol. (Diagn.)* **8**, 337

RESPIRATORY DISTRESS IN NEWBORN

Avery, M. E., Gatewood, O. B. and Brumley, G. (1966). 'Transient tachypnea of newborn; possible delayed resorption of fluid at birth.' *Am. J. Dis. Child.* **111**, 380

Fawcitt, J. (1956). 'Radiological findings in the lungs of premature infants.' *Archs Dis. Childh.* **31**, 119

Finnegan, L. P., McBrine, C. S., Steg, N. L. and Williams, M. L. (1970). 'Respiratory distress in the newborn; value of roentgenography in diagnosis and prognosis.' *Am. J. Dis. Child.* **119**, 212

Hodgman, J. E., Mikity, V. G., Tatter, D. and Cleland, R. S. (1969). 'Chronic respiratory distress in the premature infant: Wilson—Mikity syndrome.' *Pediatrics, Springfield* **44**, 179

Northway, W. H. and Rosan, R. C. (1968). 'Radiographic features of pulmonary oxygen toxicity in the newborn—broncho-pulmonary dysplasia.' *Radiology* **91**, 49

Steiner, R. E. (1954). 'The radiology of respiratory distress in the newborn.' *Br. J. Radiol.* **27**, 491

Wilson, M. G. and Mikity, V. G. (1960). 'A new form of respiratory disease in premature infants.' *Am. J. Dis. Child.* **99**, 489

INFLAMMATORY DISEASES

Feinberg, S. B., Lester, R. G. and Burke, B. A. (1961). 'The roentgen findings in *Pneumocystis carinii* pneumonia.' *Radiology* **76**, 594

Field, C. E. (1961). 'Bronchiectasis: a long-term follow up of medical and surgical cases from childhood.' *Archs Dis. Childh.* **36**, 587

Joffe, N. (1960). 'Cavitating primary pulmonary tuberculosis in infancy.' *Br. J. Radiol.* **33**, 430

Knyvett, A. F. (1966) 'The pulmonary lesions of chicken-pox.' *Q. Jl Med. N. S.* **35**, 313

Sutcliffe, J. and Chrispin, A. R. (1970). 'Chronic granulomatous disease.' *Br. J. Radiol.* **43**, 110

Weber, A. L., Bird, K. T., and Janower, M. L. (1968). 'Primary tuberculosis in childhood with particular emphasis on changes affecting the tracheobronchial tree.' *Am. J. Roentgl.* **103**, 123

AIRWAY OBSTRUCTION

Franken, E. A. (1970). 'Pneumomediastinum in newborn with associated dextroposition of the heart.' *Am. J. Roentgl.* **109**, 252

Gillam, G. L., McNicol, K. N. and Williams, H. E. (1970). 'Chest deformity, residual airways obstruction and hyperinflation and growth in children with asthma. II. Significance of chronic chest deformity.' *Archs Dis. Childh.* **45**, 789

Scott Dunbar, J. (1970). 'Upper respiratory obstruction in infants and children.' *Am. J. Roentgl.* **109**, 227

Theander, G. (1970). 'Motility of diaphragm in children with bronchial foreign bodies.' *Acta Radiol. (Diagn.)* **10**, 113

Wittenborg, M. H., Gyepes, M. T. and Crocker, D. (1967). 'Tracheal dynamics in infants with respiratory distress, stridor and collapsing trachea.' *Radiology* **88**, 653

CYSTS AND TUMOURS

Craig, J. M., Kirkpatrick, J. and Neuhauser, E. B. D. (1956). 'Congenital cystic adenomatoid malformation of the lung in infants.' *Am. J. Roentgl.* **76**, 516

Ellis, F. H. and Dushane, J. W. (1956). 'Primary mediastinal cysts and neoplasms in infants and children.' *Am. Rev. Tuberc.* **74**, 940

Rogers, L. F. and Osmer, J. C. (1964). 'Bronchogenic cyst; a review of 46 cases.' *Am. J. Roentgl.* **91**, 273

Spittle, M. F., Heal, J., Harmer, C. and White, W. F. (1968). 'The association of spontaneous pneumothorax with pulmonary metastases in bone tumours of children.' *Clin. Radiol.* **19**, 400

MISCELLANEOUS

Hamman, L. and Rich, A. R. (1944). 'Acute diffuse interstitial fibrosis of the lungs.' *Bull. Johns Hopkins Hosp.* **74**, 177

Hodson, C. J. and France, N. E. (1962). 'Pulmonary changes in cystic fibrosis of the pancreas: a radiopathological study.' *Clin. Radiol.* **13**, 54

Livingstone, J. L., Lewis, J. G., Reid, L. and Jefferson, K. E. (1964). 'Diffuse interstitial pulmonary fibrosis.' *Q. Jl Med. N. S.* **33**, 71

Reilly, B. J., Featherby, E. A., Weng, T-R, Crozier, D. N., Duic, A. and Levison, H., (1971). 'The correlation of radiological changes with pulmonary function in cystic fibrosis.' *Radiology* **98**, 281

Rose, G. A. and Spencer, H. (1957). 'Polyarteritis nodosa.' *Q. Jl Med. N.S.* **26**, 43

Rosenow, E. C., O'Connell, E. J. and Harrison, E. G. (1970). 'Desquamative interstitial pneumonia in children: Report of two cases.' *Am. J. Dis. Child.* **120**, 344

Wilkinson, R. H., Blanc, W. A., and Hagstrom, J. W. C. (1968). 'Pulmonary alveolar proteinosis in three infants.' *Pediatrics, Springfield* **41**, 510

6 GASTRO-INTESTINAL TRACT

METHODS

CONTRAST MEDIUM STUDIES

Radiological investigation of the alimentary tract necessarily involves the use of a contrast medium because the bowel has no inherent contrast and calcification resulting from disease is rarely distinctive. Swallowed air results in a natural contrast medium which outlines the lumen of the stomach, small bowel and colon in normal individuals. Its absence from the whole or part of the alimentary canal is usually indicative of disease, commonly obstructive, which prevents it reaching the distal part of the bowel. However, the information obtained by utilizing the normal air content is incomplete and an adequate demonstration of the anatomical changes resulting from disease is not provided. For this purpose the use of a positive contrast medium is needed. Barium sulphate has long been the material of choice for this purpose because it has considerable radiographic density, as well as being insoluble and inert. Barium has disadvantages however in the investigation of certain conditions in children. It can become inspissated by the absorption of water from the bowel and by so doing may convert a partial into a complete obstruction. Also, if barium leaks through a perforation into the peritoneum or mediastinum, or spills into the trachea and enters the lung, it is not absorbed and may give rise to local irritation or bronchial obstruction.

Water soluble contrast media

To overcome these difficulties the use of water soluble contrast media has been advocated. A special preparation of meglumine diatrizoate (Gastrografin) for oral use which contains a wetting agent and flavouring to disguise the unpalatable taste is available. Because of their high osmolarity the use of such substances may be dangerous to very young infants, particularly those who may be already dehydrated from continued vomiting or diarrhoea. A rise in the serum osmolarity and in haematocrit value, and also a fall in pulse rate and cardiac output, following the administration of such contrast media either by mouth or as an enema has been demonstrated in experimental work in puppies (Rowe *et al.*, 1971). Diatrizoate (Hypaque, Urografin) is also harmful if it enters the lungs. As its viscosity is low, it can reach the alveoli easily and induce pulmonary oedema of rapid onset. Less soluble and more viscous contrast media, such as barium or propyliodone (Dionosil) do not enter the alveoli but cause a mechanical obstruction in the bronchioles. Therefore the latter medium is preferred for examination of the oesophagus when there is a likelihood of spill into the trachea. The surface tension of the contrast medium may be of importance when it is desired to evaluate disorders of swallowing, especially in newborn infants. Oily contrast media, owing to their low surface tension, are more liable to be aspirated into the trachea than is a barium suspension. In spite of the above objections, if used with caution, water soluble contrast media have a place in the examination of the alimentary tract, especially in suspected obstruction, and in the investigation of sinuses and fistulae where the low viscosity is an advantage. Given as an enema in conditions such as meconium ileus and the milk inspissation syndrome (*see* pages 227, 228), they may have a therapeutic value.

Dangers of contrast enema in children

In contrast to the hypertonicity of diatrizoate solutions, barium suspended in water and given as an enema is hypotonic. It may, therefore, in certain circumstances, lead to excessive absorption of water from the colon. This is likely to occur only when the colon is markedly dilated and, in order to fill it, large quantities of barium are introduced. This may be the case in gross megacolon, either due to Hirschsprung's disease or secondary to long-standing severe constipation. In such circumstances severe shock, or even death, has been reported (Steinbach et al., 1955). Haemodilution and cerebral oedema are the most likely causes of death and it is a simple precaution to add 10 g of salt to every litre of enema fluid in order to ensure that the enema solution is isotonic. Complete filling of the colon should also be avoided when megacolon is present or if there is cardiac or renal failure with tissue oedema.

Barium suspension should not be allowed to reflux in large quantities into the small intestine through the ileocaecal valve, because in small infants this can rapidly result in filling of the whole small bowel and stomach. It may even lead to massive aspiration into the lungs (Castellino et al., 1968).

The use of a self-retaining catheter with an inflatable balloon for barium enemas should be avoided because it is possible to perforate the anterior wall of the rectum in small infants. This is because of the short distance between the anal margin and the rectosigmoid junction and the relatively narrow lumen in this area.

Contrast examination of the small intestine

Examination of the small intestine is less satisfactory than that of either the stomach or the colon. Barium is the most useful contrast medium for this purpose because neither air nor the water soluble contrast media give adequate radiographic detail of the mucosal surface. However, flocculation and clumping of the barium due to aggregation of the particles of the suspension, can interfere seriously with the demonstration of small intestinal anatomy. This is produced by the effect of excess mucus within the bowel, combined with the relatively long period during which the barium remains in contact with the mucus during its passage along the small intestine. The rate of passage of the barium along the small bowel is dependent upon peristalsis and can be controlled only to a limited extent. Although flocculation may be present in most cases of intestinal malabsorption, it can also occur in a wide variety of other diseases of the small intestine. In addition, it is also quite common in normal infants, though its occurrence in the absence of disease diminishes with increasing age. These factors have led to attempts to develop a preparation of barium which is stable in the presence of mucus. There is no doubt that they have been successful to some extent, but no preparation is completely non-flocculable. The use of accelerators, which have the effect of reducing the time of transit through the small intestine, can also improve the quality of the examination. Small quantities of water soluble contrast medium have an accelerating effect when mixed with the barium and, although its mode of action is unknown, it has been claimed that it is more effective than drugs such as Prostigmin and metoclopramide which have been recommended for the same purpose (Goldstein et al., 1971).

Compression of the ileal loops by the use of a non-opaque pad in the prone position and fluoroscopy of areas of the small bowel may enhance the value of the examination. There is a need to control the amount of barium passing through the bowel to ensure that each loop is adequately outlined. The addition of a disaccharide to the barium in the investigation of the disaccharidoses is discussed elsewhere (see page 236).

CINERADIOGRAPHIC STUDIES

The use of fluoroscopy in the course of contrast examinations of the alimentary tract has long been accepted as an essential part of the technique and one which allows an appreciation of the dynamic as well as the static features of the organs being studied. Cineradiography provides a permanent record of such fluoroscopic studies and allows a more detailed analysis of any normal and abnormal movements occurring in the different parts of the alimentary tract.

Unfortunately the use of cineradiography, especially in children, is restricted by the relatively high level of radiation involved. This disadvantage may be offset by recording the fluoroscopic image on videotape. This reduces the radiation dose compared with cineradiography but there is some reduction in quality of the image. The high cost of the equipment has also meant that this method is not yet universally available.

One sphere in which cineradiographic examination is of particular value is in the study of disorders of swallowing, especially in small infants. It enables a precise diagnosis of the mechanism of the dysphagia to be made. It may be the only way in which an organic lesion such as a tracheo-oesophageal fistula can be delineated because of the difficulty of timing standard radiographic exposures.

The importance of conventional films as adjuncts to cineradiographic studies has been stressed (Ardran and Kemp, 1956). These may give information about the anatomy which is not available on the dynamic studies where the detail is necessarily less perfect. It has been estimated the radiation received from cineradiographic runs of 3–4 seconds, at 25 frames a second, is of the order of 1 roentgen.

CHOLECYSTOGRAPHY AND CHOLANGIOGRAPHY

Both oral and intravenous cholecystography are easily carried out in children but require a proportional reduction in the dose of contrast medium compared with that used in adults. There is no greater liability to side effects and, as is the case with urographic media, the cholangiographic contrast media may be better tolerated in young children than in adults. Excretion of intravenous contrast media such as Biligram by the liver tends to be rather more rapid in the child. Tomography may be very valuable in overcoming the tendency for the bile ducts to be obscured by overlying bowel gas shadows. A dose of 1 ml of Biligram per 2 kg bodyweight injected slowly intravenously over a period of 10–15 minutes is advisable.

The direct injection of contrast medium into the gall

bladder at operation may be valuable in cases of suspected biliary atresia in order to demonstrate the patency or lack of patency of the cystic, hepatic and common bile ducts. This method has also been used to show anomalies in the bile ducts in cases of choledochal cyst.

ANGIOGRAPHY

This examination finds its main application in the investigation of abdominal masses, particularly cysts and tumours of the liver, spleen and kidney. There are a few reports of its use in the study of inflammatory diseases of the intestine. Angiography should always be regarded as complementary to other methods of investigation such as barium studies, urography, lymphography and isotope scanning, since more information will be obtained from a combination of several such methods than from any one method alone.

The transfemoral approach using the Seldinger technique is generally adopted and will allow selective catheterization of the hepatic, coeliac, renal, superior or inferior mesenteric arteries. The location of the catheter tip in main stream aortography should be high enough to ensure filling of the coeliac axis. A rapid serial changer should always be used because the arterial, capillary and venous phases of the angiogram need to be studied. The arterial phase will demonstrate the blood supply of the mass and the displacement of vessels and surrounding structures by it. The capillary and venous phases will show organ or tumour opacification ('tumour blush') and the presence of tumour vessels. If the tumour is avascular, there will be no tumour flush nor will tumour vessels be shown.

Complications are infrequent, but there may be a greater risk of thrombosis in the femoral artery than in adults, particularly where selective catheterization is employed. It has been suggested that adequate aortograms can be obtained in infants by rapid injection of contrast medium in large doses (2 ml/kg) into the femoral vein, thus avoiding the possible risks of arterial catheterization at this age. (Cecile *et al.*, 1972). There seems no doubt, however, that the quality of the aortograms so obtained will be less good. In most cases direct aortography is the method of choice, though the former technique may have a place in demonstrating those lesions such as renal or suprarenal tumours which are likely to invade or displace the inferior vena cava.

In the newborn infant, catheterization of the umbilical artery is a practicable method of performing aortography; e.g. for the study of renal or hepatic tumours or other abdominal masses.

Portovenography

The injection of contrast medium directly into the spleen in a patient with portal hypertension is a valuable method of determining the site of obstruction within the portal system of veins. Provided that the spleen in large enough to be easily palpable, the technique carries no great risk or difficulty.

Umbilical catheterization

Catheterization of the umbilical vein or artery in the neonate is a method now used more frequently for administering fluid or even nutriment to sick or immature infants. There is, however, an increasing realization that possible adverse sequelae such as portal phlebitis or arterial thrombosis, may follow this procedure, particularly if the placement of the catheter is faulty. For this reason the use of radio-opaque catheters is a wise precaution because their position can be easily checked radiographically.

ISOTOPE AND ULTRASONIC SCANNING

As in the case of angiography, organ scanning in the investigation of abdominal disease has been relatively infrequently used in children. However, it may be a useful method for localizing hepatic masses, such as hepatoblastomas, metastatic tumours, congenital and parasitic cysts and abscesses. Two different techniques can be employed. The first is the use of I^{131}- tagged rose bengal which is taken up by the liver cells and excreted in the bile; second, the use of sulphurcolloid containing technetium 99^{m} which accumulates in the reticulo-endothelial system and which will outline both the liver and spleen.

Ultrasound can also be used to localize space-occupying lesions, differentiate between solid tumours and cysts and may also give evidence of the presence of cirrhosis of the liver.

CONGENITAL LESIONS

ATRESIA OF OESOPHAGUS AND TRACHEO-OESOPHAGEAL FISTULA

Although these two congenital abnormalities need not necessarily both be present in the same individual, in the majority of cases they are associated and the radiological features in such cases reflect the presence of both anomalies. The fistulous track can be situated either within the neck at the level of the seventh cervical vertebra, or at the level of the second to fourth thoracic vertebra. It runs obliquely upwards from the oesophagus to the trachea and is demonstrable only in the lateral projection, when the trachea and oesophagus are not superimposed upon each other. Occasionally the fistula takes the form of a window between the closely apposed walls of the trachea and oesophagus and in such cases is very difficult to demonstrate.

Plain film appearances

The most frequent combination is atresia of the oesophagus with a fistula between the trachea and the oesophageal lumen distal to the atresia. In such cases all that is needed to make a pre-operative diagnosis radiologically are plain films of the chest, neck and abdomen in the anteroposterior and lateral projections.

The portion of the oesophagus above the atresia is very commonly distended with air and this enables its

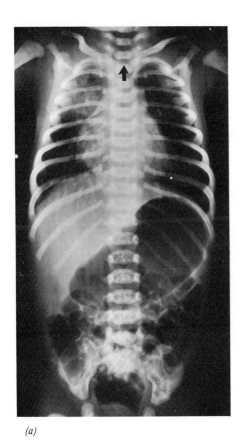

(a)

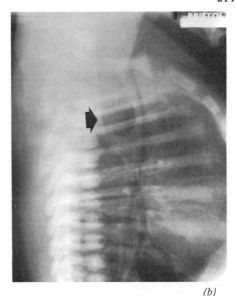

(b)

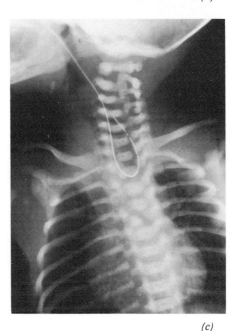

(c)

Figure 6.1. Oesophageal Atresia with Fistula between the Trachea and the Oesophagus below the Atresia: (a) The stomach and intestinal loops are somewhat distended by air which has passed through the fistula. The part of the oesophagus above the atresia is also distended by air, (arrowed) but is obscured by the spine. An opacity in the upper zone of the right lung is due to inhalational pneumonitis which has resulted from food spilling into the trachea during swallowing. (b) Lateral view of the thorax with the upper portion of the oesophagus above the atresia distended with air (arrowed) (c) An opaque catheter has been passed into the upper portion of the oesophagus and has coiled upon itself, so outlining the level of the atresia

size and, in particular, the lower limit of its extension to be determined on the lateral film without the use of a positive contrast medium (*Figure 6.1a*). The latter should be avoided because of the likelihood of aspiration into the lungs. However, if a more precise delineation of the extent of the level of the atresia is required, this can be achieved by passing an opaque flexible catheter through the mouth and allowing it to coil upon itself at the level of the atresia (*Figure 6.1c*). The stomach and intestine will contain air which has entered them through the fistula into the distal oesophagus, but the latter may not contain enough air to be accurately visualized (*Figure 6.1b*). The chest radiograph may show areas of pneumonitis due to inhalation of food or secretions into the lungs from the oesophagus (*Figure 6.1a* or *6.2*). It may also demonstrate associated congenital heart disease which may be present in about 25 per cent

of cases. Skeletal anomalies of the spine and of the upper limbs are also not infrequently seen.

Cases where an oesophageal atresia occurs without associated tracheo-oesophageal fistula constitute the next most frequent group. The plain film appearances will be similar to those described above except that there is complete absence of any air in the gastro-intestinal tract (*Figure 6.2*).

Demonstration of a tracheo-oesophageal fistula

A much more difficult radiological problem is provided by those cases in which a tracheo-oesophageal fistula occurs in the absence of atresia or connects the trachea with the upper oesophagus above an atretic segment (*Figure 6.3*). In such cases the fistula may be unsuspected

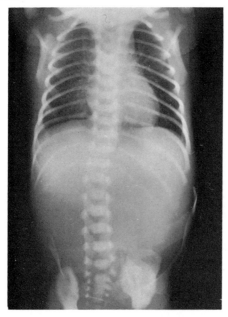

Figure 6.2. Oesophageal Atresia without Fistula: Anteroposterior view of chest and abdomen. No gas is present below the atresia. An opacity in the right lower zone is indicative of an inhalational pneumonitis

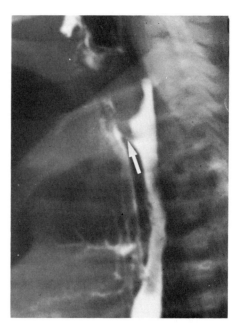

Figure 6.4. Tracheo-oesophageal Fistula ('H' type): Contrast medium (Dionosil) fills the oesophagus, the trachea and the fistulous track (arrowed) between them

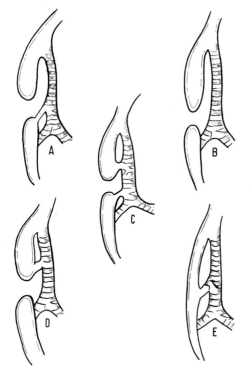

Figure 6.3. Oesophageal Atresia and Tracheo-oesophageal Fistula: A. Type in which an atresia is combined with a fistula between the trachea and the oesophagus below the atresia. This accounts for about 70 per cent of cases. B. Oesophageal atresia without associated fistula. This accounts for about 20 per cent of cases. C. Atresia with fistulae to both parts of the oesophagus. D. Fistula to the upper portion of the oesophagus only. E. Tracheo-oesophageal fistula without atresia (H-type fistula)

until persistent dysphagia, choking during feeds or the presence of pneumonitis unresponsive to treatment draws attention to the possibility. Such cases require the use of a contrast medium to demonstrate the fistula directly (*Figure 6.4*). Because inhalation of contrast medium is unavoidable, aqueous propyliodone is the type to be preferred. A flexible catheter preferably with side-holes, but no end-hole, is placed with its tip at the lower end of the oesophagus. The contrast medium is injected as the catheter is withdrawn to a point just below the junction of the pharynx and oesophagus, avoiding spill into the larynx. Passage of the contrast medium through a fistula depends on the use of gravity when the infant is placed prone or on a forcible injection through it. In older children, in whom a fistula has been missed or has recurred, barium can be swallowed in the prone position. Because of the abnormal peristalsis which accompanies tracheo-oesophageal fistulae the barium tends to remain in the upper oesophagus. When the child is asked to cough, the barium may be sucked through the fistula and up into the larynx and pharynx from where it is again swallowed. Cineradiographic studies may demonstrate this very characteristic cyclical movement (Sauvegrain *et al.*, 1969). Failure to show a fistula is no proof that it does not exist. A repeat examination in a few days time may be required because some fistulae appear to open or transmit only intermittently. If no tracheal spill occurs with propyliodone, barium may be given from a bottle to exclude other possible causes of dysphagia.

Complications

Radiology in the postoperative period may be required if complications are suspected. If pneumonitis persists

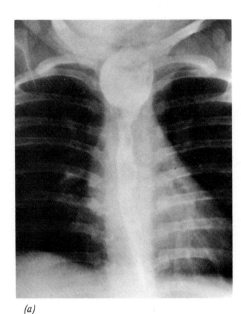

(a)

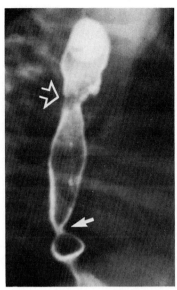

(b)

Figure 6.5. Strictures Following Primary Anastomosis for Oesophageal Atresia (a) A stricture at the site of the anastomosis. (b) Two strictures, one at the site of the anastomosis and the other in the lower third of the oesophagus (arrowed)

after operative treatment of an atresia the suspicion of a fistula to the upper pouch should be entertained. An effusion arising after operation suggests a leakage from the site of the anastomosis, which can result from respiratory distress in the postoperative period. The leak at the anastomosis may be shown by the spread of water soluble contrast medium from the oesophagus into the mediastinum or a recurrent fistulous tract may be shown. Stenoses may occur in the lower segment of the oesophagus as well as at the site of the anastomosis (*Figure 6.5*). Pyloric stenosis or atresias elsewhere in the alimentary canal may coexist and give rise to symptoms.

In cases where a primary anastomosis has not been possible owing to the extent of the atretic segment, a gastrostomy may be performed. Contrast medium introduced via the gastrostomy will usually reflux into the lower segment of the oesophagus. It may help to delineate its upper limit and the extent of the gap between the lower and upper segments.

HIATUS HERNIA

It is now accepted that the incidence of vomiting due to hiatus hernia is relatively high in the first few months of life. However, the radiological demonstration of hiatus hernia at this age may be a matter of some difficulty, partly due to the intermittent nature of the condition and partly due to the confusion that exists as to the criteria necessary for its recognition.

Two types occur in children: (1) the 'sliding' oesophagogastric type, in which the oesophagus enters at the apex of the intrathoracic portion of the stomach and (2) the para-oesophageal type, in which the gastric fundus herniates through the diaphragmatic hiatus alongside the lower end of the oesophagus (*Figure 6.6*). A third has been described in infants, under various names such as 'chalasia' (Neuhauser and Berenberg, 1947) and 'lax cardia' (Forshall, 1955) (*Figure 6.8*). There has been some controversy as to whether this type

is properly to be regarded as a true hiatus hernia or merely a neuromuscular imbalance which leads to a persistent state of relaxation of the cardia. While the former view is supported by many of the more experienced workers on the subject, there seems little doubt that the clinical features, prognosis and response to treatment differ in this type from those of classical hiatus hernia. The condition known as 'rumination' in which an infant regurgitates a feed and swallows it again has also been regarded as due to hiatus hernia because the radiological appearances are similar and because of the good response to treatment by maintaining an erect posture.

Radiological features

Of the various radiological features seen in cases of hiatus hernia, the presence of a portion of stomach above the disphragm would seem to be an essential diagnostic criterion (*Figure 6.7*). That this is not necessarily always the case is due to the fact that the recognition of a supradiaphragmatic gastric pouch may not be an easy matter. It is not a permanent feature. It is only intermittently present, moving up and down through the widened hiatus according to variations in posture and intra-abdominal pressure. It is important to ensure that the lower oesophagus is well filled with barium so that an intrathoracic gastric pouch, if present, will be distended. This can be achieved as a rule if the infant can be induced to suck from a bottle through a teat with a wide hole, while counter pressure is applied to the abdomen. Various criteria have been proposed to determine whether such a pouch is really part of the stomach but they have mostly been shown to be unreliable. A hernia with a large gastric pouch has a characteristic purse-like shape and is separated off from the oesophagus by a slight constriction. On the other hand a gastric pouch may be tubular, with no visible distinction from the oesophagus above it. This appearance may account for some of the cases of 'chalasia' (Husfeldt

214

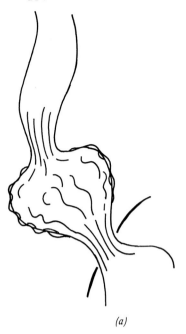
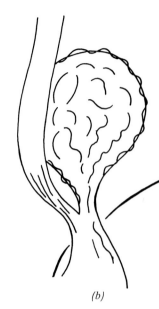

Figure 6.6. Hiatus Hernia: (a) 'Oesophago-gastric' type in which the oesophagogastric junction lies at the apex of the intrathoracic gastric pouch. (b) 'Para-oesophageal' type in which the oesophagus enters the stomach below the apex of the pouch and often below the diaphragm

(a)   (b)

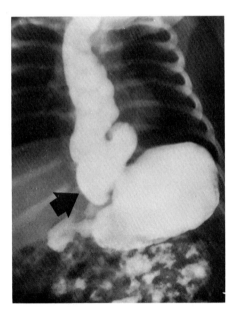

Figure 6.7. Hiatus Hernia in Infancy: oesophagogastric type with a well marked intrathoracic gastric pouch (arrowed) and a wide, rather redundant oesophagus entering the stomach at the apex of the pouch

et al., 1951). Gastric mucosal folds (if demonstrated) may be a helpful feature in diagnosing a hiatus hernia and may be recognized because their irregular and often transverse direction contrasts with the longitudinal oesophageal folds. However, in infants they are seldom obvious enough to be very useful in diagnosis. Observation of oesophageal peristalsis may reveal that it stops short above the diaphragm and does not pass through the gastric pouch thus differentiating between

oesophagus and stomach. However, in cases of 'lax cardia', peristalsis tends to be irregular and of diminished intensity and is associated with a widened, rather flaccid oesophagus.

Gastro-oesophageal reflux

Another important radiological feature in hiatus hernia is gastro-oesophageal reflux. It can be argued that the demonstration of reflux is of more importance than the presence of an intrathoracic gastric pouch, because it is the action of the acid gastric juice with its high enzyme content on the oesophageal mucosa which is responsible for most of the symptoms and serious sequelae, such as anaemia, inhalational pneumonitis and oesophageal stricture. However, confusion is again caused by difficulties in defining exactly what is meant by reflux. It is well known that infants can regurgitate their feeds as a result of over-rapid ingestion or air swallowing, and vomiting is a symptom which can result from a large variety of causes during the first few months of life. If reflux is strictly defined as the passive flow of gastric contents through the cardia into the oesophagus, the problem becomes less difficult. Reflux occurs as soon as, and whenever, the child is placed in a recumbent position or when the intra-abdominal pressure is raised by crying, struggling or sudden movement. Reflux as defined in this way very rarely occurs in normal children. It can usually be differentiated from regurgitation on the one hand, which is transient and not constantly reproducible and from vomiting on the other hand, which is an active process, accompanied by gastric contractions.

The radiological demonstration of reflux requires that the stomach should be moderately full of barium, but not over-distended to an unphysiological degree,

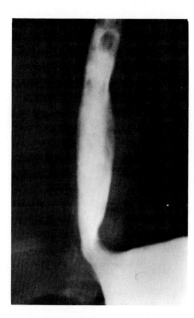

Figure 6.8. Hiatus Hernia ('chalasia' or 'lax cardia'): Free gastro-oesophageal reflux occurring in the absence of a well-defined intrathoracic gastric pouch. A hiatus hernia was subsequently repaired surgically

with active contraction of the stomach wall. This should not lead to difficulty in interpretation if it is observed that the process is initially a passive one, and is constantly provoked in response to change of position. The occurrence of reflux in the absence of a demonstrable gastric pouch above the diaphragm is a frequent finding and is responsible for the concept of 'chalasia' or 'lax cardia' (*Figure 6.8*). Although, there may be a difference in natural history and prognosis between such cases and those with a well defined pouch, the two groups of cases probably reflect a difference of degree rather than of kind. It should be recognized that hiatus hernia in the infant may be intermittent, and may be obvious on one occasion and absent on another. For this reason, in any doubtful case, it is advisable to repeat a barium meal more than once before excluding hiatus hernia as a possible cause for the child's symptoms.

In the rare, large, para-oesophageal type of hernia there may be absence of reflux, but the pouch may be clearly visible on a well penetrated chest film by virtue of its gas and fluid contents. A barium meal will readily demonstrate the lesion (*Figure 6.9*).

Complications

The complications that may arise from hiatus hernia are pneumonitis, oesophagitis (with or without stricture formation) and peptic ulceration.

Pneumonitis should always be sought for in a chest film. This occupies the characteristic site of inhalational pneumonitis in the infant, being commonest on the right side and in the upper and middle lobes. Sometimes cavitation is present, indicating the development of a lung abscess.

Oesophagitis is not detectable radiologically, the ulceration which it causes being superficial and leading to no constant abnormality of outline.

Peptic ulcer is shown as a small rounded or pointed projection from the lumen of the oesophagus. True

and that the oesophagus should be empty. It is also an advantage to have the infant quiet. Crying and struggling can undoubtedly provoke reflux, but crying especially may result in such a powerful contraction of the diaphragm that it prevents reflux occurring, at least during the prolonged expiratory phase. Furthermore, passive reflux which occurs spontaneously when the infant is quiet, is more likely to be the result of a pathological condition than the sudden intermittent flow of barium up the oesophagus which occurs during the inspiratory gasps of a crying infant. It should be noted, however, that reflux may sometimes actually induce vomiting

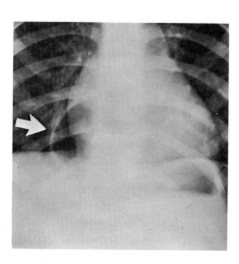

(a)

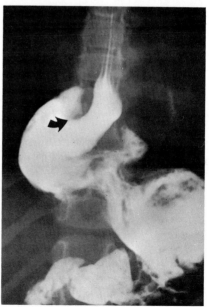

(b)

Figure 6.9. Para-oesophageal Hiatus Hernia: (a) Plain chest film in which the intrathoracic gastric pouch is visible by virtue of its gas content and lies in the right cardiophrenic angle (arrowed). (b) Barium meal of the same child as in (a) showing that the gastro-oesophageal junction (arrowed) lies below the apex of the gastric pouch

216

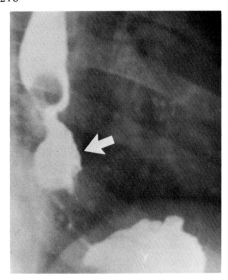

Figure 6.10. Peptic Stricture of the Oesophagus Complicating Hiatus Hernia: The Intrathoracic gastric pouch (arrowed) may often be inconspicuous in the presence of a stricture

peptic ulcer of the oesophagus is very rare, but may occur where the oesophagus is lined by gastric epithelium. Peptic ulcer of the supradiaphragmatic gastric pouch can be misinterpreted as an oesophageal ulcer where the pouch is tubular in shape and in consequence is poorly differentiated from the lower oesophagus.

Stricture of the oesophagus resulting from peptic oesophagitis occurs in 38 per cent of cases of hiatus hernia in which a definite gastric pouch is demonstrable, and in 7 per cent of the 'lax cardia' type (Forshall, 1955). Such a stricture is situated characteristically within 2 or 3 inches of the hiatus and is usually relatively short (*Figure 6.10*). Long strictures, or those occurring in the upper or middle third of the oesophagus, are likely to be due to other causes such as swallowing caustic liquids, or the presence of gastric mucosa lining the oesophagus (columnar lined oesophagus). The latter condition is probably a congenital abnormality, but one which tends to be overlooked in childhood. In the series described by Pierce and Creamer (1963) all the cases showed either a stricture or reflux due to an associated hiatus hernia. Careful observation may be required to identify early stricture. In these the degree of obstruction to fluid barium may be minimal, though more solid food may be held up. In doubtful cases cineradiographic studies may be useful. Progressive shortening of the oesophagus can occur due to spastic retraction or fibrosis; this may elongate the gastric pouch into a tubular structure, whose resemblance to a normal oesophagus is increased by the relative lack of filling and distension due to the stricture.

Unlike other types of diaphragmatic hernia, hiatus hernia is not often associated with other congenital abnormalities. There is, however, a well established association between hiatus hernia and congenital hypertrophic pyloric stenosis. For this reason the pylorus should always be examined in any infant suspected of hiatus hernia. It is important that this is done before the stomach is filled with barium which may obscure the detail of the antral region.

Radiological examination may also be required following either conservative or surgical treatment of hiatus hernia in order to assess their effectiveness in controlling reflux. In the case of the former it should be remembered that while reflux will disappear after a few months of postural treatment in the majority of cases of 'lax cardia', this may not be the case where a well defined pouch is present. These cases could become free of symptoms and still show virtually unchanged radiological findings in about 66 per cent of cases (Carré and Astley, 1960; Sorensen, 1967).

OTHER TYPES OF DIAPHRAGMATIC HERNIA

A hernia through the pleuroperitoneal canal (Bochdalek type) or through a defect in the tendinous portion of the diaphragm anteriorly (Morgagni type) may give rise to severe respiratory distress in the neonatal infant. Radiology will demonstrate the presence of such a hernia and enable it to be distinguished from other causes of respiratory distress, such as hyaline membrane disease, aspiration syndrome or pneumonia. Operative repair of the hernia to relieve compression and collapse of the lung from the presence of abdominal organs within the thorax, may be life-saving and constitutes a surgical emergency.

The radiological appearance of loops of bowel within the thorax are multiple small translucent areas surrounded by thin curvilinear walls of soft tissue density (*Figure 6.11a*). An additional feature which helps to confirm the diagnosis is marked displacement of the heart and mediastinum to the opposite side in the pleuroperitoneal type, or towards the spine in the Morgagni type. There is relative absence of bowel gas shadows in the abdomen or they may be in an abnormal position. The latter feature can be particularly helpful in the diagnosis of right-sided hernia, in which bowel loops may occur high up in the right hypochondrium. The loops of bowel within the thorax are not limited by any defined border unless there is a hernial sac present. This may be the case in about a third of the Bochdalek type hernias and in the majority of Morgagni hernias (*Figure 6.11b*). In such cases the extent of the hernia can appear to vary from day to day and differentiation from eventration where the diaphragm, though much thinned, is intact may not be possible.

The state of the lung on the side of the hernia is an important factor in the ultimate prognosis. There is often significant hypoplasia which leads to a slow and incomplete expansion after repair of the hernia. Such de-aeration may be quite extensive and be misinterpreted as 'pneumonia'. Conversely, a chest infection occurring on the same side as a diaphragmatic hernia may lead to confusion and the intrathoracic bowel may be regarded as an area of emphysema or even cystic disease of the lung.

A further very important complication is the development of a pneumothorax, which may readily be precipitated by attempts to inflate the hypoplastic lungs. Some parts may have a high resistance to inflation, whereas other parts may have a lower resistance, the latter rupturing at the pressure necessary to inflate the

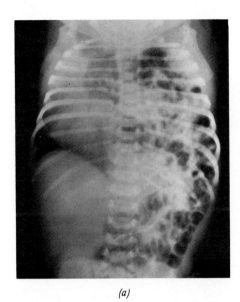

(a)

Figure 6.11. Diaphragmatic Hernia: (a) Bochdalek type with defect in the posterolateral part of the diaphragm; multiple loops of bowel are present within the thorax and the mediastinum is displaced to the right. (b) Morgagni type with defect in the anteromedial part of the diaphragm; the bowel loops are separated from the lungs by the hernial sac which is shown as a smooth, well-defined curved border (arrowed)

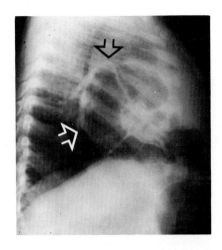

(b)

former. If the pneumothorax occurs before repair of the defect in the diaphragm, it will give rise to a pneumoperitoneum as well.

After surgical treatment, radiology may be required not only to follow the re-expansion of the lung and the return of the mediastinal structure to their normal position, but to exclude the presence of a residual sac or of a recurrence of the hernia. Contrast medium given by mouth may be helpful, though it should be remembered that these latter complications may lead to incarceration of bowel loops and obstruction.

CONGENITAL HYPERTROPHIC PYLORIC STENOSIS

In the majority of cases, the diagnosis of this condition is clinical and radiology is not required. However, in some cases, the characteristic tumour may not be easily palpable owing to the high position of the pylorus, or may be ill-defined or softer than usual. In such cases radiology may provide confirmatory evidence of the presence of pyloric stenosis.

Plain films may reveal dilatation of the stomach with little or no bowel gas shadows distal to it. However, if the gas distribution is normal, barium by mouth is required to elicit the diagnostic features of the condition. These consist of the visualization of the pyloric tumour, which indents the barium both in the body of the stomach and in the duodenum. The lumen of the stomach at the site of the tumour is represented by a thin streak of barium, concave upwards and shown as a double or even triple line due to the barium remaining in the clefts between the oedematous mucosal folds. The first part of the duodenum is crescentic in shape resulting from the protrusion of the tumour into its base (*Figure 6.12* and *6.13*). Gastric emptying may be delayed, but obstruction is rarely complete. Barium starts to leave the stomach early in the examination, especially if the infant is allowed to remain prone with the left side raised slightly from the table top and is given a dummy teat to suck. Too much barium in the stomach may obscure the pyloric region. It may be necessary to

aspirate gastric contents before starting the examination. The presence of hyperperistalsis is helpful in differentiating infants with pyloric stenosis from those in whom gastric emptying is delayed from psychogenic inhibition of gastric motility. Pylorospasm may mimic true pyloric stenosis in many of its features. It may be differentiated by the fact that peristaltic waves are observed to traverse the narrowed antrum, if followed carefully over a sufficient period of time. It should also be remembered that the surgical treatment of pyloric stenosis does not abolish the 'tumour' and the radiological signs may persist for several months afterwards (*Figure 6.14*). It follows from this that radiological examination as a means of assessing the cause of continued vomiting after treatment is unlikely to be very helpful.

Acquired pyloric stenosis is rare in childhood but it has been described after ingestion of ferrous sulphate. It develops about 4 weeks after the acute gastritis provoked by the iron compound. Congenital obstructive lesions may occur in the region of the pylorus, such as true atresia and antral mucosal diaphragm; these are all rare lesions. They may be confused with congenital pyloric stenosis, but they lack the string-like lumen and the evidence of the projection of the tumour into the stomach and duodenum.

DUODENAL OBSTRUCTION

This may be either intrinsic or extrinsic, partial or complete, and the radiological appearances will vary accordingly.

Complete duodenal obstruction is commonly due to *atresia of the duodenum* but it may occasionally be produced by extrinsic pressure. The radiological appearances are dilatation of the stomach and of the first part of the duodenum, together with absence of gas distally in the intestine (*Figure 6.15*). The appearance is usually diagnostic, but if doubt arises, the diagnosis may be confirmed by the passage of a tube into the stomach, aspiration of fluid contents and injection of air or barium. Either of these contrast media passes very rapidly through the pylorus. The pylorus may be

218

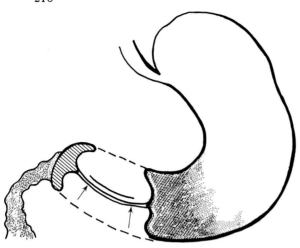

Figure 6.12. Congenital Hypertrophic Pyloric Stenosis: The 'tumour' may be recognized both by the narrowing of the lumen (arrowed) and by the crescentic indentations on the barium in the body of the stomach and the first part of the duodenum

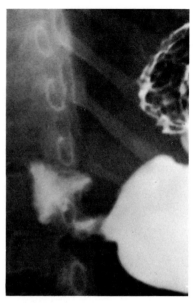

Figure 6.14. Congenital Hypertrophic Pyloric Stenosis: Residual deformity of the pyloric antrum shown in a child aged 4 years, in whom the condition had been treated by conservative measures. A similar residual deformity can persist for several months following pyloromyotomy

atresias elsewhere in the alimentary tract. There may be a history of hydramnios in the pregnancy. These features make the distinction of duodenal atresia from other causes of high obstruction such as congenital hypertrophic pyloric stenosis relatively easy. Some cases can present however with a palpable mass and without bile in the vomit and radiology may, in such cases, be very useful. Rarely in cases of duodenal atresia there is a bifid pancreatic duct with one orifice opening into the duodenum above and one below the atretic segment. Thus gas may bypass the atresia through this duct and be present in the distal small intestine (Astley, 1969).

Malrotation and volvulus

Extrinsic obstruction of the duodenum is commoner than atresia and is frequently associated with malrotation of the intestine. The latter condition may give rise to volvulus of the upper small bowel, because the fixation of the duodenum, the ascending and the descending colon to the posterior abdominal wall is abnormal. The entire intestine may be suspended from a single point of attachment in the region of the root of the mesentery; it can easily undergo twisting, with the production of a complete obstruction. The signs on the plain film may be indistinguishable from those in duodenal atresia, but after giving barium by mouth a characteristic spiral or corkscrew-like appearance in the proximal jejunum may be seen (*Figure 6.16*).

Complete obstruction from congenital bands can occur at any level in the small intestine. It is most commonly seen in the duodenum, which is crossed by a band ('Ladd's band') connecting the caecum to the posterolateral abdominal wall. Obstruction of the duodenum from extrinsic causes is, however, more commonly incomplete and intermittent. It may therefore

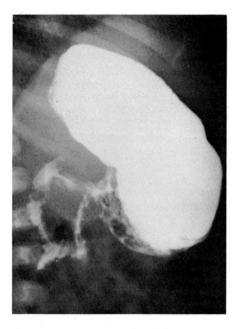

Figure 6.13. Congenital Hypertrophic Pyloric Stenosis: Barium meal showing a triple line of barium within the narrow lumen of the pyloric antrum and the 'tumour' indenting the base of the first part of the duodenum

inconspicuous because of the fact that it is dilated together with the stomach and first part of the duodenum. In cases in which there is a diaphragm across the duodenum, there may be a sharply defined curved termination to the duodenal loop, an appearance which has been graphically described as the 'windsock' duodenum.

In most cases of duodenal obstruction, there is bilious vomiting and a high incidence of associated congenital anomalies which include mongolism, heart disease and

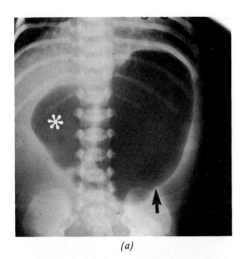

(a)

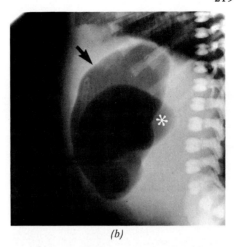

(b)

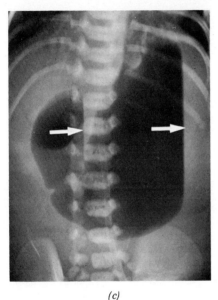

(c)

Figure 6.15. Duodenal Atresia: The dilated stomach (arrowed) and first part of the duodenum (*) are clearly shown separate from each other and gas is absent from the rest of the bowel. (a) Supine anteroposterior film. (b) Lateral film taken with the child lying on the left side so that gas fills the dilated duodenum. (c) Horizontal beam film with the child on left side; two fluid levels (arrowed) are present, one in the stomach and one in the duodenum

present in later childhood or give rise to recurrent vomiting and abdominal colic which can be misdiagnosed as 'cyclical' or 'psychogenic' vomiting. In such cases, especially if examined in between the attacks of vomiting, there may be a normal appearance on the plain film and barium meal; however, the barium meal examination may provide evidence of the condition by showing the abnormal position of the duodenojejunal flexure, the presence of jejunal loops on the right side of the abdomen and a mobile caecum lying high up in the epigastrium. However, proof of the cause of such intermittent obstruction must be sought by examination during an attack, at which time the dilated duodenal loop will usually be easy to identify and the site of obstruction may be demonstrated by a barium meal. These features may be more obvious in the supine position than in the prone or erect positions, particulalry when the cause of the partial obstruction is related to compression of the fourth part of the duodenum between the aorta and the superior mesenteric artery. The use of a barium enema has been advocated to reveal malrotation, because in complete non-rotation, the colon lies in the left side of the abdomen with the ileum entering the caecum

from the right side. A barium enema is in general less valuable than a barium meal, especially if the latter is followed through to the caecum. Duodenal obstruction may be caused by a relatively minor degree of malrotation, often amounting to no more than malfixation, and a barium enema is unlikely to show the site and cause of such obstruction.

The vascular congestion associated with volvulus or incarceration of bowel loops may lead to signs of a generalized ileus, thickening of the wall of the small bowel and free fluid in the peritoneal cavity which may be visible in a plain radiograph of the abdomen. Occasionally a prenatal volvulus may lead to necrosis and calcification of the bowel wall.

It should be remembered that extrinsic and intrinsic causes of duodenal obstruction may occasionally coexist. This may result in a volvulus or an atresia of the more distal part of the bowel being overlooked, because the radiological picture only reveals the duodenal obstruction.

Annular pancreas

In about 20 per cent of patients who have complete obstructions of the duodenum owing to atresia there is an associated annular pancreas. Such cases present within the first week of life. Annular pancreas not associated with duodenal atresia may, however, remain unsuspected until middle age. The radiological signs may be those of complete obstruction and in this event the condition will only be diagnosed at operation. If, however, the obstruction is partial, a barium meal may show a concentric stricture of the second part of the duodenum or an indentation of the right lateral border of the loop. Dilatation is often present proximal to the site of obstruction, but this may be intermittent (*Figure 6.17*) (Free and Gerald, 1968).

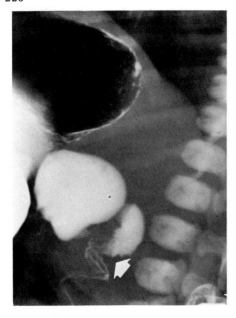

Figure 6.16. Extrinsic Obstruction of the Duodenum with Malrotation and Volvulus: The proximal duodenum is dilated. Distal to this the lumen is narrowed with a spiral appearance (arrowed) at the point where the volvulus of the mesentery occurs

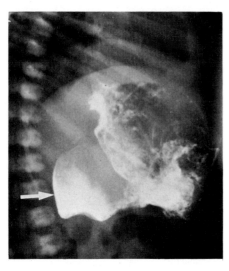

Figure 6.17. Annular Pancreas: Although barium has not passed beyond the dilated first part of the duodenum (arrowed), gas is present in the distal intestinal loops, showing that the obstruction is incomplete

RECTAL AGENESIS AND IMPERFORATE ANUS

The distinction between lesions in which the rectum ends above the levator ani and those in which it extends below this level is an important one. The site of termination of the rectum indicates whether an anal sphincter is likely to be present and the type of surgical treatment which is to be adopted. The method of taking a lateral film of the abdomen with the patient inverted and an opaque marker on the site of the anal dimple, has been

widely used for this purpose, but recently considerable doubt has been cast upon the reliability of the results obtained (*Figures 6.18* and *6.19*) (Berdon *et al.*, 1968). Complete filling of the blind end of the rectum with gas may fail to occur, either owing to insufficient time elapsing since the birth of the infant to allow swallowed air to reach the rectum, or to the presence of meconium occupying its most distal part (*Figure 6.20*). Faulty positioning or crying may also give rise to inaccuracies in the estimation of the distance between the rectum and the skin. Gas may fail to accumulate in the rectum if a large fistula is present through which it can escape. Furthermore, it is usual to relate the level of the rectal pouch to various bony landmarks in order to determine which type of lesion is present, but these landmarks possess no constant relationship to the soft tissue structures upon which the distinction is based. Of the landmarks used to distinguish 'high' lesions from 'low' ones, the pubococcygeal line joining the symphysis pubis and the sacrococcygeal joint, or the 'M' line described by Cremin (1971) are the most useful (*Figure 6.21*). However, provided these fallacies are recognized, and the technique is applied with careful attention to accurate positioning, the method is of value not only as a guide to the type of lesion present, but also as a means of demonstrating the presence of other abnormalities. These include associated spinal anomalies, particularly degree of sacral agenesis, and rectovesical or other types of fistula, which may be recognized by the presence of gas in the bladder or vagina (*Figure 6.19*).

If an external orifice is present, either in the form of an ectopic anus or a rectoperineal or rectovestibular fistula, it is desirable to attempt to inject water soluble contrast medium into it, in order to delineate the rectal pouch more clearly and to show the extent and nature of the fistulous tract (Shopfner, 1965). Retrograde urethrography in the male, or vaginography in the female, may achieve the same result. These examinations should preferably be done using a 'flushing' technique in which the tip of the catheter is inserted only just inside the orifice. If a catheter is inserted right into the orifice the results may be misleading, since the catheter may bypass the opening of the fistula.

The injection of contrast medium directly into the distal limb in an infant in whom a colostomy has been performed as the primary procedure, may also delineate fistulae and even result in filling of the ureters and renal pelves if vesico-ureteric reflux is present (*Figure 6.22*). Anomalies of the genito-urinary tract in association with rectal agenesis occur in about half the cases, particularly in those with anomalies of the sacrum. Either excretory urography, or micturating cysto-urethrography, is therefore desirable in cases with 'high' lesions and often in those with 'low' lesions as well.

The coexistence of atresias in the proximal part of the bowel is sufficiently common to give rise to difficulty in the interpretation of plain films, because in such cases gas will not reach the rectum. Rudhe (1968) suggests that percutaneous puncture of the rectal pouch may overcome this difficulty. Other skeletal anomalies, such as talipes, congenital dislocation of the hip, polydactyly and the radial aplasia syndrome (*see* page 32 *et seq*) may be present and should be investigated by the appropriate radiographs. Associated congenital heart disease is also not uncommon.

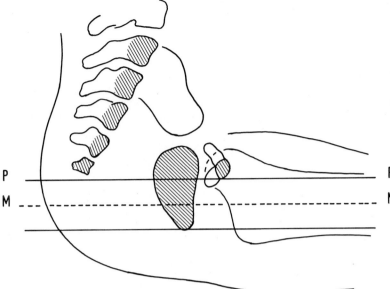

Figure 6.18. Imperforate Anus: Lines used to define the level of the most distal point reached by the rectal gas in the inverted lateral view. The pubococcygeal line (P) joins the symphysis pubis and the coccyx. The M-line (M) described by Cremin which he states indicates the plane of the levator ani. This is drawn parallel to the pubococcygeal line and half way between it and the third line passing through the lowermost point of the ossification centre for the ischium

MECKEL'S DIVERTICULUM

Although it is a common congenital malformation of the alimentary tract, occurring in between 1 and 2 per cent of all individuals at autopsy, Meckel's diverticulum is difficult to demonstrate radiologically. This is due to its situation in the ileum, where contrast media cannot be introduced without filling much of the remainder of the bowel as well, so that the diverticulum is obscured.

The importance of Meckel's diverticulum lies in the complications which may ensue from it. Bleeding or perforation from peptic ulceration may occur in heterotopic gastric mucosa. Obstruction due to bands, volvulus and internal herniae may be associated. The diverticulum may act as the predisposing cause of an intussusception; in such cases it may become invaginated and present as

a tube-like or polypoid defect on barium enema. Calcification can develop in the wall of a Meckel's diverticulum or in faecoliths within its lumen. Rarely a Meckel's diverticulum can attain a large size and be full of faeces. In this event it will be shown as a spherical mass with a mottled bubbly appearance in it due to mixed gas and faecal material.

ATRESIA OF THE BILE DUCTS

This is the commonest cause of obstructive jaundice in the newborn infant and is a condition which sometimes may be amenable to surgical correction. It has to be distinguished from other causes of jaundice. These include neonatal hepatitis, galactosaemia, infections, e.g. Toxoplasmosis, syphilis and cytomegalovirus, and

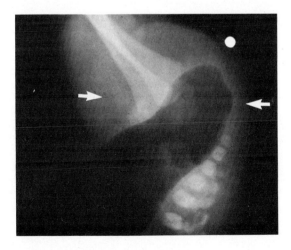

Figure 6.19. Imperforate Anus—low type: Lateral film taken with the infant inverted with an opaque marker placed over the anal dimple. The gas in the dilated rectum is shown to extend well below the plane of the levator ani (arrowed)

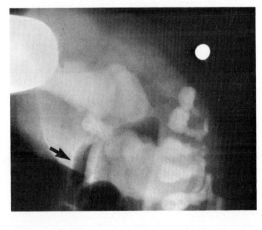

Figure 6.20. Imperforate Anus—high type: The rectal gas fails to extend beyond the plane of the levator ani, suggesting that the distal part of the rectum and the anal sphincter are absent. The presence of gas in the bladder (arrowed) (lying anterior to the dilated rectum) indicates the presence of an associated rectovesical fistula. There is also maldevelopment of the sacrum

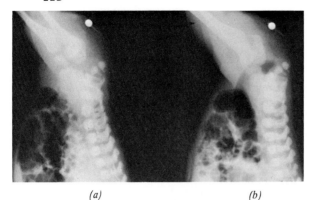

(a)   *(b)*

Figure 6.21. Imperforate Anus: These two inverted lateral films (a) and (b) were taken successively at an interval of 20 minutes during which the inverted position was maintained. The infant was 7 hours old when examined. The distal progress of intestinal gas to fill the upper part of the rectum is well shown, but it fails to extend below the plane of the levator ani

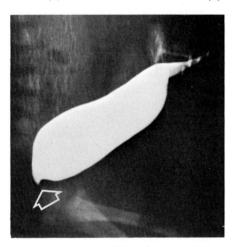
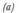

(a)

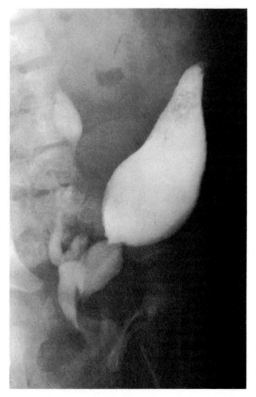

(b)

Figure 6.22. Imperforate Anus—loopogram: (a) Contrast medium injected into the distal limb of a colostomy performed for imperforate anus has delineated the blind end of the rectum. The presence of a fistula is suggested by the fine tapering of the distal end of the rectum (arrowed). Contrast medium has leaked out onto the towel beneath the infant (b) and (c) Contrast medium injected into the distal limb of a colostomy (C) has passed through a rectovesical fistula to fill not only the bladder (B), but also the vagina (V), the right ureter (UR) and an ectopic right renal pelvis (P)

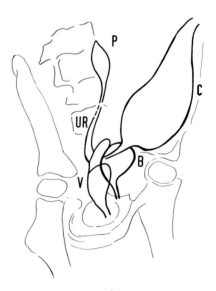

(c)

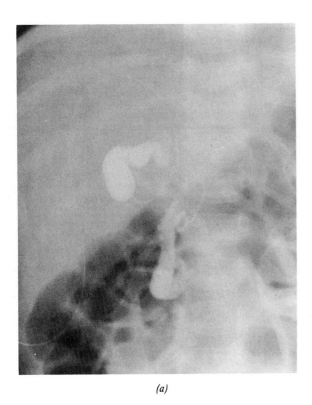

(a)

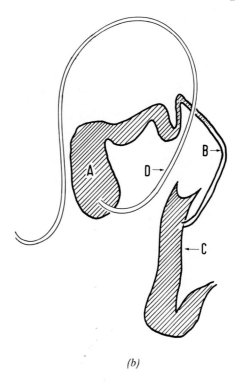

(b)

Figure 6.23. Operative Cholangiogram: Contrast medium injected via a catheter (D) into the gall bladder (A) at laparotomy has demonstrated patency of the cystic duct and common bile duct, (B) with passage of the contrast medium into the second part of the duodenum (C). Atresia of the bile ducts suspected as being the cause of obstructive jaundice has been excluded

bile inspissation. Operative cholangiography may be necessary in order to make this distinction. It should be carried out as soon as practicable, certainly before 8 weeks of age, lest irreversible cirrhosis should develop. 10 ml of water soluble contrast medium injected into the gall bladder at laparotomy should normally opacify the hepatic and common bile ducts and enter the duodenum (*Figure 6.23*). This will not be the case if the bile ducts are atretic. A liver biopsy can be taken at the same time. The distinction between congenital atresia of the bile ducts and neonatal hepatitis may be difficult. In the latter the hepatic ducts may not fill and the common bile duct may be very small due to a 'disuse atrophy' which is potentially reversible after recovery from the hepatitis. (Hays *et al.,* 1967). However, in such doubtful cases, contrast medium is usually seen to enter the duodenum. If the gall bladder is absent or very small, radiology is best avoided as attempts at retrograde injection from the common bile duct may be dangerous.

INTESTINAL OBSTRUCTION

GENERAL

Some congenital anomalies result in intestinal obstruction and many of these have already been discussed in a previous section. However, there are also a number of conditions in which obstruction arises as a result of acquired disease or in which the relation of the obstruction to the congenital abnormality is less immediate.

For instance, intestinal obstruction due to a strangulated inguinal or femoral hernia, although not very common in childhood, is usually not difficult to diagnose on clinical grounds. Occasionally the nature of such a case may be obscure and in this situation the presence of gas-filled bowel lying below the inguinal ligament in a plain film of the abdomen may help to suggest the cause of the obstruction.

Obstruction of the intestine is demonstrated radiologically by showing dilatation of the bowel proximal to the site of obstruction and the dilated bowel contains fluid levels on radiographs taken with a horizontal beam. It is important to realize that the presence of fluid levels alone on films taken erect or inverted does not necessarily mean that obstruction is present. For proof of this, it is necessary to establish the presence of distended gas- and fluid-filled loops proximal to the site of obstruction and of collapsed airless bowel distal to it. While theoretically this is a simple enough requirement, in practice, especially in the small infant, it may be difficult. The reason is that, at this age, loops of dilated small and large intestine resemble one another very closely, both in site and in contour. Furthermore, because of the rather restricted space within the infant's abdomen, it is very difficult to separate individual loops from one another. In this respect, the use of an inverted lateral film of the abdomen may often be very helpful. In such a projection, the gas-filled rectum may be clearly seen extending into the pelvic cavity parallel to the hollow of the sacrum and separate from the rest of the intestine (*Figure 6.24*). The presence of gas in the

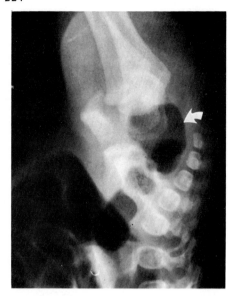

Figure 6.24. Use of Inverted Lateral View in Cases of Suspected Intestinal Obstruction: Although distended loops of bowel and gas–fluid levels in films taken with a horizontal beam may be present, the fact that gas has filled the rectum (arrowed) establishes that obstruction is not the cause

rectum in reasonable quantities affords presumptive evidence that a major degree of obstruction is not present. If the obstruction is complete however, no gas will reach the rectum.

The use of a contrast medium to outline the intestine in cases of suspected obstruction is not often required. Barium given by mouth is safe in cases of gastric or high small bowel obstruction where it is likely to be well diluted by the fluid within the bowel proximal to the obstruction. Its use is less desirable in suspected obstruction of the distal bowel because there is a risk of increasing the obstruction due to inspissation by absorption of water from the contents of the bowel. Water soluble contrast media are to be avoided in infants who may already be suffering from dehydration because owing to their hypertonicity these contrast media may withdraw fluid from the tissues. The use of a barium enema to investigate distally situated obstructions is a relatively safe procedure, and one which in certain circumstances may even have some therapeutic value.

FUNCTIONAL OBSTRUCTION IN THE NEWBORN INFANT

In children of any age who are investigated for vomiting it is common to find no organic cause. This may be the case in newborn infants, who have the classical symptoms of obstruction, i.e. repeated vomiting, abdominal distension and failure to pass a stool. Such infants are often premature and suffer from the respiratory distress syndrome (Dunn, 1963). Other causes are feeble peristalsis due to immaturity, ileus due to infections, cerebral damage, metabolic disturbances and drugs given to the mother during labour or late pregnancy.

Plain radiography of the abdomen in such cases seldom shows fluid levels and gas can usually be seen in the rectum in the inverted lateral film. Barium enema

seldom reveals the exact cause in such conditions, although the demonstration of a colon of normal calibre may exclude ileal atresia or meconium ileus.

Functional obstruction of the gastro-intestinal tract due to adrenocortical insufficiency may resemble mechanical obstruction very closely (Weens and Golden, 1955). These cases suffer from a lack of aldosterone and may present with projectile vomiting and severe dehydration and with radiological appearances indistinguishable from congenital hypertrophic pyloric stenosis or duodenal atresia. In consequence the condition has been referred to in the past as 'pseudo pyloric stenosis'.

HIRSCHSPRUNG'S DISEASE

Radiology has long played an important role in the diagnosis of colonic aganglionosis and especially in distinguishing it from secondary megacolon resulting from chronic constipation (*Figure 6.25*). The demonstration of the transition zone between the grossly dilated proximal bowel and the aganglionic segment in the well established case is not usually a difficult matter provided lateral views of the rectum, taken both during the injection of barium and after its evacuation, are included. Cases may be recognized early in life, often as a result of symptoms suggestive of intestinal obstruction in the neonatal period. It has now been found that cases occur in which the aganglionosis involves the whole colon and even the small intestine. These may be much commoner than has so far been realized; it may be that they have not been recognized because their clinical presentation and radiological appearances are different. Even the use of rectal biopsy, as the ultimate diagnostic criterion, may be misleading when normal ganglion cells are present distal to the aganglionic segment, e.g. in the 'zonal' type described recently by McIver and Whitehead (1972). For these reasons a knowledge of the variations in the radiological appearances that occur at different ages and in the various types of the disease is important (Hope *et al.*, 1965).

In the newborn infant suspected of having intestinal obstruction, a plain film of the abdomen will show that the colon is disproportionately large compared with the normal-sized small intestinal loops, in cases of Hirschsprung's disease. An inverted lateral view, which should always be obtained, will sometimes reveal fluid levels, but it will also show that little or no gas is present in the rectum (*Figure 6.25*). Such plain film appearances are never diagnostic and a contrast enema should always be undertaken. The classical transition zone may not be present at this stage and may only become visible several weeks after birth (Ehrenpreis, 1946). The response of the colon to the injection of contrast is always abnormal. There is an increased tolerance to its presence and this allows filling of the whole colon. The enema may not be evacuated as in the normal child and some may be retained for as much as 14 days in spite of attempts to remove it by lavage. For this reason, it has been considered better to use water soluble contrast media, such as Hypaque. Because these are hypertonic, the possibility of excessive and dangerous absorption of water may be avoided (*see* page 209).

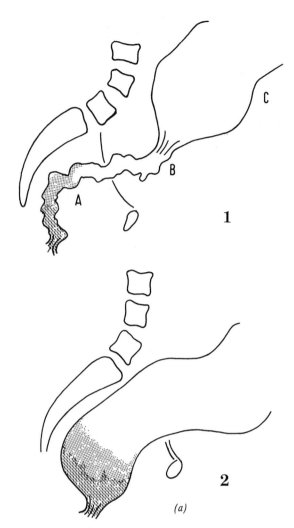

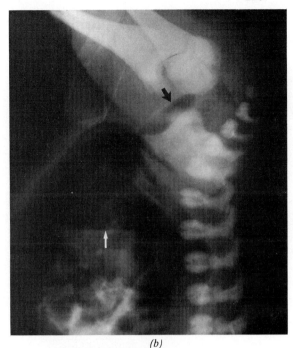

(b)

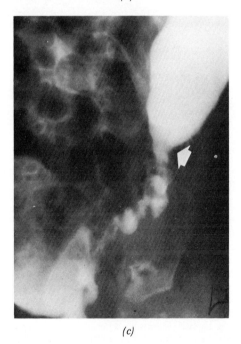

(c)

(a)

Figure 6.25. Hirschsprung's Disease: (a) In Hirschsprung's disease the aganglionic segment (A) is divided from the dilated colon proximal to it (C) by the transition zone (B). This distinction depends on the presence of a sufficient degree of dilation of the proximal colon. (a) (2) In secondary megacolon due to constipation no such distinction is present and the dilated bowel extends as far as the anal canal. (b) Inverted lateral view in a case of Hirschsprung's disease showing dilated bowel with fluid levels (white arrow) and a relatively small amount of gas extending into the rectum (black arrow). (c) Enema using water soluble contrast medium in the same case. The distinction between the aganglionic segment, the contour of which is irregular and the much wider colon proximal to the transition zone (arrowed) which contour is smooth, is well shown

As the child becomes older, the distinction between the normal and aganglionic colon will become more obvious, especially if care is taken not to overdistend the latter and delayed films are taken (*Figure 6.26*). The use of the term 'narrow segment' is to be deplored, because the calibre of the aganglionic part of the colon may be normal. It is the relative difference in calibre between the abnormal segment and the dilated colon proximal to it which constitutes the significant radiological feature of the disease (*Figure 6.25b*). The aganglionic segment may show an irregularity of outline, with projections from the lumen which do not completely encircle the whole colon. This feature can be

particularly helpful in the recognition of long segment aganglionosis where, apart from some shortening of the colon which results in the caecum being displaced upwards, it may be the only abnormality. The small bowel in this type of the disease is usually dilated and the appearance, therefore, closely resembles meconium ileus (*see* page 226) with masses of meconium filling the distal ileal loops or caecum. Contrast readily floods into the ileum and may even reach the stomach and reflux into the oesophagus. It is important to recognize the long segment type of disease because the prognosis is poor. The mortality rate is as high as 70 per cent from diarrhoea, infection and haemorrhage. Necrotizing

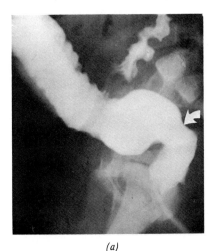

(a)

Figure 6.26. Hirschsprung's Disease: Contrast enema in a child with a very short aganglionic segment. (a) During injection of contrast medium. (b) After evacuation. The transition zone (arrowed) between the aganglionic segment and normal colon may be obscured during injection but is accentuated after evacuation because the contrast medium is held up at the transition zone

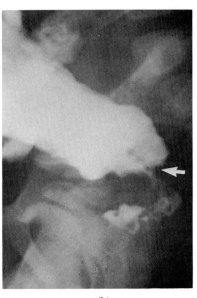

(b)

enterocolitis forms an important and sometimes fatal complication of Hirschsprung's disease (*see* page 234).

Following operative treatment, radiological investigation may be required if complications develop such as stenosis at the site of the anastomosis or fistula formation.

Associated congenital abnormalities, though not very common, may be of radiological interest. Atresia or stenosis elsewhere in the alimentary tract may be present and together with malrotation may lead to confusion as to the site of obstruction. Dilatation of the urinary tract, especially the ureters and bladder, has been described in association with aganglionosis and may be demonstrated on urography. There appears little evidence to support the view that there is a common aetiology between the two conditions. A type of skeletal dysplasia has been shown to occur in association with aganglionosis under the term 'cartilage hair hypoplasia'. The radiological appearances of the bones suggest that it is a variant of metaphyseal dysostosis (*see* page 14).

MECONIUM ILEUS

Some infants with cystic fibrosis of the pancreas develop obstruction in the neonatal period due to an abnormal stickiness of the meconium which may become impacted and plug the lumen of the bowel, usually in the proximal part of the ileum.

The radiological appearances are those of small bowel obstruction but there may be certain features which are suggestive, though not as a rule diagnostic, of the underlying cause. Thus, there is often a group of finely mottled translucencies lying across the midline in the lower abdomen, due to small bubbles of air trapped within the mass of sticky meconium in the ileum (*Figure 6.27*). This appearance, however, can occur in other conditions in which semisolid faecal matter accumulates within dilated loops of bowel, notably Hirschsprung's disease and imperforate anus.

In meconium ileus fluid levels are often scanty or absent and, when present, they form only slowly after the child is placed in the erect position, as would be expected from the nature of the bowel contents. However, when an atresia or volvulus of the ileum accompanies meconium ileus, which may be the case in over half the cases, fluid levels may be much more in evidence.

Calcification scattered over the surface of the peritoneum is occasionally seen and is due to *meconium peritonitis* (*Figure 6.28*). It has been estimated that this may occur in as many as 33 per cent of cases of Meconium ileus (Grossman *et al.*, 1966). It results from an intra-uterine perforation of the bowel which allows an escape of sterile meconium into the peritoneal cavity. The meconium undergoes rapid calcification, probably within a few days. Such calcification, when present, is very characteristic of meconium peritonitis, but does not occur solely in cases of meconium ileus; it can occur in any condition in which intestinal obstruction with perforation is present before birth, such as volvulus, internal hernias and congenital bands. It can also occur following spontaneous perforation without obstruction (Smith and Clatworthy, 1961).

The usual type of calcification consists of small plaques diffused all over the peritoneum, but occasionally, when the perforation occurs into the lesser sac or becomes localized, it may take the form of a calcified *pseudocyst* (*Figure 6.29*). Most frequently, the intestinal perforation is sealed off before birth but rarely this may not be so, in which case a pneumoperitoneum will develop when the child starts swallowing air. Swallowed amniotic fluid may leak from such a perforation with the production of *neonatal ascites*. Symmetrical, dense, horizontal bands have been described in the metaphyseal regions of the long bones and around the edges of the flat bones; they are similar to the 'lines of arrested growth' and are presumably due to the systemic disturbance caused by the disease. As they do not occur in other types of neonatal intestinal obstruction they would suggest the presence of meconium peritonitis.

If a contrast enema is undertaken, the colon is found to be narrow and slightly tortuous. This appearance is

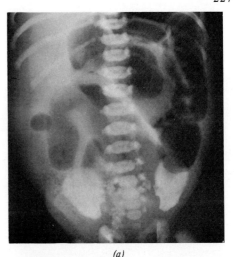

(a)

Figure 6.27. (a) Meconium Ileus: There are dilated loops of small intestine and absence of gas in the colon and distal ileum, except for fine mottled translucencies in the right iliac fossa due to small bubbles of gas within the mass of inspissated meconium. (b) Milk Inspissation Syndrome: The appearances in a plain film of the abdomen are very similar to those of meconium ileus showing dilated loops of small intestine and a mottled gas pattern in the right iliac fossa. (c) A contrast enema showing the colon to be normal in calibre or slightly distended with a mass of inspissated milk curds in the distended terminal ileum (black arrow). In meconium ileus by contrast the colon is collapsed and narrowed. (The position of the ileocaecal valve is shown by the contrast medium filled appendix) (white arrow) (by courtesy of Dr. R. H. Levick, Children's Hospital, Sheffield)

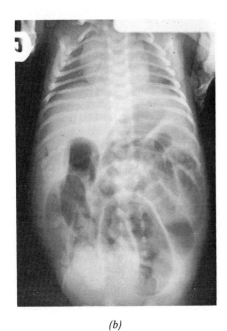

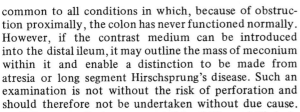

(b)

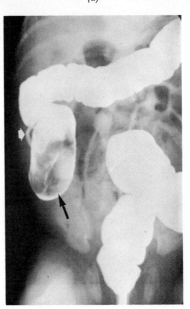

(c)

common to all conditions in which, because of obstruction proximally, the colon has never functioned normally. However, if the contrast medium can be introduced into the distal ileum, it may outline the mass of meconium within it and enable a distinction to be made from atresia or long segment Hirschsprung's disease. Such an examination is not without the risk of perforation and should therefore not be undertaken without due cause.

It has recently been suggested by Lillie and Chrispin (1972) and by Wagget *et al.* (1970) that an enema, using a hypertonic water soluble contrast medium such as Gastrografin, may be a useful therapeutic measure. The contrast medium will envelope the obstructing mass of sticky meconium, and by attracting water into the lumen of the ileum, will separate it from the bowel wall and lubricate its onward passage. This process is aided by the presence of a wetting agent in this type of contrast medium. If this method of treatment is adopted, handling of the baby should be reduced to a minimum and the time spent on the procedure should not exceed

45 minutes. An intravenous saline drip is a wise precaution to guard against the risk of excessive dehydration. The presence of complications such as volvulus, gangrene and peritonitis must be carefully excluded and atypical appearances in the plain radiograph will point to such a possibility. In successfully treated cases stools will be passed within a few minutes in some cases and certainly within an hour. In spite of the possible risks of this procedure, it is worth considering as a therapeutic agent because the mortality from surgical treatment is not negligible. In addition, according to Lillie and Chrispin (1972), it does not carry any risk of the disaccharide intolerance which has been described following operative treatment. Two conditions are found in newborn infants which may resemble meconium ileus.

(1) *The 'meconium plug syndrome'* This condition occurs in premature infants in whom spontaneous passage of the plug of meconium which normally occupies the rectum does not take place. Vomiting

228

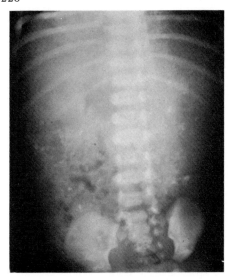

Figure 6.28: Meconium Peritonitis: Widely scattered areas of calcification are present, due to leakage of meconium into the peritoneal cavity following an intra-uterine perforation of the bowel

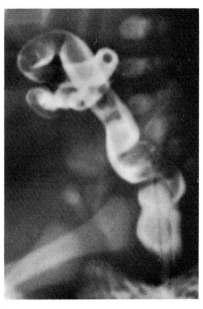

Figure 6.30. Meconium Plug Syndrome: An enema using water soluble contrast medium shows a colon of normal calibre containing a long cylindrical defect due to the meconium retained proximal to the 'plug'

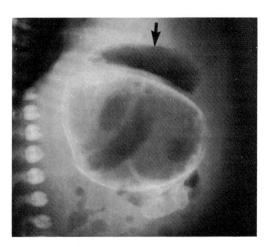

Figure 6.29. Calcified Pseudocyst: This gas-filled cystic lesion with calcification of its walls resulted from a perforation into the lesser sac proximal to atresia of the jejunum. This constitutes in effect a localized meconium peritonitis. The stomach is elevated (arrowed) and there is also calcification on the peritoneal surface of the loop of small bowel

and increasing abdominal distension may suggest obstruction but they usually respond rapidly to digital removal of the plug from the rectum. In cases where this fails a water soluble contrast enema may be both diagnostic and curative. The appearances on plain abdominal films may resemble those of meconium ileus, but the colon when outlined by the contrast enema is of normal calibre, except possibly at its extreme distal end. It may contain long continuous casts of meconium which will be outlined by contrast medium and which are readily displaced by it (*Figure 6.30*).

(2) *The 'milk inspissation' syndrome* This condition may present with an obstruction in the distal ileum closely resembling meconium ileus but the onset of the

condition is later, the infant being normal for the first week of life. It appears to be due to the formation of semisolid curds derived from artificial milk feeds. The colon is shown to be of normal calibre on contrast enema. If the enema refluxes into the distal ileum it may liquefy the inspissated milk stool, which is then passed (*Figure 27b* and *c*).

Cystic fibrosis may cause bouts of obstruction in older children, especially when there has been a change in diet or a failure to adhere to treatment. However, the condition is seldom so severe as it is in the newborn period, although cases have been described in which adherent viscid faecal material has initiated an intussusception. The mucosal pattern of the small intestine may be abnormally coarse, with a marginal nodularity which may resemble the oedematous folds occurring in intestinal lymphagiectasia (*see* page 242). The effect of the abnormal mucus on the small bile ducts is to produce biliary cirrhosis and intrahepatic portal hypertension which lead to splenomegaly, ascites and haemorrhage from oesophageal varices. In such cases portovenography may be required to differentiate the condition from splenic or portal vein thrombosis. Pancreatic calcification, though rare, may be seen with increasing frequency due to the improved prognosis resulting from the use of antibiotics in combating its pulmonary complications.

INTUSSUSCEPTION

Many cases of ileocolic intussusception are easily diagnosed from the clinical signs, but plain films are advisable to exclude complications, such as obstruction or perforation, in any case with more than a few hours history (Middlemiss, 1955). These should include a

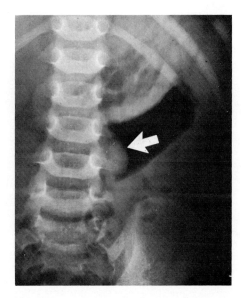

Figure 6.31. Intussusception: The head of the intussusceptum (arrowed) is shown in the transverse colon, outlined by gas which has been displaced during its passage from the ileo-caecal valve

film taken in the supine position and one with a horizontal beam, usually erect. A right lateral decubitus film (the right side up with a horizontal beam) has a possible advantage in that an absence of gas in the caecum in this position is very suggestive evidence of the presence of intussusception. It may be possible to obtain unequivocal confirmation of the diagnosis on a plain film by demonstrating the head of the intussusceptum, since this may be shown as a convex soft tissue mass directed distally, when it is outlined by gas displaced in front of it along the colon (*Figure 6.31*). This sign is stated to be present in between a third and half of the cases in various published series. Another suggestive appearance in the plain film is a dilated ileal loop lying in a curve concave to the right and terminating in a tapered point. This sign represents the loop of bowel which lies immediately proximal to the origin of the intussusception. Different opinions have been expressed as to the value of plain abdominal films in the diagnosis of intussusception. Although they are

not always productive of useful information, it is a simple procedure which may avoid the need for more elaborate investigations.

A barium enema will usually confirm the diagnosis in doubtful cases. It demonstrates the concave defect at the head of the column of barium due to the apex of the intussusceptum. The latter may be outlined by barium, which may percolate between it and the wall of the intussuscipiens (*Figure 6.32*). This appearance is made more obvious if some of the barium is evacuated from the colon distal to the apex of the intussusception. Rarely, it may be possible to visualize a primary cause for the intussusception in the form of a polyp or Meckel's diverticulum.

Reduction by barium enema

In cases in whom a barium enema is performed to confirm the diagnosis, the advisability of an attempt to reduce the intussusception under screen control should be considered (*Figure 6.32*). The advantages and disadvantages of this have been well reviewed by Girdany *et al.* (1959) and Nordentoft (1969). The present authors would consider that with certain important qualifications this is a reasonable procedure. Even if it is not successful in achieving complete reduction it will normally enable a subsequent operative reduction to be undertaken more easily and with less handling of the bowel. It does, however, carry certain well recognized dangers which must be avoided by careful selection of cases. These dangers are reduction of gangrenous or non-viable bowel perforation with the production of a chemical peritonitis from barium leaking into the peritoneal cavity and exhaustion of an already sick child. For these reasons, reduction should not be attempted in any case in whom the history is longer than 48 hours, in whom the general condition is poor, or when there are clinical or radiological signs suggestive of obstruction. The attempt at reduction

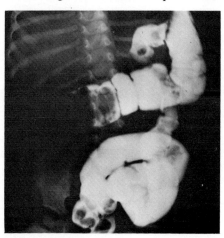

Figure 6.32. Intussusception: Barium enema during which the head of the intussusceptum has been reduced from (a) the mid-transverse colon to (b) the ileocaecal valve. Further reduction could not be achieved and a laparotomy was required to complete it

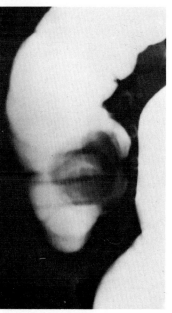

(a)

(b)

should always be preceded by a plain film of the abdomen and should be abandoned if gentle hydrostatic pressure at a height of not more than 30 cm above the table top fails to displace the intussusception after a period of 5 minutes. The surgeon in charge of the case should always be consulted and his approval sought before the procedure is undertaken. Complete reduction is likely to be achieved in about half the cases which satisfy these criteria. There is virtually no mortality and the rate of recurrence should be little higher than with surgical reduction. It is important, however, to watch the child carefully for 24 hours after the procedure, even when proof of satisfactory reduction has been obtained by filling the ileum with barium and by relief of symptoms. If doubt remains, barium can be given by mouth to demonstrate that there is a free passage into the colon.

INFLAMMATORY DISEASES

GASTRO-ENTERITIS

Non-specific infections of the alimentary tract are by no means uncommon, especially in young infants. They do not however give rise to any diagnostic radiological features. A plain film of the abdomen will often show a paucity of gas shadows due to the excess amount of fluid which fills the lumen of the bowel in this condition. If the bowel is dilated the presence of gas will lead to the formation of fluid levels shown on erect or inverted lateral films. Confusion with intestinal obstruction is thus likely to occur; this is particularly so as it is difficult to distinguish between loops of small and large bowel at the age at which gastro-enteritis is most common.

PEPTIC ULCER

Peptic ulcer in childhood is rare and the condition is often difficult to diagnose because its clinical presentation is atypical. The radiological features resemble those in adult cases. A crater or 'niche' is shown as a localized projection of barium from the outline of the stomach. In the duodenum, the crater is often seen *en face* as a dense fleck of barium surrounded by a translucent halo due to oedematous mucosa around it. The mucosal folds may converge towards the crater. The demonstration of this feature requires careful fluoroscopic examination, combined with compression. This is required in order to displace excess barium which may be obscuring the crater (*Figure 6.33*). The ulcer crater can also be well demonstrated by double contrast using air and barium. Deformity of the duodenal bulb due to spasm is another radiological feature associated with ulceration. Reliance cannot be placed on this sign. It is often absent in children or, when present, may be due to another cause (Lafferty, 1959). Tenderness may be present on palpation over an ulcer crater and may be a valuable confirmatory sign. Pylorospasm or pyloric stenosis may be present with a duodenal or pyloric ulcer.

Peptic ulcer occurs in the newborn infant (*Figure 6.34*). At this age the crater is difficult to demonstrate radiologically, not only because of the problems of examining such small infants, but also because ulcers in newborn infants are often superficial erosions and not

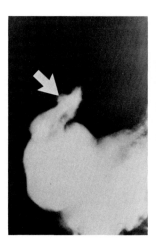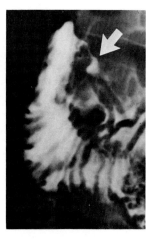

Figure 6.33. Duodenal Ulcer: An ulcer crater on the anterior wall of the first part of the duodenum is shown (a) in profile and (b) en face (arrowed) when most of the barium had been removed from the area of the ulcer by compression over it, leaving the crater still containing barium within it

the penetrating ulcers which occur in adults or older children. Perforation is not uncommon at this age, particularly in an infant in whom peptic ulcer is associated with disease of the central nervous system. This complication may be evident on plain films of the abdomen because free gas may be seen within the peritoneum.

Duodenal ulcers are relatively more common than gastric ulcers in children and 25 per cent may be post-bulbar in site (Rosenlund and Koop, 1970). Children may also develop peptic ulcers in other unusual sites, such as in a Meckel's diverticulum or in the oesophagus when lined with gastric mucosa.

APPENDICITIS

This condition is one in which radiology does not usually play an important role in diagnosis. However, the clinical signs and symptoms may sometimes be atypical in young infants. In such cases, plain films of the chest and abdomen may be helpful. In addition to excluding other conditions, such as a right-sided pneumonia with basal pleurisy they may reveal positive evidence of the presence of appendicitis or its sequelae. The radiological signs are an abnormal distribution of bowel gas shadows. They are scanty in the right lower quadrant and may be numerous in the left upper quadrant. This distribution will be especially apparent when the appendix has perforated and produced an intraperitoneal abscess. It may also be accompanied by the signs of free intraperitoneal fluid (*see* page 241). The right psoas shadow may not be visible and the peritoneal fat line on the right side may be ill-defined or obscured. If this latter feature is accompanied by localized increase in the thickness of the right side of the abdominal wall, it is very suggestive of a perforation and a pelvic abscess.

There is a strong association between appendicitis and the presence of a calcified faecolith in the right iliac fossa (*Figure 6.35*). In the series described by Wilkinson *et al.* (1969) it was found in 32 per cent

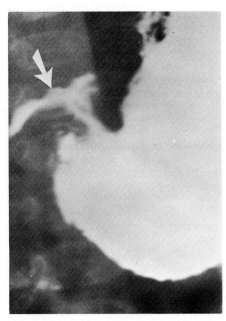

Figure 6.34. Duodenal Ulcer: Barium meal in an infant aged 6 weeks. The first part of the duodenum is flattened and deformed with an ulcer crater (arrowed) projecting from its upper surface. Perforation subsequently occurred and was repaired surgically

of cases of appendicitis, three-quarters of which had perforated. The exact cause of this relationship is not fully understood. It would seem likely that the presence of a faecolith in association with inflammation would favour perforation, presumably by the obstruction which it causes. The faecolith may come to lie free within a peri-appendicular abscess cavity and may then predispose to delay in wound healing or sinus formation if it is not removed at the time of operation. Faecoliths are rounded in shape, immobile on serial films and frequently uniform in texture, but they may occasionally be laminated. Most of the other causes of opacities in

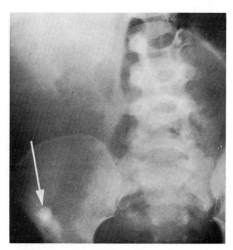

Figure 6.35. Appendicitis: The presence of a calcified 'faecolith' in the region of the appendix (arrowed) as shown in this plain film is often suggestive of perforation. The soft tissue mass and absence of intestinal gas are confirmatory signs suggesting a pelvic abscess

the right iliac fossa, such as calcified lymphnodes, calculi in the right ureter, or opaque medicinal tablets are unlikely to be confused with them (Goldman *et al.,* 1968).

REGIONAL ENTERITIS (CROHN'S DISEASE)

Crohn's disease occurs predominantly in the distal ileum. It leads to the development of stenosis and fistulae to other loops of bowel or on to the skin surface. Unaffected bowel is sharply demarcated from the diseased segment. When these signs are present the condition is not difficult to diagnose. The radiological appearances are narrowing of the lumen of the distal ileum and extrinsic pressure deformity of the medial wall of the caecum which is due to inflammatory oedema around the affected part of the small bowel (*Figure 6.36*).

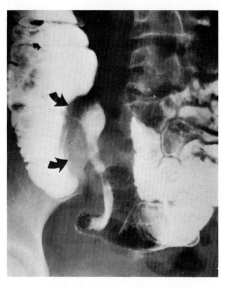

Figure 6.36. Regional Enteritis (Crohn's disease): Localized narrowing of the terminal loop of ileum is associated with wide separation from adjacent small bowel and the caecum, the medial wall of which is indented by the inflammatory mass (arrowed) surrounding the affected portion of ileum

In children, Crohn's disease occurs in a more variable form than it does in adults, and there is a greater tendency to systemic effects such as fever, anaemia, and arthralgia. There is also considerable interference with growth and physcial development. The condition may present with severe, acute abdominal pain and be suggestive of appendicitis. Radiological examination may therefore be important in the diagnosis of the condition. Barium studies should always include both a barium meal to demonstrate the small intestine and an enema to demonstrate the colon. It is now well recognized that in some cases the colon may be the predominant or even the only part of the bowel involved, whereas in others the jejunum and ileum are the only region affected. Sharply delineated segmental lesions are not uncommon, but they are not present in every case. The bowel between these lesions is normal and the appearance has been described as 'skip lesions'. In addition a similar appearance may be produced by internal fistulae from

232

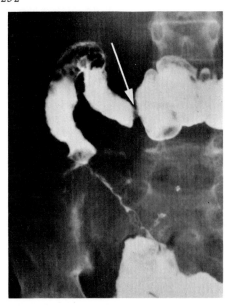

Figure 6.37. Regional Enteritis (Crohn's disease): Extensive involvement of the distal ileum, caecum, ascending colon and part of the transverse colon. The sharp demarcation between the affected part and the normal distal colon (arrowed) is well shown. The distal ileum is very markedly narrowed giving rise to the 'string sign'. Note the presence of sacro-ileitis; this is frequently an accompaniment of Crohn's disease

one part of the bowel to another. Thickening with oedema of the mucosal folds occurs in both the small intestine and the colon. In combination with deep longitudinal penetrating fissures, an appearance of the mucosal surface resembling cobblestones may be produced.

Opinions differ as to the frequency of stenosis. Moseley *et al.* (1960) found them in only 18 per cent of their series and they relate their appearance to the length of time necessary for their development. These stenoses are nearly always multiple and they may affect both small bowel and large bowel. They are most frequent in the terminal ileum and at the ileocaecal valve, where they give rise to an appearance described as the 'string sign' (Kantor, 1934) (*Figure 6.37*). Dilatation of the bowel proximal to such stenosis is variable in extent.

The radiological features of the colonic lesions of Crohn's disease may show a marked resemblance to ulcerative colitis (Sutcliffe, 1963) (*see* below and opposite). The haustral pattern may be exaggerated in the early stages of the disease, an appearance which may be confused with the sacculations seen in the colon in scleroderma; in the later stages, loss of haustration and shortening of the colon may occur, a feature which is also seen in ulcerative colitis. Ulceration in Crohn's disease may be deep and penetrating and the ulcers may undercut the mucosa, leading to a 'collar stud' effect. Associated with the delay in physical growth there is always some degree of retardation of skeletal maturation, and this is more marked the longer the disease has been present.

Crohn's disease is rare in infancy, but cases have been described which presented in the first 6 months of life with weight loss and abdominal distension, symptoms which are suggestive of some form of malabsorption

(Miller and Larsen, 1971). The radiological features in these infants are those of increasing small bowel obstruction.

ULCERATIVE COLITIS

Like Crohn's disease, ulcerative colitis in children often resembles the condition as seen in adults. Radiological investigation by barium enema is undertaken to diagnose the condition and to determine its severity. The ulceration of the colonic mucosa may be detected early in the course of the disease due to the fact that it produces a fine serrated contour to the barium-filled lumen (*Figure 6.38a*). If it is extensive the ulceration may give rise to a double contour to the bowel, the numerous small ulcer craters coalescing into a line peripheral to the barium within the lumen. This feature is indicative of severe disease with denudation of the mucosa. Large, deeply penetrating ulcers are seen only in the advanced stages. They can lead to a 'collar stud' type of appearance due to dissection beneath the mucosa or to sinus tracks within areas of pericolitis. Deep fissures appearing as thorn-like projections of barium extending several millimetres perpendicular to the lumen are rare. They are more suggestive of Crohn's disease of the colon than ulcerative colitis. Abnormalities of the haustral pattern may occur. If the haustra are lost, the colon becomes smooth and featureless in contour. Sometimes the haustrations are replaced by an irregular contour which has been described as corrugation (*Figure 6.38b*). In addition the colon may be shortened and rigid and its tubular lumen is narrowed due to the extensive fibrosis in the wall (*Figure 6.38c*). In some cases this may go on to the development of a definite stricture.

A radiological sign which is of ominous prognosis is gross dilatation of the large bowel, often referred to as toxic megacolon. It occurs either in the acute fulminating type of disease or in severe exacerbations. Such an appearance, especially if combined with a ragged irregular outline of the bowel, due to undermining of the mucosa by ulceration, may follow prolonged steroid therapy. If this abnormality is seen in a patient who is on steroids, it is an indication for stopping treatment; alternatively it should be regarded as a contra-indication to the use of steroids. The mucosal pattern may become abnormal at an early stage of the disease. The folds are illdefined and hazy and they are arranged in a longitudinal direction. In the later stages, when mucosal destruction becomes more extensive, an appearance resembling multiple polyps may be present due to the presence of islands of normal mucosa surrounded by areas where it is absent. This 'pseudopolyposis' is a sign of extensive and advanced disease; it may not be demonstrable unless the colon is distended with air following evacuation. Such air insufflation is not attended with any increased risk in ulcerative colitis (Hoeffel, 1969).

An increase in the width of the space between the sacrum and the posterior wall of the rectum, which should normally not exceed 5 mm at its narrowest part, has been found to be an early and frequent sign in ulcerative proctocolitis (Rudhe, 1960). This sign is not, however, specific and it can occur in a number of other inflammatory diseases involving the rectum,

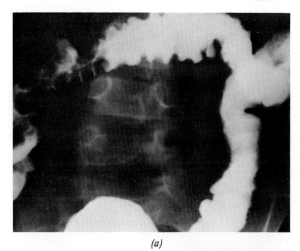

(a)

Figure 6.38. Ulcerative Colitis: (a) There is a lack of the normal haustral pattern in the descending colon where the bowel lumen has a finely serrated outline due to barium filling ulcers on the mucosal surface. In the transverse colon the folds are short, wide and irregular, the appearance being termed corrugation. (b) The rectum and sigmoid colon of this infant are uniform in calibre with loss of the normal curves and haustral folds, due to shortening and thickening of the bowel wall. Mucosal ulceration produces numerous shallow projections which give the bowel an irregular outline. The lumen of the bowel proximal to the abnormal segment is dilated. (c) The descending colon of another case showing the serrated outline of the bowel due to multiple ulcers. The colon is uniform in calibre and its border is abnormally straight

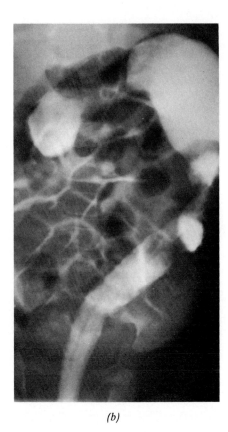

(b)

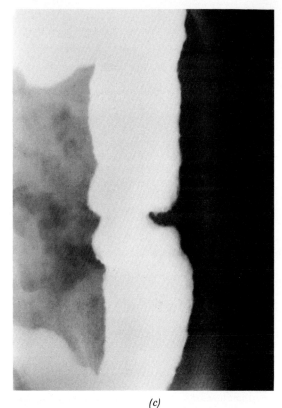

(c)

including Crohn's disease, Cushing's syndrome, or even in obesity. A lateral view of the rectum is needed to demonstrate this feature. This is a view which should always be obtained in any barium enema examination because it may also reveal early changes in the contour of the rectum. It has been estimated that between 10 and 30 per cent of children with ulcerative colitis may show normal radiological findings up to 2 years after the clinical onset of the disease (Davidson *et al.*, 1965).

Ulcerative colitis may lead to severe delay in skeletal and sexual development. Estimation of the bone age may be helpful in the assessment of the extent of such developmental delay. There is also a risk of carcinoma developing in any child who has had ulcerative colitis

for a number of years. Radiological examination is important in excluding this complication, although carcinoma is unlikely to occur until early adult life.

The differentiation of ulcerative colitis from other inflammatory diseases of the colon such as tuberculosis, amoebiasis or dysentery, may be difficult. The radiological appearances in all these conditions are very similar; however, they tend to occur in the proximal rather than in the distal colon where ulcerative colitis commonly arises. Crohn's disease of the colon may be readily distinguished in typical cases, but many of the signs may occur in both conditions. Helpful differentiating features are the dilatation of the terminal ileum, the infrequency of strictures and of deep ulceration in ulcerative colitis. The rectum and pelvic colon are

234

predominantly involved in ulcerative colitis and spared in Crohn's disease. It has been suggested recently that the arteriographic appearances are different in the two conditions and might be useful in differentiating them, but this applies only in the advanced stages.

NECROTIZING ENTEROCOLITIS OF INFANCY

This is a condition which may sometimes be confused with ulcerative colitis. It differs because it occurs in premature infants, especially in those who are not thriving and in those cases in which there is a predisposing condition leading to ischaemia of the gut wall. It has been described in cases in whom thrombosis or embolism has followed catheterization of the umbilical artery (Pochaczevsky and Kassner, 1971).

The radiological signs may be non-specific and consist only of intestinal distension. The dilatation may be quite marked. When it involves the colon, it may lead to confusion with Hirschsprung's disease; it may indeed

occur as a complication of this condition. If perforation occurs, pneumoperitoneum and ascites will be evident. There are two radiological features, however, which are particulalry characteristic of necrotising enterocolitis and because of the serious nature of the condition these signs carry an ominous prognostic significance. One sign is pneumatosis intestinalis, the presence of gas within the wall of the bowel in sufficient quantities to be detectable on plain films of the abdomen. The gas is apparent as linear translucent streaks parallel to the lumen of the gut, but separated from it by the shadow of the mucosa. If a loop of intestine is seen end-on the gas in the wall will appear in the form of a circle, giving a very characteristic 'double ring' effect (*Figure 6.39*). Pneumatosis has also been reported in other parts of the alimentary tract, i.e. the stomach and oesophagus. It may also occur in other conditions which cause intestinal distension in infancy, i.e. congenital atresias or Hirschsprung's disease. It is also likely that the condition of pneumatosis intestinalis occurring in infancy bears little relationship to the relatively benign

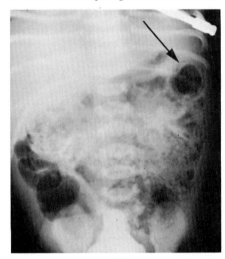

(a)

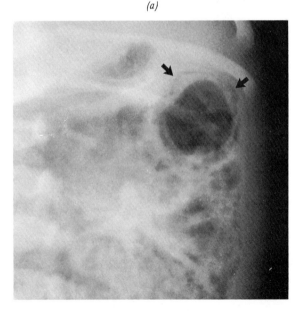

(b)

Figure 6.39. Necrotizing Enterocolitis: (a) A plain film of the abdomen showing gas in the wall of the colon (pneumatosis intestinalis) (arrowed). This may appear as a translucent ring surrounding but separate from the gas-filled lumen or as a more generalized 'mottling' obscuring the bowel loops. (b) Detailed view of the same film as (a) to show pneumatosis intestinalis in the wall of the colon (arrowed) (c) Branching linear translucencies are shown in the area of the liver due to gas within the portal vein and its branches (arrowed) (By courtesy of Professor J. H. Middlemiss, Bristol Royal Infirmary)

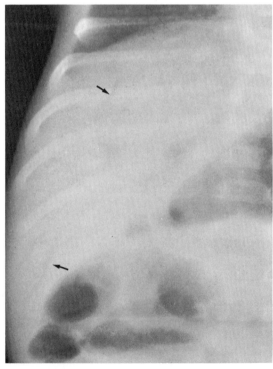

(c)

condition in adults. The other sign is the presence of gas in the portal vein. In cases of necrotizing enterocolitis this feature implies an even more serious prognosis. It has been found to be present in 22 per cent of cases (Mizrahi *et al.*, 1965). It is a sign which is not difficult to detect if it is looked for. The gas in the portal veins shows as translucent lines branching towards the periphery of the liver. The only conditions likely to be confused with it are an air bronchogram in the right lower lobe, in which the direction of the gas shadows is downward and outwards, and gas in the biliary duct system. In the latter the branching translucent lines are most marked at the hilum and they do not extend so far towards the periphery of the liver as does gas in the portal vein. Gas may also occur in the portal vein after umbilical vein catheterization, but in these circumstances its presence does not have the same bad prognostic significance.

Barium enema often reveals little abnormality. In general this examination is not advisable in these patients because of the likelihood of perforation which may lead to flooding of the peritoneum with barium.

PNEUMOPERITONEUM

Free gas within the peritoneal cavity is almost always indictative of perforation of some part of the alimentary tract. This is especially true in a child, because air introduced into the peritoneal cavity at laparotomy is absorbed extremely rapidly. It is very rare for any air to be demonstrable radiologically more than 24 hours after operation, and its presence can therefore be regarded as valid evidence of a leak from an anastomosis following abdominal surgery (Hope and Cramer, 1958). Apart from the well recognized causes of perforation such as

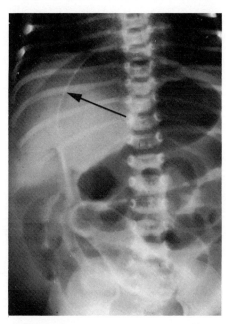

Figure 6.40. Pneumoperitoneum: In the supine film gas beneath the diaphragm has outlined the falciform ligament which appears as a thin curved linear opacity to the right of the midline (arrowed). The wall of bowel is outlined both by gas within the lumen and gas on its peritoneal aspect

peptic ulcer, trauma, appendicitis and necrotizing enterocolitis, it is known that it can occur, especially in the newborn infant, as an appararently spontaneous event. It is postulated that congenital defects in the gut wall, with or without local haemangiomata, and ischaemia related to vasospasm or to asphyxia at birth may be responsible, but in many cases no cause is apparent.

The radiological diagnosis is usually obvious on plain films of the chest and abdomen, especially if erect films are taken. The gas in the peritoneum is shown as a crescentic translucency which separates the diaphragm from the abdominal organs on films taken with the child erect. If the child is supine gas appears as an oval translucency extending into the flanks and is bisected by the linear shadow of the falciform ligament. The gas also surrounds the bowel loops centrally and outlines their walls (*Figure 6.40*).

PERFORATION OF THE OESOPHAGUS

This may give rise to dysphagia and may be revealed by swallowed contrast medium leaking into the mediastinal tissues or even into the pleural cavity. The appearances resemble a double oesophagus, and can be an unexpected finding in the newborn infant following vigorous clearing of the airway after birth or attempts at passing an excessively rigid endogastric tube. If mediastinitis occurs, this may lead to widening of the mediastinum and there may also be an associated pleural effusion. Such cases, however, will usually heal spontaneously, when the abnormal appearances are no longer visible (Eklof *et al.*, 1969).

MALABSORPTION

COELIAC DISEASE

In malabsorption resulting from the damaging effect of gluten on the mucosa of the small intestine, complete remission can be expected if the gluten is removed from the diet. Diagnosis of the condition is therefore a matter of considerable importance and for this purpose biopsy of the small intestinal mucosa has become routine procedure. Nevertheless, a barium meal and follow-through study of the small bowel is undoubtedly a simpler and less unpleasant procedure for the patient than jejunal biopsy, but it must be realized that the radiation incurred is not negligible.

The radiological signs observed in cases of coeliac disease are not specific and it is arguable that the demonstration of a radiologically normal small intestine is more useful in excluding coeliac disease then are the positive findings in making the diagnosis.

If the examination is carried out with plain barium sulphate suspension, the mucus secreted in the intestine in response to the excess of free fatty acids derived from the unabsorbed fat within the bowel lumen causes the barium to precipitate. This results in the formation of large clumps of barium which fail to delineate the contour or mucosal pattern adequately. The appearance so produced, described as flocculation, clumping or

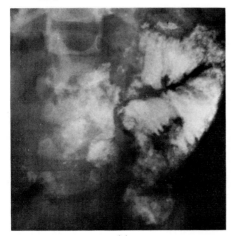

(a)

Figure 6.41. Coeliac Disease: (a) In the active stage of the disease the small intestinal loops are dilated with loss of the normal mucosal pattern; dilution and flocculation of the barium prevent complete demonstration of the outline of the bowel. (b) After treatment with a gluten-free diet, the calibre of the small intestinal loops becomes normal and the mucosal pattern is again clearly shown

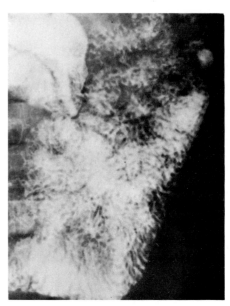

(b)

segmentation, is highly distinctive (*Figure 6.41a*). However, in infants and young children it may occur in response to many other diseases of the small bowel and it may be a normal finding in infants under 2 years of age. If a more stable preparation of barium is used which does not flocculate, the degree of dilatation of the bowel can be assessed. The degree of small intestinal dilatation correlates well with the presence of gluten enteropathy. Normal values for the average width of the jejunum at different ages have been published. These varied from 13 mm in the first year of life to 23 mm at 15 years. In coeliac disease the mean width was 2 mm above the standard value, returning to normal about 4 months after the gluten has been removed from the diet (*Figure 6.41b*) (Haworth *et al.*, 1967). In cases which relapse the diameter of the small bowel increases before clinical symptoms become apparent. The mucosal pattern in the dilated loops may also be abnormal. The feathery type of jejunal folds are replaced by transverse parallel folds as in any condition in which the calibre is increased. The transit time for the barium to reach the ileocaecal valve is increased, owing to a diminution in intestinal motility. In order to make it possible to compare examinations carried out at different times on the same patient, it is clearly an advantage to standardize the type and quantity of barium used.

The radiological findings in patients who suffer from mucoviscidosis or secondary malabsorption due to various primary diseases of the small intestine, are similar to those found in cases of coeliac disease, and radiology cannot therefore be used to differentiate them. However, anatomical abnormalities which are known to cause malabsorption, i.e. malrotation, blind loops, fistulae or Crohn's disease, may be encountered on barium meal and follow-through examination. This method of examination will also show the extent of previous surgical resection of the small bowel.

Bone changes, such as rickets or osteomalacia or simple demineralization with consequent pathological fractures, occur only in long-standing cases and are not often seen at the present time. Similarly retardation in bone growth and skeletal maturation are only present in cases in which the diagnosis and treatment has been delayed.

DISACCHARIDOSES

This group of conditions constitutes a specific type of malabsorption which arises from a congenital absence of the enzymes required to split lactose, sucrose or maltose into the corresponding monosaccharides. Only the latter are capable of being absorbed by the intestinal mucosa. A transient diminution in the amount of enzyme may occur following infections.

A specific radiological test for these conditions has been devised in which the result of the barium meal and follow-through examination using barium alone is compared with that obtained when barium is mixed with 25 g of the suspected disaccharide (Laws and Neale, 1966). The positive findings are dilution of the barium from excessive fluid within the bowel lumen, decreased transit time for the barium to pass from the stomach to the caecum and mild dilatation of the bowel loops. These findings are not present in the control examination without disaccharide.

McNeish and Sweet (1968) have applied this method to children and conclude that it is more reliable than any other test except faecal pH values. Although secondary disaccharidase deficiency can occur in some cases of coeliac disease, the dilution effect and decreased transit time may help to differentiate the two conditions effectively. In coeliac disease the transit time is increased and the barium precipitated rather than diluted.

INTRA-ABDOMINAL CYSTS AND TUMOURS

The kidney and suprarenal gland are discussed elsewhere (*see* page 268). The present section is concerned with cysts and tumours related to the alimentary canal, the liver, spleen and pancreas. These are conveniently grouped together because they may present clinically as a mass in the abdomen. Individually they are rare conditions but collectively they provide an important diagnostic problem of differential diagnosis.

Radiology may contribute to the solution of the problem of differentiating between abdominal masses by defining their shape, size and position, by showing their relationship to the other abdominal organs, their blood supply or lack of it, and whether there is calcification in them. Plain films of the abdomen taken in different positions can be supplemented by barium studies, urography, cholecystography, retroperitoneal pneumography, myelography, cyst puncture or sinus injection as appropriate. These space-occupying lesions may sometimes be demonstrated well by isotope examination, and their solid or fluid contents determined by the use of ultrasound.

ENTEROGENOUS CYSTS (DUPLICATION CYSTS)

Localized duplication of any part of the alimentary canal may present as a cystic mass and may, in some cases, also communicate with the subarachnoid space surrounding the spinal cord. Enterogenous cysts occurring in relation to the oesophagus present as cystic masses in the neck or thorax and they are discussed elsewhere (*see* page 202). The majority of these cysts occur within the abdomen and are derived from stomach, colon or small intestine, the latter being the commonest site of derivation. Occasionally they are multiple. Communication with the lumen of the gut is not present in the majority of cases. Owing to their close proximity to the wall and their tendency to enlarge progressively, these cysts may obstruct the part of the gut involved.

On plain films of the abdomen the cyst is usually well shown as a soft tissue mass. It is often situated anteriorly in the right lower quadrant. There may be

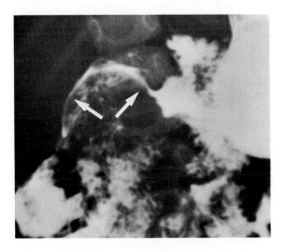

Figure 6.42. Duplication Cyst of Duodenum: The large cyst indents the first and second parts of the duodenum from below reducing its lumen to a narrow channel (arrowed). The rest of the duodenal loop is of normal calibre

calcification in the cyst wall but this is uncommon. A fluid level within the cyst indicates that a communication with the gut lumen is present. Barium studies are valuable even if such a communication is not present. The close relationship of the cyst to the wall of the bowel may produce indentation of the outline of the barium within the stomach or intestine (*Figure 6.42*) and if the extrinsic pressure is marked the cyst may produce a stenosis, the appearances of which may resemble those seen in Crohn's disease (Hammer, 1967). Signs of obstruction, volvulus or intussusception may also be present.

Duplication of the colon may be associated with duplication or other anomalies of the urinary tract (Kottra and Dodds, 1971). These cases are likely to present in early childhood. Urography or cystourethrography may be indicated. In order to define the extent of the associated anomalies in those cases in which spinal dysraphism coexists, either with or without a communication with the spinal theca, views of the spine or myelography may be required.

MESENTERIC CYSTS

This type of cyst resembles the enterogenous cyst in being frequently subumbilical and anterior in situation but it differs in that the bowel lumen is not as a rule compressed or indented. Intestinal obstruction is also rare. They are commonly lymphatic in origin but they do not communicate with lymphatic channels. The diagnosis is usually made by exclusion.

OMPHALOMESENTERIC DUCT CYSTS

These cysts arise from a persistent part of the omphalomesenteric duct which connects the ileum with the umbilicus. They may be of radiological interest because some of them communicate either with the skin surface or with the gut. In the former case there is a sinus at the umbilicus, and contrast medium injected along it may fill the cyst. Those cases which communicate with the ileum do so through a Meckel's diverticulum; a gas fluid level may be visible within the cyst. Small bowel obstruction may sometimes occur.

PANCREATIC CYSTS

These can be either true cysts of the pancreas or pseudocysts arising from a localized encysted area of peritonitis around the pancreas, usually in the lesser sac. The latter may result from trauma, perforation or acute pancreatitis. Both types are rare in children and resemble each other in their radiological features.

Pancreatic cysts present as a mass in the upper abdomen and they vary considerably in their relation to and displacement of adjacent organs. Widening of the duodenal loop and elevation of the pyloric antrum of the stomach are rare in children (Wilson, 1955). More commonly the mass lies between the stomach and transverse colon; the former is displaced forwards and upwards, and the latter is depressed. However, the colon may be elevated if the cyst lies below it, and

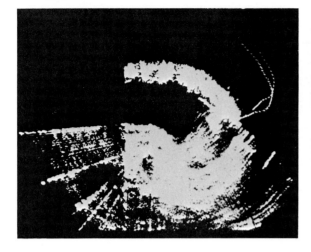

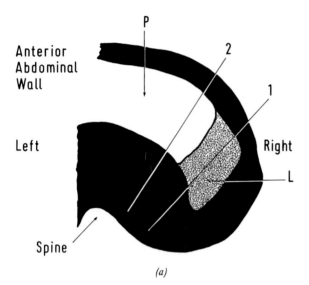

Anterior
Abdominal
Wall

Left

Right

L

Spine

(a)

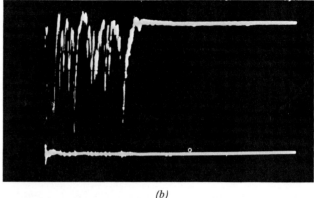

(b)

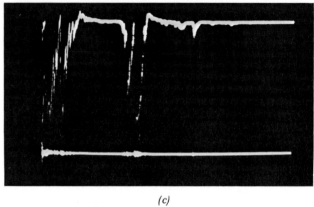

(c)

Figure 6.43. Pancreatic Pseudocyst: Ultrasonic scans in a child. (a) Transverse B-scan with line drawing. The large fluid-filled transonic pseudocyst (P) compresses the liver (L). (b) A-scan through the liver along line 1 in the drawing shows multiple echoes throughout the liver. (c) A-scan through the pseudocyst along line 2 demonstrated no echoes where the ultrasound beam passes through the fluid in the cyst

the stomach may be depressed or displaced to the right if the mass is above it or between it and the spleen. Occasionally, when the lesser sac is involved in an inflammatory reaction, there is elevation of the left hemidiaphragm or an area of collapse or pneumonitis at the base of the left lung. Calcification may occur within a pseudocyst which has derived from an intra-uterine perforation, and this occurrence may be regarded as a localized area of meconium peritonitis (*see* page 226). Pancreatic cysts do not displace the kidney or ureter. This allows a distinction to be made on urography from retroperitoneal tumours or enlarged glands in the upper para-aortic area. Pancreatic cysts may be diagnosed by ultrasound (*Figure 6.43*).

CHOLEDOCHAL CYSTS

Dilatation of and obstruction to the distal part of the common bile duct may give rise to an upper abdominal mass known as a choledochal cyst. They usually lie slightly to the right of the midline and present with pain and jaundice, sometime during the first decade. On plain films of the abdomen a choledochal cyst may be seen as a well defined soft tissue mass and it is rarely calcified. Faint opacification of the cyst is sometimes obtained on oral or intravenous cholecystography, but more commonly the cyst is not demonstrated, especially if jaundice is present. On barium meal the first part of the duodenum is displaced forwards; if the cyst becomes very large the second part may also be displaced downwards and to the right side. Such displacement of the retroperitoneal portion of the duodenum is characteristic; it does not occur in other upper abdominal masses except for duplication cysts of the duodenum itself, which usually displace it upwards.

A pre-operative diagnosis of choledochal cyst may be valuable. This may be obtained by direct puncture of the cyst, followed by injection of contrast medium in order to opacify it. The procedure, however, carries a risk of producing a biliary leak and consequent peritonitis (Wilson, 1955; Han *et al.*, 1969). It has therefore been suggested that, if such a method is contemplated, it should always be done directly prior to surgery and contrast medium should not be injected until the cyst has been decompressed by aspirating its contents.

SPLENIC CYSTS

Like pancreatic cysts, cysts of the spleen may be true cysts derived from endothelial or epithelial tissues, or pseudocysts which arise as a result of trauma or localized inflammation.

The mass can usually be easily defined because such cysts often attain a large size (Forde and Finby, 1961); the stomach and colon are displaced downwards and medially.

Aortography has proved a useful method for providing a definitive diagnosis because the branches of the splenic artery are displaced in a regular manner around the avascular cyst. Direct injection of contrast medium into the cyst by the technique employed for portal venography may also be undertaken. The cyst may be shown clearly by ultrasound.

CYSTS AND TUMOURS OF THE LIVER

These may be of varying histological types. Radiologically they all present as an upper abdominal mass inseparable from the liver. Calcification is not uncommon, particularly in the malignant hepatoblastoma, in the more benign haemangio-endothelioma and also in hydatid cysts.

Displacement of the stomach and colon is almost always present but its direction depends upon the location of the lesion within the liver. Those masses in the right lobe of the liver displace the stomach downwards and slightly to the left, and the hepatic flexure downwards. Those masses in the left lobe displace the stomach to the left and forwards. The duodenum, especially in the region of the duodenojejunal flexure, is displaced downwards by left lobe masses but much less markedly, if at all, by masses in the right lobe (*Figure 6.44*). Urography may show compression of the right renal pelvis by the mass lying anteriorly to it and the kidney is often displaced downwards. Relatively avascular masses, such as cysts, can be demonstrated

as negative defects in the liver within the 'total body opacification' which results when films are exposed at the end of the intravenous injection of relatively high doses of contrast medium. This will not show lesions under 5 cm in diameter (Griscom, 1965).

Selective arteriography of the hepatic artery is the most useful investigation in suspected hepatic tumours (Fredens, 1969). Not only may the extent and location of the tumour be shown, but the presence of abnormal vessels and a tumour blush when present will indicate the malignant nature of the lesion. Haemangioendotheliomata share with the malignant tumours an increase in the size and number of the arteries supplying the lesion, and early filling of the draining hepatic veins. This evidence of arteriovenous shunting in these latter tumours accounts for their tendency to present with a high output cardiac failure. Differentiation between primary and metastatic malignant tumours of the liver may be impossible. Portal venography is usually not of great use in diagnosing hepatic masses because it may merely show obstruction of the portal vein. A chest film should always be taken in order to determine whether pulmonary metastases are present. Hepatic tumours do not frequently metastasize to bone but all forms may show a severe generalized osteoporosis with pathological fractures in some cases.

OVARIAN TUMOURS AND TERATOMATA

Ovarian cysts in children are most frequently teratomata or dermoid cysts. They are usually diagnosed radiologically because they contain dense localized calcification derived from the dental or bony elements. Such lesions present as pelvic masses, and they may be outlined by a thin translucent fat line (*Figure 6.45*). They may have a sacrococcygeal element which provides clinical evidence of their presence. Rarely such teratomatous cysts may contain more highly organized skeletal elements which represent an included maldeveloped

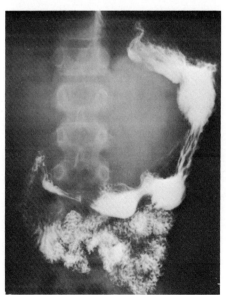

(a)

Figure 6.44. Cyst of Left Lobe of Liver: (a) The mass displaces the stomach and duodenum downwards and to the left in the anteroposterior view. (b) The stomach is displaced forwards in the lateral view

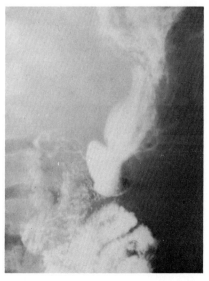

(b)

240

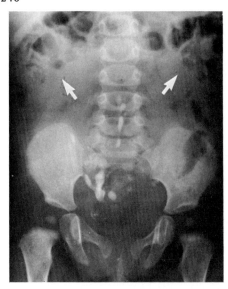

Figure 6.45. Dermoid Cyst (teratoma): There is a large lower abdominal mass (arrowed) containing dense calcified opacities representing bone and dental elements within the tumour

twin of the fetus in fetu type, although presenting initially as a pelvic cystic mass.

Teratomata may be confused with other ovarian tumours or with pelvic masses such as sarcoma of the bladder or prostrate (*see* page 274) or anterior sacral meningocele (*see* page 309). The highly distinctive radiological appearance of most pelvic teratomata, however, usually enables the correct diagnosis to be made. The malignant ovarian tumours commonly cause hypergonadism and sexual precocity. In such cases estimation of skeletal maturity may reveal significant acceleration of the bone age.

TUMOURS OF THE GASTRO-INTESTINAL TRACT

The only tumours of the bowel which are common in childhood are *polyps*. These tumours are of clinical importance, as a source of haemorrhage, as a basis for intussusception, or in the case of multiple polyposis as a premalignant condition. They may be of various histological types, but the most common variety is the juvenile retention polyp of the colon. This type of polyp is usually solitary but occasionally may be multiple. They predominantly occur in the rectosigmoid colon and they are commonest between 3 and 5 years of age. (Duhamel and Bauche, 1965). They are difficult to demonstrate radiologically owing to their small size and their site. They occur in most cases in a region of the colon where they may be obscured by overlap between loops of bowel. Unless the colon has been adequately cleared, they may also be confused with small masses of faecal material. In addition, they are liable to be obscured by the density of the barium filling the lumen of the bowel. It is essential therefore to employ a double air contrast technique when performing the barium enema and it is advisable to include views taken with a horizontal beam. Films taken after

evacuation of the barium, in order to show the details of the mucosa, are also helpful.

Apart from the secondary effects they may produce, such as bleeding or intussusception, simple polyps are benign, and they often disappear spontaneously before adolescence by a process of 'auto-amputation'. A much more serious condition is hereditary multiple polyposis because of the tendency in such cases for the development of carcinoma during adolescence or early adult life. Fortunately radiological diagnosis is seldom difficult, because of the large number of polyps which are present. On barium enema the whole surface of the colonic mucosa is shown to be carpeted with innumerable rounded filling defects, an appearance more striking in the post-evacuation mucosal pattern and air contrast films than in the early films following the injection of barium (*Figure 6.46*). Multiple polyposis may be detected as early as 2 years of age, but most cases do not become apparent before late childhood. Routine examination of the children in affected families is advised at 2 to 3 years intervals from the age of 10 years onwards, if the patient remains asymptomatic.

A variant of multiple polyposis, in which osteomata of the cranial vault and jaws and fibromata of the skin occur, is known as Gardner's syndrome. Because there is the same liability to malignant transformation as in other types of polyposis, any case in whom cysts or bony tumours of the skull and facial bones are discovered, should be referred for a barium enema to detect whether multiple polypi are present.

The Peutz—Jeghers syndrome is another variety of multiple polyposis in which the polyps are much less numerous than in the former types and are distributed throughout the whole of the alimentary tract. In this condition the polyps are probably of the nature of hamartomata and therefore do not carry the same risk of malignant transformation. The associated buccal and facial pigmentation makes the diagnosis easy. Barium studies of the stomach and small intestine will be required in addition to examination by barium enema, in order to demonstrate the full extent of the polyposis (*Figure 6.47*). Compression of the abdomen to separate the loops of small intestine is helpful (Godard *et al.*, 1971). This

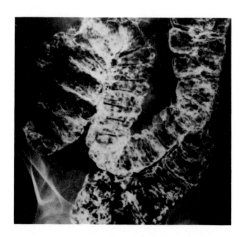

Figure 6.46. Hereditary Multiple Polyposis of the Colon: Double air contrast technique showing numerous small rounded filling defects due to polyps

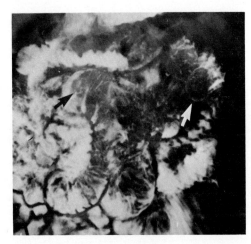

Figure 6.47: Peutz–Jeghers Syndrome: A barium small bowel examination shows a number of rounded filling defects due to the polyps (arrowed)

may conveniently be effected by lying the patient prone over a non-opaque pad. The use of an accelerator such as Gastrografin added to the barium is also an advantage in showing the mucosal pattern. The presence of polyps in the small intestine may lead to the development of intussusception and obstruction, and these complications may be demonstrated by a plain film of the abdomen.

Carcinoma of the colon, although very rare, is not unknown in childhood. It may occur in patients either with multiple polyposis or long-standing ulcerative colitis. The radiological features of these tumours, i.e. concentric narrowing or polypoid filling defects, do not differ from those seen in adults.

ASCITES

The presence of excess fluid within the peritoneal cavity gives rise to radiological appearances which are not difficult to recognize. These features are:

(1) General haziness of the whole abdomen.
(2) Bulging of the flanks in the supine position.
(3) Greater density in the lower abdomen and pelvis on the erect films because the gas-filled loops of bowel float into the upper abdomen.
(4) Separation of the loops of bowel by wide bands of increased density.
(5) A wider than normal gap between the lumen of the ascending or descending colon and the extraperitoneal fat. These structures should normally be in close contiguity.
(6) Obliteration of the outline of the inferolateral angle of the liver in the right flank, a border which is usually clearly defined.
(7) A trans-sonic area in each flank on ultrasound examination.

Ascites in the newborn infant may be particularly important to recognize and differentiate from other causes of abdominal distension. It may arise from peritonitis with or without perforation, from leakage of blood or chyle into the peritoneum, from diseases of the liver, from obstruction to the lower urinary tract, and in severe haemolytic disease due to blood group incompatibilities. A number of these types of ascites are of particular radiological interest.

PORTAL HYPERTENSION

The cause of portal hypertension may be prehepatic, hepatic and posthepatic. The prehepatic type is due to obstruction in the portal system of veins, commonly from thrombosis or hypoplasia of the portal vein. The former results, in many cases, from portal phlebitis secondary to umbilical infection in the neonatal period. Among the causes of the hepatic type are hepatitis and consequently cirrhosis, other intrinsic diseases of the liver such as cystic disease, angiomatosis, Wilson's disease, and biliary cirrhosis consequent upon atresia of the bile ducts or cholangitis. The posthepatic type may be due to stenosis of the hepatic veins (Budd–Chiari syndrome).

Portovenography is required in order to determine the state of the splenic and portal veins, and on this information possible operative treatment may be planned. The distribution and extent of the collateral circulation will also be shown.

'CHYLOUS' ASCITES

This is due to a leakage of chyle from the mesenteric lymphatics. It may be due either to local abnormalities in the lymphatic channels themselves or to obstruction or injury to the cisterna chyli or thoracic duct. In order to try to determine the cause of the condition, lymphangiography may be of value. The most suitable site for the injection of the contrast medium is into the lymphatics of the foot. By this method generalized lymphangiectasia may be shown and thoracic duct obstruction demonstrated. Occasionally there may be retrograde flow into the mesenteric lymphatics (Craven *et al.*, 1967).

'URINE' ASCITES

This condition has been described in newborn infants who are suffering from some congenital obstructive lesions of the lower urinary tract. It may occur in the absence of any perforation of the bladder or ureters and it then arises merely from transudation of urine into the peritoneal cavity. Excretory urography or micturating cysto-urethrography will be required to demonstrate the site of the obstructive lesion and its effect on the upper urinary tract.

HAEMOPERITONEUM

In the newborn infant this most commonly occurs in haemorrhagic disease of the newborn associated with vitamin K deficiency. Plain films of the abdomen may help to localize the source of the bleeding. There may be an opaque mass in the area of the source of bleeding and this may displace adjacent viscera (Cywes and Cremin, 1969).

PROTEIN-LOSING ENTEROPATHY

Oedema due to hypoproteinaemia may occur either from loss of protein through the kidneys, e.g. in nephrosis, or from protein loss through the wall of the gut. This results from a wide variety of diseases, all of which cause an increase in the permeability of the bowel wall. It has been recognized with increasing frequency since a simple test using isotope-labelled polyvinylpyrolidone (PVP) has been available, to detect the presence of serum protein in the faeces.

Radiological investigation may be helpful in two ways. Firstly, in the majority of cases it may demonstrate the presence of primary intestinal disease such as Crohn's disease, ulcerative colitis, coeliac disease, mucoviscidosis, Hirschsprung's disease, tuberculous enteritis, lymphoma and lymphoid hyperplasia. Secondly, radiological investigation may show distinctive appearances which are due to primary protein-losing enteropathy. On barium meal the mucosal pattern of the small intestine and especially of the jejunum may be abnormal. There may be numerous transverse parallel folds, resembling those found in dilatation from any cause. In protein-losing enteropathy they are coarser and when seen end-on at the periphery of the bowel lumen they appear club-shaped. Other less constant features are dilution of the barium by hypersecretion of fluid into the lumen and separation of the loops due to oedema of the bowel wall or ascites (*Figure 6.48*). Flocculation does not occur, and this is in contrast to the appearances in coeliac disease (Pock-Steen, 1966; Marshak *et al.*, 1967). These changes are often associated with intestinal lymphangiectasia.

DISORDERS OF INTESTINAL MOTILITY

It is usual to record the time taken for the transit of barium from the stomach to the ileocaecal valve during follow-through studies in order to determine whether intestinal hurry or delay is occurring. It should be emphasized, however, that the transit time through the small bowel will vary with the technique employed: it may be increased if food is mixed with the barium and it may be decreased if accelerators such as sorbitol or Gastrografin are used. It is essential, therefore, that a standard technique be employed so that the results of the different examinations may be comparable. The limits of the normal range are wide and vary from just less than an hour up to about 4 hours.

The emptying time of the stomach is a measurement in which it is difficult to define precise limits. The time between ingestion of barium and the first bolus to pass the pylorus is variable, especially in infants; it often depends more on psychogenic factors which can inhibit gastric motility than on spasm or obstruction at the pylorus. The amount of barium remaining in the stomach after a fixed interval, such as 4–6 hours, is a more reliable indicator of pyloric obstruction, but this only applies if no further food has been given by mouth.

DYSPHAGIA

This is a symptom which frequently occurs in the infant. It arises not only from a large number of structural abnormalities but also from neurogenic disorders which can interfere with normal swallowing. The reflux pathways on which swallowing depends are not fully organized at birth. This is especially true in premature infants. This type of failure of development may be a cause of respiratory distress in the newborn infant, and also of recurrent aspiration pneumonitis in infants of all ages (Frank and Gatewood 1966).

Examination of the process of swallowing carried out by fluoroscopic examination or by cineradiographic studies may be of considerable help in determining its efficiency, and in analysing the exact part of the mechanism which may be at fault (Adran *et al.*, 1965). However, it may be desirable not to undertake cineradiography too early, since many neonates who have

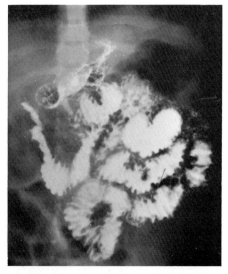

Figure 6.48. Protein-losing Enteropathy: Small bowel studies in intestinal lymphangiectasia. (a) The mucosal folds in the jejunum are coarse and clubbed where they are seen in profile. The wide separation of the loops is due to oedema of their walls. (b) The barium in the distal jejunal loops has become diluted by the excess fluid content within the lumen

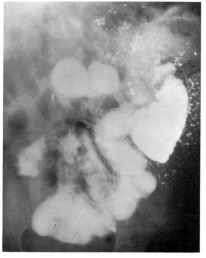

(a)

(b)

difficulty in swallowing may recover spontaneously during the first weeks of life. In the type of dysphagia due to immaturity of the swallowing mechanism, there was always some degree of paresis of the constrictor muscles and often ineffective sucking and weak tongue movements as well. Green (1959), studying the effect of cleft palate on swallowing and phonation, both before and after operation, was able to assess the degree of impairment of the normal process of nasopharyngeal closure.

Radiological examination may reveal the presence of many organic lesions which are likely to be present in infants with dysphagia. These include the micrognathos of the Pierre—Robin syndrome, choanal atresia, tracheo-oesphageal fistula, vascular rings, abnormalities of the temporomandibular joints, tumours and cysts in the neck, pharynx or larynx. The features of these conditions are discussed elsewhere.

FAMILIAL DYSAUTONOMIA (RILEY—DAY SYNDROME)

This is a condition which has attracted some attention recently because of the widespread radiological abnormalities associated with it. It is considered to be a hereditary dysfunction of the autonomic nervous system which leads to episodic hyper- and hypotension, sweating, lacrimation, diminished sensation and decreased reflexes. Dysphagia, dysarthria and muscular incoordination are also prominent features. Cineradiographic studies of swallowing have shown that the defect is a failure of the cricopharyngeus to relax and not a weakness in the constrictor muscles. This may lead to variable degrees of spill into the trachea with consequent pulmonary changes (Margulies *et al.*, 1968). Other radiological

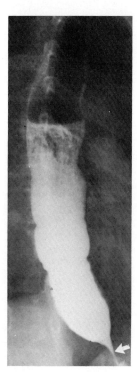

Figure 6.49. Achalasia of the Cardia: The oesophagus is markedly dilated but tapers to a narrow point at its lower end (arrowed). The barium is held up above this and fails to enter the stomach

features associated with the condition are: abnormalities of oesophageal and gastric motility; abnormal peristaltic activity; a thoracic scoliosis; dysplastic hip joints; generalized demineralization of the skeleton with pathological fractures; metaphyseal lesions resembling those of osteochondritis and possibly related to the diminished pain sensation; and a retardation of skeletal maturation.

ACHALASIA OF THE CARDIA

Although rare in childhood, this may occasionally lead to vomiting and regurgitation in infants. It commonly presents as recurrent 'pneumonia' which is due to aspiration of food into the lungs, possibly during sleep.

The radiological features are similar to those found in adults. There is dilatation of the oesophagus which may be marked. It may be visible as a mediastinal mass containing a fluid level in plain chest films. On barium meal there is retention of barium within the oesophagus, the lower end of which is symmetrically tapered (*Figure 6.49*). Passage of the barium into the stomach occurs slowly under the influence of gravity in the erect position and it may be accelerated by the use of amyl nitrite. In the stage before the oesophagus becomes too dilated, abnormal contractions with reversed peristalsis will occur.

REFERENCES

METHODS

Ardran, G. M. and Kemp, F. H. (1956). 'Radiologic investigation of pharyngeal and laryngeal palsy.' *Acta Radiol.* **46**, 446

Castellino, R. A., Verby, H. D., Friedland, G. W. and Northway, W. H., (1968). 'Delayed barium aspiration following complete reflux small bowel enema.' *Br. J. Radiol.* **41**, 937

Cecile, J. P., Fournier, A., Lelong, M., Bayart, M. and Regnier, G. (1972). 'Phlebo-arterio-urography in the diagnosis of abdominal masses in children.' *Clin. Radiol.* **23**, 340

Goldstein, H. M., Poole, G. J. Rosenquist, C. J., Friedland, G. W. and Zboralske, F. F. (1971). 'Comparison of methods for acceleration of small intestinal radiographic examinations.' *Radiology* **98**, 519

Rowe, M. I., Furst, A. J., Altman, D. H. and Poole, C. A. (1971). 'The neonatal response to Gastrografin enema.' *Pediatrics, Springfield* **48**, 29

Steinbach, H. L., Rosenberg, R. H., Grossman, M. and Nelson, T. L. (1955). 'The potential hazard of enemas in patients with Hirschsprung's disease.' *Radiology* **64**, 45

CONGENITAL LESIONS

Astley, R. (1969). 'Duodenal atresia with gas below the obstruction.' *Br. J. Radiol.* **42**, 351

Berdon, W. E., Baker, D. H., Santulli, T. V. and Amoury, R. (1968). 'The radiologic evaluation of imperforate anus.' *Radiology* **90**, 466

Carre, I. J. and Astley, R. (1960). 'The fate of partial thoracic stomach ('hiatus hernia') in children.' *Archs Dis. Childh.* **35**, 484

Cremin, B. J. (1971). 'The radiological assessment of anorectal anomalies.' *Clin. Radiol.* **22**, 239

Forshall, I. (1955). 'The cardio-oesophageal syndrome in childhood.' *Archs Dis. Childh.* **30**, 46

244

Free, E. A. and Gerald, B. (1968). 'Duodenal obstruction in the newborn due to annular pancreas.' *Am. J. Roentgl.* **103**, 321

Hayes, D. M., Wooley, M. M., Snyder, W. H., Reed, G. B., Gwina, J. L. and Landing, B. H. (1967). 'Diagnosis of biliary atresia: relative accuracy of percutaneous liver biopsy, open liver biopsy and operative cholangiography.' *J. Pediat.* **71**, 598

Husfeldt, E., Thomsen, G. and Wamberg, E. (1951). 'Hiatal hernia and short oesophagus in children.' *Thorax* **6**, 56

Neuhauser, E. B. D. and Berenberg, W. (1947). 'Cardio-esophageal relaxation as a cause of vomiting in infants.' *Radiology* **48**, 480

Pierce, J. W. and Creamer, B. (1963). 'The diagnosis of the columnar lined oesophagus.' *Clin. Radiol.* **14**, 64

Rudhe, U. (1968). 'Rontgenological examination of anal and rectal anomalies in the newborn male infant.' *Annls Radiol.* **11**, 429

Sauvegrain, J. Borde, J. and Mareschal, J-L. (1969). 'Atresies de l'oesophage avec fistule du bout superieur.' (Oesophageal atresia with fistula of the upper end: radiologic diagnosis). *Annls Radiol.* **12**, 145

Shopfner, C. E. (1965). 'Roentgenologic demonstration of the "Ectopic Anus" associated with Imperforate Anus.' *Radiology* **84**, 464

Sorensen, B. M. (1967). 'Hiatus Hernia in Infancy.' *Acta Paediat. Scand.* **56**, 513

INTESTINAL OBSTRUCTION

Dunn, P. M. (1963). 'Intestinal obstruction in the newborn with special reference to transient functional ileus, associated with respiratory distress syndrome.' *Archs Dis. Childh.* **38**, 459

Ehrenpreis Th. (1946). 'Megacolon in the newborn—a clinical and roentgenological study with special regard to the pathogenesis.' *Acta Chir. Scand.* **94**, Suppl. 112

Girdany, B. R., Bass, L. W. and Sieber, W. K. (1959). 'Rontgenological aspects of hydrostatic reduction of ileocolic intussusception.' *Am. J. Roentgl.* **82**, 455

Grossman, H., Berdon, W. E. and Baker, D. H. (1966). 'Gastrointestinal findings in cystic fibrosis.' *Am. J. Roentgl.* **97**, 277

Hope, J. W., Borns, P. F. and Berg, P. K., (1965). 'Roentgenological manifestations of Hirschsprung's disease in infancy.' *Am. J. Roentgl.* **95**, 217

Lillie, J. G. and Chrispin, A. R. (1972). 'Investigation and management of neonatal obstruction by Gastrografin enema.' *Annls Radiol.* **15**, 237

McIver, A. G. and Whitehead, R. (1972). 'Zonal colonic aganglionosis, a variant of Hirschsprung's disease.' *Archs Dis. Childh.* **47**, 233

Middlemiss, J. H. (1955). 'Intussusception in childhood. Radiological appearances on plain radiography.' *Br. J. Radiol.* **28**, 257

Nordentoft, J. M. (1969). 'The significance of hydrostatic pressure level in the non-operative reduction of intussusception in children.' *Annls Radiol.* **12**, 191

Smith, B. and Clatworthy, H. W. (1961). 'Meconium peritonitis: prognostic significance.' *Pediatrics, Springfield* **27**, 967

Wagget, J., Johnson, D. G., Borns, P. and Bishop, H. C. (1970). 'The non-operative treatment of meconium ileus by Gastrografin enema.' *J. Pediat.* **77**, 407

Weens, H. S. and Golden, A. (1955). 'Adrenal cortical insufficiency in infants simulating high intestinal obstruction.' *Am. J. Roentgl.* **74**, 213

INFLAMMATORY DISEASE

Davidson, M., Bloom, A. A. and Kugler, M. M. (1965). 'Chronic ulcerative colitis of childhood.' *J. Pediat.* **67**, 471

Eklöf, O., Löhr, G. and Okmian, L. (1969). 'Submucosal perforation of the esophagus in the neonate.' *Acta Radiol.* **8**, 187

Goldman, W., Perl, T. and Sarason, E. L. (1968). 'Postappendectomy fistula due to residual fecolith.' *Am. J. Roentgl.* **103**, 351

Hoeffel, J. C. (1969). 'Aspects radiologiques de la recto-colite ulcero-haemorragique chez l'enfant.' (Radiological Aspects of ulcero-hemorrhagic rectocolitis in children). *Annls Radiol.* **12**, 205

Hope, J. W. and Cramer, H. R. (1958). 'The significance of postoperative pneumoperitoneum in infants and children.' *Radiology* **74**, 797

Kantor, J. L. (1934). 'Regional (terminal) ileitis—its Roentgen diagnosis.' *J. Am. med. Ass.* **103**, 2016

Lafferty, J. O. (1959). 'Duodenal ulcers in children; with notes on their etiology.' *Radiology* **73**, 374

Miller, R. C. and Larsen, E. (1971). 'Regional enteritis in children.' *Am. J. Dis. Child.* **122**, 301

Mizrahi, A., Barlow, O., Berdon, W., Blanc, W. A. and Silverman, W. A. (1965). 'Necrotizing enterocolitis in premature infants.' *J. Pediat.* **66**, 697

Moseley, J. E., Marshak, R. H. and Wolf, B. S. (1960). 'Regional enteritis in children.' *Am. J. Roentgl.* **84**, 532

Pochaczevsky, R. and Kassner, E. G. (1971). 'Necrotizing Enterocolitis of infancy.' *Am. J. Roentgl.* **113**, 283

Rosenlund, M. L. and Koop, C. E. (1970). 'Duodenal ulcer in childhood.' *Pediatrics, Springfield* **45**, 283

Rudhe, U. (1960). 'Roentgenologic examination of the rectum in ulcerative colitis.' *Acta Pediat. Stockh.* **49**, 859

Sutcliffe, J. (1963). 'Crohn's disease of the colon.' *Br. J. Radiol.* **36**, 27

Wilkinson, R. H., Bartlett, R. H. and Eraklis, A. J. (1969). 'The diagnosis of appendicitis in infancy—The value of abdominal radiographs.' *Am. J. Dis. Child.* **118**, 687

MALABSORPTION

Haworth, E. M., Hodson, C. J., Joyce, C. R. B., Pringle, E. M., Solimano, G. and Young, W. F. (1967). 'Radiological measurement of small bowel calibre in normal subjects according to age.' *Clin. Radiol.* **18**, 417

Laws, J. W. and Neale, G. (1966). 'Radiological diagnosis of disaccharidase deficiency.' *Lancet* **2**, 139

McNeish, A. S. and Sweet, E. M. (1968). 'Lactose intolerance in childhood coeliac disease: assessment of its incidence and importance.' *Archs Dis. Childh.* **43**, 433

INTRA-ABDOMINAL CYSTS AND TUMOURS

Duhamel, J. and Bauche, P. (1965). 'Polyps of the colon beyond the reach of the sigmoidoscope.' *Archs Dis. Childh.* **40**, 173

Forde, W. J. and Finby, N. (1961). 'Splenic cysts.' *Clin. Radiol.* **12**, 49

Fredens, M. (1969). 'Angiography in primary hepatic tumours in children.' *Acta Radiol (Diagn.)* **8**, 193

Godard, J. E., Dodds, W. J., Phillips, J. C. and Scanlon, G. T. (1971). 'Peutz-Jeghers syndrome: clinical and roentgenographic features.' *Am. J. Roentgl.* **113**, 316

Griscom, N. T. (1965). 'The roentgenology of neonatal abdominal masses.' *Am. J. Roentgl.* **93**, 447

Hammer, J. W. (1967). 'Duplication of the small bowel simulating regional enteritis.' *Am. J. Roentgl.* **99**, 52

Han, S. Y., Collins, L. C. and Wright, R. M. (1969). 'Choledochal cyst: report of five cases.' *Clin. Radiol.* **20**, 332

Kottra, J. J. and Dodds, W. J. (1971). 'Duplication of the Large Bowel.' *Am. J. Roentgl.* **113**, 310

Wilson, J. W. (1955). 'The diagnosis of abdominal cysts in infants and children.' *Radiology* **64**, 178

ASCITES

Craven, C. E., Goldman, A. S., Larsen, D. L., Patterson, M. and Hendrick, C. K. (1967). 'Congenital chylous ascites: lymphangiographic demonstration of obstruction of the cisterna chyli and chylous reflux into the peritoneal space and small intestine.' *J. Pediat.* **70**, 340

Cywes, S. and Cremin, B. J. (1969). 'The roentgenological features of hemoperitoneum in the newborn.' *Am. J. Roentgl.* **106**, 193

PROTEIN-LOSING ENTEROPATHY

Marshak, R. H., Khilnani, M., Eliasoph, J. and Wolf, B. S. (1967). 'Intestinal edema.' *Am. J. Roentgl.* **101**, 379

Pock-Steen, O. Ch. (1966). 'Roentgenologic changes in protein-losing enteropathy.' *Acta Radiol (Diagn.)* **4**, 681

DISORDERS OF INTESTINAL MOTILITY

Ardran, G. M., Benson, P. F., Butler, N. R., Ellis H. L. and McKendrick, T. (1965). 'Congenital dysphagia resulting from dysfunction of the pharyngeal musculature.' *Devel. Med. Ch. Neurol.* **7**, 157

Frank, M. M. and Gatewood, O. M. B. (1966). 'Transient pharyngeal incoordination in the newborn.' *Am. J. Dis. Child.* **111**, 178

Green, R. I. (1959). 'The radiological appearances of the soft palate with reference to the treatment of cleft palate.' *J. Fac. Radiol.* **10**, 27

Margulies, S. I., Brunt, P. W., Donner, M. W. and Silbiger, M. L., (1968). 'Familial dysautonomia: a cineradiographic study of the swallowing mechanism.' *Radiology* **90**, 107

7 URINARY TRACT

METHODS

UROGRAPHY

The basic principles of excretory urography in children differ little from those underlying the investigation in adults. However, certain problems and difficulties are encountered, especially in the small infant, consequent upon the age of the subject.

Excretion of contrast medium

Older children excrete urographic contrast media in a concentration which is as good as, and sometimes even better than, in adult patients. This is not true of infants, especially in the neonatal period. There seems little doubt that the kidney of the newborn infant handles contrast media injected into the bloodstream in a different way from older children. If urograms in babies under 1 month of age are compared with those in infants between 1 and 2 years of age, it is apparent that the density in the pelvis builds up relatively slowly and does not reach its maximum until between 30 minutes and 3 hours after the injection (Nogrady and Scott Dunbar, 1968). In the older infants on the other hand the maximum density is reached within the first 10 minutes and is more rapidly attained than in adult patients. It is not an uncommon experience to find a dense urogram on films taken 24 or even 48 hours after an angiocardiogram on very young infants. In view of the foregoing observation it is surprising that the appearance of a nephrogram, in which the contrast medium outlines the kidney by opacifying its parenchyma occurs as promptly in neonates as in older children (*Figure 7.1a*). It may however be the production of the nephrogram as part of a total body opacification that

is one of the reasons for the slow build-up of the pyelogram. This could be because the contrast medium is deviated into the extra vascular compartment and from there it is only very slowly reabsorbed into the vessels whence it can be excreted through the glomeruli. The kidney of the newborn infant may be immature, with a glomerular filtration rate of only 10 per cent of the adult kidney. This could clearly also contribute to the effects described above.

Factors concerned in production of an adequate pyelogram

In addition to the production of a nephrogram, the objects of excretory urography are to produce sufficient concentration of contrast in the renal pelvis in order to give a pyelogram of adequate density, and distension of the pelvicalyceal system sufficient to provide an adequate demonstration of the calcyeal structure and pattern, but without distortion or over-distension (*Figure 7.1b*) (Saxton, 1969). The factors which influence the attainment of these criteria are the same in the child as in the adult. The concentration of contrast medium in the renal pelvis is enhanced by increasing the dose, and also by dehydration. Adequate distension of the renal pelvis and calyces is produced by increasing the flow of urine resulting from diuresis and by compressing the ureters.

Dehydration

Of these factors, dehydration in the small infant is highly undesirable. The blood volume at this age is small and it may be depleted easily. Moreover, the size of the renal pelvis in small infants will mean that the volume of urine containing contrast medium within it is small. It

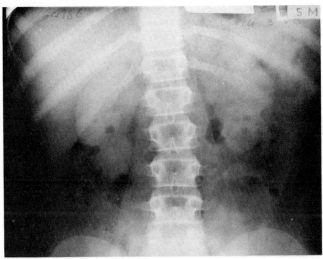

(a)

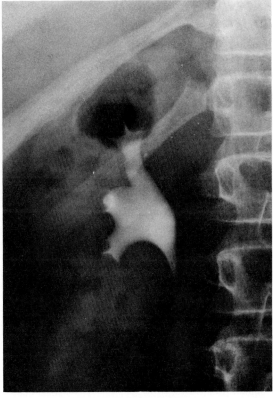

(b)

*Figure 7.1. Normal Urography: (a) Nephrogram. In the early
stages of urography, the contrast medium being excreted by the
kidney leads to an opacification of the renal parenchyma and a
clear definition of the outline of the kidney. (b) Pyelogram.
Concentration of the contrast medium in its passage down the
renal tubule leads to a dense opacification of the calyces and
body of the renal pelvis. The cup shape of the minor calyces
depends upon the pyramid and fornices being shown in profile
and this in turn depends upon the direction in which the calyces
are facing*

is therefore particularly important to ensure that the renal pelvis and calyces are distended. There is good reason to employ hydration of the young infant rather than dehydration as the desirable preparation for excretory urography.

Ureteric compression

Although perfectly practicable in the older child, this is difficult to apply efficiently in infants and very young children. It has been suggested that a similar distension of the renal pelvis and calyces may be brought about by ensuring that excretory urography is always carried out in the presence of a full bladder. This is however only effective in a small proportion of cases.

Dosage of contrast medium

In all age groups the most effective way of ensuring good quality of the urograms is to inject a higher dose of contrast medium than has been used in the past. Those contrast media which are commonly used at the present time are sodium or methyl glucamine diatrizoate and the corresponding iothalamates. They contain three iodine atoms in their molecules and are relatively more opaque than the earlier types of contrast medium. It is the authors' practice to give 2.5 ml/kg bodyweight to infants weighing less than 8 kg and to give 20 ml to all children between 8 and 30 kg. Over the age of six years, the adult dose is used. In cases in whom renal failure is suspected, double these quantities may be used; thus, an

infant in the first few months would receive 5 ml/kg bodyweight. In most cases this dosage will ensure that opacification of the renal pelves and ureters occurs and some useful information is obtained. In both the prerenal and postrenal types of azotaemia, excellent results can often be obtained and it has been shown that there is no increased risk of reactions. Some workers have suggested that better results may be obtained if the dose of contrast medium is given in two separate injections, instead of the whole quantity being given at once. It is however preferable to avoid the need for more than one venepuncture in small children. The use of the drip infusion technique has not been generally accepted in children. Dilution of the contrast with 5 per cent dextrose or saline makes no appreciable difference to the quality of the urogram and the advantages of this technique are due entirely to the high dosage of contrast medium given.

Reactions to contrast medium

As stated above, there is no evidence that reactions to the administration of contrast medium are a serious problem in small infants. This applies even when high dosage techniques are used, provided that the injection rate is kept slow (not less than 1 minute for completion of the injection) and prior dehydration is avoided. However, Ansell (1970) has recently reported a fatal outcome in two infants which he ascribes to overdosage. He stresses the danger that over-confidence in the lack of toxicity of contrast media may lead to an increase in the dose above safe levels in inexperienced hands. Attention has also been drawn to the possibility of untoward reactions resulting from an increase in serum osmolality in neonates if these precautions are not observed (Standen *et al.*, 1965). Haemorrhagic renal cortical necrosis following the rapid injection of large doses of contrast medium for angiocardiography has been reported and is associated with renal intravascular thrombosis (Gilbert *et al.,* 1970). Dehydration and hypoxia may increase the risk of serious renal damage from such doses of contrast media. Renal failure as such, on the other hand, does not increase the risk of reactions to the injection of contrast medium. It is a sensible precaution to give antihistamines prior to the injection of contrast medium if there is a history of allergy either in the patient or his family. However, antihistamines should not be mixed with the contrast medium in the same syringe as the two drugs may be incompatible and therefore ineffective. Minor reactions to contrast medium such as nausea, vomiting or an urticarial rash subside rapidly and require no special treatment. Very rarely, more serious reactions may be encountered and in our experience their occurrence cannot be predicted from a prior history of allergy nor are they related to the dose employed. These reactions fall into two main types; those leading to asphyxia as a result of laryngeal oedema and bronchospasm and those resulting in hypotension and circulatory collapse which ultimately may lead to cardiac and respiratory arrest. The former type of reaction should be treated by re-establishing a patent airway, oxygen and adrenaline. The latter reaction which is potentially more serious may require treatment by intravenous fluid and hydrocortisone and possibly a noradrenaline drip. Cardiac massage and artificial ventilation, in order to maintain cardiac and respiratory function, may occasionally be required. Fortunately, these serious reactions are rare and they are even less frequent in young children than in adults.

Intravenous injection

The small size and inaccessibility of superficial veins in infants may occasionally be a problem, particularly when previous intravenous therapy has led to thrombosis in the veins. The use of scalp veins in babies is often easier than the conventional sites for venepuncture, particularly if a scalp vein type of needle is employed with a flexible polythene tube interposed between the needle and the syringe. The use of the femoral or external jugular veins has been advocated by some workers. The latter route is inadvisable because of the possibility of inducing a pneumothorax by accidentally puncturing the apical pleura. This event is a real danger in a struggling infant. It is even more important to avoid injection into the superior longitudinal sinus through an open fontanelle. This procedure may lead to intracranial extravasation of blood or contrast medium.

Subcutaneous urography

In patients in whom a vein cannot be punctured for the injection, the subcutaneous route is well worth considering. If the technique is adequately carried out, the chances of obtaining a diagnostic urogram are good. The main disadvantage is that the dose that can be given is necessarily limited and the maximum density of the urogram is attained more slowly than by the intravenous route. Dilution of the contrast medium to a concentration of about 10−15 per cent is necessary in order to avoid local irritation. The use of hyaluronidase and massage of the site after injection are essential to speed up absorption. Our practice for a baby of up to 6 months of age is to give a total of 12 ml of 45 per cent sodium diatrizoate, and this is diluted with 36 ml of sterile water. The dose is divided into two equal portions; each portion is mixed with ½ ml of hyaluronidase and injected into the suprascapular region of each side. This region has the advantage of being well clear of the urinary tract and therefore avoids the possibility of producing confusing shadows overlying it.

Intestinal gas shadows

Small infants tend to have large amounts of gas present in the intestine. This may lead to much difficulty in interpretation of the appearances of the pelvis and ureters and they may be completely obscured. Preparation designed to clear the bowel of faecal matter is relatively ineffective in overcoming this problem, but mild sedation may be helpful by reducing crying. Similarly, giving a feed just before the examination may produce a contented infant and if the interval between the feed and the urography is kept short enough, it will not diminish the concentration of contrast medium in the renal pelvis. In spite of these measures the amount of bowel gas frequently leads to a very real difficulty in interpretation and various methods such as the use of the prone position with compression have been suggested to overcome this problem. The authors' experience has indicated two other methods to be particularly helpful.

First, inflation of the stomach with gas may enable the renal pelvis to be seen against a more uniform background; as it were through the window of the gas-filled stomach (*Figure 7.2*). This is most effective in demonstrating the left kidney. Oblique views may however be needed to show the kidneys clearly, particularly the right one. The stomach may be filled, either by the passage of an intragastric tube and injection of air by a syringe, or with less trouble and probably greater safety by the administration of a carbonated beverage. The efficacy of this method depends, however, on the position of the stomach relative to the kidneys and its relative size compared with the intestines and these are less favourable in the older child than in the young infant. Moreover, the child may refuse to take a sufficient amount quickly enough to distend the stomach to a sufficient degree or may get rid of the gas before the film has been taken.

Secondly the use of tomography may be helpful by blurring out the shadows of the bowel loops while leaving the renal pelves and ureters in sharp focus (*Figure 7.3*). Selection of the correct plane for the tomographic 'cut' may be difficult. This can be made easier by the use of a 'multisection' cassette, which allows cuts at three or more levels to be obtained with a single x-ray exposure. The thickness of the plane of tissue in focus may also be increased by reducing the arc of movement of the tube and

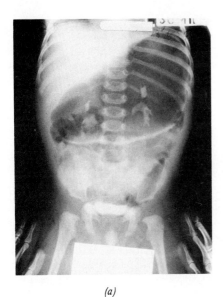

(a)

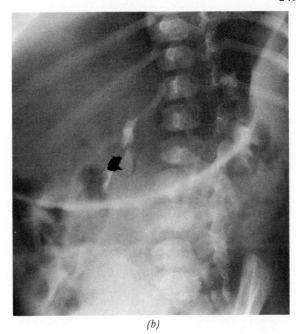

(b)

Figure 7.2. Use of Gastric Inflation: After administration of a carbonated beverage the distended stomach displaces other bowel shadows and permits a clear view of the renal pelves. (a) Anteroposterior projection showing the left renal pelvis well. (b) Right posterior oblique projection showing the right renal pelvis

film, but the degree to which this may be done is limited by the need for adequate elimination of the confusing bowel shadows. This will mean that respiratory and other movements which cannot be controlled in small infants will blur detail of the urogram. In a survey of both these methods in order to assess their effectiveness, it was observed that whereas gastric inflation alone was completely successful in only 40 per cent and tomography alone was successful in only 49 per cent of the cases, when both methods were used in combination, the proportion of successes increased to 70 per cent and they failed to provide some diagnostic information in only 7 per cent. It is advocated, therefore, that both methods should be used in combination in cases in which the presence of bowel gas obscures the detail of the urogram.

Radiographic technique

Details of radiographic technique will not be considered here other than to say that, as in all paediatric work, it must be flexible in order to obtain the best results.

Uses and indications

The chief uses of excretory urography in children are the demonstration of anatomical and structural abnormalities in the calyces, renal pelves, ureters and bladder due to congenital or acquired disease and also for the assessment of renal function. As regards the former, excretory urography is generally accepted as a reliable and indispensable method in the investigation of urinary disease in children. The latter use is more controversial.

Whereas it is true that renal function is directly related to the concentration of contrast medium in the glomular filtrate and therefore in the renal tubule and renal pelvis, this is not the only factor concerned. Indeed this relationship is not of the same degree in the different types of renal failure. Thus, azotaemia due to prerenal causes or to obstructive disease may not be associated with any appreciable diminution in the density of the urogram. However, factors such as the degree of hydration and variations in the urinary flow rate which may result from diuresis, obstruction, renal ischaemia and other causes may affect it to a very considerable degree. For these reasons, it has been suggested that other techniques, such as isotope renography, may be more effective and preferable in assessing renal function.

There is also the possibility that with the increasingly high doses employed for excretory urography, the detection of early renal failure may be made more difficult (Saxton, 1969). This is a reasonable price to pay for the improvement in anatomical information so obtained, especially as there are alternative ways in which renal function can be assessed.

CYSTO-URETHROGRAPHY

Investigation of the lower urinary tract by the introduction of contrast medium into the bladder and urethra has been more frequently requested in the past few years, because a relationship between vesico-ureteric reflux and irreversible renal damage, particularly in the presence of urinary tract infection, has been established (Hodson and Edwards, 1960).

250

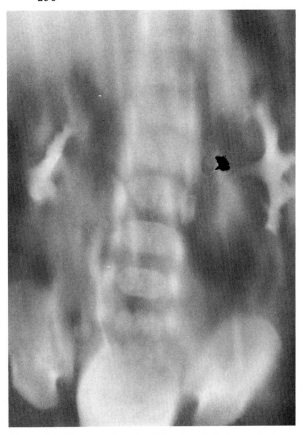

Figure 7.3. Tomography: Overlying bowel shadows which may obscure detail of the renal pelvis may be blurred out leaving the urogram in sharp focus provided that respiratory movement can be controlled

Technique

Contrast medium can be injected retrogradely into the urethra, when the object of the examination is to study the anatomy of the anterior urethra, and to demonstrate diverticula, acquired strictures and similar lesions. Abnormalities of the bladder, ureteric orifices and the posterior urethra are better studied by micturating cysto-urethrography, for which contrast medium is introduced into the bladder by urethral catheter. Studies of the urethra are made during micturition (*Figure 7.4*).

Following catheterization, the bladder is emptied and a catheter specimen of urine obtained for pathological examination. Sodium diatrizoate 10 per cent is run in from an intravenous drip bottle through the catheter until the bladder is sufficiently full to provoke a desire to micturate or until ureteric reflux is seen to occur on fluoroscopy. The quantity of contrast medium required is very flexible, and it depends on the size of the child and on the tolerance of the bladder to distension. It is usually of the order of 75–100 ml for infants, 200–250 ml for older children, up to 400 or 500 ml for adolescents. Films are exposed at the end of filling, during micturition and after complete emptying of the bladder. It should be emphasized that the latter film is important as it may be the only one to show reflux. It is also important that the renal areas should be included on these films as well as

the bladder, because otherwise the extent and severity of the reflux cannot be assessed.

Some authors have advocated the use of a sterile suspension of barium sulphate instead of water soluble medium. This use of barium suspension cannot be recommended because of the possibility that insoluble barium particles carried by reflux into the renal pelvis could act as a nidus for calculus formation. Different types of contrast media have been compared in respect of their liability to produce pain, uncontrolled voiding, mucosal irregularities or even transient vesico-ureteric reflux due to mucosal oedema. It has been concluded that concentrations of sodium or meglumine diatrizoate below 20 per cent are satisfactory from this point of view (Shopfner, 1967a).

It is usually not difficult to induce micturition with the child in the supine position, provided the bladder has been adequately filled and sedation has not been too heavy. Infants may be stimulated to void by gentle pressure on the abdomen or by applying a cold object to the skin. In cases of difficulty, it is worth trying to obtain films in the standing or sitting position. If the ureteric orifices are incompetent the intravesical pressure is more than sufficient to force contrast medium up the ureters into the renal pelves even against the force of gravity. A triggering device can be used to expose the film as soon as urine comes into contact with it; infants can then be left in position until micturition occurs spontaneously (Scott Dunbar et al., 1961). Some workers insist that continuous fluoroscopy is essential throughout micturition in order to be certain of not missing minor degrees of reflux. Others have used cineradiography for the same reason and also because they consider interpretation of the appearances in the region of the bladder neck and posterior urethra to be more reliable than they are with fluoroscopy. It is felt, however, that these methods are unnecessary for routine use. They will also increase the radiation dosage, which is inevitably high in terms of gonad dose no matter which technique is used. Cineradiographic studies are inferior to spot films taken on a serial changer in showing fine detail and are no better in detecting transient reflux (Shopfner, 1965). In view of the increasing use of micturating cysto-urethrography for the investigation of all cases of recurrent or persistent urinary infection, it is considered that the radiation dosage should be kept to as small a level as possible.

Catheterization and infection

Catheterization of the urethra has been criticized on the grounds that infection may be introduced into the bladder or that irritation of the urethra may lead to inability to void. Suprapubic puncture has been suggested as an alternative means of introducing contrast medium into the bladder. The bladder in the small infant is an abdominal organ and the technique is not difficult. The puncture can be performed under local anaesthetic after distending the bladder by means of oral or intravenous fluid. This method has a place in the rare cases where urethral obstruction makes catheterization impracticable. That it is possible to introduce a fresh

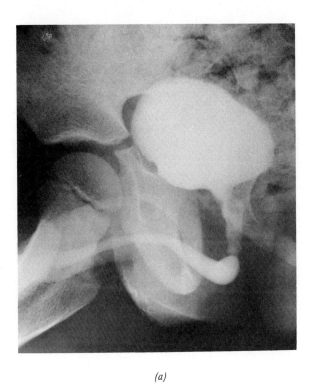

(a)

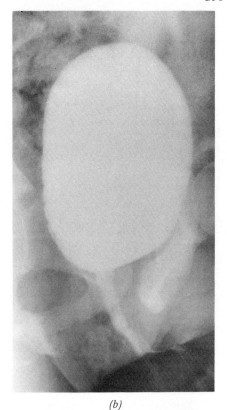

(b)

Figure 7.4. Cysto-urethrography: (a) Normal male urethra shown on a film exposed during voiding. (b) Normal female urethra. (c) Filling of the vagina may occur when voiding occurs in the supine position and this may lead to confusion by the super-imposition of the vaginal (white arrow) and urethral (black arrow) shadows

(c)

infection by urethral catheterization was shown by Glynn and Gordon (1970). However, they concluded that this was relatively infrequent (8 per cent). It usually occurred in cases of gross hydronephrosis and hydro-ureter with stasis and vesico-ureteric reflux. Provided that the urethral catheter was not allowed to remain *in situ* for more than a short time before or after the investigation, the infection was only transient and was easily controlled. This danger has also been reported in cases of meningomyelocele in whom there was an incidence of infection in 42 per cent of patients (Cooper, 1967).

It has been claimed that micturating cysto-urethro-graphy performed at the end of excretory urography is useful for studying the lower urinary tract. It may demonstrate obstruction or anatomical abnormalities. It may even identify reflux by showing refilling and distension of the lower ureters during and after mictur-ition (Hope *et al.,* 1960). Our own experiences would confirm the first of these claims, but would indicate that the demonstration of vesico-ureteric reflux is not sufficiently reliable by such a combined method.

Apart from mild sedation for particularly nervous children and an anaesthetic and antiseptic lubricant applied to the catheter, anaesthesia has not been found necessary. Indeed, it may lead to error by causing transient reflux in children whose ureters are otherwise competent.

Uses and indications

Much the most common indication at the present time for micturating cysto-urethrography is the detection of vesico-ureteric reflux in cases of recurrent or persistent urinary infection. In such cases it will usually be combined with excretory urography. If these two examinations are to be carried out on the same day, micturating cysto-urethrography should be performed first. The importance of detecting vesico-ureteric reflux has inevitably resulted in a great increase in the number of these investigations. They are time consuming and expensive in terms of irradiation dosage. These facts have led to a search for some alternative screening procedure which might reduce the number of cases in which the full investigation was necessary. At the present time, however, it has not been possible to devise such a test and the importance of preventing irreversible renal damage from the combination or reflux and infection must justify the large numbers subjected to urography and micturating cysto-urethrography. It is, however, common practice to use them only in those children who have failed to respond to adequate treatment or who have had more than one attack or urinary infection.

In those cases in whom the problem is solely that of demonstrating abnormalities in urethral or vesical anatomy, the use of high dosage urography may render it economical to obtain micturating films at the end of excretory urography or may make the use of retrograde urethrography advisable.

The use of micturating cysto-urethrography in the investigation of enuresis has been shown to be relatively unprofitable in demonstrating abnormalities of the urinary tract (Hallgren *et al.*, 1961). The authors' experience would support this view.

Difficulties in interpretation in female children

The interpretation of the outline of the bladder neck and urethra in the female child is a matter of considerable difficulty. Clayton *et al.* (1966) have investigated the variations which may occur in apparently normal individuals and they have attempted to correlate these with the intra- and extra-luminal pressures during micturition. They conclude that the appearance of constriction at either end of the female urethra and of dilatation of the intermediate portion show very little correlation with local obstruction or increase in resistance to urine flow. It is likely that cineradiography might be helpful in determining the range of normal variation and in differentiating pathological appearances from those due to physiological variations. It is not uncommon for contrast medium to fill the vagina in girls when they micturate in the supine position (*Figure 7.4c*). This is considered to have no significance but it may produce confusing opacities overlying the urethra.

ANGIOGRAPHY

Angiography is not used as widely in the investigation of diseases of the urinary tract in children as it is in adults. There are however three situations in which it can afford useful information. These are the investigations of suspected tumours of the kidney or suprarenal, the diagnosis of the cause of hypertension, particularly when this is suspected to be due to renal ischaemia or phaeochromocytoma, and the investigation of unexplained haematuria (*Figures 7.5 and 7.37*).

The use of the transfemoral approach by the Seldinger method allows the opportunity for selective renal arteriography. It can also be used for the simultaneous catheterization of the inferior vena cava via the femoral vein, which has widened the scope of the available information that can be obtained by this method.

Indications and uses

It has been maintained that in the case of childhood tumours which are invading the kidney or arising within it as determined by excretory urography, it is not justifiable to delay operative treatment by performing arteriography. This is because nephrectomy is inevitable and should be carried out as soon as possible if a permanent cure is to be achieved. However, with the advent of chemotherapy and with the greater use of radiotherapy, it is likely that the importance of establishing the nature and extent of the tumour as accurately as possible will increase. This is particularly the case when a tumour occurs in a horseshoe or other abnormal type of kidney or when no function is demonstrable on urography. With modern techniques the risk of angiography to the patient is negligible.

Renal arteriography and phlebography of the inferior vena cava are used in the localization of tumours and in detecting invasion of the retroperitoneal tissues or obstruction of the vena cava. Their role in this respect has recently been discussed (McDonald and Hiller, 1968); Tucker, 1965). Misinterpretation of the appearances shown on inferior vena caval phlebograms may occur owing to unsuspected abnormalities in the venous drainage of the lower limbs and to the effects of non-contrast-containing blood forming a layer separate from the contrast medium. These pitfalls can be reduced by taking anteroposterior and lateral films and by catheterizing the inferior vena cava via the femoral vein, instead of by injecting contrast medium into the saphenous vein in the leg.

Renal ischaemia, though not very common in children, should not be forgotten as a possible cause of unexplained hypertension. This is discussed in detail on page 282.

Unexplained haematuria in a child is sometimes a difficult diagnostic problem, especially when all routine investigations are essentially negative. In these circumstances, renal arteriography may be justifiable in order to exclude haemangiomata or other renal tumours which because of their small size are not detected by excretory urography. However, it must be admitted that the frequency with which abnormalities are shown by arteriography is low, and unless the haematuria is very

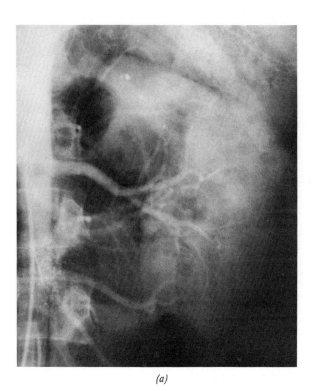

(a)

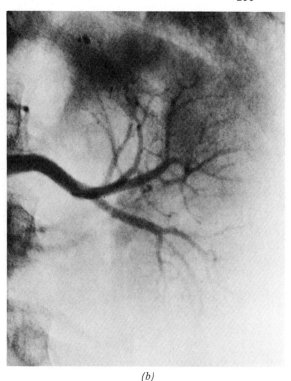

(b)

Figure 7.5. *Renal Arteriography: (a) Opacification of normal renal artery and its branches as a result of a free aortic injection. Although selective catheterization may give a view of the renal artery unobscured by other vessels, the existence of accessory renal arteries supplying the poles of the kidney may be overlooked. (b) The detail of the arterial branches may be enhanced by the use of a 'subtraction' technique, whereby the shadows of the bones and other soft tissues are reduced or eliminated. (c) Normal inferior vena cava opacified by injection of contrast medium into a leg vein for the purpose of excretory urography.*

Two undissolved opaque tablets are present in the bowel

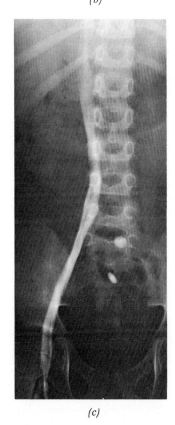

(c)

profuse or persistent, it is probable that this investigation is seldom justified.

Phlebography of the inferior vena cava may be helpful in establishing the presence of renal vein thrombosis. Filling of the renal veins may however not occur even though they are normally patent unless measures are taken to obstruct the flow in the upper part of the inferior vena cava. This can be achieved when the patient is under general anaesthetic by compressing the anaesthetic bag at the moment when the contrast medium is injected.

RETROPERITONEAL PNEUMOGRAPHY AND NEPHROTOMOGRAPHY

In cases where it is desired to obtain a clear picture of the outline of the kidneys or suprarenal glands, it has been the practice in many centres to use either gaseous contrast medium in the perirenal tissues or positive contrast medium in the renal parenchyma for this purpose. Gas is injected into the perirenal space either from the lumbar region posteriorly or from the presacral space, a procedure termed retroperitoneal pneumography. Nephrotomography is performed by giving a rapid intravenous injection of a large volume of urographic contrast medium followed by tomography of the renal areas within a few seconds of the end of the

254

injection. The use of high dosage techniques for routine urography and of renal arteriography has resulted in these methods becoming less frequently used than they were a few years ago. This is because the density of the nephrogram produced, particularly by arteriography, is considerably better than that obtained by nephrotomography and the delineation of the renal outline as good as that produced by perirenal gas insufflation. The latter method may, however, still have a use in demonstrating the size and shape of the suprarenal glands in cases in which localization of a tumour may be required prior to surgery. Such cases are rare, however, in children and arteriography is probably the investigation which should be tried first, because most suprarenal tumours are vascular and are likely to be opacified. If carbon dioxide is used as the contrast medium instead of air, retroperitoneal pneumography is quite a safe procedure. It has the disadvantages associated with dissection of the tissue planes by the injected gas, in that bizarre appearances may be produced if the gas surrounds masses of fat as well as the gland or tumour being investigated. This may readily lead to error in interpretation and may produce both false negative as well as false positive results.

TRANSLUMBAR (ANTEGRADE) PYELOGRAPHY AND RENAL PUNCTURE

These methods, used for many years in adults, have recently been applied to young infants. The opacification of the renal pelvis and ureter by contrast medium injected directly through the back under fluoroscopic control may be very useful. This is especially so in cases of obstructive uropathy in whom excretory urography has failed to opacify the whole or part of the renal pelvis and ureter (*Figure 7.6*) (Lalli, 1969). A very similar technique has been used in the investigation of various types of renal cysts or cystic anomalies of the kidney. Individual cysts are opacified by contrast medium injected into them (Saxton *et al.*, 1973).

GENITOGRAPHY AND GYNAECOGRAPHY

Abnormalities of the lower urinary tract and the internal and external genitalia are often associated. Investigation by the injection of contrast medium into abnormal genital passages from their external orifices may be carried out in very much the same way as in retrograde urethrography. Such a procedure is termed *genitography* (*Figure 7.7*). The internal genitalia in the female may also be visualized by inducing a pneumoperitoneum and positioning the patient in such a way that the air or gas ascends into the Pouch of Douglas to surround the ovaries, uterus and broad ligaments. This investigation is known as *gynaecography* (*Figure 7.8*). Such procedures may be of considerable value when the sex of an infant is indeterminate, and may, in conjunction with chromosome studies and biochemical tests, enable an accurate determination of the infant's sex to be made. They may also give an indication of the extent and nature of the abnormalities of the genitalia, which may be essential if surgical treatment is to be undertaken.

The use of genitography has been well reviewed by

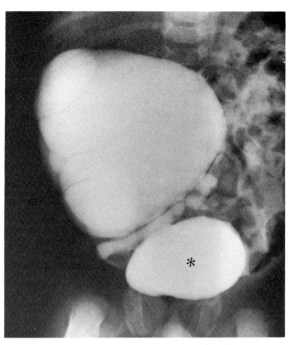

Figure 7.6. Translumbar Pyelography. Injection of contrast medium through direct needle puncture from the back has opacified a large hydronephrotic renal pelvis and has passed into the ureter. The bladder (*) was opacified by urethral catheterization

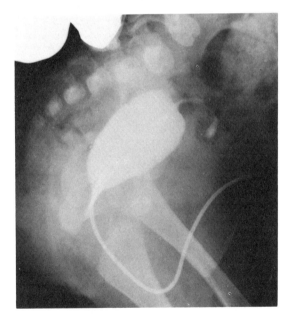

Figure 7.7. Genitography: Contrast medium injected into an abnormally placed genital orifice has outlined the vagina and passed through the cervix into the cavity of the uterus

Shopfner (1967b). A viscous contrast medium, either aqueous or oily, is used and must be introduced in such a way that it fills all the genital and urinary cavities which open externally. This is best achieved by the use of a Knutsson's rubber-tipped nozzle or by a catheter of a diameter slightly wider than that of the perineal orifice. An air-tight seal between the syringe or nozzle

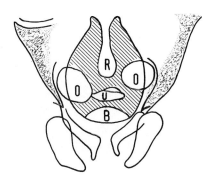

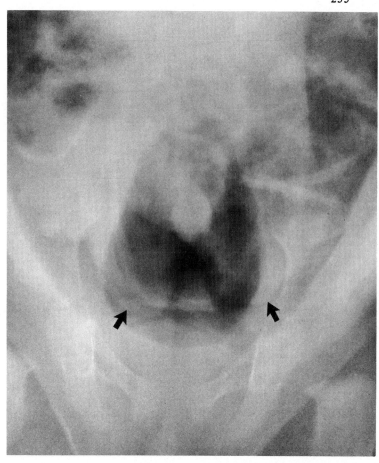

Figure 7.8. Gynaecography: After the injection of 200 ml of carbon dioxide into the peritoneal cavity of an infant with abnormal external genitalia, the presence of the uterus (U) and both ovaries (O) are revealed (arrowed). The rectum (R) and the bladder (B) are also shown but it is important that the bladder should be emptied prior to the investigation because it may obscure the uterus and ovaries

and the perineal opening is essential and, if more than one opening is present, multiple catheters may be required. A lateral view is the most useful in demonstrating the anatomy, but should always be supplemented by an anteroposterior view, because the contrast may pass into unexpected viscera; a single view may not allow all of these to be identified. An excretory urogram with a micturating film or contrast medium in the rectum may sometimes be required in puzzling cases, in order to demonstrate the relationship of a genital cavity to the bladder, urethra and rectum. The procedure is without risk, apart from the remote possibility of inducing a salt-losing syndrome in cases of adrenal cortical hyperplasia. The investigation may demonstrate the following structures:

(1) *The urethra and bladder.* These are usually easily opacified except when the catheter or nozzle is passed straight into the vagina and bypasses or obstructs the urethral meatus; this is likely to happen when the urethra and vagina open into a common urinogenital sinus which itself opens by a single orifice onto the surface of the perineum.

(2) *The vagina.* This can be difficult to demonstrate when it opens high up on the posterior urethra as it may do in highly virilized girls. In such cases the more the bladder is distended, increasing the resistance to injection, the better the chance of filling the vagina is likely to be. Even if the vagina is not completely filled, the point of junction with the urethra is usually easy to demonstrate.

(3) *The uterus.* Occasionally the presence of the uterus is demonstrated either by the filling of its cavity by contrast medium or by the presence of a filling defect in the vagina due to the cervix.

(4) *The ureters and renal pelvis.* Rarely, filling of an ectopic ureter and renal pelvis may occur when the opening of the ureter is into the urethra or vagina.

(5) *Fistulae.* Rectovesical or recto-urethral fistulae may be demonstrated by the passage of contrast medium into the rectum and in this way the blind end of the rectosigmoid colon may be opacified in cases of rectal atresia.

Gynaecography may supplement the information gained by genitography, in cases in whom it is desired to demonstrate the internal genitalia. Provided that carbon dioxide is used, the procedure is free from the risk of air embolism and causes little disturbance to the child. It can be carried out under sedation and local anaesthetic and is usually not technically difficult even in small infants. The amount injected varies from 20–30 ml in newborn infants, to 600–800 ml in adolescents. The films are taken with the child prone and tilted 40–70 degrees head down in order to ensure that the gas rises into the pelvis.

The uterus, broad ligaments and the two ovaries may usually be visualized and the degree to which they are developed can be assessed in cases of female pseudo-hermaphroditism or true hermaphroditism. In cases of Turner's syndrome the effect of hormonal treatment in stimulating uterine development may be followed. Malformation of the uterus and vagina may be well demonstrated by combining a pneumoperitoneum with hysterosalpingography. Finally, advantage may be taken of the fact that patency of the processus vaginalis in the first few months of life allows gas to pass into the scrotum and thus demonstrate the presence of testes in cases of male pseudohermaphroditism.

CINERADIOGRAPHY

Many workers have advocated the use of cineradiographic studies in the investigation of disorders of the lower urinary tract in children. It can be used in children with urinary tract infection to obtain records of the whole of micturition. It may also be used in studying the different types of mega-ureter (*see* page 279). Finally, it may be useful in confirming the presence of bladder neck hypertrophy, which may be demonstrated more clearly in the terminal phases of voiding. Detail is, however, inferior in cineradiographic films to that obtained by spot films, and these latter should always be obtained in order to secure an adequate demonstration of the anatomy. This implies that cineradiographic studies must be additional to the conventional methods of investigation. The average level of radiation dosage received during the cineradiographic studies has been estimated to be of the order of 2 roentgens and that the maximum dose never exceeds 50 roentgens (Benjamin *et al.*, 1955). However, this is not to deny that in the difficult or doubtful case in which conventional spot films had dailed to establish the diagnosis with certainty, or in which additional information relating to the dynamic and functional aspects of the urinary tract would be desirable, cineradiography may not be of value. It should however be used with discretion with a clear idea of the information which it is likely to afford and of how this can assist in the management of the case. An alternative to cineradiography is provided by videotape recording. In cases in whom fluoroscopy is undertaken, videotape affords a persistent record which can be studied repeatedly without increasing radiation dosage to the patient.

USE OF ISOTOPES AND ULTRASOUND

Isotopes

Radioactive isotopes can be applied to the investigation of the urinary tract in children in several different ways. These have been well summarized by Winter (1966). The two methods which have been most generally used are *isotope renography* and *renal scintiscanning*.

Isotope renography involves the intravenous injection of hippuran into which I^{119} or I^{127} has been incorporated. This substance is taken up by the kidney and excreted into the renal pelvis where it can be detected by collimated counters placed over the lumbar regions. The degrees of radioactivity from each kidney is recorded

separately in the form of a tracing covering the period of the test which normally lasts about 30 minutes. After an initial rise due to the presence of the isotope in the blood, the activity increases more slowly as the kidney removes it from the blood into the renal tubules and pelves. A peak value is reached after about 10 minutes, at which time the increase in activity due to renal excretion is balanced by the removal of the isotope by the drainage of urine from the renal pelvis down the ureter. The latter reduces the level of activity progressively so that it falls to less than half the peak value within 10 or 20 minutes. This characteristic curve (renogram) may be used to assess renal function (*Figure 7.9*). This is measured by the rapidity with which the radioactivity

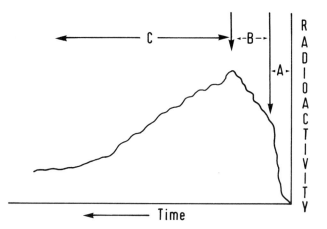

Figure 7.9. Isotope Renography: The curve represents the changes in the intensity of radiation over the area of the kidneys with time. Immediately after the injection (at the right of the diagram) activity rises rapidly due to the presence of isotope in the blood vessels (A). Following this there is a slower rate of increase in activity due to concentration and excretion of the isotope by the kidney (B). After the peak level has been reached there is a relatively slow fall in activity as the isotope is drained into the bladder (C). If obstruction to flow of urine from the pelvis or vesico-ureteric reflux is present, the fall in activity may occur only very slowly

reaches its peak and the height of the curve at this point. It may also afford an indication of the effectiveness of the drainage of urine from the renal pelvis which may be impaired both by obstructive disease and by vesico-ureteric reflux.

Radioactive isotopes may also be used to produce a renal scan when the variation in intensity of radioactivity is recorded in space rather than time. This permits a visual picture of the renal size and shape, i.e. a scintiscan. It should detect a non-functioning intrarenal mass of more than 3 cm in diameter. The nature of such lesions will not, however, be determined by this method. These methods do not replace excretory urography, to which they should be regarded as complementary. It is considered that they afford a more sensitive index of renal function particularly in unilateral renal disease, in which the pathological kidney can be directly compared with the normal one. They are much less accurate in delineating anatomical structure than conventional radiography, but they have the advantage that the radiation dosage involved is negligible in amount compared to that received during excretory urography or cysto-urethrography. This is a consideration which must carry considerable weight in the paediatric age range, especially when repeated examinations are required.

Ultrasonic scanning

High frequency sound waves can also be employed to scan the area of the kidney (Wells, 1972). They may be useful not only in detecting the presence of intrarenal masses, but also in determining whether they are solid or cystic. The latter, by virtue of their fluid content will not reflect the sound waves and will appear as a transsonic 'space' within the normal renal tissues. This method is as yet comparatively new and its reliability and potential have still to be fully assessed. It has the advantage of being non-invasive and does not involve the use of ionizing radiations (Mountford *et al.*, 1971).

INFLAMMATORY DISEASES

PYELONEPHRITIS AND VESICO-URETERIC REFLUX

Indications for radiological investigation

There is an increasing awareness of the fact that urinary tract infection in children may, if persistent or recurrent, lead to progressive renal damage and ultimately to death from renal failure, especially when the condition is associated with vesico-ureteric reflux. This has resulted in a great increase in the use of radiology for investigation and assessment of such cases. However, there is a wide variation in the indications for the use of the different investigations that radiology can offer. To subject all children with a urinary tract infection to a full radiological investigation will impose a considerable burden upon radiodiagnostic departments and a not inconsiderable radiation dosage to the patients. Nevertheless, a good case has been made for such a policy. Hodson (1967) and Smellie *et al.* (1964) advise that both excretory urography and micturating cysto-urethrography should be performed on all children once the existence of a urinary infection has been proven and controlled by suitable treatment. They do not consider that it is desirable to wait for a further attack to occur, because there is always doubt as to whether a given infection is in fact the first attack, and also because focal scarring may begin at any age between 2 and 10 years. It is then progressive. Moreover, if this process is bilateral it is likely to lead to a fatal outcome in the majority of cases, often during the second decade.This view is, however, not universally accepted. The present authors believe that it is reasonable to await the result of treatment. If this is effective, radiological investigation may be postponed until it is decided that infection is persisting in spite of adequate therapy. Nevertheless, each case should be considered individually; certain classes of patient known to be particularly liable to develop renal damage should be investigated without delay. Among these are boys under the age of 2 years with obstructive lesions in the lower urinary tract and children

with neurogenic disorders. Early recurrence of infection in girls after control of the initial attack is also considered to be a factor conducive to the onset of progressive renal damage and warrants early radiological investigation.

At whatever stage it is decided that radiological investigation is called for, both excretory urography and micturating cysto-urethography should be undertaken, because the two methods are complementary to one another and each may contribute information of value in the assessment of the case.

Acute pyelonephritis

The radiological changes in the urogram in the acute stages of urinary tract infection are variable and usually of little importance. In a series of many infants examined by excretory urography at this stage, 38 per cent were found to have normal appearances (Reilly, 1967). In some instances there was a prolonged nephrogram, a feature which has also been described in renal tubular obstruction due to some forms of proteinuria (Berdon *et al.*, 1969). Of children with acute urinary infection 77 per cent were shown to have dilated, atonic renal pelves and ureters with ineffective or reversed peristalsis, and vesico-ureteric reflux occurred in half the cases. These changes disappeared after treatment and were not present in a control series of uninfected patients (Shopfner, 1966).

Chronic pyelonephritis

The radiological features resulting from chronic pyelonephritis are of much greater importance and they have been well described by Hodson (1967) (*Figure 7.10a*). These are abnormalities in the size and shape of the renal outlines: the outer margin of the kidney is locally indented in one or more places and there is a reduction in the thickness of the renal parenchyma relative to the size of the renal pelvis at the sites of indentation. There is also some reduction in the size of the kidney as a whole, which has been ascribed to a failure of growth; this is characteristically asymmetrical on the two sides, affecting one kidney more than the other. It has been suggested that there is little correlation between the reduction in the size of the kidney and its function, as measured by the glomular filtration rate. The indentation of the renal outline is always found at the same level as a calyx and the latter is deformed due to shrinkage of the renal papilla. In consequence of this, the calyx loses its normal lateral concavity and becomes convex or 'clubbed'. The outline of the affected calyx is always smooth and regular, never ragged or ill defined. One or more calyces may be affected; unaffected calyces retain their normal appearance. These changes may occur anywhere in the kidney but are most common at the poles, the right upper pole being most frequently affected. The density of the pyelogram is normal both in the diseased and in the unaffected kidney. These radiological signs are focal in distribution and this is one of the characteristic features of chronic pyelonephritis. It results from the localized damage to the kidney with

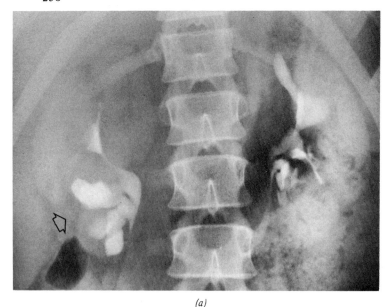

(a)

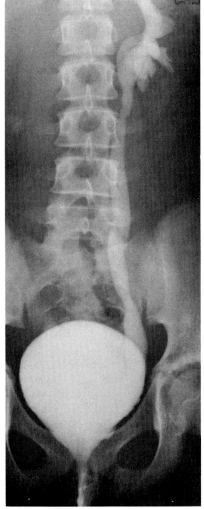

(b)

Figure 7.10. Chronic Pyelonephritis and Vesico-ureteric Reflux:
(a) Urogram showing clubbing and distortion of the minor
calyces with reduction of renal tissue particularly at the upper
pole on the left side and at the lower pole on the right. The
renal outline in addition is indented as a result of local fibrosis
and scarring (arrowed) (b) the same case; on micturating cysto-
urethrography severe vesico-ureteric reflux (Grade III) has
occurred on the left side

consequent scarring produced by the underlying pathological process. However, in some cases the radiological
features are less characteristic. This may be the case
when there is an associated obstructive lesion which
leads to the superimposition of obstructive atrophy of
the kidney on the signs of chronic pyelonephritis. The
former is essentially a diffuse process, and one which
causes enlargement rather than reduction in size of the
kidney. It may also be necessary to differentiate between
the classical type of chronic pyelonephritic kidney as
described above, and a small evenly contracted kidney
resembling renal hypoplasia and associated with dwarfism
and renal failure. Excretory urography may reveal, in
addition to the signs of chronic pyelonephritis, the
presence of associated congenital abnormalities and there
is no doubt that the incidence of these is considerably
higher than in cases without urinary infection.

Vesico-ureteric reflux

Vesico-ureteric reflux is very common in chronic pyelonephritis, being found in 85 per cent of cases (*Figure
7.10b*) (Weber and Weylman, 1966). Because it is now
generally accepted that vesico-ureteric reflux, if present

in combination with active urinary tract infection, is
the main factor responsible for the development of the
progressive renal damage described above, it is clear
that the demonstration of its presence is a matter of
considerable importance. It is essential that it should
be detected before there has been time for irreversible
changes to occur in the kidney.

INCIDENCE

Estimation of the overall incidence of vesico-ureteric
reflux is difficult, because the figures obviously vary
according to the selection of cases subjected to micturating cysto-urethrography. The incidence reported
in large series of investigations carried out for all types
of urinary condition ranged from 14 to 31 per cent. It
cannot be proven conclusively that reflux never occurs
as a normal phenomenon. This is particularly so in the
small infant where the uretero-vesical junction may be
immature. However, the bulk of the available evidence
is against this possibility of reflux being a normal occurrence (Rooney, 1961; Iannaccone, 1966).

SEVERITY

Vesico-ureteric reflux is classified in terms of increasing severity (*see* Table).

TABLE

Grade of reflux

I	Part or whole of one ureter filled.
II	Ureter and renal pelvis filled.
III	Ureter and renal pelvis filled and dilated.

Hodson (1967) considers Grade I as probably not significant, but regards Grade II as sufficient to convey infection to the renal pelvis and to cause the infection to persist. There is general agreement that Grade III reflux is of serious import and in the presence of persistent infection will inevitably lead to the development of chronic pyelonephritis and progressive renal damage.

INTRARENAL REFLUX

It has also been observed that during micturating cysto-urethrography the contrast medium may opacify not only the ureters and renal pelves but part of the renal parenchyma as well. This is shown either as linear striations radiating from a calyx or as a more uniform opacification of a segment of renal substance. It resembles pyelotubular backflow resulting from the use of excessive pressure during retrograde pyelography. When occurring during micturating cysto-urethrography it has been termed 'intrarenal reflux' and has been shown by Rolleston *et al.* (1974) to be most common under the age of 1 year. It is only seen in the presence of moderate or severe reflux and is often followed by focal scarring in the affected part of the kidney. It may therefore be a sign of serious prognostic significance.

AETIOLOGY

It is still a matter of speculation, whether vesico-ureteric reflux arises as a consequence of urinary infection, or whether the reflux is the primary factor which favours persistence or recurrence of the infection. In favour of the former contention some authorities consider that urinary infection may impair the competence of the uretero-vesical junction, at any rate temporarily, due to the local oedema which may accompany the cystitis. It is likely that there is a considerably higher incidence of reflux in cases with infection than in those in whom the urine is sterile. However, Forsythe and Wallace (1958) report that reflux occurs in 50 per cent of cases in whom there is no infection at the time of investigation. Many of these may have had a urinary infection which has since cleared up, but it is likely that some may never have been infected. The concept that the vesico-ureteric reflux may be the primary factor has been increasingly favoured in recent years. Those who hold this view suggest that a congenital defect in the uretero-vesical junction, either lateral ectopia or a small para-ureteric diverticulum may be an important aetiological factor.

Obstruction at the bladder neck or in the urethra are other factors which many believe may predispose to reflux, especially in young boys. The incidence of reflux in several large series of cases of bladder neck obstruction is of the order of 67 per cent. Similarly, in cases of neurogenic bladder, reflux is a frequent finding, especially in the infant with meningomyelocele. The incidence of reflux in cases of meningomyelocele has been estimated as 26 per cent. It is much more likely to occur in those cases with a large, atonic bladder than in those with a hypertrophied, sacculated bladder wall (Williams and Verrier Jones, 1968).

Demonstration of reflux

It is generally accepted that micturating cysto-urethrography is the only method by which the presence of vesico-ureteric reflux can be unequivocally demonstrated. While irradiation, particularly of the gonads, is the chief disadvantage of micturating cysto-urethrography, there is also another disadvantage in the possible introduction of infection during the performance of catheterization. In view of the large number of children who require investigation attempts have been made to devise alternative methods which are either less time-consuming or involve less exposure to radiation. These attempts have centred in the first place on a search for an alternative method of demonstrating reflux. This may be carried out by detecting activity over the kidney after a radioactive isotope is injected into the bladder. Isotope cystography has not however proved reliable and has not so far gained general acceptance.

The appearances on excretory urography, while not diagnostic of the presence of reflux, may be sufficiently suggestive to serve as a screening test. Signs suggestive of vesico-ureteric reflux on excretory urography are:

(1) Dilatation of the lower third of the ureter persistent in several films and especially on a postmicturition film.
(2) The presence of a small para-ureteric vesical diverticulum.
(3) The presence of excess residual urine for which no other cause is apparent.
(4) Unexplained hydronephrosis and hydro-ureter.
(5) Poor initial density of the pyelogram which improves in the later films.
(6) Where a duplex renal pelvis or ureter is present, vesico-ureteric reflux is also common and usually occurs in the ureter supplying the lower moiety.
(7) Striations within the renal pelvis or upper ureter (*Figure 7.11*).

However, there is no doubt that reflux may occur in patients who have a normal excretory urogram. According to Rooney (1961) this was the case in 75 per cent of all cases of reflux, but other series report normal findings in only about 10 per cent of those cases where the reflux was severe enough to warrant surgical treatment. It has been suggested therefore that if excretory urography is normal in children over the age of 4 years, it is justifiable to treat the infection with antibiotics and delay micturating cysto-urethrography until either the infection

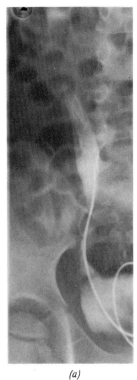 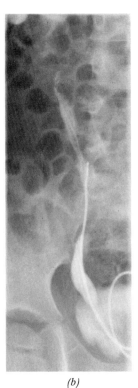

(a)   *(b)*

Figure 7.11. Retrograde Ureterogram: two films (a) and (b) showing longitudinal folds in the mucosa of the dilated ureter. These are frequently associated (as in this case) with urinary tract infection and with vesico-ureteric reflux

recurs or the urogram becomes abnormal (Haran *et al.,* 1967).

The frequency with which micturating cysto-urethrography should be repeated in cases in whom vesico-ureteric reflux has been treated either by medical or surgical methods is also a matter of controversy. Each case must obviously be judged individually. It is however important to weigh up the cumulative effect of irradiation dosage to the gonads against the need to be sure that treatment has been effective and the need to assess the progress of any renal damage that may have occurred. An average time of about 12 months between successive radiological investigations would be a reasonable interval.

Differential diagnosis

It may be difficult to distinguish the radiological picture of chronic pyelonephritis from a large number of other conditions which may resemble it. Some of these are as follows.

FETAL LOBULATION

The lobulated or indented normal variant of the renal outline sometimes seen in young children may be confused with the indentation due to focal scarring. However, fetal lobulation is much more regular in its pattern, never involves one pole to the exclusion of the rest of the kidney and the indentations are situated in between and not opposite the calyces.

URINARY TUBERCULOSIS

Several inflammatory conditions, particularly those which are chronic in type, tend to produce focal damage to the kidney and therefore a radiological picture which may resemble chronic pyelonephritis closely. Of these conditions, the most important is renal tuberculosis. Although much less common now than it used to be 20 years ago, it still occurs with sufficient frequency to be a possible alternative diagnosis. The calyces may be more severely dilated and distorted in tuberculosis with a ragged outline, due to the necrosis of the papillae, which are destroyed and not merely atrophied as in chronic pyelonephritis. Furthermore, tuberculosis may produce widespread effects on the urinary tract as a whole. with abnormalities not only in the renal pelves but also caseous lesions of the renal parenchyma which may calcify. Fibrosis of the ureters and bladder may occur and produce radiological deformity. Nevertheless, in many cases, radiology will only suggest the probability of the tubercle bacillus as the cause, and it is necessary to await its identification by the bacteriologist to prove the diagnosis.

RENAL CARBUNCLE

Haematogenous infection by pyogenic organisms will produce cortical abscesses which can displace or distort the calyces, but which do not lead to permanent scarring, except in the most severe cases.

PAPILLARY NECROSIS

In patients with diabetes or following over-dosage with phenacetin, the papillae may become necrotic and be sloughed off. The resulting deformity of the calyces resembles that of tuberculosis more than the smooth 'clubbing' of chronic pyelonephritis.

FIBROSIS OF THE KIDNEY

Infarcts or radiation damage may produce a shrinkage of the kidney with evidence of focal scarring, but these conditions are very rarely seen in children. The papillae are not destroyed and the normal cupped shape of the calyces will be preserved.

OBSTRUCTIVE UROPATHY

This produces back pressure atrophy of the kidneys, resulting in thinning of the renal parenchyma and dilatation of the calyces. It is, however, a diffuse process and, except when the neck of one calyx is obstructed—for instance, by a calculus impacted in it—it should not be difficult to differentiate from chronic pyelonephritis. However, as stated above, it is by no means uncommon for chronic pyelonephritis to occur in association with obstructive atrophy and in that case the radiological picture may have the features of both conditions.

Other conditions in which the kidney is reduced in size may be difficult to differentiate from chronic pyelonephritis. Differentiation may not in fact be possible and in any case not infrequently renal hypoplasia is associated with infection and subsequent pyelonephritic changes. However, where there is a small but anatomically normal pelvis with no disproportion between its size and that of the kidney as a whole, the diagnosis may be less difficult.

GLOMERULONEPHRITIS AND RENAL FAILURE

Glomerulonephritis

Glomerulonephritis and the nephrotic syndrome are conditions in which there are diffuse lesions of the renal parenchyma without involvement of the collecting system. Radiology therefore contributes little to the diagnosis or management of these conditions, Nevertheless, an estimation of the size of the kidney may give an indication of the stage which the condition has reached, and help in determining prognosis (Olsson, 1954). If the power of the kidneys to concentrate is diminished, the density of the nephrogram and the pyelogram is as a consequence reduced. Nevertheless, the use of high dosage techniques (*see* page 247) may allow an adequate assessment of the overall renal size and also a comparison between the relative sizes of the renal parenchyma and the renal pelvis. A demonstration of the size, shape and position of the kidneys may also be of assistance in the performance of needle biopsy of the kidney, a procedure which is useful in the diagnosis of this group of renal diseases. The technique of assessment of renal size and the range of normal variation have been discussed elsewhere (*see* pages 362, 363).

Renal failure

The assessment of renal function by urography is subject to considerable errors and this has been noted elsewhere (*see* page 249). There may be only poor correlation between renal size and other tests for renal function (Berg *et al.,* 1970). In spite of this, urography may be justified in the assessment of cases in which renal failure is present because of the additional anatomical information which it can provide. The increasing use of high dosage urography has made this aspect more effective, but it has decreased the usefulness of urography as a means of assessing renal function. There are, however, many better methods available for the latter purpose, and even within the field of radiodiagnosis, isotope renography or scintiscanning have a greater value in this respect.

Pulmonary changes in renal disease

The incidence of abnormalities in the lungs in glomerulonephritis is high, especially in the acute stage. Various authors have quoted figures of between 50 and 60 per cent (Kattamis and Nicolaides, 1967). These abnormalities are:

Changes in the pulmonary vasculature

These are either an increase in the calibre of the pulmonary arteries and veins, especially those in the hilar regions, an increase in the number of visible arteries, especially in the periphery of the lung fields, or a loss of definition in the outline of the intrapulmonary vasculature.

The presence of fluid in the pleural cavities

This may either take the form of interlobar effusions or free intrapleural fluid. The effusions may be quite small and only demonstrable in films taken using a horizontal beam with the patient lying on his side (lateral decubitus).

Pulmonary oedema

This occurs in about 30 per cent of all cases with positive findings in the chest. It can take the form of a diffuse haziness of the whole lung or of confluent densities resembling areas of inflammatory consolidation. However, they clear more rapidly than in the latter condition. Symmetrically placed shadows in both perihilar zones, known as 'batswing shadows', are less common than is often suggested (*Figure 7.12*).

Areas of segmental consolidation or collapse

These may persist after the vascular changes have disappeared.

Oedema of the chest wall

This may be detected as a loss of the clear definition of the fat planes in the lateral chest wall.

Cardiomegaly

This may persist for as long as several months and is related to the development of systemic hypertension. It is therefore not seen in the nephrotic syndrome, except when a pericardial effusion is present.

The lung changes are frequently symmetrical and bilateral; they may occur however on one side only and in such cases are found commonly on the right side. They are related most closely to the presence of generalized oedema, and not to the level of the blood urea or the blood pressure.

Skeletal lesions

Chronic renal disease leading to diminution in renal function may produce effects upon the skeleton, which are conveniently referred to under the generic term of renal osteodystrophy. These are described in greater detail elsewhere (*see* page 83 and *Figure 3.27*) and are summarized briefly as follows.

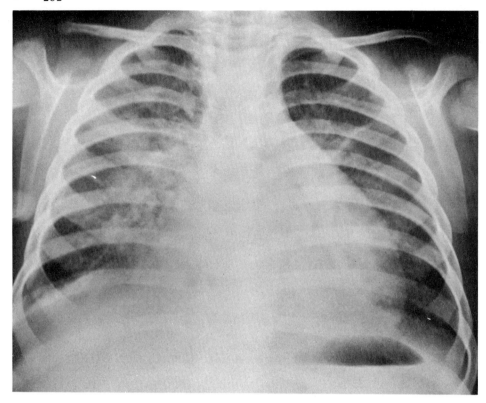

Figure 7.12. Pulmonary Oedema in Acute Nephritis: Bilateral ill-defined peri-hilar opacities indicative of alveolar pulmonary oed-ema with associated cardiac enlargement in a boy with acute glomerulonephritis

Rickets or osteomalacia

The exact cause of this feature is debatable. It may be related to the acidosis which occurs with failing kidneys, though there is an increasing awareness that an acquired resistance to the action of vitamin D may be involved.

Osteitis fibrosa

This is due to secondary hyperparathyroidism. The parathyroid glands are stimulated to over-activity by the low serum calcium and high serum phosphate levels.

Osteosclerosis

This occurs especially in the lumbar vertebral bodies ('rugger jersey' spine), but also in the metaphyses of the long bones. The cause of this feature is also obscure, but recent opinion has favoured excess calcium or vitamin D given in treatment or some osteoblast-stimulating hormone, such as calcitonin, as possible aetiological factors.

CONGENITAL ABNORMALITIES

INTRODUCTION

In children, congenital abnormalities are a relatively common finding arising from radiological investigation of the urinary tract. However, many of the individual lesions are rare, and have less practical importance than

might be assumed from their often striking appearances.

Congenital stenosis occurring at various levels of the collecting systems are discussed in the section on obstructive uropathy. However, many lesions which are not directly obstructive in nature impair the efficacy of drainage through the collecting ducts and in this way may predispose to urinary infection. The adverse consequences of such infection afford a reason why the detection and recognition of congenital abnormalities is of importance (*see* page 257). Finally, the function of the kidney as an organ of excretion depends to a large extent upon its normal development. Although congenital maldevelopment may take second place to acquired disease as a cause of renal failure even among children, the presence of maldevelopment of the kidney may reduce its reserve capacity. This may render it less able to compensate for the presence of acquired disease, or make the treatment of such disease by nephrectomy hazardous or impracticable.

Congenital anomalies of other systems

Congenital abnormalities of the urinary tract may also be commonly associated with congenital malformations elsewhere in the body. In this way they may form part of more extensive syndromes, and their presence may then have a significant influence upon the prognosis.

In particular, an association between congenital heart disease and abnormalities of the genito-urinary tract is not infrequent and, for this reason, it has been suggested that the contrast medium injected for the purpose of angiocardiography should be utilized to obtain a demonstration of the urinary tract which may exclude or reveal such associated abnormalities (*see Figure 4.1* and page 100).

Single umbilical artery

It has also been noted that abnormalities of the genito-urinary tract may be commonly associated with a single umbilical artery. For this reason excretory urography and, where appropriate, micturating cysto-urethrography should be carried out on all cases with this anomaly in order to permit early surgical correction of those lesions which are amenable to treatment. Thirty-four per cent of cases were found to have abnormalities of the genito-urinary tract and these are sometimes severe. Obstructive lesions of the lower urinary tract with hydronephrosis and vesico-ureteric reflux are the commonest (Feingold, Fine and Ingall, 1964).

RENAL APLASIA

The congenital absence of one kidney is not very un-common, the incidence being 1 in 500 individuals (Ashley and Mostofi, 1960). It is more frequent in males than in females. It is chiefly of importance where the contralateral kidney becomes diseased or injured and the possibility of nephrectomy has to be considered. In such cases one of the most important functions of excretory urography is to demonstrate the existence of a normally functioning kidney on the opposite side.

RENAL HYPOPLASIA

It is considered that the cause of small kidneys in a number of patients is congenital hypoplasia. It may be difficult however to distinguish such kidneys from small kidneys which result from acquired disease, especially chronic pyelonephritis. One feature, however, which may be of particular help in making this distinction is that the proportion between the size of the renal pelvis and calyces, and that of the renal parenchyma is preserved and in true hypoplasia the renal cortical index is normal (*see* page 363). The small renal pelvis is normal in shape, but the calyces may be reduced in number and they may be distributed either regularly or in an irregular manner towards one or both poles (*Figure 7.13*). The latter type is commoner in males and the former 'pseudominiature' type in females. Dysplastic kidneys can also be small and under-developed but their function is always severely impaired and their structure grossly abnormal. In unilateral renal hypoplasia, the contralateral kidney is usually hypertrophied; if it is not, the probability is that the hypoplasia is bilateral but unequal in degree on the two sides. Associated congenital abnormalities are uncommon in simple hypoplasia. If present, they would suggest the possibility of renal dysplasia.

FUSED KIDNEYS

Fusions of the two kidneys may occur in several forms. The commonest type is the horseshoe kidney, where the

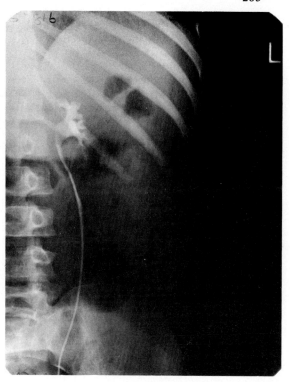

Figure 7.13. Renal Hypoplasia: A small renal pelvis in which the calyces are neither deformed nor distorted and where the kidney is reduced in size to a degree proportionate to the size of the renal pelvis

fusion occurs between the two lower poles, so that a bridge of renal tissue crosses the spine. On plain films, the renal outlines are lower in position, nearer the mid-line, and their long axes are more vertical than in the normal child. On excretory urography the lowermost calyces point medially and the ureters arise from the inferolateral aspect of the two renal pelves, giving the characteristic flower-vase appearance (*Figure 7.14*). Fusion of the two upper poles or the presence of a single renal mass consisting of renal tissue from both kidneys are very much less common. Crossed ectopia results in fusion of the lower pole of the normally placed kidney with the upper pole of the ectopic kidney, giving rise to the characteristically S-shaped renal pelves ('sigmoid kidney') (*Figure 7.15*).

The importance of all these types of fused kidney lies in their increased liability to complications, mainly hydronephrosis, infection, calculi and trauma. The frequency with which these conditions may be found as incidental findings in adult life suggests that such sequelae may not be as common as is sometimes supposed. They are readily diagnosed because of their distinctive appearances on excretory urography. In the cases in which calculi are present, the position of the radiographic opacity may be unusual. In the rare instances of Wilm's tumour arising in a horseshoe kidney, the urographic appearances may be so bizarre as to require arteriography to elucidate them. When a nephrogram is obtained this will often reveal the isthmus of functioning renal tissue joining the two kidneys.

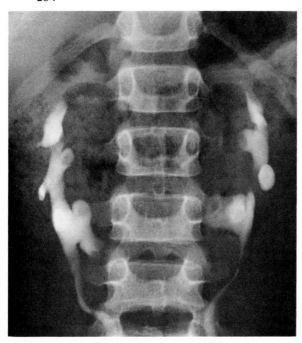

Figure 7.14. Horseshoe Kidney: The two kidneys are fused at the lower poles with the result that the lower minor calyces are rotated on their long axes; the ureters arise from the infero-lateral aspect of the pelves and deviate towards each other as they cross the isthmus of renal tissue which joins the two lower poles

DUPLEX PELVIS

This is the commonest congenital anomaly of the kidney and may, or may not, be associated with a partial or complete duplex ureter. It is found in 3–4 per cent of all urograms. In most cases it does not produce morbidity. However, it is an important lesion to detect, especially because of serious complications that may develop when infection of the urinary tract is also present, and because of the other anomalies that may be associated with it, The incidence of associated anomalies is estimated to be as high as 42 per cent. The commonest of these are ectopic ureteric orifices, ureterocele, congenital stenoses, malrotated and fused kidney, renal hypoplasia and ectopia vesicae.

The size and shape of the kidney with a duplex pelvis differs from those of a kidney which is drained by a single pelvis. The length of the abnormal kidney will be increased from 1 to 3 cm (*Figure 7.16*). If the two kidneys are of equal length in a patient who has a unilateral duplex pelvis, this kidney is probably pathologically small. The thickness of the renal parenchyma may vary along the length of the kidney. It may be reduced over both poles and increased in the part intermediate between the two pelves. In this situation an appearance of 'pseudotumour' may be produced with consequent difficulty in excluding a true tumour. The size and shape of each moiety of the renal pelvis may also vary from case to case according to the proportion of the affected kidney drained by each pelvis. Where one moiety drains a portion of the kidney which is functioning poorly and is therefore not opacified on excretory urography, it is important to recognize the presence of

the duplex pelvis from the shape and position of the other moiety. This situation is particularly likely to arise if one ureter opens ectopically (*see* below), or is associated with a ureterocele. The following features may be helpful when the lower moiety alone is opacified (Innes Williams, 1954).

(1) The number of calyces will be fewer than normal.
(2) The uppermost calyx may be shortened and may point outwards or downwards instead of upwards. This may give the whole renal pelvis a characteristic 'drooping flower' shape.
(3) The renal pelvis and ureter will be asymmetrically placed in relation to the renal outline as a whole, an appearance which may however be difficult to assess when the nephrogram is of poor density. However, if the renal outline is well seen, this can be a most helpful sign.
(4) The pelvis may be rotated on its horizontal axis so that its upper part is displaced away from the spine (*Figure 7.17*).

Poorly functioning moieties of a duplex pelvis are often hydronephrotic, but it has been pointed out that in only a small proportion of these can an organic obstruction be found. The development of hydronephrosis may be related to the undoubtedly high incidence of vesico-ureteric reflux, estimated by various authors to be between 25 and 45 per cent of complete duplex ureters. Reflux is three times more common in the ureter draining the lower moiety. This is ascribed to the fact that it always has a shorter intramural course which renders its valve-like action less efficient (Hartman and Hodson, 1969). In partially duplex ureters, the phenomenon of uretero-ureteral reflux may occur. This is produced when a normal peristaltic wave travels down one ureter and, at the point of junction, moves in a reverse direction up the other ureter, instead of continuing down the common ureter. The high incidence of vesico-ureteric reflux combined with an increased liability to urinary tract infection carries a risk of progressive renal damage from chronic pyelonephritis. It is therefore advised that micturating cysto-urethrography should always be carried out where duplex pelves are associated with infection (Hartman and Hodson, 1969).

ECTOPIC URETERS

Of the various congenital anomalies commonly associated with duplex pelvis, ectopic ureteric orifices may often be suspected from the radiographic signs described in the previous paragraphs. This is particularly so in a patient who suffers from continuous dribbling incontinence and in whom only one moiety of a duplex pelvis is opacified. It is especially important that this condition should be recognized, because it is easily cured by appropriate surgical treatment. It must, however be recognized that it is not often possible to identify directly the site at which the ectopic ureter opens and the indirect signs may be the only radiological evidence of this condition. The contralateral renal pelvis may be duplex or single. If the latter is the case the existence of the ipsilateral duplex pelvis may be overlooked unless

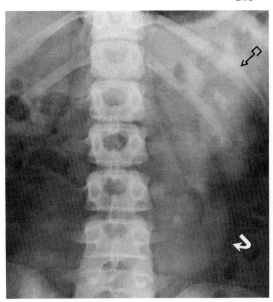

(a)

Figure 7.15. Crossed Ectopia of the Kidney: (a) Nephrographic phase of an excretory urogram showing the two kidneys lying one above the other on the left side of the spine (arrowed). (b) Later stage of the urogram; both renal pelves are dilated but the calyces of the lower (ectopic) kidney face medially and its ureter (arrowed) crosses the midline at the level of the fifth lumbar vertebra and continues its descent on the right side of the pelvis. (c) Diagram of anatomy of renal pelves and ureters

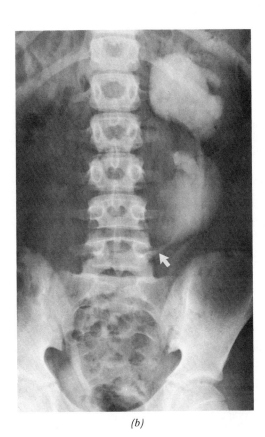

(b)

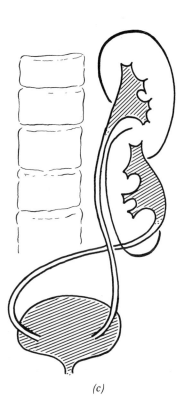

(c)

extreme care is taken to recognize the characteristic appearances (*Figure 7.18*).

Although the commonest site for an ectopic ureteric orifice is in the urethra, it may be situated in any structure arising from the cloaca, urogenital sinus, Wolffian or Müllerian ducts, including the vestibule, vagina, seminal vesicles or vas deferens. The uterus and rectum are rare sites. An infant in whom an ectopic ureter drains into the vagina may present with a hydrometrocolpos and may in rare instances develop vaginal calculi (*see Figure 7.26* on page 275). Delayed and postmicturition films taken after excretory urography may be helpful in making the diagnosis. Sufficient contrast may then have been excreted to opacify the dilated hydronephrotic pelvis. Alternatively reflux may occur into it from the bladder following micturition, in cases in which the ureter opens into the urethra above the external sphincter.

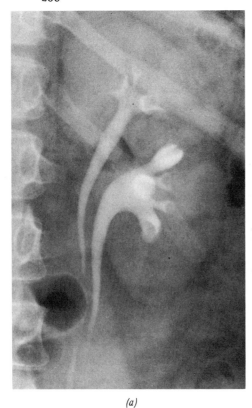

(a)

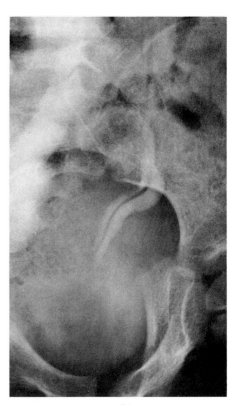

(b)

Figure 7.16. Duplex Pelvis and Ureter: (a) The two halves of the renal pelvis are of unequal size and there is also an indentation in the lateral border of the kidney. (b) The ureters may be separate through their whole length as in this example or may join at any point above their orifice into the bladder

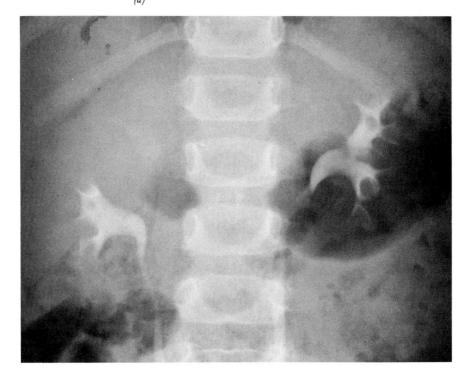

Figure 7.17. Duplex Pelvis with Ectopic Ureter: In such cases the upper moiety of the duplex pelvis is often not opacified due to lack of function of the portion of kidney drained by it. The existence of such a non-functioning upper moiety can be inferred from the eccentricity of the opacified moiety in relation to the renal outline and from its size and shape as compared with the single pelvis on the opposite side

URETEROCELE

Ureterocele is commonly associated with a duplex pelvis, and it almost always involves the ureter which drains the upper moiety. Ureteroceles vary considerably in size from patient to patient and even in the same patient at different times. Their radiological appearance also varies with the function of the kidney or part of the kidney drained by the abnormal ureter. If function is inadequate, sufficient contrast medium may not be excreted into the ureterocele to opacify it. The uretero-cele will then appear as a filling defect with a smooth,

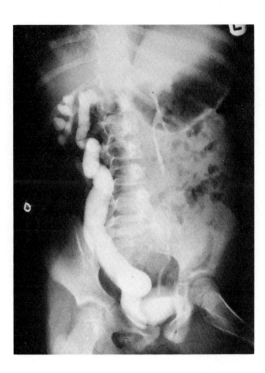

Figure 7.18. Ectopic Ureter: Opacification of an ectopic ureter draining the upper moiety of a right duplex pelvis as a result of passing a urethral catheter into it instead of into the bladder in the course of an attempted micturating cysto-urethrogram. The right lower moiety, the left renal pelvis and the bladder are opacified as a result of excretory urography

round, elliptical or heart-shaped outline within the contrast medium filled bladder at the expected site of entry of the ureter (*Figure 7.19*). On the other hand when contrast medium opacifies the ureter and the ureterocele, the wall of the ureterocele will appear as a thin linear defect separating it from the contrast medium in the bladder surrounding it. This produces the characteristic 'cobra head' effect (*Figure 7.19b*). The distinction between ureteroceles associated with normal or ectopic ureters is not as a rule easily made on the radiological appearances. The latter tend to be larger and to have a broader base. They are the common type found in infancy and are more likely to give rise to serious sequelae than the ureteroceles arising at normally sited ureteric orifices (Friedland and Cunningham, 1972). The ureter and renal pelvis associated with a ureterocele are hydronephrotic in 85 per cent of cases. The other ureter and renal pelvis may also show evidence of obstruction because the ureterocele if large enough may compress or displace the orifice of an adjacent ureter. In girls it may even produce obstruction by prolapsing into the urethra.

Vesico-ureteric reflux may also be demonstrable on micturating cysto-urethrography, especially if the ureterocele has ruptured or has been treated surgically Occasionally calculi may develop within ureteroceles. The diagnosis is not usually difficult if the possibility is considered. Care has to be taken to avoid confusion with rectal gas shadows, calculi impacted in an oedematous ureteric orifice, or the rare tumours of the bladder such as neurofibroma or rhabdomyosarcoma, the latter occasionally having a smooth outline. Ectopic ureteroceles when collapsed can easily be missed.

CONGENITAL ABNORMALITIES OF THE BLADDER AND URETHRA

These are considered in more detail elsewhere. A few of these lesions which do not cause obstruction are of radiological interest and are considered here.

CONGENITAL FISTULAE

Fistulae between the rectum, bladder, urethra or vagina are commonly associated with imperforate anus or rectal agenesis (*see Figure 6.22*). They may require treatment together with the more obvious presenting condition. Excretory urography or retrograde cystography may not only delineate such fistulae, but may also reveal other, more extensive, abnormalities of the genito-urinary tract which may have considerable bearing on the ultimate outcome.

INTERSEX

Vesical or urethral abnormalities may also be of importance in the different varieties of intersex. Such conditions pose a difficult diagnostic problem whose solution may be a matter of considerable importance for the future management of the child. The methods which may be employed in such cases have been described elsewhere (*see page 254*). They aim at the demonstration of the abnormal genital and urinary passages by the injection of contrast medium into them or by inducing a pneumoperitoneum in an attempt to delineate the internal genitalia.

The degree of virilization in female pseudohermaphroditism has been related to the ratio between the length of the horizontal and the vertical part of the urethra. This can vary from a value of 0 in the normal female to 1.6 in the male with hypospadias, but it showed an average of 0.89 in one series of female pseudohermaphrodites (Fauré *et al.*, 1969). These cases are often due to the adrenogenital syndrome. They may show a uterus and vagina which join the posterior urethra above its external orifice and may be associated with other anomalies such as fused or ectopic kidneys, imperforate anus or fistulae. If a vagina arises from the urethra in cases of male pseudohermaphroditism, it may be possible to distinguish these cases from the female pseudohermaphrodite by the fact that there is no defect within the vagina due to the cervix, because the uterus is usually absent.

The use of micturating cysto-urethrography has been recommended in cases of male pseudohermaphroditism. If the urethral orifice is occluded during the course of micturition, contrast medium may be forced into the vagina and uterus if these are present and communicate with the urethra (Marcinski and Grzybowska, 1970). Similar results on micturating cysto-urethrography may be obtained in highly virilized female pseudohermaphrodites but retrograde injection up the urethra may force contrast medium into the bladder and not into the vagina opening into the urethra.

The true hermaphrodite, who has gonads of both types, is very rare. There may be considerable variation in the pattern of the external genitalia, and there is also

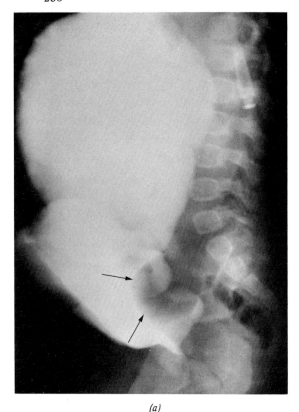
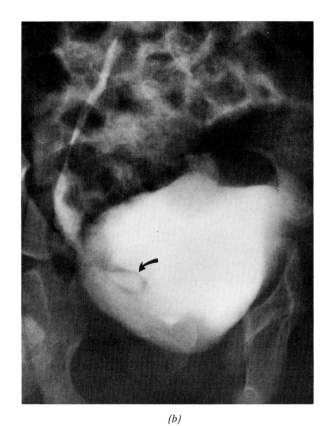

(a)   (b)

Figure 7.19. Ureterocele: (a) A rounded filling defect is shown projecting into the posterior aspect of the bladder due to the dilated lower end of the ureter. In this case the ureterocele (arrowed) contains no contrast medium and was of the ectopic type associated with an ectopic ureter draining a grossly hydronephrotic renal pelvis (shown filled with contrast medium injected by the translumbar route, see page 254). (b) A simple ureterocele where the cavity of the ureterocele (arrowed) is filled by contrast medium following an excretory urogram. This is surrounded by a linear defect due to the wall of the uterocele which projects into the contrast medium filled bladder

an increased incidence of other anomalies. A uterus, Fallopian tubes and gonads within the abdominal cavity are present in most cases.

The existence of a characteristic pattern of skeletal abnormalities in some of the disorders of the sex chromosomes, such as Turner's syndrome and the tetra XY syndrome, is referred to elsewhere (*see* pages 23, 24). In such cases radiological examination of the bones is a helpful procedure. These conditions, in so far as they produce gonadal dysgenesis, may also be investigated by pneumoperitoneum. The effects of hormonal treatment in stimulating growth of the internal genitalia may be followed by the same method.

TUMOURS AND CYSTS INVOLVING THE URINARY TRACT

LESIONS OF THE KIDNEY

It is proposed to discuss under this heading lesions of the kidney and bladder, and of the adrenal gland. Owing to its intimate anatomical relationship to the kidney, tumours arising in the adrenal glands manifest themselves largely by the effects they may produce upon renal structure and function.

Introduction

Radiology may provide information upon the following features in respect of tumours and cysts involving the urinary tract:

(1) The size and site of the mass. It is usually possible to obtain an accurate assessment of the site of origin of tumours or cysts, of the degree to which they extend into or displace adjacent structures, and whether they are single or multiple.

(2) The nature of the lesion. This may often be determined with a considerable degree of accuracy.

(3) The effect of lesions on the rest of the urinary tract. This may be readily assessed, particularly as concerns renal function or obstruction to drainage from the collecting system.

(4) The presence of metastases—especially when these are situated in the bones or in the thorax.

(5) The presence of associated congenital abnormalities. These may be of some importance in the management of the case.

(6) The result of treatment, i.e. the effect of radiotherapy and chemotherapy on the size of tumours can easily be followed.

(7) Renal cysts can be punctured and the fluid which they contain removed under fluoroscopic control. This may have a therapeutic as well as a diagnostic value (Frimann-Dahl, 1964).

Among neoplasms arising within the kidney, nephroblastoma or Wilms' tumour is the most common type seen in children. Renal cell carcinoma, leukaemia or lymphosarcoma involving the kidneys are all very rare in children. Tumours of suprarenal origin may, on occasion, arise within the kidney or invade it by direct extension.

Nephroblastoma (Wilms' tumour)

These tumours cause enlargement of the kidney, and this frequently in an anteromedial direction. The renal pelvis and calyces are displaced to one side of the kidney. They are compressed or splayed and usually not invaded by the tumour (*Figure 7.20a*). Occasionally the renal pelvis is occupied by numerous filling defects in a similar manner to the pelvic carcinoma in an adult (*Figure 7.20b*). The lateral projection is often a useful supplementary view to the standard antero-posterior films because it frequently shows the renal pelvis and ureter displaced anteriorly (Eklöf and Lundin, 1969). Rarely the affected kidney fails to excrete sufficient contrast medium to opacify the pelvis (Cope *et al.*, 1972). When this occurs, it may indicate that the tumour has invaded the renal vein. Occasionally the opposite kidney may be the site of a similar tumour, either simultaneously or after removal of the original tumour.

Metastases are most commonly seen in the lungs (*Figure 7.21*). They have been reported in as many as 50 per cent of cases in various series. They may be present when the patient first comes to hospital and

therefore a chest film is essential early in the investigation. Skeletal metastases are much less common than pulmonary involvement, but their incidence is not negligible (3–15 per cent). All parts of the skeleton may be involved, but the skull, spine and pelvis are commoner sites than the limb bones. The bone lesions are always purely destructive and are always associated with pulmonary metastases (Rudhe, 1969).

On renal angiography the aorta may be displaced away from the tumour. The renal artery supplying the affected kidney may be dilated, elongated and stretched with its branches splayed by the tumour. The angiogram will also show tumour vessels, pooling of contrast medium in lakes and relatively avascular areas within the tumour showing as ill-defined irregular areas of translucency. Phlebography of the inferior vena cava will usually show displacement of this vessel, but occasionally partial or complete occlusion may follow extension of tumour into its lumen from the affected renal vein (*see* page 253).

Neuroblastoma of adrenal gland

Neuroblastoma is the most frequent type of tumour of the adrenal gland which may produce radiological abnormality of the kidney in children. This tumour is also stated to be the commonest solid tumour in childhood. Rarely, it may affect both adrenals at the same time or even occur remote from the adrenal gland along the sympathetic chain.

The tumour mass is usually clearly visible on a plain film of the abdomen. A lateral view may reveal that the kidney is displaced anteriorly by the tumour. Occasionally, however, the tumour may extend down in front of the kidney which is then either not displaced or is

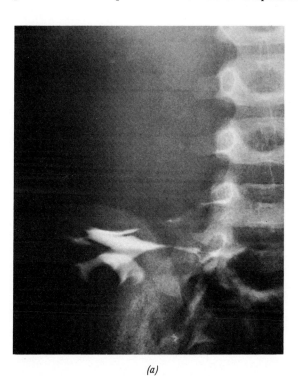

(a)

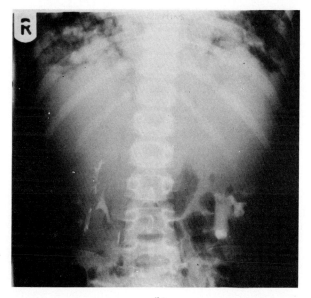

(b)

Figure 7.20. Nephroblastoma: (a) Urogram of a case of nephroblastoma, showing a large tumour of the upper pole of the right kidney compressing, distorting and displacing the renal pelvis. Function of the remaining part of the kidney is not impaired and concentration remains sufficiently good to allow a dense pyelogram to be produced. (b) Another case of nephroblastoma of the left upper pole in which the renal pelvis has been invaded by the tumour

270

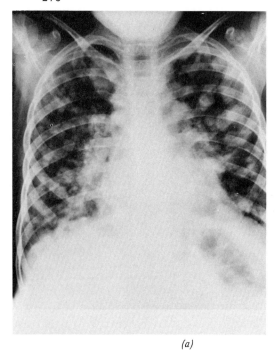

(a)

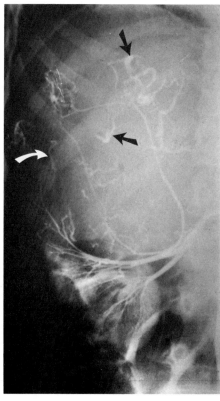

(b)

Figure 7.21. Nephroblastoma: (a) The same child as in Figure 7.20b with multiple metastatic tumours in both lungs. (b) Renal arteriogram showing displacement of the renal artery and its branches by the relatively avascular tumour, within which are tortuous abnormal vessels (arrowed) and pooling of contrast medium (By courtesy of Dr. J. R. Cope and Messrs. John Wyeth, Publishers)

flattened. The soft tissue mass in the radiograph may represent not only the primary tumour but metastases in adjacent para-aortic glands or liver as well. Calcification within the tumour is not uncommon (in 33–60 per cent of cases, according to different authorities). It is usually stippled or in the form of confluent homogeneous calcified masses; rarely it may take the form of a crescentic shell on the periphery of the mass. It is only found in the primary growth, where it may occur without an otherwise distinguishable mass and it may thus be the sole sign of the presence of the tumour. Usually the kidney as a whole is displaced but not invaded by neuroblastomas. Invasion of the kidney may however be present in a third of cases (Barrett and Toye, 1963). The individual calyces may then be distorted or displaced (*Figure 7.22*). Rarely the kidney fails to excrete contrast medium and when this occurs it is due to interference with the renal blood supply. Because neuroblastomas can originate anywhere along the sympathetic chain, the ureters or bladder may be displaced or obstructed. On arteriography, displacement of the renal vessels is frequently seen and a tumour circulation is present in 46 per cent of cases (McDonald and Hiller, 1968). The nephrogram in the majority of cases shows the renal substance to be intact. On phlebography of the inferior vena cava, this vessel is displaced and narrowed but never completely obstructed.

Metastases from neuroblastoma occur characteristically to the skeletal system or intracranially. The former occur in the long bones, pelvis, spine and cranial vault, are often symmetrical and are commoner in the proximal than in the distal bones of the limbs. Though sometimes purely osteolytic, they often show periosteal new bone formation around them and occasionally radiating spicules of bone extending into the adjacent soft tissues. When involving the cranial vault metastases tend to be multiple and give rise to numerous irregular osteolytic areas with rather indistinct margins. Sutural diastasis was formerly held to indicate intracranial metastases, with a rise of intracranial pressure. However, it has been suggested that since such deposits tend to form plaques between the inner table and the dura, the tumour tissue may extend between the sutures causing separation of the adjacent bones (Carter *et al.*, 1968).

The presence of a wide mediastinal shadow, seen most commonly on the left side, is evidence of spread of tumour to the para-aortic and mediastinal tissues. This sign has a bad prognostic significance, because 70 per cent of the cases in which it was present survived less than 6 months as compared with 31 per cent of those where it was not present (Eklöf and Gooding, 1967). The primary tumour was not always on the same side as the mediastinal widening (*Figure 7.23*).

Other adrenal tumours

These are much less common in children and usually present in the adolescent age group, with hyperadrenalism, Cushing's syndrome or hypertension. Radiological investigation may follow a similar pattern to that outlined for neuroblastoma. Many of the tumours are relatively small and therefore produce little or no abnormality of the pyelogram and on arteriography may show little evidence of abnormal vessels or tumour blush. For this reason many authors advocate retroperitoneal pneumography as a complementary form of investigation, especially when arteriography is negative. Adrenal carcinoma and many cases of phaeochromocytoma are revealed on arteriography by abundant abnormal tumour vessels and tumour blush, often with a characteristic central translucency in phaeochromocytoma. Arteriography is not however without risk in the case of the latter tumours because it may provoke a hypertensive crisis. For this reason, it should always be carried out by the transfemoral, rather than the translumbar route, with intravenous Rogitone available for use if such a complication ensues. Selective adrenal artery catheterization may be very informative but it should always be supplemented by an intraluminal aortic injection to exclude extra-adrenal tumours.

Adrenal venography has recently been practised with success in the diagnosis of adrenal tumours based on the fact that these tumours distort the veins to a greater extent than the arteries.

The results of retroperitoneal pneumography have been compared with those of arteriography. It is stated to be accurate in 80 per cent of cases, though it may give both false positive results due to adrenal hyperplasia, fat pads or postinflammatory masses, and false negative results when the tumours are small or extra-adrenal in site. The presacral route is advocated for the injection of the gas because this will allow both sides to be examined with only one needle puncture (Boijsen et al., 1966). This has the disadvantage, however, of the gas taking longer to travel to the desired situation. The risk of air embolism has been virtually eliminated by the use of carbon dioxide as the contrast medium. Before surgical

removal of the tumour is undertaken, it is important to demonstrate the contralateral adrenal because if it is atrophic or hypoplastic, replacement therapy with cortisone will be needed during and after the operation.

Excretory urography may fail to provide diagnostic signs in over 50 per cent of cases because of the small size of the tumour. Nevertheless, it has an important function in cases which present with hypertension in that it may exclude other renal causes for this complication.

Renal cysts

Cysts of the kidney may occur in a large number of different disease processes and radiology may provide a valuable indication as to the nature of many of these.

SIMPLE CORTICAL CYST

Although common in adults, these are rarely seen in children because they are slow-growing and asymptomatic. Occasionally a cyst may present as a very large renal mass in the newborn infant or be discovered as an incidental finding on excretory urography carried out for other reasons. In such cases the cyst will be shown as a smooth rounded mass arising from the kidney and outlined by the displaced and compressed calyces. This type of cyst is probably of little importance clinically. The cyst may be difficult to differentiate from neoplasm, especially when it is very large. In an attempt to solve this problem ultrasound is the investigation of first choice. If this investigation demonstrates a cystic lesion, then the next logical examination is cyst puncture.

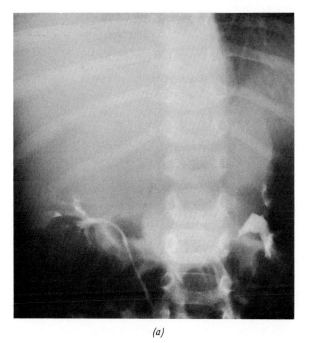

(a)

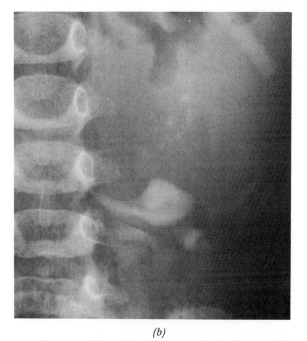

(b)

Figure 7.22. Suprarenal Neuroblastoma: (a) A large tumour situated above the right kidney which is displaced downwards and rotated but not invaded by the tumour. (b) Neuroblastoma of left suprarenal containing punctate calcification within it. The renal pelvis is not only displaced but also deformed. At operation the tumour was found to have extensively invaded the kidney

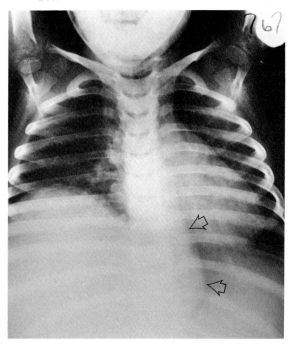

Figure 7.23. Chest film from same child as in Figure 7.22a, showing metastatic tumour extending upwards in the left para-vertebral region (arrowed). It is to be noted that this has occurred on the contralateral side to the primary tumour. Metastasis is also present in the neck of the right humerus

Alternatively, if ultrasound demonstrates a solid lesion, renal arteriography should be the next examination to be performed. On arteriography most tumours in children are vascular and will therefore be disclosed by the existence of tumour blush or tumour vessels. If an avascular area is shown at the site of the abnormality on excretory urography the probability of a cyst is increased. Tumour however is not entirely excluded. A very large cystic mass in the renal area in an infant is more commonly due to a large pelvic hydronephrosis from congenital obstructive disease in the lower urinary tract than to a renal cyst. The former can however often be differentiated by the use of delayed films, because contrast medium will in time outline the dilated pelvis and ureter, provided renal function has not been completely lost.

CALYCEAL CYST (DIVERTICULUM)

This is a condition of little importance in children. It is seen as a small diverticulum from a calyx on excretory urography.

URAEMIC SPONGE KIDNEY

Appearances similar to the condition of medullary sponge kidney as seen in adults have been described in infants and young children, first, in association with a type of polycystic disease (Potter Type III) for which the term 'uraemic sponge kidney' has been used to emphasize the liability to progressive renal failure, and, second, in association with congenital hepatic fibrosis (Kerr *et al.,* 1962). Both these conditions are generally considered to be separate entities from the medullary sponge kidney of the adult from which they have significant differences both in outcome (uraemia or portal hypertension) and in age and sex incidence. Radiologically, they are shown

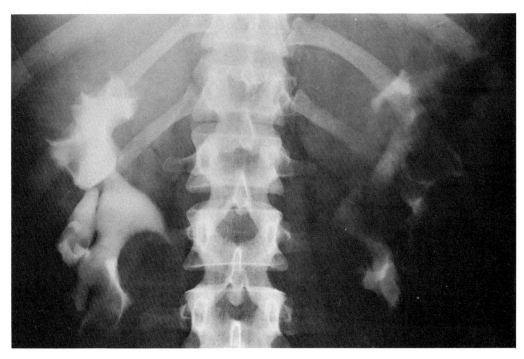

Figure 7.24. Polycystic Disease of the Kidney: Both kidneys are enlarged and the renal pelves deformed by multiple rounded filling defects

on excretory urography as beaded lines of contrast medium within the papillae and related to the calyces.

RENAL DYSPLASIA (MULTICYSTIC KIDNEY)

This condition usually presents with prominent clinical features. Radiologically it is shown as a renal mass with no demonstrable function on excretory urography. A retrograde pyelogram may reveal the ureter ending blindly or a very rudimentary renal pelvis. This procedure carries a special risk of perforating the ureter by the catheter in this condition. However, by virtue of the fact that in surviving cases of renal dysplasia, the condition must necessarily be unilateral, radiology has an important part to play in demonstrating the condition of the contralateral kidney which may be hydronephrotic or hypoplastic (Pathak and Innes Williams, 1964). Radiology may also reveal any associated congenital anomalies in the heart, lungs and gastro-intestinal tract which occur in about 15 per cent of cases.

POLYCYSTIC DISEASE OF THE KIDNEY

This condition has an unfavourable outlook due to the liability to develop renal failure and hypertension which may not be discovered until middle age. It may however present in childhood and lead to deformity of the renal pelves and calyceal pattern due to stretching, compression and distortion by the numerous cysts of different sizes (*Figure 7.24*). On arteriography the branches of the renal artery are similarly displaced and stretched around the cysts and in the nephrogram the latter may show as multiple rounded translucent defects. It is however only in the 'adult' form that renal function is sufficiently good to produce a diagnostic appearance on excretory urography. In the 'infantile' type, inherited as a recessive rather than a dominant gene and therefore a distinct genetic entity, retrograde pyelography may result in the demonstration of the pelvic and calyceal abnormality, though this is never so marked as in the adult type.

Multiple congenital abnormalities in the rest of the body are relatively common, particularly in the skeleton and the central nervous system and some of these may be demonstrated radiologically, These may be important for both their diagnostic and prognostic significance.

The value of different methods of radiological investigation of renal masses

The plain film of the abdomen may occasionally afford good evidence as to the nature of the condition and will always demonstrate the extent and localization of the mass if it is large enough. A lateral film is very useful in this respect, particularly when an extrarenal mass overlies the kidney in the anteroposterior projection, Calcification, if present, will strongly suggest neuroblastoma of the adrenal gland although it may occur in the wall of a cyst. Calcification in a renal cyst is a slow process and is therefore hardly ever seen in childhood; if present it would favour an acquired cystic lesion such as hydatid disease or a tuberculous cavity. Similarly, the characteristic pattern of calcified opacities indicative

of medullary sponge kidney in the adult does not develop before the end of childhood. It is also desirable to examine the bones for evidence of metastases from neuroblastoma. These tumours may rarely extend into the spinal canal and produce erosion of one or more vertebral foramina, the latter being shown in the lateral projection. Loss of the psoas shadow on the side of the mass and widening of the mediastinal shadow are signs suggestive of tumour spread beyond the organ in which the tumour originated.

The value of excretory urography has already been sufficiently emphasized in the description of the pyelographic features of the various lesions, but the additional information which may be obtained by the use of high dosage techniques and by tomography should again be emphasized. Retrograde pyelography may thus be avoided, which is desirable in view of the possible risks of perforating the ureter or the tumour mass with the catheter. Renal arteriography, particularly where selective catheterization is employed, may be of great value in delineating tumours and if these are vascular, in differentiating them from cysts and other avascular lesions. However, the need for surgical treatment to be undertaken as rapidly as possible and the fact that some tumours cannot be clearly differentiated from cysts has resulted in this method being employed less readily than in adults, but as stated on page 252, now that the technical difficulties have been largely overcome, its use should become more general in the future. However, the problem of the differentiation of tumours from cysts and other space-occupying lesions may be a very difficult one. There is no doubt that, in such cases, the use of other methods of investigation, such as cyst puncture, scintiscanning and ultrasound may increase the likelihood of obtaining the correct diagnosis. For instance, ultrasound will demonstrate polycystic kidneys with considerable accuracy. Inferior vena caval phlebography and presacral pneumography may also help in individual cases, and their use has been more fully discussed elsewhere (*see* page 253).

Differential diagnosis

Tumours and cysts of the kidney have to be distinguished both from other causes of enlargement or deformity of the kidney and from similar lesions arising in adjacent organs. The complete list of conditions which can be confused with them is very large. It is only possible to mention here a few of the more important ones.

Among lesions of the kidneys it should be remembered that pelvic hydronephrosis is the commonest cause of a 'cystic' renal mass and its differentiation from renal tumours or cysts may be difficult, especially when there is a hydronephrotic, non-functioning moiety of a duplex pelvis and ureter. The so-called 'crescent' sign, where contrast medium accumulates in the compressed renal parenchyma surrounding dilated calyces, may also occur around a cyst. In this condition is may often be seen to extend around the whole circumference of the lesion instead of only in an arc around individual hydronephrotic calyces. The appearance of a stenosis of the pelvi-ureteric junction on retrograde pyelography may also resemble the blindly ending ureter of unilateral multicystic kidney. In this

274

situation ultrasound may be helpful in making the diagnosis.

Renal vein thrombosis may present with a renal mass and haematuria in infancy and, if bilateral, may resemble polycystic kidney. A localized protuberance due to the splenic impression may occur on the outer border of the normal left kidney and this may be confused with an intrarenal mass. However, when this 'bulge' is due to a normal variation there is usually an elongated calyx corresponding to it, whereas in the case of a 'tumour' the adjacent calyx will be displaced and probably compressed.

Extrarenal masses are usually not difficult to differentiate radiologically from the kidney because they may be seen to lie above, below or in front of the kidney, either on the plain film or in the urogram. When a mass displaces or indents the kidney outline, the renal pelvis rotates as a whole. If the mass is intrarenal it will compress and distort the pelvis as well as displacing it. In infants, congenital cysts of the mesentery and of the biliary passages, or those arising from ectopic portions of gut, and also tumours of the liver or retroperitoneal tissues, are the chief extrarenal lesions to be differentiated. Enlarged lymph glands in the pre-aortic tissues may displace the kidneys laterally. Teratomata, although commonly situated in the pelvis, may sometimes be very large and appear as a mass in the loin; their characteristic dense opacities will be helpful in differentiating them.

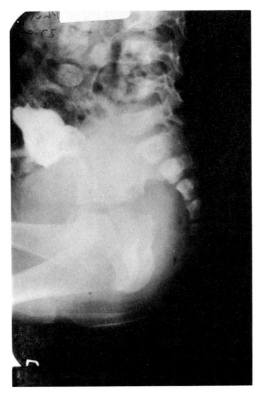

Figure 7.25. Sarcoma of Prostate: Contrast medium injected into the bladder through a suprapubic catheter shows it to be reduced in size, irregular in outline and to be displaced upwards out of the pelvis by a large soft tissue mass lying beneath it

LESIONS OF THE BLADDER AND PROSTATE

Both benign and malignant tumours occasionally occur in the bladder, in the region of the prostate in boys or the vagina in girls. Those referred to as botryoidal sarcoma, rhabdomysarcoma or embryoma are highly malignant, and they usually present in the first 4 years of life with rapidly increasing outflow obstruction of the bladder or haematuria. The extent and location of the tumours may be demonstrated either by excretory urography or retrograde cystography. The bladder wall is irregular, often with a lobulated filling defect at the site of the tumour. The base may be greatly elevated in those tumours arising from the region of the prostate, and the lower ends of the ureters are also elevated in a J-shaped course. Renal function may be impaired and the renal pelves or ureters dilated as a result of the obstruction. The urethra may be distorted and displaced as well (*Figure 7.25*).

Benign tumours of the bladder and urethra are also rare and if large enough will give rise to filling defects without the distortion and displacement associated with the malignant lesions.

Differential diagnosis of bladder tumours is from ureteroceles, extrinsic pressure defects on the bladder due to loaded bowel, pelvic abscesses or enlarged lymph glands. Prostatic or para-urethral abscesses can sometimes give a very similar appearance on urethrography. Congenital absence of the anterior abdominal wall is also a condition which may be associated with bizarre abnormalities in the shape of the bladder.

HYDROMETROCOLPOS

Although not strictly a lesion of the urinary tract, cystic dilatation of the vagina in newborn girls may occasionally present as a large pelvic mass closely resembling an enormously distended bladder. This is due partly to an imperforate hymen preventing the secretion from the genital tract from escaping, but it is especially likely to present in this way when it is associated with an ectopic ureter draining into the vagina.

The function of radiology in such cases is to demonstrate the shape and extent of the mass and to determine the degree to which renal function is impaired. It should also enable the degree of dilatation of the upper urinary tract caused by the pressure of the mass on the bladder and ureters to be assessed (*Figure 7.26*). Ultrasound may also be helpful in showing the cystic nature of the lesion.

OBSTRUCTIVE UROPATHY

Radiology has two main functions in the investigation of cases presenting with obstructive lesions of the urinary tract. First, it should demonstrate the effect of such lesions on the structure and function of the upper urinary tract and, second, demonstrate the site and nature of the obstructing lesion.

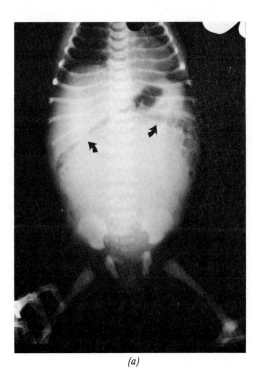

(a)

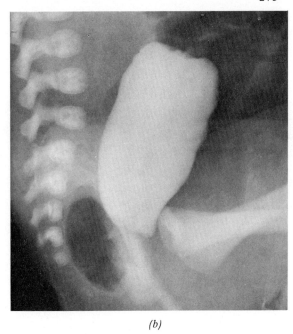

(b)

Figure 7.26. Hydrometrocolpos: (a) Plain film of a newborn infant with a large soft tissue mass in the lower part of the abdomen, representing the fluid-filled vagina (arrowed) (b) After drainage, contrast medium has been injected into the vagina which remains enlarged though much less markedly than in (a)

HYDRONEPHROSIS AND HYDROURETER

The effect of obstructive lesions of the urinary tract is to produce hydronephrosis and, if sufficiently prolonged, to cause progressive interference with renal function. The latter effect may impair the concentrating power of the kidney and this, combined with the dilution of the contrast medium by the urine already present in the dilated renal pelvis, may make the radiological demonstration of the renal pelvis and ureter more difficult. However, there is no doubt that, with the use of higher doses of contrast medium and of delayed films taken an hour or more after the injection, it is usually possible to obtain an adequate demonstration of the calyces, renal pelvis and ureters without recourse to retrograde pyelography. This may be achieved either by the production of a nephrogram in which the dense rim of renal parenchyma outlines the relatively translucent calyces ('negative pyelogram') (*Figure 7.27*) or by the accumulation of sufficient quantities of contrast medium in the calyces and renal pelvis to overcome the dilution. Even if the whole of the renal pelvis is not filled with contrast medium, the use of prone as well as supine positions may displace the contrast-medium-laden urine sufficiently to demonstrate the calyceal structure, the pelvi-ureteric junction and the upper ureter satisfactorily (*Figure 7.28*).

If the obstruction is infravesical, there is likely to be vesico-ureteric reflux into the dilated incompetent ureters. Translumbar pyelography (*see* page 254) may, in some cases, be the only method of obtaining radiological delineation of a large closed hydronephrosis which will have presented clinically as a renal mass (*see Figure 7.6*). Although ultrasonic scanning may confirm the

cystic nature of such a mass and isotope renography reveal impairment of drainage from the renal pelvis, these methods offer a less comprehensive demonstration of its exact size and structure.

The severity of hydronephrosis may be assessed from the size of the renal pelvis and calyces or from its effect on renal function as shown by the density of the excreted contrast medium and the thickness of the renal parenchyma.

Four grades of increasing severity have been described in the infant (Berdon *et al.*, 1970).

Grade I: Acute ureteral obstruction. A dense persistent nephrogram outlines radiolucent calyces which are later well opacified.

Grade II: Long-standing incomplete obstruction from which the kidney may still be salvaged. The nephrogram shows thinning of the renal parenchyma with a dense scalloped outline to the calyces followed later by opacification of the calyces and renal pelves.

Grade III: Long-standing more severe obstruction. The nephrogram shows a greater degree of thinning of the renal parenchyma and localized dense 'crescents' surrounding the translucent dilated calyces (*see Figure 7.29*). This effect is produced by the contrast medium in the compressed collecting tubules which have been rotated through 90 degrees so that they lie parallel to the surface of the calyx. The subsequent opacification of the calyces and renal pelvis is very faint.

Grade IV: Long-standing irreversible hydronephrosis often originating before birth. Although no glomerular filtration takes place, delineation of the remaining renal substance may still be achieved due to the presence of the contrast within the blood vessels, as occurs in 'total body opacification' (*see Figure 7.27a*). The renal substance may be seen as a thin linear soap-bubble-like

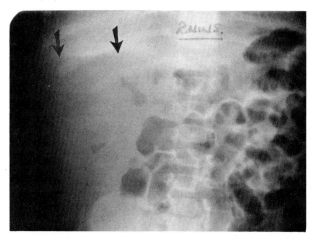

Figure 7.27. Hydronephrosis: Early film from a urogram of a child with a very large hydronephrosis. The dilated pelvis can be seen as a negative shadow (arrowed) outlined by the 'total body opacification' due to the contrast medium given in high dosage being still present in the more vascular tissues surrounding the hydronephrotic renal pelvis. (see Figure 7.6 where the renal pelvis of the same child has been filled with opaque contrast medium)

appearance outlining the enormously dilated calyces. No subsequent opacification of the calyces and renal pelvis occurs.

The progressive reduction in the thickness of the renal parenchyma has been referred to as 'obstructive atrophy' (Hodson, 1967). It is distinguished by its diffuse rather than localized character from focal scarring due to chronic pyelonephritis. The size of the kidney, though increased at first, will ultimately become smaller than normal due to subsequent impairment of renal growth.

OBSTRUCTION AT THE PELVI-URETERIC JUNCTION

Hydronephrosis in the infant due to obstruction at the pelvi-ureteric junction often has an appearance in which the calyces are flattened and 'coin-like' and are grouped to one side of the enormously distended, balloon-like pelvis. In such cases the ureter may either appear to arise abruptly from the medial wall of the renal pelvis well above its most caudal point, or to arise from the lowest point of the pelvis. It may then turn medially and upwards and form an abrupt bend before passing downwards. This latter appearance is particularly seen in cases in whom a separate lower polar artery is present. Retrograde injection of contrast medium into the ureter in such cases may often give a good demonstration of the stenotic area, through which the relatively dense contrast medium passes in a jet, before it becomes rapidly diluted in the dilated pelvis above it (*see Figure 7.28b*). The demonstration of the structure and function of the contralateral kidney is of considerable importance, because it may not infrequently prove to be abnormal in infants with 'giant' hydronephrosis. Only 35 per cent of these cases has a completely normal kidney on the opposite side. This kidney can either be the site of a similar obstructive lesion or of multicystic disease, or it may even be absent (Uson *et al.,* 1969). Nephrectomy

for such hydronephrotic kidneys should clearly not be contemplated unless excretory urography demonstrates a normal contralateral kidney.

Apparent narrowing or kinking of the ureter should not be too readily assumed to be the cause of an obstructive uropathy, particularly if this appearance has only been demonstrated on excretory urography. Such kinking may be a normal appearance or result from tortuosity and redundancy due to obstructive lesions in the lower urinary tract. Retrograde ureterography may be very useful in doubtful cases in securing a controlled demonstration of the calibre and contour of the ureter, particularly when the injection is made under fluoroscopic control with an image intensifier or television.

LOWER URINARY TRACT OBSTRUCTION

The determination of the site of obstructive lesions in the lower urinary tract requires the use of techniques which permit not only an anatomical demonstration of the bladder and urethra, but which also allow an assessment of their functional activity during the act of micturition. Ideally this could be achieved by the combination of retrograde urethrography, micturating cysto-urethrography and cineradiographic studies of micturition. However, in most instances such a battery of investigations is too costly in time and personnel and involves too much irradiation to the gonads to be justifiable. The choice of more limited types of investigation, however, calls for great care in the interpretation of the radiological features, if false positive or false negative results are to be avoided. This is particularly the case in the assessment of the significance of variations in the shape and calibre of the female urethra and in the assessment of obstructive lesions of the bladder neck. Variations in calibre at the bladder neck or urethral meatus are in most cases related to the force and velocity of the stream during micturition rather than to organic stenosis.

BLADDER NECK OBSTRUCTION AND NEUROGENIC BLADDER

The radiological investigation of obstructive lesions at the bladder neck should include films taken either in the lateral or a markedly oblique projection, because the most reliable feature of bladder neck obstruction is a posterior, or, more rarely, an anterior indentation at the vesico-urethral junction. This should be constant throughout micturition but it may be more obvious in the later stages. The authors' view is that for reasons of economy in irradiation, cineradiographic studies should only be employed when the site of obstruction is still in doubt after a full conventional radiological and urological investigation. Cystoscopy will often provide conclusive confirmation or disprove the diagnosis, rendering the use of cineradiographic studies unnecessary. There are a few cases, however, in which it may be rewarding and there is no doubt that it allows a better understanding of the significance of the features seen in conventional radiographs. Other radiological features which may occur in bladder neck obstruction are trabeculation and thickening of the bladder wall, but

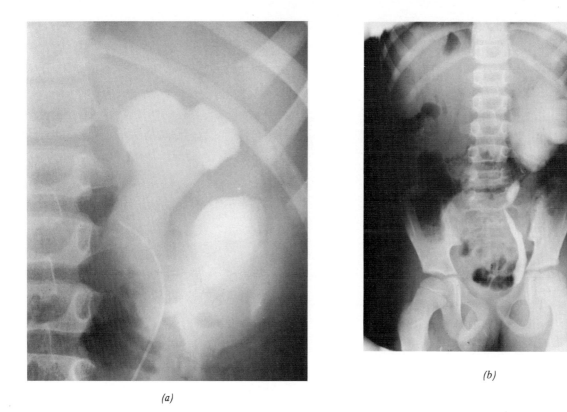

(a)

(b)

Figure 7.28. Hydronephrosis due to Obstruction at the Pelvi-ureteric Junction: (a) Supine view following injection of contrast medium via a ureteric catheter. Some of the calyces are outlined but the body of the pelvis and in particular the site of the obstruction are not shown. (b) Prone view of the same child after withdrawal of the catheter below the stenosis and injection of further contrast medium. The narrowed and distorted segment of the upper ureter and the dilated body of the renal pelvis are now well demonstrated (arrowed)

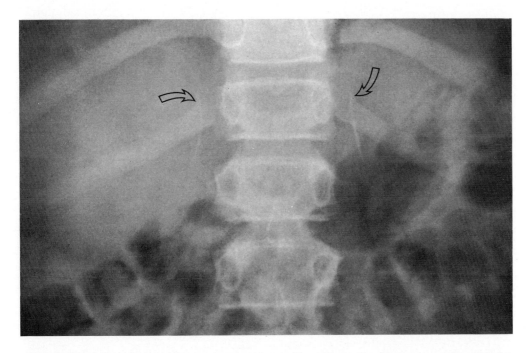

Figure 7.29. Urograms from a Child with a Very Gross Hydronephrosis: No opacification of the renal pelvis has occurred, but a thin linear opacity (arrowed) represents contrast medium in the compressed renal parenchyma surrounding the dilated calcyes (crescent sign) (by courtesy of the Editor of Clinical Radiology)

278

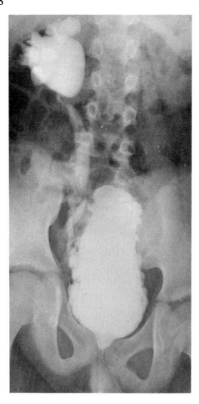

Figure 7.30. Neurogenic Bladder: A micturating cysto-urethro-gram of a boy with a meningomyelocele showing gross vesico-ureteric reflux on the right side (Grade III); the bladder is elongated vertically and has an irregular outline with numerous sacculations ('pine tree' bladder)

these are never as gross as those seen in neurogenic bladder. In cases of neurogenic bladder in which the spinal centres are involved, the trabeculation and thickening of the bladder wall may produce a cone-shaped irregular outline, graphically described as a 'pine-tree' bladder (*Figure 7.30*). However, in assessing trabeculation from irregularity of the bladder outline, care must be taken to ensure that the bladder is moderately full and at rest. Puckering of the mucosa can occur during contraction of the bladder wall, and also arise as the result of irrigation from concentrated solutions of contrast medium or from infection. Residual urine is a common finding, but it is an unreliable sign in children who may not void completely on request. Finally, there is no doubt that cases with unequivocal endoscopic evidence of bladder neck hypertrophy can give normal appearances on radiological examination.

The incidence of vesico-ureteric reflux in obstruction due to hypertrophy of the bladder neck is estimated by several authors as about 67 per cent, but in neuro-genic bladder the figures quoted are more variable, ranging from 13 to 60 per cent. In cases of meningo-myelocele, reflux occurs more commonly in those cases in whom the bladder is large and smooth in outline, than in those who have the 'pine tree' type of bladder. This observation may account for the variations in its incidence (Williams and Verrier Jones, 1968).

URETHRAL VALVES AND OTHER OBSTRUCTIVE LESIONS OF THE URETHRA

Obstructive lesions situated distal to the bladder neck, though mostly rare, may give rise to severe hydronephrosis and impairment of renal function in male infants. Valves of the posterior urethra most commonly take the form of folds extending distally from the apex of the verumontanum to the lateral wall of the urethra. It is possible to demonstrate these as thin linear defects in the contrast medium filling the urethral lumen during micturating urethrography. However, it is not sufficient merely to demonstrate such folds, because they may exist as an anatomical feature in normal children and be of no clinical significance. In addition to their presence it is also necessary to establish the fact that they are a cause of obstruction. This may be inferred when some of the following features are present.

(1) Associated dilatation and elongation of the posterior urethra.
(2) Little or no contrast in the urethra distal to the valves.
(3) Indentation of the bladder neck due to secondary hypertrophy.
(4) Trabeculation or diverticula of the bladder.
(5) Vesico-ureteric reflux, which is also very common (*Figure 7.31*).

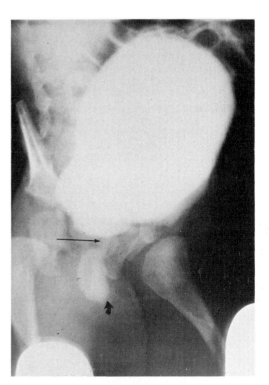

Figure 7.31. Valves of the Posterior Urethra: Micturating cysto-urethrogram showing a dilated posterior urethra with a rounded distal border (thick arrow) beyond which the anterior urethra is visible as a narrow channel. The bladder neck also appears narrow and eccentrically placed relative to the rest of the posterior urethral (thin arrow). This is due to the associated hypertrophy of the detrusor muscle of which the bladder neck forms a part

Urethral valves must also be differentiated from the normal narrowing at the level of the perineal membrane. Considerable distal displacement of urethral valves can occur, but the narrowing produced by them must be shown to be separate from the narrowing at the perineal membrane. Films taken during micturition are essential, because the valves may fail to show either on retrograde urethrograms or on urethroscopy. These may, at least in small children, be obtained with advantage as part of excretory urography, and this will permit assessment of the state of the upper urinary tract as well as demonstrating the urethral lesion. However, when renal function is impaired or micturition cannot be obtained, the bladder must be filled retrogradely.

Other urethral lesions which may lead to obstruction with hydronephrosis or reflux are meatal stenosis, which may occur in both sexes, and a flap valve of the anterior urethra. The latter occurs in boys in whom an incomplete duplication of the urethra communicates with the urethral lumen, and allows micturition to occur into the accessory urethra which then dilates to cause obstruction by compressing the anterior urethral lumen. Such cases may often be convincingly demonstrated by a combination of retrograde and micturating urethrography. Acquired strictures of the urethra are relatively rare in childhood, being mostly of traumatic origin. These are best studied by a combination of retrograde and micturating urethrograms in order to show the site and length of the strictures. They are common at, or just proximal to, the membranous urethra and in this site may be difficult to distinguish from urethral valves. The distal end of the dilated posterior urethra is commonly tapered in the case of a stricture, but it is frequently convex and bulging when urethral valves are present (Innes Williams, 1954).

Obstructive lesions of the urethra, especially bladder neck hypertrophy, are present in as many as 25 per cent of enuretic children (Mitchell and Andrews, 1953). Although this high figure may reflect a bias in the selection of cases, it raises the question of the importance of radiological investigation of such children. It is the authors' opinion that such investigation should not be undertaken in cases of enuresis unless there is evidence of persistent infection, neurological abnormality, or

clinical signs which would point to the likelihood of obstructive uropathy or congenital abnormalities of the urinary tract.

MEGAURETER–MEGACYSTIS SYNDROME

One of the more difficult problems in evaluating the radiological evidence of obstructive disease of the urinary tract lies in the distinction between mild hydronephrosis and the effects of over-filling or ureteric compression produced by the techniques employed during the examination of excretory urography. It has been pointed out that a full bladder can occasionally produce sufficient distension of the upper tract for an obstructive lesion to be diagnosed (Nogrady *et al.*, 1963). However, if these effects are thought of, it should be possible to avoid such errors. Cases in whom the renal pelves and ureters are dilated and in which no obstructive cause can be found are not infrequently seen. These are discussed by Innes Williams (1954) under the term 'megaureter–megacystis syndrome'. Such cases, in addition to the dilatation, very often show vesico-ureteric reflux and on fluoroscopy or cineradiographic studies, vigorous but incoordinated peristaltic activity, with waves travelling in both an upward and downward direction. The ureters may be elongated and tortuous. They usually have a relatively abrupt narrowing at the lower end and this is conical, tapering to a point (*Figure 7.32*). The analogy with achalasia of the cardia and the fact that there may be an association with Hirschsprung's disease of the distal colon has led some authorities to postulate an abnormality of the autonomic nerve supply or ganglia in these patients. Such an abnormality has never been proved histologically. Infection leading to paralysis or hypotonia of ureteric muscle has been postulated by Shopfner (1966) as a cause and he found dilated ureters in 77 per cent of acute urinary infection who did not have demonstrable obstruction. There is no doubt that infection is a common sequel to dilatation of the urinary tract. In some children the bladder has an abnormally large capacity and will tolerate large volumes of urine without discomfort or desire to void, but the amount of residual urine after

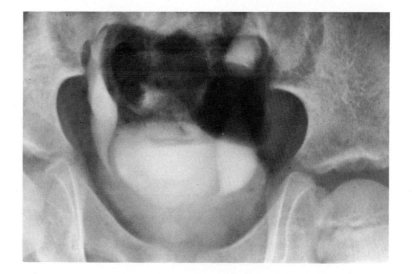

Figure 7.32. Idiopathic Megaureter: Excretory urogram in which the dilated ureters are shown to taper towards their lower ends

micturition is negligible. In many of these children, the ureters are also dilated and infection, chronic pyelonephritis and renal failure, or retardation of growth are more likely to occur. Micturating cysto-urethrography, in addition to excretory urography, will allow assessment of the capacity of the bladder and the presence of reflux. Cineradiographic studies may also be a valuable adjunct, both in establishing the diagnosis and assessing the effectiveness of operative treatment.

URINARY CALCULUS AND NEPHROCALCINOSIS

The deposition of solid material within the renal tissues and within the collecting system is less frequent in children than in adults. Nevertheless, when it does occur it may have far-reaching effects upon the whole of the urinary tract. It is a significant cause of morbidity and even mortality. It is moreover a condition in which radiology has an important part to play in the diagnosis and in the management of the condition.

Urinary calculi

The incidence of urinary calculi has decreased and there is evidence that the type of calculi have changed over the past 30 years. The male predominance reported by most authors has become less marked (Myers, 1957). Calculi may occur at any age, even in infants, but there is a peak frequency between 2 and 4 years. Urinary tract infections and congenital abnormalities, particularly those causing obstruction to the drainage of the collecting system, are commonly associated with

them. Metabolic and other primary causes of urinary calculi are only apparent in a minority of cases.

The radiological demonstration of calculi depends upon a number of factors of which the most important is the radio-opacity of the calculus, due basically to its chemical content (*Figure 7.33a*). The great majority of calculi found in childhood are to some extent radiopaque, even those largely composed of non-opaque materials such as cystine and uric acid. The radio-opacity of the calculus may be related to the frequent presence of infection, especially infection with *B. proteus*, which renders the urine alkaline. This leads to deposition of calcium phosphate, which is radiopaque, upon any nidus which may be present (*Figure 7.35*). However, in small children, the chief factor governing the visibility of a calculus on a radiograph may be the presence of gas and especially faecal matter in the intestine. Superimposition over the bone of the spine and pelvis may also make it difficult to detect calculi. It is virtually impossible to avoid bowel shadows even with the most assiduous use of purgatives and other means. As in the case of excretory urography, the demonstration of urinary calculi or nephrocalcinosis may require the use of measures such as tomography or gastric inflation (*Figure 7.34b*), as already described in the section on urography (*see* page 248). Movement may also prevent small calculi from being detected. This is difficult to avoid completely in the younger children, but the use of modern radiographic techniques makes this a less serious problem by allowing shorter exposures. Completely nonopaque calculi will of course not be detectable except as defects within the opacified renal pelvis and ureters on excretory or retrograde pyelography (*Figure 7.33b*). Excretory urography should always be carried out in any child

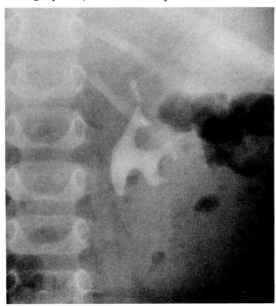

(a)

Figure 7.33. Renal Calculus: (a) A large staghorn calculus in the left renal pelvis. Densely opaque, this type of calculus forms a cast of the renal pelvis and calyces. (b) A non-opaque calculus (arrowed) lying in the body of the renal pelvis shown by virtue of the surrounding contrast medium which has been injected via a ureteric catheter

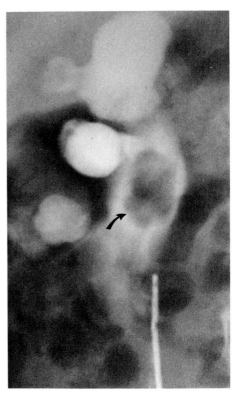

(b)

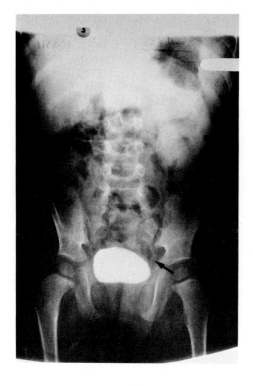

(a)

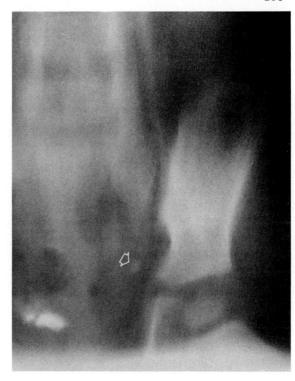

(b)

Figure 7.34. Ureteric Calculus: (a) Excretory urogram in which the calculus in the lower end of the left ureter is hardly visible (arrowed) but the presence of which is strongly suggested by the dense 'obstructive nephrogram' outlining the left kidney. (b) Tomogram of the same case showing the calculus more clearly (arrowed)

suspected of having a calculus as it will not only localize the calculus but will also enable the effects produced on renal structure and function to be assessed. In this respect the condition of the contralateral kidney may also be of importance in management. Associated obstructive uropathy or congenital abnormalities may also be demonstrated and in those cases in whom urinary infection is present, focal scarring due to chronic pyelonephritis may be excluded (*Figure 7.34*).

Accurate localization of calculi may require the use of oblique or lateral projections to demonstrate that the shadow of the calculus coincides with that of the renal pelvis or ureter in more than one plane. Ureteric catheterization using an opaque catheter may also be helpful in this respect. Although retrograde pyelography is less essential since high dosage urography has been employed, it may still be valuable in certain circumstances, especially when it is desired to demonstrate ureteric lesions such as strictures or stenoses which may be related to the development of calculi.

Micturating cysto-urethrography has only a small place in the investigation of urinary calculi, but when infection is present, it may be essential to demonstrate or exclude vesico-ureteric reflux.

Calculi may often be passed spontaneously and radiology has an important part to play in demonstrating whether this has occurred or whether calculi have moved to a different position. Even after passage or removal

of the calculus, regular radiological examination may be required to exclude recurrence.

Differentiation of calculi from other abdominal opacities is less difficult than in adults, because many of those likely to be confused are not seen in children. The most common opacities resembling a calculus in a child are small dense objects within the faecal matter in the colon but these will usually be easy to identify from their mobility in subsequent films. A diagnostic problem in a child is more often posed by the presence of haematuria or abdominal colic, the cause of which is undetermined. Calculi are a relatively infrequent cause of such symptoms. Radiological examination, particularly excretory urography, will almost certainly identify a calculus as a cause if it is present. In a case of acute renal colic excretory urography may only demonstrate an obstructive nephrogram, but this, together with the absence of opacification of the renal pelvis or ureter, will point to the presence of a calculus (*Figure 7.34a*).

Nephrocalcinosis

The incidence of calcification within the renal tissues demonstrable by histological methods either in biopsy or autopsy specimens is much greater than that of radiologically demonstrable calcification. This is partly due to the technical difficulty of differentiating small

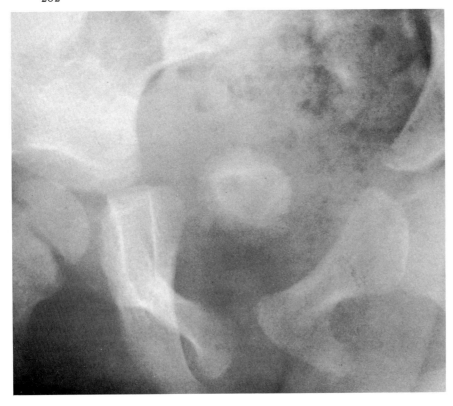

Figure 7.35. Vesical Calculus: The oval calculus lying within the bladder shows lamination with a layer of greater opacity surrounding a less opaque centre

opacities within the renal parenchyma through the bowel pattern in small children. Nevertheless, it may be a very important condition to diagnose, in view of the unfavourable effect it may have upon renal function. Nephrocalcinosis occurs especially in two circumstances. Firstly, when a renal tubular enzyme defect is present which interferes with the ability of the kidney to conserve base and which leads therefore to a renal tubular or hyperchloraemic acidosis. Secondly, it occurs in the presence of hypercalcaemia, either when this is of the idiopathic type, or when it occurs as a result of over-dosage with vitamin D. Nephrocalcinosis has also been described in children in relation to oxalosis, in hypothyroidism and after prolonged administration of steroids. These conditions are so rare as to be curiosities.

The radiological investigation is very similar to that already detailed in the case of urinary calculi except that excretory urography is less likely to be helpful. If calcification is visible, however, its symmetrical distribution in relation to the renal pyramids makes it easy to distinguish from other opacities (*Figure 7.36*). The only condition that is likely to be confused with nephrocalcinosis is medullary sponge kidney (*see* page 272). In this disease, small calculi develop within the cystic dilatations of the collecting tubules. However, this is a process which occurs only slowly, so that it rarely presents in childhood.

RENAL VASCULAR DISEASE

Disease of the renal vascular system is less frequent and less important in children than in adults. However, hypertension is not particularly rare in children and when due to renal lesions may be considerably more amenable to treatment than in adults. In a recent series renal disease was by far the commonest cause, being responsible for 84 per cent of the cases (Chrispin and Scatliff, 1973). Hypertension due to non-renal causes such as phaeochromocytoma and Cushing's disease may require radiological investigation of the urinary tract. Of the renal lesions causing hypertension, those due to direct involvement of the renal artery, such as stenosis, thrombosis and endarteritis from irradiation, form only a minority, the remainder being due to conditions such as pyelonephritis, obstructive uropathy, polycystic disease, renal dysplasia or tumours of the kidney or suprarenal gland. In most of these conditions there will be radiological signs by which their presence may be detected.

RENAL ARTERY STENOSIS

Because the chance of finding a potentially curable condition is relatively much higher in children, it is always desirable to investigate each case thoroughly. Excretory urography should be the basic examination and, although the results are frequently disappointing, due to absent or diminished renal function, it may be useful by indicating which kidney is likely to be involved. It may also determine the need for further specialized investigations.

A reduction in length of a kidney of more than 1 cm is regarded by some authors as a significant radiological abnormality suggestive of renal artery stenosis. However, the determination of absolute values for the renal length

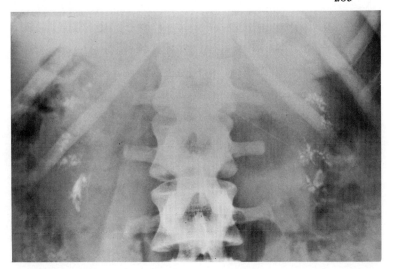

Figure 7.36. Nephrocalcinosis: Plain film of the renal areas in an adolescent girl with renal tubular acidosis. Numerous opacities are present in the region of the renal pyramids of both kidneys. Initially these are punctate in size, but in older children they may become larger and less uniform in size and may then be extruded into the renal pelvis to form calculi

is much less useful than comparison with a normal kidney owing to the wide range of normal variation (*see* page 363). Delay in the appearance of the contrast medium in the renal pelvis or differences in the opacification of the two pelves may also be suggestive signs of renal artery stenosis. In order to appreciate the former, several films should be taken during the first 5 minutes after injection of the contrast medium. The density of the contrast medium in the calyces and renal pelvis is often greater on the side of the stenosis than on the normal side. However, it may be decreased on the affected side; this occurs in 20 per cent of cases according to Scott *et al.* (1961). There may also be delay in the appearance of the contrast medium; this is not a very reliable sign on its own, but it is more significant if accompanied by a disparity in density of the pyelograms. A 'water load' urogram may be a useful method of confirming which kidney is abnormal when there is doubt on this point in a case of hypertension. The principle on which the use of water load urography depends is that the diuresis produced after ingestion of a large quantity of fluid will wash out the contrast medium already in the normal kidney. The ischaemic kidney however is 'protected' by the vascular lesion and the pelvis remains densely opacified.

Rarely, opacities due to vascular calcification may be present, particularly when thrombosis has occurred or if an aneurysm of the renal artery is present. Clubbing, or distortion of the calyces, and localized indentation of the renal outline may be indicative of focal scarring due to chronic pyelonephritis or to the presence of renal infarction. Hydronephrosis or hydroureter due to obstructive lesions, or distortion and displacement of calyces due to the presence of renal cysts or tumours will be significant indications of a possible underlying cause for the hypertension. Suprarenal tumours, by displacing the whole kidney, may likewise be demonstrated on excretory urography.

It has been suggested that isotope renography may be a more sensitive indicator of the presence of unilateral renovascular disease, giving a positive result in 90 per cent of cases, as compared to 54 per cent on excretory urography (Levitt *et al.,* 1968). The renogram is, however, quite non-specific and affords little indication of the probable response to treatment. A combination of isotope renography and excretory urography may give better results than either method used separately. Hypertension due to primary chronic pyelonephritis is usually accompanied by vesico-ureteric reflux. Micturating cysto-urethrography has therefore a place in the investigation of hypertension in children. It may also have a value in its prevention, because it may encourage more efficient treatment and hence lead to a reduction in the number of cases which develop hypertension. The indicence of hypertension in chronic pyelonephritis is estimated to be of the order of 40—60 per cent (Guntheroth *et al.,* 1963).

Direct demonstration of abnormalities of the renal artery will require arteriography. As has been pointed out elsewhere (*see* page 252) this technique is technically not difficult even in the youngest children, but it is a method which is expensive in terms of time and staff. For this reason some means of selecting the cases which are likely to profit from it is very desirable. Any child with serious and sustained hypertension should have an arteriogram. This is especially the case if the hypertension is associated with an audible bruit, where there is asymmetrical renal function, when the kidneys are unequal in size or when tetra-ethyl ammonium chloride fails to produce a significant fall in blood pressure. However, this is not indicated in children with mild hypertension and a positive family history, or whose response to tetra-ethyl ammonium chloride is typical of a neurally mediated hypertension. Stenosis in the main renal artery is usually easily demonstrated (*Figure 7.37*), but if the stenosis is situated at the origin of the artery from the aorta it may be missed because the catheter tip may pass through it. It may then only be revealed by the detection of poststenotic dilatation. The frequency of multiple renal arteries, estimated to be as high as 20 per cent (Scott *et al.,* 1961), should be kept in mind espcially when selective renal arteriography is employed. Because of these two possibilities which may lead to failure to recognize a curable cause for the hypertension it is important to make a free injection into the aorta before the catheter is removed. Aneurysms and narrowing of the renal arteries from extrinsic pressure are not difficult to demonstrate.

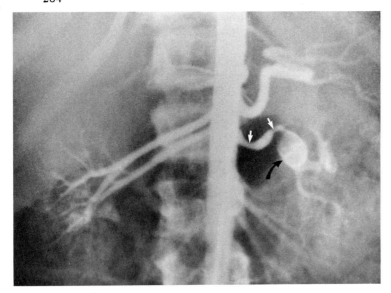

Figure 7.37. Renal Artery Stenosis: Aortogram showing two stenoses of the left renal artery (white arrows), proximal to an aneurysmal dilatation (black arrow) in a boy with neurofibromatosis, a condition known to be associated with renal vascular abnormalities. The presence of two right renal arteries is noteworthy and emphasizes the value of a free aortic injection of contrast medium as complementary to selective catheterization

RENAL ARTERY THROMBOSIS

Thrombosis of the renal artery in neonates may lead to haematuria, heart failure and azotaemia. It may possibly be related to the processes of circulatory readjustment in the neonatal period, in particular to closure of the ductus arteriosus. Excretory urography will show a non-functioning kidney in such cases. Thrombosis of segmental renal arteries may often be suggested by the presence of a defect in the nephrogram. It is conceivable that arteriography or aortography could play a part in elucidating the cause of this.

RENAL VEIN THROMBOSIS

Thrombosis of the renal vein is a condition which is particularly liable to occur in the newborn period, especially in relation to dehydration and increased blood viscosity during attacks of gastro-enteritis. Fifty per cent of cases are bilateral (McFarland, 1965). Of the unilateral cases the right kidney is stated to be affected more commonly than the left. The clinical presentation may be fairly characteristic with haematuria, proteinuria, fever and the sudden development of a renal mass. Radiology has little part to play at the time of the acute incident. By the use of excretory urography, radiology may be helpful in the follow-up of a case, because continued impairment of renal function may be an indication for nephrectomy to prevent the development of hypertension later.

The direct demonstration of the thrombus in the renal vein can only be achieved by phlebography and this is not an easy examination as is indicated by the number of techniques for performing it which have been suggested by various authors. The chief difficulty lies in the fact that non-filling of the renal vein need not necessarily imply that it is thrombosed. To overcome this Chait *et al.* (1968) suggest that the venous phase of a selective renal arteriogram will give a more reliable result than attempts at retrograde filling from the inferior vena cava. However, the use of adrenaline to produce a temporary arrest in the blood flow through the affected kidney may assist in obtaining a complete retrograde filling of the normal renal venous system (Gyepes *et al.*, 1969). Contra-indications to renal phlebography are a very ill patient, a history of recent thrombo-embolism and the presence of significant uraemia. Indirect evidence of the presence of renal vein thrombosis may be obtained from the plain film or urogram. In addition to absence of function on the affected side, there may be fine granular calcification present, and when opacification of the collecting system is obtained there may be pressure defects on the calyces due to parenchymal oedema, pyelovenous backflow and ureteral notching due to dilated tortuous collateral veins.

Renal vein thrombosis may also occur secondarily to thrombosis of the inferior vena cava. This type may occur at any age and will show signs of vena caval obstruction as well as those related to the kidney. Harrison *et al.* (1956) therefore suggest that phlebography should be carried out when unexplained proteinuria and oedema are accompanied by dilated veins in the abdominal wall, when there is evidence of malignant disease in the region of the vena cava or renal veins and in cases of the nephrotic syndrome resistant to steroids.

NECROSIS OF THE KIDNEY

Necrosis may occur in three separate sites within the kidney in the young infant. It may be predominantly cortical involving a thin layer of renal tissue just under the renal capsule together with the columns of Bertin. Alternatively, it may involve the renal tubules or it may be confined to the papillae of the renal calyces, which then undergo sloughing. The radiological features of these three types are different and may be quite characteristic.

In cases of *renal cortical necrosis*, there may be failure or delay in concentration of the contrast medium on excretory urography. Calcification may occur and it is linear, bilaterally symmetrical and parallel to the renal surface. It often forms a double line with extensions at right

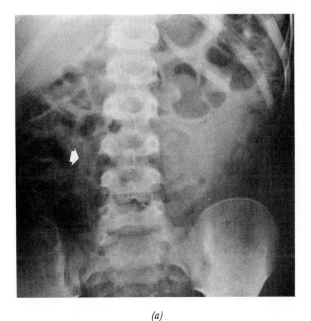

(a)

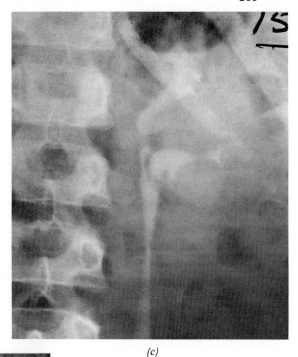

(c)

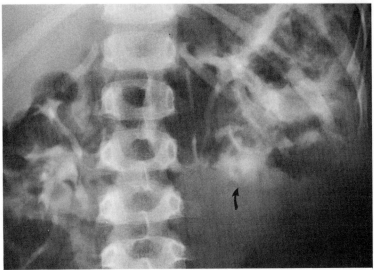

(b)

Figure 7.38. Renal Trauma: (a) Plain film following injury to the left loin. There is absence of bowel gas over the injured kidney and the left psoas shadow has been obliterated. Compare normal right psoas shadow (arrowed). (b) On excretory urography, contrast medium is shown to leak from the lower part of the renal pelvis into the surrounding soft tissues (arrowed) indicating a rupture of the kidney and renal pelvis. The right kidney is shown to be functioning and to be structurally normal. (c) The same case as in (b), 4 years later showing persistent deformity of the renal pelvis due to scar formation

angles to the surface due to the involvement of the columns of Bertin. The kidneys, at any rate in the early stages, are enlarged in contrast to the small kidneys of renal artery occlusion.

Tubular necrosis may result in a persistence of the nephrographic phase of the excretory urogram, for up to 2 hours more after the injection of contrast medium. This is considered to be due to tubular obstruction with leakage of contrast medium into the renal parenchyma analoguous to that seen in Tamm—Horsfall proteinuria in which condition the tubules are plugged by protein casts (Chrispin and Lillie, 1971).

Papillary necrosis is much less common in children than in adults, in whom it is a well recognized sequel to phenacetin overdose or to diabetes. In all age groups it gives a very similar radiological appearance. The sloughed papillae may be visible as rounded filling defects within the renal pelves or calyces, the latter being abnormal in shape, the normal concavity being replaced by an irregular convexity where the papillae have separated. Subsequently the appearances may be associated with focal scarring and become indistinguishable from chronic pyelonephritis.

INJURIES OF THE URINARY TRACT

Trauma of the urinary tract in childhood may involve the kidney as part of severe abdominal injuries resulting from falls from a height or road traffic accidents. The urethra may be injured after falling astride a hard object or in association with fractures of the pelvis.

RENAL INJURIES

Suspected injuries of the kidney call for investigation by excretory urography which may establish the fact that a normal kidney which functions well is present on the opposite side to that which is thought to have been injured. It will also, however, give information as to the extent and severity of the damage to the injured kidney, and reveal the presence of associated fractures.

Contrast medium may fail to be excreted in sufficient concentration to opacify the renal pelvis of an injured kidney, but if it is, the calyces may be displaced or deformed, or contrast medium may leak from a rupture of the renal pelvis into the renal sinus or perirenal space (*Figure 7.38*). Haemorrhage into the perirenal space or within the psoas sheath may lead to a loss of the renal or psoas outlines on the affected side. Bleeding into the renal pelvis may cause an irregular filling defect due to the presence of a blood clot. There may also be a scoliosis concave towards the injured kidney, due to spasm of the lumbar muscles.

Renal arteriography also has a place in the investigation of renal injuries, because it may give a more accurate picture of the extent of the damage to the renal parenchyma, and of the condition of the vascular supply to the injured parts of the kidney. Ischaemic areas may be identified as striped or spotty translucencies within the nephrogram, and the boundary between renal cortex and medulla may be blurred or the renal outline obscured.

The value of urography subsequent to an injury to the kidney has been emphasized. Information may be obtained as to whether there have been permanent effects on renal function and structure (Palavatana *et al.*, 1964). In the majority of cases the long-term results are good in spite of considerable radiological abnormality at the time of the original injury. In a minority of cases evidence of renal cortical atrophy and scarring may be obtained from the distortion or displacement of the minor calyces and from an irregularity of the renal outline, similar to that seen in chronic pyelonephritis except that the calyces are not clubbed.

URETHRAL INJURIES

Injuries to the urethra may be demonstrated by urethrography in the acute stage. Contrast medium injected retrogradely may leak into the tissues of the pelvic floor through the urethral tear. Provided that the contrast medium used is not too concentrated or too viscous such a procedure is well tolerated, but it is seldom essential because the information it affords can be more readily obtained by clinical or other means.

A more important function of urethrography is to demonstrate the presence of a stricture developing as a sequel to urethral rupture or of false passages produced either by the original injury or by subsequent instrumentation (*Figure 7.39*). Both retrograde and micturating urethrograms are desirable to demonstrate the length and extent of strictures and the degree to which they cause obstruction to the passage of fluid in both directions. If a catheter cannot be passed, or is likely to become impacted in a false passage, a micturating urethrogram may be obtained quite satisfactorily

in children by utilizing contrast medium collected in the bladder as a result of excretory urography. In distinction to urethral valves, a stricture tends to show a gradual tapering, rather than a dilated bulging, of the urethral lumen proximal to the obstructing lesion.

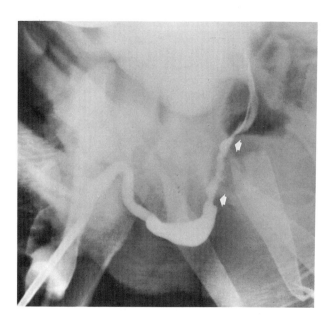

Figure 7.39. Urethral Injury: Micturating urethrogram showing a long irregular stricture of the posterior urethra (arrowed) which had resulted from a rupture of the urethra some years previously

REFERENCES

METHODS

Ansell, G. (1970). 'Fatal overdose of contrast medium in infants.' *Br. J. Radiol.* **43**, 395

Benjamin, J. A., Joint, F. T., Ramsay, G. H., Watson, J. S., Weinberg, S. and Scott, W. W. (1955). 'Cinefluorographic studies of bladder and urethral function.' *J. Urol.* **73**, 525

Clayton, C. B., Dee, P. N., Scott, J. E. S. and Simpson, W. (1966). 'The micturating urethrogram in female children.' *Br. J. Radiol.* **39**, 771

Cooper, D. G. W. (1967). 'Urinary tract infection in children with myelomeningocele.' *Arch. Dis. Childh.* **42**, 521

Gilbert, E. F., Khoury, G. H., Hogan, G. R., and Jones, B. (1970). 'Haemorrhagic renal necrosis in infancy: relationship to radiopaque compounds.' *J. Pediat.* **76**, 49

Glynn, B. and Gordon, I. R. S. (1970). 'The risk of infection of the urinary tract as a result of micturating cystourethrography in children.' *Annls Radiol.* **13**, 283

Hallgren, B., Larsson, H. and Rudhe, U. (1961). 'Nocturnal enuresis in twins—II. Urethro-cystographic examination.' *Acta Paediat. Scand.* **50**, 117

Hodson, C. J. and Edwards, D. (1960). 'Chronic pyelonephritis and vesico-ureteric reflux.' *Clin. Radiol.* **11**, 219

Hope, J. W., Jameson, P. J. and Michie, A. J. (1960). 'Voiding urethrography: an integral part of intravenous urography.' *J. Pediat.* **56**, 768

Lalli, A. F. (1969). 'Translumbar pyelography in the child.' *Pediatrics, Springfield* **44**, 1016

McDonald, P. and Hiller, H. G. (1968). 'Angiography in abdominal tumours in childhood with particular reference to neuroblastoma and Wilms' tumour.' *Clin. Radiol.* **19**, 1

Mountford, R. A., Ross, F. G. M., Burwood, R. J. and Knapp, M. S. (1971). 'The use of ultrasound in the diagnosis of renal disease.' *Br. J. Radiol.* **44**, 860

Nogrady, M. B. and Scott Dunbar, J. (1968). 'Delayed concentration and prolonged excretion of urographic contrast medium in the first month of life.' *Am. J. Roentgl.* **104**, 289

Saxton, H. M. (1969). 'Urography.' *Br. J. Radiol.* **42**, 321

– Cameron, J. S., Chantler, C. and Ogg, C. S. (1973). 'Renal puncture in infancy.' *Br. med. J.* **3**, 267

Scott Dunbar, J., Goldbloom, R. B., Pollock, V. and Radford, R. (1961). 'An automatic device for voiding urethrography in infants and small children.' *Radiology* **76**, 467

Shopfner, C. E. (1965). 'Cystourethrography: An evaluation of method.' *Am. J. Roentgl.* **95**, 468

– (1967a). 'Clinical evaluation of cystourethrographic contrast media.' *Radiology* **88**, 491

– (1967b). 'Radiology in pediatric gynecology.' *Rad. Clins. N. Am.* **5**, 151

Standen, J. R., Nogrady, M. B., Dunbar, J. S. and Goldbroom, R. B. (1965). 'The osmotic effects of methylglucamine diatrizoate (Renografin 60) in intravenous urography in infants.' *Am. J. Roentgl.* **93**, 473

Tucker, A. S. (1965). 'The Roentgen diagnosis of abdominal masses in children.' *Am. J. Roentgl.* **95**, 76

Wells, P. N. T. (1972). *Ultrasonics in Clinical Diagnosis.* Edinburgh & London; Churchill-Livingstone

Winter, C. C. (1966). 'Pediatric urological tests using radio-isotopes.' *J. Urol.* **95**, 584

PYELONEPHRITIS AND VESICO-URETERIC REFLUX

Berdon, W. E., Schwartz, R. H., Becker, J. and Baker, D. H. (1969). 'Tamm–Horsfall proteinuria.' *Radiology,* **92**, 714

Forsythe, W. I. and Wallace, I. R. (1958). 'The investigation and significance of persistent and recurrent urinary infection in children.' *Br. J. Urol.* **30**, 297

Haran, P. J., Darling, D. B. and Fisher, J. H. (1967). 'The excretory urogram in children with ureterorenal reflux.' *Am. J. Roentgl.* **99**, 585

Hodson, C. J. (1967). 'The radiological contribution toward the diagnosis of chronic pyelonephritis.' *Radiology* **88**, 857

Iannaccone, G. (1969). 'Ureteral reflux in normal infants.' *Annls Radiol.* **9**, 31

Reilly, B. J. (1967). 'Infantile pyelonephritis; a preliminary report.' *Annls Radiol.* **10**, 268

Rolleston, G. L., Maling, T. M. J. and Hodson, C. J. (1974). 'Intrarenal reflux and the scarred kidneys.' *Archs Dis. Childh.* **49**, 531

Rooney, D. R. (1961). 'Vesico-ureteral reflux in children.' *Am. J. Roentgl.* **86**, 545

Shopfner, C. E. (1966). 'Non-obstructive hydronephrosis and hydroureter.' *Am. J. Roentgl.* **98**, 172

Smellie, J. M. Hodson, C. J., Edwards, D. and Normand, I. C. S. (1964). 'Clinical and radiological features of urinary infection in childhood.' *Br. med. J.* **2**, 1222

Weber, A. L. and Weylman, W. T. (1966). 'Evaluation of vesico-ureteral reflux by intravenous pyelography and cinecystography.' *Radiology* **87**, 489

Williams, J. E. and Verrier Jones, E. R. (1968). 'The radiological investigation of the renal tract in spina bifida cystica, in the first month of life.' *Annls Radiol.* **11**, 445

GLOMERULONEPHRITIS AND RENAL FAILURE

Berg, U., Aperia, A., Broberger, O., Ekengren, K. and Ericsson, N. C. (1970). 'Relationship between glomerular filtration rate and radiological appearance of the renal parenchyma in children.' *Acta paediat., Stockh.* **59**, 1

Kattamis, C. A. and Nicolaides, X. (1967). 'Acute glomerulonephritis. I. Radiological changes of the lungs, (incidence, types and relation to oedema, hypertension and uraemia).' *Acta Paediat., Stockh.* **56**, 132

Olsson, O. (1954). 'Some radiological problems connected with Bright's disease.' *Br. J. Radiol.* **27**, 86

CONGENITAL ABNORMALITIES

Ashley, D. J. B. and Mostofi, F. K. (1960). 'Renal agenesis and dysgenesis.' *J. Urol.* **83**, 211

Fauré, C., Fortier-Beaulieu, M. and Josso, N. (1969). 'La Genitographie dans les états intersexués. A propos de 86 cas.' ('Genitography in intersex conditions: 86 cases'). *Annls Radiol.* **12**, 259

Feingold, M., Fine, R. N. and Ingall, D. (1964). 'Intravenous pyelography in infants with single umbilical artery. A preliminary report.' *New Engl. J. Med.* **270**, 1178

Friedland, G. W. and Cunningham, J. (1972). 'The elusive ectopic ureteroceles.' *Am. J. Roentgl.* **116**, 792

Hartman, G. W. and Hodson, C. J. (1969). 'The duplex kidney and related abnormalities.' *Clin. Radiol.* **20**, 387

Innes Williams, D. (1954). 'The ectopic ureter: diagnostic problems.' *Br. J. Urol.* **26**, 253

Marcinski, A. and Grzybowska, B. (1970). 'Cysto-uretrovaginographie dans le pseudohermaphrodisme masculin.' ('Cystourethrovaginography in male pseudohermaphroditism'). *Annls Radiol.* **13**, 277

TUMOURS AND CYSTS

Arida, E. J. and Goldstein, P. J. (1964). 'Diagnosis of congenital renal cyst in the newborn. An application of the concept of total body opacification.' *Radiol.* **83**, 999

Barrett, A. F. and Toye, D. K. M. (1963). 'Sympathicoblastoma: Radiological findings in forty-three cases.' *Clin. Radiol.* **14**, 33

Boijsen, E., Williams, C. M. and Judkins, M. P. (1966). 'Angiography of pheochromocytoma.' *Am. J. Roentgl.* **98**, 225

Carter, T. L., Gabrielson, T. O. and Abell, M. R. (1968). 'Mechanism of split cranial sutures in metastatic neuroblastoma.' *Radiology* **91**, 467–470

Cope, J. R., Roylance, J. and Gordon, I.R.S. (1972). 'The radiological features of Wilms' tumour.' *Clin. Radiol.* **23**, 331

Eklöf, O. and Gooding, C. A. (1967). 'Intrathoracic neuroblastoma.' *Am. J. Roentgl.* **100**, 202

– and Lundin, E. (1969). 'Renal pelvis appearances in nephro- and neuroblastomas; diagnostic value of true lateral projections.' *Acta Radiol. (Diagn.)* **8**, 209

Frimann-Dahl, J. (1964). 'Radiology in renal cysts, particularly on the left side.' *Br. J. Radiol.* **37**, 146

Kerr, D. N. S., Warrick, C. K. and Hart-Mercer, J. (1962). 'A lesion resembling medullary sponge kidney in patients with congenital hepatic fibrosis.' *Clin. Radiol.* **13**, 85

McDonald, P. and Hiller, H. G. (1968). 'Angiography in abdominal tumours in childhood with particular reference to neuroblastoma and Wilms' tumours.' *Clin. Radiol.* **19**, 1

Pathak, I. G. and Innes Williams, D. (1964). 'Multicystic and cystic dysplastic kidneys.' *Br. J. Urol.* **36**, 318

Rudhe, U. (1969). 'Skeletal metastases in Wilms' tumour; a roentgenologic study.' *Annls Radiol.* **12**, 337

OBSTRUCTIVE UROPATHY

Berdon, W. E., Levitt, S. B., Baker, D. H., Becker, J. A. and Uson, A. C. (1970). 'Hydronephrosis in infants and children—value of high dose excretory urography in predicting renal salvageability.' *Am. J. Roentgl.* **109**, 380

Hodson, C. J. (1967). 'Obstructive atrophy of the kidney in children.' *Annls Radiol.* **10**, 273

Innes Williams, D. (1954). 'The radiological diagnosis of lower urinary obstruction in the early years.' *Br. J. Radiol.* **27**, 473

Mitchell, J. P. and Andrews, G. S. (1953). 'Symposium on bladder neck obstruction; clinical aspects and pathology of bladder neck obstruction.' *Proc. R. Soc. Med.* **46**, 549

Nogrady, M. B., Dunbar, J. S. and McEwan, D. W. (1963). 'The effect of (voluntary) bladder distension on the intravenous pyelogram.' *Am. J. Roentgl.* **90**, 37

Shopfner, C. E. (1966). 'Non-obstructive hydronephrosis and hydroureter.' *Am. J. Roentgl.* **98**, 172

Uson, A. C., Levitt, S. B. and Lattimer, J. K. (1969). 'Giant hydronephrosis in children.' *Pediatrics, Springfield* **44**, 209

Williams, J. E. and Verrier-Jones, E. R. (1968). 'The radiological investigation of the renal tract in spina bifida cystica, in the first month of life.' *Annls Radiol.* **11**, 445

URINARY CALCULUS

Myers, N. A. A. (1957). 'Urolithiasis in childhood.' *Archs Dis. Childh.* **32**, 48

RENAL VASCULAR DISEASE

Chait, A., Stoane, L., Moskowitz, H. and Mellins, H. Z. (1968). 'Renal vein thrombosis.' *Radiology* **90**, 886

Chrispin, A. R. and Lillie, G. (1971). 'Acute kidney damage with tubular necrosis and papillary necrosis in young infants.' *Annls Radiol.* **14**, 199

— and Scatliff, J. H. (1973). 'Systemic hypertension in childhood.' *Pediat. Radiol.* **1**, 75

Guntheroth, W. G., Howry, C. L. and Ansell, J. S. (1963). 'Renal hypertension: a review.' *Pediatrics, Springfield* **31**, 767

Gyepes, M. T., Desilets, D. T., Gray, R. K. and Katz, R. M. (1969). 'Epinephrine-assisted renal venography in renal vein thrombosis. Report of two adolescents with nephrotic syndrome.' *Radiology* **93**, 793

Harrison, C. V., Milne, M. D. and Steiner, R. E. (1956). 'Clinical aspects of renal vein thrombosis.' *Qt. Jl. Med. N. S.* **25**, 285

Levitt, J. I., Amplatz, K. and Loken, M. K. (1968). 'Renovascular hypertension. Correlation of surgical results with certain predictive tests. *Radiology* **91**, 521

McFarland, J. B., (1965). 'Renal venous thrombosis in children.' *Qt. Jl. Med. N.S.* **34**, 269

Scott, R., Morris, G. C., Scott, F. B., Selzman, H. M. and Feste, J. R. (1961). 'The diagnostic approach to renovascular hypertension.' *J. Urol.* **86**, 31

INJURIES OF THE URINARY TRACT

Palavatana, C., Graham, S. R. and Silverman, F. N. (1964). 'Delayed sequels to renal injury in childhood.' *Am. J. Roentgl.* **91**, 659

8 CENTRAL NERVOUS SYSTEM

METHODS

RADIOGRAPHIC EXAMINATION OF THE SKULL

As with any methods involving the use of contrast media, preliminary films are essential, but these are perhaps more important in the case of examination of the central nervous system than of other parts of the body. This is because of the close relationship that exists between the brain and spinal cord and the bony envelope which invests them and which is involved at an early stage in many disease processes which may be present. Furthermore, diseases primarily affecting the skull may affect the growth and development of the brain. A study of the size and shape of the cranial vault and also of the width and depth of the bony spinal canal may be of great value in directing attention to the likelihood of disease in the brain and spinal cord. The presence of expansion or destruction of the bony structures of the base of the skull, and in particular a study of the foramina through which the nerves and blood vessels emerge from the skull and from the spinal canal, may help in the localization of these disease processes. Finally, calcification, which is visible in a plain film of the skull, is not uncommon in disease of the central nervous system, or it may be shown in normal structures which may undergo displacement by expanding or contracting lesions within the brain. It should be recognized that the appearance of the skull in the newborn infant may differ from that in the older child since this may lead to misinterpretation (*see Figure 8.1*).

ENCEPHALOGRAPHY AND VENTRICULOGRAPHY

A direct demonstration of the brain or spinal cord may be achieved by the use of contrast medium injected into the fluid-filled cavities within and around these structures (*see Figure 8.2*). Of the media available, the most extensively used is air or some other gas such as oxygen which is not toxic to nervous tissue. Such gas may be injected into the spinal theca either by a lumbar or cisternal puncture, a method referred to as pneumo-encephalography, or by direct puncture into the lateral ventricles. This may be performed either through the anterior fontanelle in the infant in the first few months of life or through a burr hole through the cranial vault in the older child. This latter method is referred to as ventriculography. Which route is adopted depends chiefly on whether the intracranial pressure is raised or not. If the pressure is raised, encephalography involves some risk that 'coning' of the medulla may occur, and this risk can be avoided with ventriculography (*see Figure 8.30d* and *e* on page 321). Encephalography by the lumbar or cisternal route avoids the need for directing the needle or catheter through cerebral tissue. Direct ventricular injection through the fontanelle in hydrocephalic infants may lead to the subsequent development of porencephalic cysts of the brain along the track of the needle puncture (Lorber and Grainger, 1963). The likelihood of serious sequelae, or of unpleasant after-effects from pneumo-encephalography, is reduced by injecting as small a volume of gas as possible and by the use of the fractional method as described by Lindgren (1949). In this method separate small injections of between 6 and 10 ml of gas are made and lateral films taken after each injection in order to determine whether the gas is passing into the ventricles. Every effort should be made to avoid a fall in the pressure within the spinal theca, and this is ensured by injecting the gas before allowing cerebrospinal fluid to escape. A fall in intrathecal pressure will not only predispose to 'coning' of the medulla, but it will militate against successful filling of the ventricular system by causing collapse of the cisterna magna and blockage of the basal foramina.

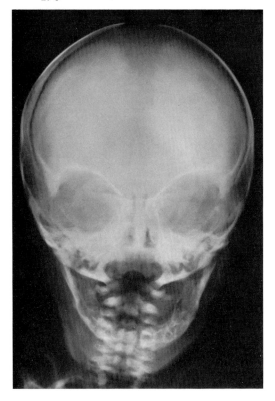

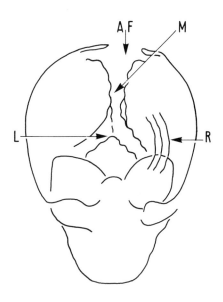

(a)

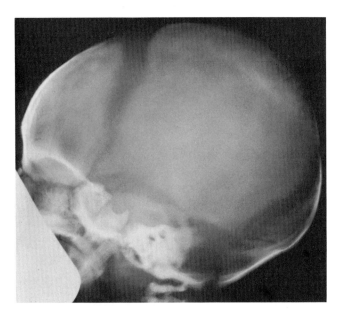

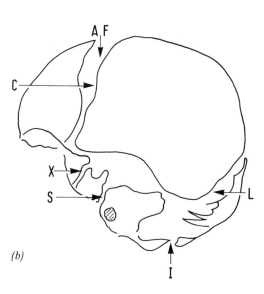

(b)

Figure 8.1. Skull of a Normal Newborn Infant: (a) Anteroposterior view. The widely open anterior fontanelle (AF) and the metopic suture between the two halves of the frontal bone are prominent features. 'Ripple marks' (R) due to corrugation of the scalp are present above the left orbit. These are not uncommon particularly when the skin is inelastic and should not be interpreted as evidence of disease. L–lambdoid suture (b) Lateral view. The coronal suture (C) is considerably wider than in the skull of older children. There are also gaps in the base of the skull due to the innominate synchondrosis (I) and the spheno-occipital synchondrosis (S). A thinner translucent line crossing the body of the sphenoid anterior to the pituitary fossa represents the intersphenoid synchrondrosis (X) but this is only visible in 15 per cent of newborn infants. It is due to an embryonic cleft (cont.)

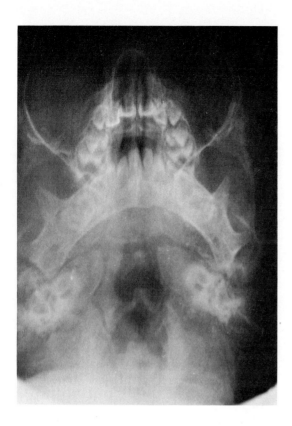

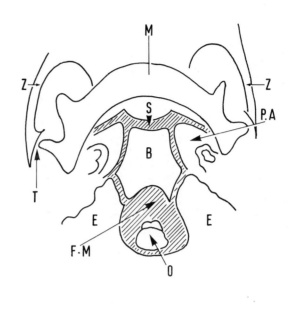

(c)

Figure 8.1. (cont.) (c) Submentovertical projection. The bones forming the base of the skull are separated by cartilage or fibrous tissue which appear as translucencies. M—mandible; Z—zygomatic arches; F.M—foramen magnum; S—spheno-occipital synchondrosis; B—basi-occipital; E—exoccipitals; O—odontoid process; T—temporo-mandibular joint

Absence of ventricular filling

Failure to obtain filling of the whole or part of the ventricles after injection by the lumbar or cisternal route may be due to obstructive lesions blocking the basal foramina or the cerebrospinal fluid pathways between them and the choroid plexus. It is however more commonly the result of purely technical factors. The position of the head relative to the neck and the maintenance of normal tension in the cisterna magna are considered to be most important. As regards the former, the optimum position is usually one of slight flexion, but there is undoubtedly considerable individual variation from case to case. Another cause of failure to obtain ventricular filling is injection of the gas into the subdural instead of the subarachnoid space and this may occur even when the lumbar puncture needle has been positioned so that cerebrospinal fluid drips from it (*Figure 8.3*). It is suggested that this situation is due to the use of a needle with too long a bevel, which has been positioned so that the lumen at its tip lies half out of the subarachnoid space. The presence of gas in the subdural space is easily recognized from its position over the convexity of the hemispheres and beneath the tentorium and by the absence of the characteristic pattern formed by subarachnoid gas filling the cerebral sulci. It has been suggested that passage of gas into the

subdural space is facilitated by the presence of subdural effusions. This presumably results from the maintenance of an actual, instead of a potential, space between the dura and arachnoid membranes (Boudreau and Crosby, 1958). The frequency with which gas fails to fill the ventricular system has been stated to be between 1.5 and 7 per cent. In a large series of pneumo-encephalograms in patients of all ages, an organic cause was found in only 15 per cent of the cases in which no filling of the ventricles was obtained. Of the rest, in 16 per cent the gas filled the subdural space, and in over half the cases in which the examination was subsequently repeated, satisfactory filling was obtained on the second occasion. The use of general anaesthesia was also considered to be a possible contributory factor (Moller, 1970).

Anaesthesia

It is considered that the investigation is best carried out under general anaesthesia, at any rate in small children, and use should be made of a special chair and head support in order to maintain the unconscious patient in the desired position. Comparison of general anaesthesia and basal sedation for performing pneumo-encephalography in children has shown that complications and

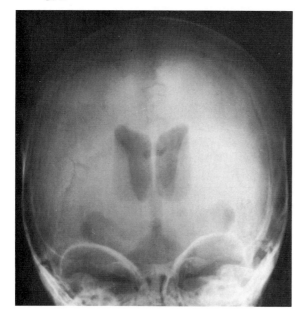
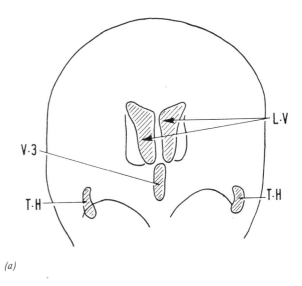

(a)

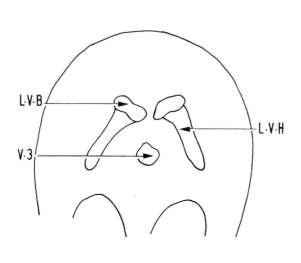
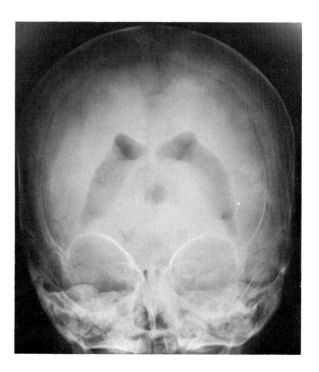

(b)

Figure 8.2. Normal pneumo-encephalogram: (a) Anteroposterior view taken supine. In this position the gas fills the body and frontal horns (LV), the two temporal horns (TH) of the lateral ventricles and the anterior part of the third ventricle (V3). (b) Postero-anterior view taken prone. In this position the gas fills the body and occipital horns of the lateral ventricles (LV) and the suprapineal recess of the third ventricle (V3) (cont.)

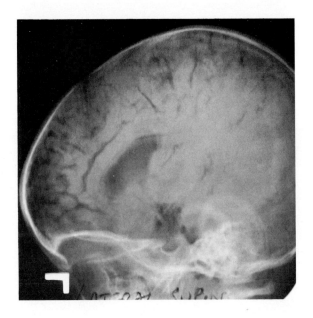
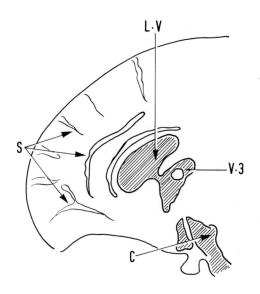

(c)

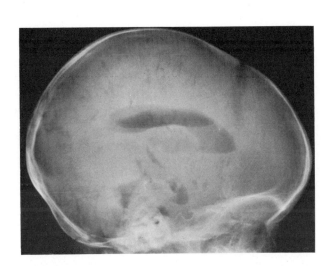
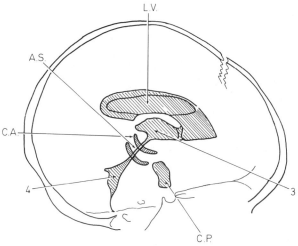

(d)

Figure 8.2. (cont.) (c) Lateral view taken supine. In this film the gas outlines the frontal horns of the lateral ventricles (LV) and the anterior part of the third ventricle (V3). It is also present in the basal cisterns above the pituitary fossa (C) and in the subarachnoid space over the convexity of the cerebral hemispheres where it outlines many of the sulci (S). (d) Lateral view taken erect during injection of gas. 3—third ventricle; 4—fourth ventricle; AS—aqueduct of Sylvius; CA cisternae ambientes; CP—cisterna interpeduncularis. LV—lateral ventricles

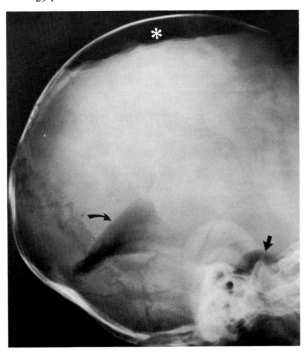

Figure 8.3. Gas in the Subdural Space: The subdural spaces over the convexity of the cerebral hemispheres, (*) beneath the tentorium (curved arrow) and over the dorsum sellae (straight arrow) are outlined. The relatively smooth contour of the subdural spaces compared with that of the subarachnoid space or basal cisterns is helpful in distinguishing between them (Figure 8.2b)

sequelae are less severe and that less time is spent on the investigation with the use of basal sedation. There was no difference in the proportion of cases in which the ventricles failed to fill in the two groups of cases (Groover *et al.*, 1966). The use of general anaesthesia may mask the occurrence of minor after-effects and the frequency of these is in consequence difficult to assess in children. Serious reactions, especially respiratory or cardiac arrest due to 'coning', may be minimized by careful technique and by avoiding the lumbar or cisternal route. This applies particularly in patients in whom the intracranial pressure is raised or in whom there is a likelihood that symptoms are due to a space-occupying lesion in the posterior fossa. It should not be forgotten that these serious sequelae may be delayed for some hours after the investigation and all cases should be kept under observation for at least 12 hours after the examination.

Effect on cerebrospinal fluid

Changes may occur in the cerebrospinal fluid following encephalography. There is a significant rise in the cell count from 3 to 30 mononuclears per mm^3 and a fall in the protein content. The latter change is due to displacement of intraventricular cerebrospinal fluid irrespective of whether gas has been injected or not. If it is desired to collect cerebrospinal fluid for laboratory

examination at the same time as pneumo-encephalography is being performed, it should ideally be collected before any gas has been injected. As has been pointed out, however, this practice is undesirable on other grounds and, provided the pathologist is aware of the effects produced, it should be possible to allow for them. Alternatively cerebrospinal fluid for laboratory examination may be collected on a separate occasion. However, a lumbar puncture for this purpose should not be carried out during the period immediately prior to encephalography because this may lead to difficulty in obtaining a free flow of cerebrospinal fluid before injecting the gas. Emphasis has been placed on the importance of ventricular filling, and it is certainly true that a study of the size, shape and position of the ventricles affords a most important part of the information obtainable from this technique. Nevertheless, a demonstration of the basal cisterns and of the subarachnoid space over the convexity of the hemispheres should not be neglected, and may, in certain conditions, be of considerable importance. In cases in whom there has been failure to fill the ventricles, some information as to the relative size of the cerebral hemispheres and the presence of displacement of midline structures will be afforded by the gas in the subarachnoid space.

Indications

In view of the potential dangers involved and the relatively time-consuming nature of the investigation, it is desirable to limit the use of air studies of the brain in children to cases in whom it is likely to provide information essential to diagnosis, prognosis and management. It is generally agreed that in cases of suspected space-occupying lesions, which in children are predominantly situated in the posterior fossa, encephalography and ventriculography are of great value. However, they should only be carried out when easy access to a neurosurgical team is possible, in order that rapid decompression may be carried out should 'coning' occur. Likewise, in cases of hydrocephalus, it may be useful, in order to assess the degree of ventricular dilatation and the site of the obstruction, if present, and to determine whether a shunting procedure is needed. It is less justified in cases of 'epilepsy', cerebral palsy or mental retardation. In the first-named condition encephalography should be restricted to the following groups of cases.

(1) Those in whom the fits are focal in type.
(2) Those in whom there is electro-encephalographic evidence of a focus from which the fits arise:
(3) Those in whom the fits have followed injury to the brain.

In these cases there may be an underlying tumour or a focal scar, the removal of which may relieve the fits. Encephalography may often demonstrate the localization of such lesions. In cerebral palsy or mental retardation, encephalography is seldom of practical value, but it is possible to justify carrying out the investigation in order to demonstrate the presence of severe developmental abnormalities of the brain, cerebral hypoplasia or atrophy. In this way, a more rational assessment of the prognosis may be made and this may be helpful in allowing the parents of a mentally or neurologically handicapped child to come to terms with the situation. There may also be cases in which the signs and symptoms are suggestive of disease of the brain but are not of themselves sufficient to indicate the nature and aetiology of the condition. In such cases encephalography may be used as a means of excluding remediable conditions or of establishing that appearances are normal.

POSITIVE CONTRAST MEDIUM VENTRICULOGRAPHY

The delineation of the aqueduct and third ventricle with gas may be inadequate, especially when obstruction is present. Even the use of tomography may fail to show minor degrees of displacement or deformity. In such cases the use of a positive contrast medium, such as ethyl iodophenylundecylate (Myodil), injected by direct ventricular puncture, may give a better demonstration of these structures and, provided only a small quantity is used, no harmful sequelae have been recorded (*see Figure 8.26c*). The greater density of the contrast medium relative to the cerebrospinal fluid allows it to be directed into the third ventricle and aqueduct by changing the position of the patient's head. The use of an emulsified mixture of Myodil and cerebrospinal fluid, as described by Calderon-Gonzales (1967), or of water-soluble contrast medium such as 'Conray 60', as used by Raimondi *et al.* (1969), is not entirely free from unpleasant or even dangerous sequelae.

ANGIOGRAPHY

The opacification of the cerebral vessels by water soluble contrast medium has now become generally accepted as a practicable method in children. This examination in many cases is complementary to encephalography and carries a smaller risk of complications and sequelae. However, the standard technique of percutaneous carotid puncture as applied in adults suffers from the disadvantage that, in children, intracranial disease is more often situated in the posterior fossa. It is also frequently bilateral or the indication of the side of the lesion is not evident. Bilateral carotid and vertebral artery injections are practicable (*see Figures 8.4 and 8.32*); however, they are time-consuming and they require considerable skill. For this reason, an alternative method has been suggested, by which contrast is injected into the thoracic aorta in order to fill all four cerebral arteries. This can be achieved either by percutaneous catheterization of the femoral artery by the Seldinger method, the injection being made as for an arch aortogram, or by a retrograde injection into the brachial artery with a pressure injector. Newton and Gooding (1968) prefer selective catheterization of the carotid and vertebral arteries. Films of both the arterial and venous phases should be obtained (*Figure 8.4*).

Complications

Sequelae are very few, but they may be increased by the practice of employing compression of the opposite carotid artery in an attempt to secure bilateral filling after injection of one side. The formation of a haematoma around the puncture site is potentially more dangerous in children owing to the proximity and small size of the larynx and trachea. This is avoided by methods employing brachial or femoral arterial catheterization. An increase in the volume of contrast medium used does not result in any significant rise in complications.

Indications

The chief indications for cerebral angiography in children are vascular diseases and space-occupying lesions within the skull, including tumours, abscesses and subdural haematoma. This is especially the case in those conditions in which the intracranial pressure is raised, because in such cases, as has been stated above, encephalography may be not be devoid of risk. The frequency of infratentorial tumours in childhood makes vertebral angiography a desirable accompaniment to carotid angiography. In the group of vascular diseases, in addition to arteriovenous malformations and vascular tumours, cases of acute hemiplegia in children may be due to obstruction of the carotid arteries by embolism or thrombosis. Early localization of the site of such obstruction is important in order to allow curative surgery to be undertaken with success. Although the majority of such obstructions occur in the intracranial arteries, there are a significant minority due to obstruction in the neck which may be overlooked unless the injection is made low down in the common carotid or from the aorta.

In cases of cerebral palsy in general, however, particularly in the more chronic stages, angiography is of less value and encephalography may give more information. Nevertheless, angiography may be valuable in cases of recent origin, in those presenting with focal fits, or to exclude the possibility of some other associated condition.

BRAIN SCANNING

Radioactive isotopes may be useful in the investigation of intracranial disease in children. When there is a suspicion of a focal lesion such as a tumour, abscess or haematoma, the lesion may take up a sufficient amount of the isotope to allow its demonstration by scanning. For this purpose ^{203}Hg or ^{197}Hg in the form of Chlormerodrin is used. The uptake is highest in lesions with an increased vascularity and high cellular activity, but the site of the lesion also affects the ease with which lesions can be detected, because those near the base of the brain and in the posterior fossa may be hidden by the high level of normal activity in this region. In another method the radioisotope may be injected into the ventricular system or subarachnoid space and used to evaluate the flow pattern of the cerebrospinal fluid in the assessment of hydrocephalus. For this purpose, radioiodinated serum albumen is used and scanning carried out at intervals after the injection for as long as 24 or even 72 hours if the flow is very slow. This is not found to be a reliable method of making the primary diagnosis or of obtaining anatomical details, for which purposes contrast medium studies are preferable. However, it does not carry any risk of upsetting the equilibrium of the cerebrospinal fluid flow or of reactivating a hydrocephalus, and where a shunt is present, it avoids the possibility of air passing through the shunt and entering the heart. Radioiodinated serum albumen may be injected into subdural haematomas or effusions in infants, when it is desired to assess the size and location of such effusions.

ULTRASOUND

The use of ultrasound probes to determine the position of midline structures such as the falx cerebri and pineal gland in cases of suspected displacement by tumours or

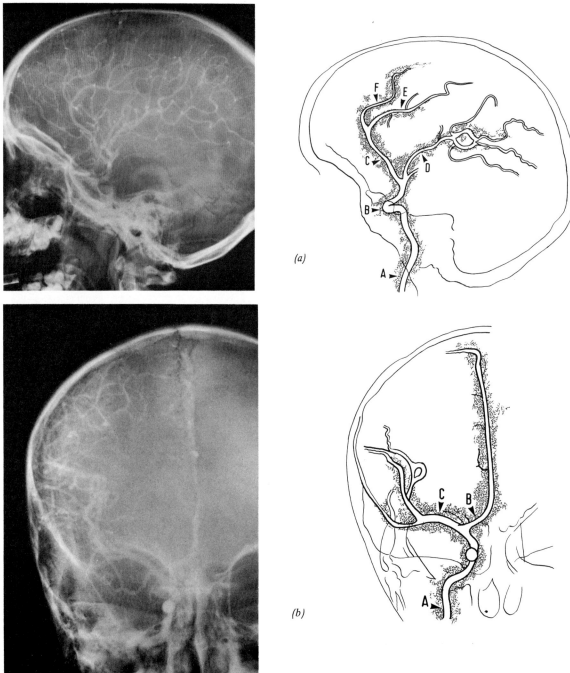

(a)

(b)

Figure 8.4. See facing page for caption

other space-occupying lesions is well established as a safe, convenient and harmless technique, and it has been shown to be practicable in children. Such A-scan methods are unreliable and inaccurate in determining ventricular size, according to Sjögren (1970). However, they may possibly be useful as a method of follow-up study in order to assess the effect of treatment in hydrocephalus. The accuracy of the A-scan method has been considerably improved by the recent introduction of automatic midline computerized techniques.

MYELOGRAPHY

This investigation is usually carried out by using between 2 and 4 ml of ethyl iodophenylundecylate (Myodil) according to age (*Figure 8.5*). This is manipulated by gravity along the length of the spinal canal. In most cases, the injection is made by the lumbar route. In some situations the cisternal route is required to delineate the upper border of a tumour or other lesion causing a spinal block. It may also be used when there is a possibility that the spinal cord is tethered at an abnormally low level, as may occur in diastematomyelia or other forms of spinal dysraphism. In such cases there is a possibility that the lower end of the cord may be injured by the lumbar puncture needle. However, cisternal injection should be avoided for similar reasons when there is any likelihood of an Arnold-Chiari type of malformation at the craniocervical junction (Gryspeerdt, (1963).

Delineation of abnormalities may be impaired by the excessive density of the contrast medium or by the contrast medium being broken up into numerous small globules in its passage up and down the spinal canal. The use of a more dilute concentration, or of an emulsion of the Myodil with cerebrospinal fluid, has been suggested to overcome these disadvantages, but the latter method appears to be liable to produce unpleasant after-effects, and it has not gained acceptance.

The use of gas as a contrast medium for examination of the spinal canal has long been popular in Scandinavia, largely on the ground that it is difficult to remove Myodil completely once it has been injected and the fear that residues of this substance within the spinal and cerebral subarachnoid spaces may, in the long term lead to foreign-body granulomas or arachnoiditis. However, there is no doubt that fine details are much less well demonstrated with gas than with positive contrast medium, even with the help of tomography, though it has been claimed that filling of the sac of a meningocele may be achieved more readily with gas than with Myodil, unless the latter is used in excessive amounts. Water soluble contrast media have not yet proved to be generally acceptable, because a spinal anaesthetic is required for their administration owing to the pain caused by irritation of the meninges and nerve roots; if the contrast medium is allowed to pass higher than the lumbar region, dangerous sequelae may ensue. It must be admitted that Myodil is not the ideal contrast medium; but, until a better one has been developed, its use is justified by the importance of detecting lesions which if untreated may cause severe and prolonged disability or even death. However, it should be limited to such cases which show either clinical signs of neurological abnormality or plain film evidence of intraspinal disease.

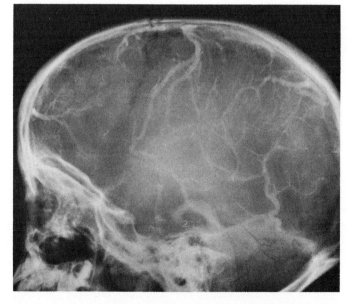

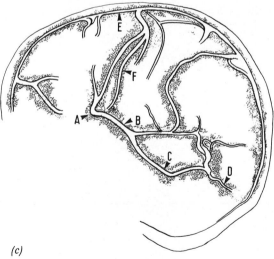

(c)

Figure 8.4. Normal Carotid Angiography: (a) Lateral view of the arterial phase. The internal carotid artery and its main branches are opacified but the vertebral artery and its branches are not normally opacified (see Figure 8.32 for an example of a vertebral arteriogram). A—Internal carotid artery; B—carotid siphon; C—Anterior cerebral artery; D—middle cerebral artery; E—pericallosal branch; F—callosomarginal branch. (b) Anteroposterior view of the arterial phase. A—internal carotid artery; B—anterior cerebral artery; C—middle cerebral artery. (c) Lateral view of the venous phase. A—'venous angle'; B—internal cerebral vein; C—great vein of Galen; D—straight sinus; E—superior longitudinal sinus; F—vein of Labbe. The venous angle is a useful landmark since it is close to the position of the foramen of Monro

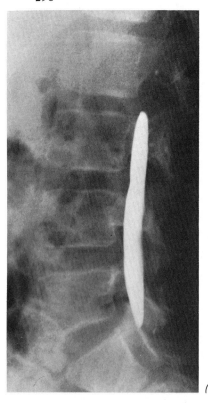

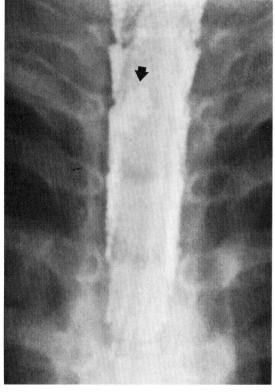

Figure 8.5. Normal Myelography: (a) Lateral view of the lumbar region with the patient prone. The contrast medium in this position outlines the anterior surface of the theca. (b) Lateral view of the cervical region, with the patient prone. In this position the contrast medium outlines not only the anterior surface of the theca, but also the anterior surface of the spinal cord (arrowed). (c) Antero-posterior view of the upper thoracic region. The notches in the lateral border of the column of contrast medium are due to the spinal nerve roots; the spinal cord is shown as a slightly translucent zone in the centre of the contrast medium. Some globulation of the oily contrast medium has occurred (arrowed)

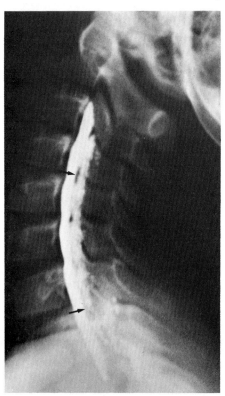

COMPUTERIZED AXIAL TOMOGRAPHY (EMI SCANNING)

A technique has been recently introduced for the tomographic scanning of the head in the transverse axial plane (Hounsfield, 1973; Ambrose, 1973). The method employs a narrow beam of x-rays which pass through the head at a number of different angles. The intensity of the emergent beam is estimated by detectors coupled to the x-ray tube. The absorption of the x-rays by the tissues of the skull and brain is calculated for a large number of positions in the selection plane by the help of a computer. The accuracy of this estimation is sufficiently great to allow differentiation between normal and abnormal structures and the result can be presented in a pictorial form.

This method is becoming more widely applied for the diagnosis of diseases of the brain in children and seems likely to reduce the number of cases in which pneumo-encephalography and angiography are required. The cost of the apparatus is however considerable, and has delayed the installation of the machines in more than a few centres, but these will soon be increased in number.

The method has the advantage of being non-invasive and free from subsequent morbidity and mortality, but since it is essential for the patient to remain perfectly still for 4 minutes, sedation or a general anaesthetic may be needed in younger children. Serial examinations can be undertaken to study the progress of the disease without fear of complications.

The size and position of the ventricular system and of the subarachnoid space over the cerebral hemispheres are well demonstrated owing to the marked difference in density between the cerebrospinal fluid and normal

owing to the proximity of denser bony masses in the skull base, but further flexion of the patient's head and the use of smaller cones provide increased detail.

Cerebral tumours are demonstrated as areas of increased or diminished density or a combination of the two depending upon whether they are solid or cystic,

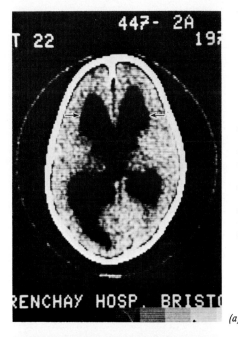

(a)

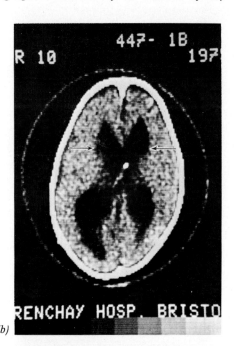

(b)

Figure 8.6. Computerized Axial tomo-graphy—Hydrocephalus: To show the effect of drainage on the size of the lateral ventricles (arrowed). (a) Original examination. (b) Follow-up examination 6 months after the insertion of a drainage tube which can be seen entering from the left side. (By courtesy of Dr. J. L. G. Thomson, Frenchay Hospital, Bristol)

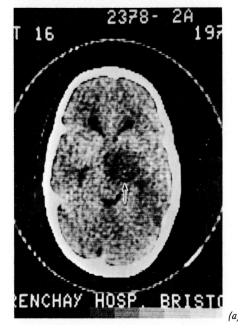

(a)

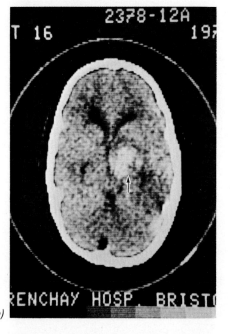

(b)

Figure 8.7. Computerized Axial Tomography—Glioma: This tumour (arrowed) is in the region of the right thalamus adjacent to the third ventricle. To illustrate enhancement after intravenous sodium iothalamate (20 ml). (a) Before contrast medium injection. (b) After contrast medium. (By courtesy of Dr. J. L. G. Thomson, Frenchay Hospital, Bristol)

brain tissue. The method is therefore valuable in the diagnosis of cerebral atrophy and hydrocephalus and is useful for following the progress of treatment in the latter disease (*Figure 8.6*). The tomographic scans are made in different horizontal planes parallel to, or slightly angled to, the orbitomeatal line. Structures in the posterior fossa may be more difficult to visualize

together with distortion or displacement of the ventricles. The contrast between solid tumours and the surrounding brain tissue can be enhanced by the injection of a contrast medium intravenously (*Figure 8.7*) as this is retained for a time by the tumour. Sodium iothalamate 20–40 ml has been used for this purpose, scans being made up to 20 minutes after the injection.

Haematomas following cerebral injury are similarly distinguished as dense areas either within the substance of the brain or at the periphery of the cortex in the case of subdural or extradural bleeding. Simple contusion of the brain or a subdural effusion on the other hand will result in areas of diminished density. A cerebral abscess produces a low density area (*Figure 8.8*) which may be enhanced peripherally by contrast medium injection and the mass is accompanied by displacement of contiguous structures.

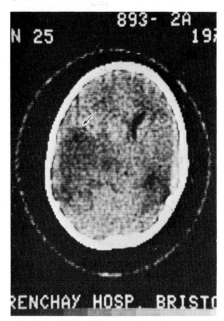

Figure 8.8. Computerized Axial Tomography—Cerebral abscess: Extensive area of low density in the left temporal region (arrowed) and displacement of lateral ventricles to the right. (By courtesy of Dr. J. L. G. Thomson, Frenchay Hospital, Bristol)

The size of a lesion which can be demonstrated by this method depends upon its density. In the case of dense areas of calcification it may be quite small, but is larger in lesions that are ill defined and whose density approximates to that of the surrounding brain. The method is especially valuable in revealing unsuspected disease in children with epilepsy or focal lesions or those thought to have diffuse cerebral disorders. It can also be used together with a plain skull film and an isotope brain scan to determine whether air studies or angiography or both are likely to be useful in a given case. A review of the results obtained with this method has been given by Paxton and Ambrose (1974).

INTRACRANIAL CALCIFICATION

Intracranial calcification is a frequent feature of many diseases of the brain in children. It arises as a result of healed inflammatory disease, neoplasms, and in mentally retarded children of various types. Very rarely, massive generalized calcification may occur throughout the superficial layers of the cerebral cortex and cerebellum (Harwood-Nash *et al.*, 1970). The cause of this is not known, but an intra-uterine encephalitis due to rubella or a similar virus is a possibility.

Calcification is more commonly localized and is only rarely physiological. Such 'normal' calcification is much less common in the child, than in the adult. The pineal gland only occasionally calcifies in childhood. Calcification within the normal choroid plexus is rather more frequent (*Figure 8.9*). It has to be differentiated from that occurring in tumours arising in this situation and from the more extensive calcification affecting the whole of the choroid plexus of the temporal horns of the lateral ventricles which has been described in children with neurofibromatosis (Zatz, 1968). 'Normal' calcification can also occur in the parasellar ligaments of children, especially in the interclinoid ligaments and in the falx cerebri.

The majority of instances of localized calcification in and around the brain may be ascribed to definite local lesions such as meningitis, encephalitis, ependymoma, papilloma of the choroid plexus, lipoma of the corpus callosum, arteriovenous malformations, especially in the Sturge—Weber syndrome, haematomas and parasitic infestations such as cysticercosis.

However, there is a group of cases in which bilateral symmetrical calcification occurs in the region of the basal ganglia, and in which the exact cause is uncertain (*Figure 8.10*). It seems likely that about half of these are due to disturbances in the metabolism of calcium and phosphate due to parathyroid dysfunction. Postoperative or idiopathic hypoparathyroidism accounts for the majority of these, but a few cases are due to pseudo-hypoparathyroidism. These types should be easily distinguishable by the abnormality in the calcium and phosphate levels in the blood.

Some cases of intracranial calcification are due to toxic causes such as carbon monoxide or lead poisoning and a few others are familial. About 30—40 per cent of all cases of calcification in the region of the basal ganglia are sporadic and have no defined cause. Some cases are associated with other disorders of the nervous system, such as amaurotic familial idiocy, epilepsy, extrapyramidal syndromes and the Hallervorden—Spatz syndrome. As stated on page 303 calcification in the basal ganglia may also be associated with mental defect as in Fahr's disease, in which it is thought to occur on the basis of deposits of protein or lipoid in or around the cerebral blood vessels (*Figure 8.10*). A characteristic round midline calcification of about 33 mm diameter has been described in the anterior parietal region in children with congenital agyria (lissencephaly). This is said to be diagnostic of this condition and to be related to persistence of the paraphysis, an embryonic structure which normally disappears after the third month of fetal life.

CONGENITAL ABNORMALITIES

MICROCEPHALY AND CEREBRAL ATROPHY

Congenital malformations of the brain may be of two main types: one comprises generalized failure of the brain to develop, which results in microcephaly and generalized cerebral atrophy; and the other includes the major deformities which result from errors arising

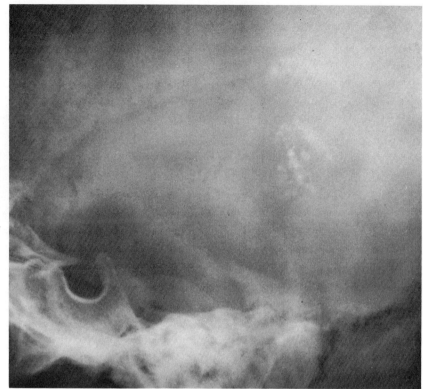

Figure 8.9. Calcification in Choroid Plexus: (a) Plain film of skull showing the characteristic type of calcification above and behind the dorsum sellae. (b) Prone postero-anterior pneumo-enceph-alogram; the choroid plexuses are shown as soft tissue masses within the body of the lateral ventricles

(a)

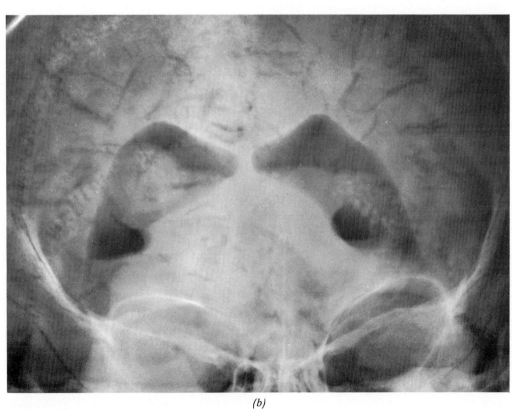

(b)

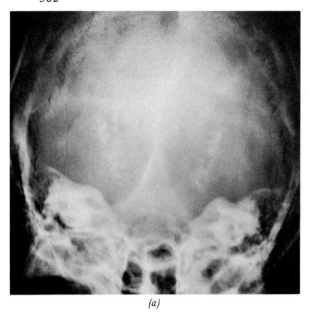
(a)

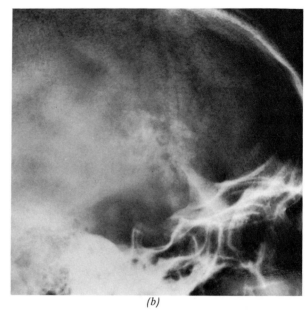
(b)

Figure 8.10. Calcification in the Region of the Basal Ganglia: Opacities situated symmetrically above and lateral to the pituitary fossa in a microcephalic mentally retarded girl. No primary cause was found for this which is probably an example of 'Fahr's disease' (a) Anteroposterior view. (b) Lateral view

early in embryonic life. These disorders often produce severe mental defect and are seldom amenable to effective treatment. Radiology plays a relatively minor part in their investigation. Nevertheless, even if the benefit to the individual from radiographic investigation may be small, the impact of such conditions on the family and the need for genetic counselling may justify an attempt to obtain accurate information of the nature and extent of the brain lesions present. In particular, this information may enable the prognosis to be assessed with authority and may help the parents to accept and adjust more readily to the fact of the child's condition.

Cranial capacity

Plain films of the skull will allow estimation of the size and shape of the cranial vault, both of which features may be of importance in determining the state of the underlying brain. The technique of such measurement has been discussed elsewhere (*see* page 347). Although it is obvious that measurement of the head circumference, or other external dimensions, will afford an equally good means of determining the presence of microcephaly, the additional information provided by skull radiography will often make it a necessary part of the investigation of any child suspected of cerebral maldevelopment. This being so, it is clearly desirable to estimate cranial size, together with any other abnormal features that may be present. There is no doubt that the size of the cranial vault is closely related to that of the brain contained within it, but at the same time, cranial vault size is not the only factor concerned. The dimensions of the rest of the body must also be taken into account. A disproportion between a small cranial cavity and the normal size of the facial bones, or of the rest of the skeleton, may be of considerable significance

in relation to brain development. Moreover, it has to be recognized that the range of normal variation in skull size is wide, and therefore deviation from the mean value must be considerable before it becomes significant. Variation of skull size with age, and to a much lesser extent with the sex of the child, must also be taken into account and the difference between two estimations at different times, defining the rate of change with time, may also be more valuable than the result of a single examination.

Abnormalities in the shape of the skull

In addition to abnormalities in the size of the cranial vault, its shape may be abnormal. This is most obvious in the localized types of brain damage to be considered later; many authors, however, have suggested that in generalized microcephaly there is a characteristic abnormality in skull shape. Thus, in many mentally retarded children with small heads the cephalic index may be low, indicating a dolichocephaly (Penrose, 1972). On the other hand, it has been reported that in certain specific types of case, such as Down's syndrome, the cephalic index is high and the cranium is brachycephalic. This may also be true of children with mental defect secondary to brain damage in the perinatal period. This view is not shared by all authorities, but it may serve to draw attention to the importance of recording abnormalities in skull shape. An abnormally small anterior fossa and a ridge-shaped vertex with inwardly sloping parietal bones have also been regarded as important signs of microcephaly. A flattening of the occipital pole has been noted in many cases, but this feature is by no means specific to microcephaly because it is also common in hypotonic and relatively immobile infants who lie predominantly on their backs.

Other features on plain films of the skull

Microcephalic children show an abnormal thickening of the bones of the vault and a smooth featureless inner table which lacks the normal indentations produced by an actively growing brain (*Figure 8.11*). The sutures between the bones of the vault are narrow but they do not, in most cases, fuse prematurely. In some types of chromosomal abnormality such as trisomy, however, microcephaly may be associated with abnormally wide sutures and fontanelles. The paranasal sinuses and mastoid air cells are often unusually large and the base of the skull abnormally short and narrow with hypotelorism. The pituitary fossa is usually normal in shape and of correct proportional size to the rest of the skull. An exception to this is in Hurler's syndrome in which the 'Omega or J-shaped sella', due to a deepening of the chiasmatic sulcus lying anterior to the pituitary fossa, is especially common. Calcification within the skull may occasionally provide a characteristic feature of some specific types of mental defect (*Figure 8.10*). Perhaps the best known of these is tuberose sclerosis although, as stated later (*see* page 327), the extent of the calcification has no close relationship with the degree of mental defect. Infections, such as tuberculosis, toxoplasmosis and cytomegalovirus encephalitis may also give rise to calcification. Finally, a symmetrical calcification in the region of the basal ganglia may be present in association with mental defect in 'Fahr's disease'.

Pneumo-encephalography

In microcephaly, pneumo-encephalography may demonstrate enlargement of the ventricles (*Figure 8.11*) and widening of the basal cisterns and subarachnoid space. The sulci between the cerebral convolutions may be abnormally prominent, especially in the frontal and parietal regions. Filling of cystic spaces (porencephalic cysts) within the cerebral tissues, although commoner in local brain damage due to vascular disease, may occur in a proportion of cases of cerebral maldevelopment. The 'cysts' are lined by ependymal cells and appear to be of developmental origin.

Relation of radiological signs to mental defect

Correlation between the radiological signs of cerebral atrophy and the clinical evidence of impaired intelligence or neurological defect has been attempted by several authors. The results have been variable and the impression is given that this correlation is, in general, not clearly demonstrated. Vesterdal *et al.* (1954) conclude that the value of penumo-encephalography in mentally retarded children is in most cases small. However, it may be useful in cases who have persistent and localized epilepsy and in those with vague neurological symptoms such as hypotonia or even in infants who are failing to thrive. In such cases it may reveal unsuspected cerebral atrophy or a localized lesion such as a fibrotic scar. Moreover, microcephaly is not always due to lack of brain growth and it may occasionally be merely an expression of a general defect in growth as a whole. In such cases it is compatible with normal intelligence. Craniostenosis (*see* page 25) may also lead to a small head and the distinction between these other causes of microcephaly and cerebral atrophy may be assisted by radiography (Gordon, 1970).

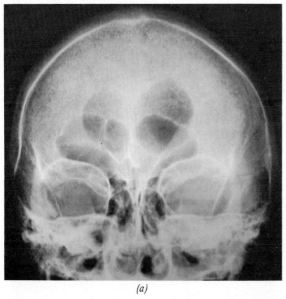

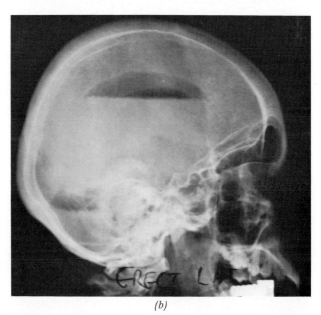

(a)　　　　　　　　　　　　　　　　*(b)*

Figure 8.11. Generalized cerebral atrophy and microcephaly: pneumo-encephalogram in a severely microcephalic boy aged 15 years. The cranial vault is thickened with an unusually smooth inner table; the facial bones and paranasal sinuses are large compared with the small cranial vault; the lateral ventricles are both enlarged ('compensatory hydrocephalus'). (a) Lateral view in the erect position. (b) Anteroposterior view with the patient supine in which the gas outlines the frontal horns but shows little distinction between them and the body of the ventricles

LOCALIZED ATROPHY

Unilateral cerebral atrophy

Asymmetrical growth of both the vault and the base of the skull results from failure of one cerebral hemisphere to develop normally. The effect of this is that one hemicranium is smaller than the other. The

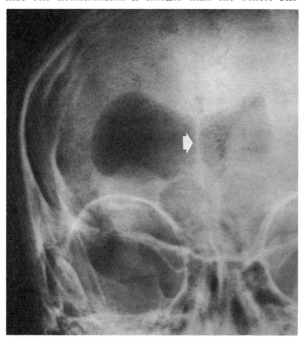

Figure 8.12. Unilateral cerebral atrophy: Pneumo-encephalogram in a child with a left hemiplegia. This antero-posterior view taken with the child supine shows dilatation of the right lateral ventricle and a shift of the septum pellucidum (arrowed) to the right shown by its relationship to the outline of the orbits. This is due to the small size of the undeveloped right cerebral hemisphere. The left lateral ventricle is normal in size

bones of the vault on the abnormal side are thicker and the sutures asymmetrically placed. The base of the skull is elevated on the affected side and this is particularly obvious in the lesser wing of the sphenoid and the petrous ridge. These latter features tend to be apparent earlier than the abnormalities of the vault and the latter may not be present until after 6 or 7 years of age. The lateral ventricle on the side of the atrophic hemisphere is larger than the opposite ventricle and the septum pellucidum and third ventricle are displaced towards the abnormal side (*Figure 8.12*). Porencephalic cysts are more common in atrophy of one hemisphere, such cases being often the result of trauma at birth and consequent intracerebral haemorrhage.

Cerebellar atrophy

Localized atrophy of the cerebellum may give rise to radiological signs which enable the condition to be recognized. These are demonstrated by pneumo-encephalography. The fourth ventricle and the cisterna magna are enlarged and the intervening density due to the normal cerebellum may be absent or abnormally small (*Figure 8.13*). It has been suggested that a direct demonstration of widening of the sulci over the cerebellar hemispheres, which may be achieved by special positioning, is a more reliable diagnostic criterion.

AGENESIS OF THE CORPUS CALLOSUM

Of the many different types of structural abnormality of the brain due to errors in development, agenesis of the corpus callosum has long been known to produce specific radiological abnormalities. These are best demonstrated on pneumo-encephalograms because plain skull films are either normal or show only a small cranial vault. The lateral ventricles are dilated and they have a strikingly abnormal shape in the anteroposterior

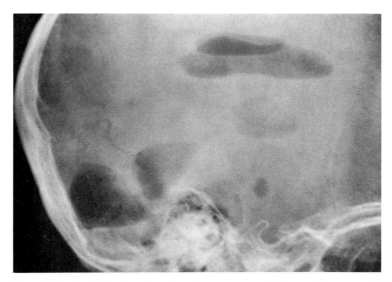
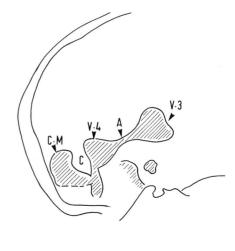

Figure 8.13. Cerebellar Atrophy: Lateral pneumo-encephalogram taken erect. The fourth ventricle (V4) is disproportionately enlarged and elevated and the cisterna magna (CM) is also large. The atrophic cerebellum (C) is represented by the soft tissue density lying between them. (V3—third ventricle; A—aqueduct of Sylvius). Compare with normal appearances shown in Figure 8.2d

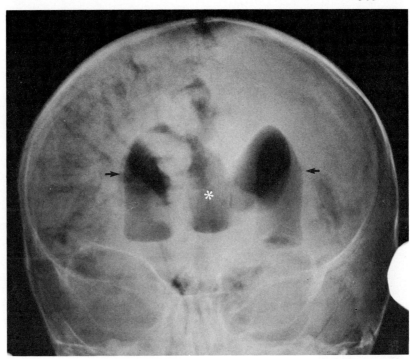

Figure 8.14. Agenesis of the corpus callosum: Pneumo-encephalogram in which the lateral ventricles (arrowed) are widely separated from each other by the dilated and elevated third ventricle (*). The pointed roof of the lateral ventricles and the widened sulci above the third ventricle are also characteristic of this condition (see text) (By courtesy of Dr. J. L. G. Thomson, Frenchay Hospital, Bristol)

projection, their medial borders being concave and their upper borders sharply pointed. The lateral ventricles are also widely separated from each other by the third ventricle which is dilated and considerably elevated and lies at the same level as the lateral ventricles. The foramina of Monro are elongated and the sulci on the medial aspects of the hemispheres are arranged in a radial fashion (*Figure 8.14*). Although these features are usually diagnostic, Bull (1967) considers that angiography has an essential part to play in the diagnosis of this condition. He enumerated the following features which may help to elucidate the pathology in greater detail. The pericallosal artery in the lateral projection takes an irregular course instead of the normal semicircular sweep around the genu and rostrum of the corpus callosum. In the anteroposterior projection the two pericallosal arteries are widely separated. The internal cerebral veins are splayed apart and often elevated by the high position of the third ventricle. The great vein of Galen does not show its normal U-shaped curve around the splenium of the corpus callosum. In 30 per cent of cases the corpus callosum may be only partially developed. On the other hand, absence of the whole corpus callosum may be accompanied by other types of cerebral maldevelopment or by anomalies elsewhere in the body such as cleft palate, spina bifida or abnormalities of the kidneys or suprarenal glands. These may often be detected by radiological means.

HOLOPROSENCEPHALY AND MIDLINE CYSTS

The other anomalies of the brain found in association with agenesis of the corpus callosum may be relatively unimportant, such as cysts of the septum pellucidum or a cavum vergae, or comprise such severe defects as arrhinencephaly or holoprosencephaly. The latter type of defect is associated with severe deformity of the face and orbits and it seldom requires radiological investigation. It may be detected by antenatal radiography of the mother undertaken because of hydramnios or high parity. It can also occur as part of a trisomy 13–15 (Patau's syndrome). The condition can be difficult to diagnose *in utero*, even in the most severe types with a single midline orbit, and the skull may merely appear small or be suspected of being abnormal without the possibility of visualizing the defect itself. In cases without severe facial deformity, or in cases in whom it is desirable to ascertain whether a median facial cleft syndrome is associated with a corresponding severe brain defect, radiology may have a greater part to play. In such cases Kurlander *et al.* (1966) have stressed the value of measuring the interorbital distance because cases with hypertelorism are unlikely to have an associated brain defect or mental impairment, whereas in those with hypotelorism the reverse is true. However, when severe microcephaly is present, such measurements must be interpreted with caution. Other radiographic features likely to indicate fusion of the cerebral hemispheres or absence of the olfactory lobes are a 'keel-shaped' frontal bone (trigonocephaly) especially when associated with absence or hypoplasia of such midline facial structures as the vomer, ethmoids, cribriform plates and nasal septum. On pneumo-encephalography, a 'dorsal cyst' representing the fused lateral ventricles, may be present high up in the midline above the third ventricle, with or without absence of the falx cerebri or corpus callosum (*Figure 8.15*). On angiography there are abnormalities of the anterior cerebral arteries which can either be single or arise from the middle cerebral arteries above the normal site of bifurcation of the internal carotid artery.

Hydranencephaly is a severe brain defect in which the cerebral hemispheres do not develop, but the falx

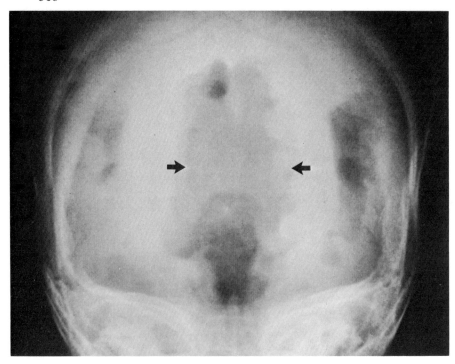

Figure 8.15. Holoprosencephaly: This is shown as a large midline cavity (arrowed) filled with gas on pneumo-encephalography

cerebri is always present. Absence of the septum pellucidum may give rise to what appears to be a single midline ventricle, but apart from this they retain their normal shape and position. It should also be emphasized that simple trigonocephaly is very much commoner than the severe cerebral defects described above and that this finding alone does not necessarily imply that any such defects are present.

Cysts of the septum pellucidum (cavum septi pellucidi), the cavum vergae and the interventricular cistern, are of little clinical importance but they may lead to confusion and suspicion of more serious lesions when they communicate with the ventricular system and therefore fill with gas on encephalography. They may, however, sometimes be a cause of failure to fill one lateral ventricle by pressing on the foramen of Monro.

ENCEPHALOCELE

A midline bony defect in the frontal or occipital bone may be associated with a palpable cystic swelling and be the site of a herniation of the meninges or of cerebral tissue (*Figure 8.16a*). The appearance on the plain skull film is of an oval defect with a smooth corticated margin which is unlikely to be confused with other conditions. However, confusion may arise with the less common condition of encephalocele of the base of the skull, because the resulting defect in the skull base may be difficult to detect without special views or tomography. This type of encephalocele commonly presents as a soft tissue mass in the nasopharynx, the nasal cavity, the face, orbits and sinuses and it may be mistaken for a polyp. If excised after this misdiagnosis disastrous results may ensue.

The axial or basal projection is required to demonstrate both the bony defect, which occurs in the body of the sphenoid, the superior orbital fissure or cribriform plate and also the soft tissue mass. In difficult cases tomography may be of great help. Hypertelorism, with an increase in the interorbital distance up to 10 mm above the average value for the age may also be a helpful sign. Encephalography may demonstrate the passage of gas into the encephalocele and this may be especially well shown in tomograms (*Figure 8.16b*).

SPINAL DYSRAPHISM

Definition

A variety of congenital abnormalities of the spinal canal and spinal cord, which result from failure of fusion of the midline embryonic tissues lying dorsal to the alimentary tract, have been described under the term spinal dysraphism. Confusion in terminology does, however, arise as some authors exclude meningomyelocele because it originates in a different manner. This view is supported by the fact that there is no female preponderance as occurs in the other types of spinal dysraphism. The degree of the abnormality may vary considerably from a simple spina bifida occulta of no clinical importance to severe defects of the type described as the 'split notochord' syndrome, which are associated with visceral and enteric malformations.

Abnormalities on plain films of the spine

Most of these lesions present because they have a limp, sphincter troubles or a local cutaneous lesion at the base of the spine such as a tuft of hair, a fistula or a sinus. Plain films of the spine may be normal or show merely

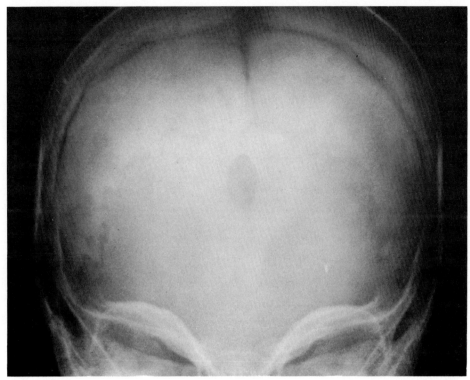

(a)

Figure 8.16. Encephalocele: (a) Plain film of skull with an oval midline defect in the frontal bone. It is through such a defect that the meninges protrude to form a 'cystic' swelling, representing the encephalocele. (b) Lateral pneumoencephalogram in the supine position showing gas within a basal encephalocele which projects through a defect in the body of the sphenoid (arrowed) anterior to the pituitary fossa

an unfused neural arch. More significant abnormalities comprise extensive bony defects, vertebral fusion and hemivertebrae, anterior spina bifida and the presence of a midline bony spur dividing the spinal canal into two halves, indicative of diastematomyelia. It should, however, be emphasized that minor degrees of posterior spina bifida are extremely common, being estimated to occur in over 80 per cent of children in general. This is a normal finding in infancy because the neural arches fuse only during the first and second years of life. Measurement of the width of the spinal canal in both the coronal plane (interpedicular distance, see page 352) and in the sagittal plane may be very helpful. A localized increase in these dimensions at the site of the lesion is common. This may also occur when a spinal tumour is present. In spinal dysraphism the pedicles retain their convex, rounded contour and are never flattened or eroded as with a tumour (Figure 8.17). Such widening points especially to the likelihood of diastematomyelia or intraspinal lipomata and, in the case of the latter, may be accompanied by local scalloping of the posterior surface of the vertebral bodies. Defects in the body of the sacrum, as opposed to the neural arches, are associated with anterior meningocele in this region. The resulting appearance is often very striking, because the remaining part of the sacrum forms a sickle-shaped bony mass which encircles the neck of the meningocele.

Myelography

When difficulty is encountered in the interpretation of these plain film findings due to lack of bone density or

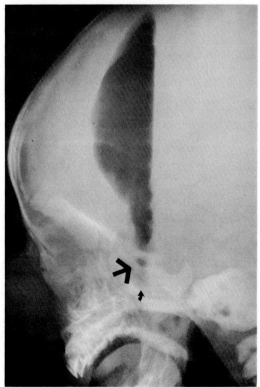

(b)

overlying bowel shadows, as may be the case in the very young infant, tomography may sometimes prove valuable. In most cases however, it is unnecessary in view of the much greater information afforded by myelography, and this latter investigation is of most value in these cases. Myelography should be carried out on any patient in whom a defect in the neural arch or lamina is associated with neurological signs or a suspicious skin lesion such as a tuft of hair or midline sinus or lipoma (Gryspeerdt, 1963). The cisternal route may be preferable to the normal lumbar puncture for injecting the contrast medium in view of the likelihood of an abnormally low position of the conus medullaris of the spinal cord or of an intrathecal lipomatous mass interfering with the free injection. However, it should be borne in mind that the association of meningomyelocele with an Arnold–Chiari malformation may make cisternal puncture inadvisable except in occult spinal dysraphism. It is important to examine the whole length of the spinal canal during myelography because lesions may be present at more than one level. The important points to be detected in myelography in this group of conditions are:

(1) The detection of space-occupying masses within the spinal canal, either intra- or extrathecally.
(2) The detection of midline septa and the determination of their length.
(3) The detection of bands and adhesions.
(4) The identification of the level of the conus medullaris.

The last named is important because it may indicate whether the cord or the cauda equina is involved in the congenital malformation and likely to be subject to stretching due to the greater growth rate of the bony spinal canal. At birth the lower end of the spinal cord lies at the upper border of the body of the third lumbar vertebra. By the age of 5 years it reaches the adult level which is opposite the lower border of the body of the first lumbar vertebra. If the conus medullaris is identified below the lower border of the body of the third lumbar vertebra, it is abnormal in position. It should be remembered that in cases in whom a meningocele is present, the conus medullaris may lie within the sac and be tethered in this position. In cases where difficulty is experienced in determining the level of the conus medullaris with certainty, the identification of the anterior spinal artery or its branches as linear defects in the myelogram may be helpful.

Diastematomyelia

It is usually obvious when a septum is present from the fact that the column of Myodil splits into two, one on either side of the septum (*Figure 8.17*). However, only one side may fill and the appearances may then resemble a unilateral filling defect. Occasionally the spinal cord may be split (diplomyelia) without a midline septum being present. Traction bands and adhesions may be confused with septa, but they are always posteriorly situated, unlike septa, which are anterior in position.

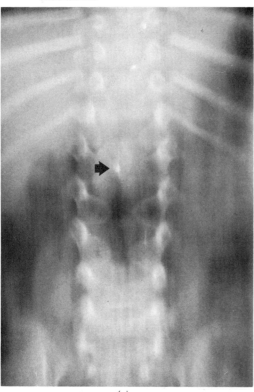

(a)

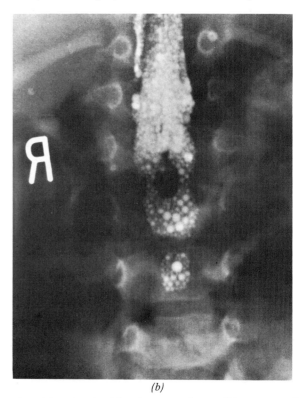

(b)

Figure 8.17. Diastematomyelia: (a) Tomography of the thoracolumbar region of the spine. A midline bony spur (arrowed) is present and is associated with widening of the interpedicular distances and a posterior spina bifida. (b) Myelography of the same case. The contrast medium lies on both sides of the midline septum dividing the spinal theca into two halves. Globulation of the contrast medium has occurred during its passage along the spinal canal

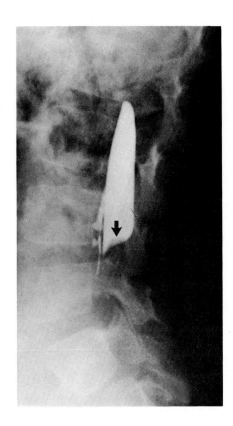

Other types of spinal dysraphism

Lipomata are shown as rounded intrathecal defects or, if they are extradural, may distort and compress the column of Myodil (*Figure 8.18*). In some cases they may not be visualized on myelography. Fistulae or sinuses may be investigated by introducing contrast medium into them and, if extensive, they may show passage of contrast medium into the gut. In cases of anterior sacral meningocele, cystography or a barium enema may serve to demonstrate the relation of the sac to the bladder or rectum. Contrast medium may also be made to pass into the sac of a meningocele. This may be of particular value in the differentiation of anterior meningoceles situated either in the thorax or in the pelvis, in which position the nature of the mass can be obscured (*Figure 8.19*). Some authorities advocate gas as a useful contrast medium for this purpose, in view of the large capacity of some meningoceles.

Figure 8.18. Lipoma of the Spinal Canal: A myelogram shows a space-occupying lesion (arrowed) which prevents the contrast medium from filling the lower part of the theca. The lesion has the features of an intradural extramedullary tumour with a sharply pointed angle at the point where the contrast medium projects between the mass and the wall of the theca

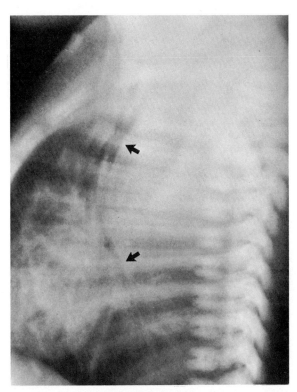

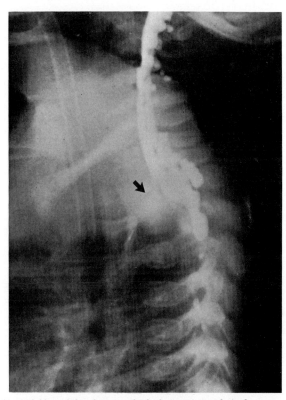

Figure 8.19. Anterior Meningocele of the Cervicothoracic Region: (a) Lateral film of the chest in which the meningocele is shown as a mass in the posterior mediastinum (arrowed), displacing the trachea forwards. (b) Myelogram in the prone position with contrast medium in the cervical part of the spinal theca. A minute track (arrowed) is outlined by the contrast medium extending downwards and forwards from the spinal canal towards the meningocele which has been treated surgically

MENINGITIS AND ENCEPHALITIS

Pyogenic meningitis

Radiology is not contributory in the acute stage of this condition. A proportion of children, especially infants, suffer from serious sequelae of pyogenic meningitis; in particular, hydrocephalus due to meningeal adhesions in the region of the basal foramina or tentorial hiatus. The incidence of the development of hydrocephalus is about 30 per cent (Lorber and Pickering, 1966). The head circumference is not necessarily increased. Pneumo-encephalography will reveal the degree of hydrocephalus and demonstrate the obstruction to the passage of gas from the spinal theca to the ventricles or from one lateral ventricle to the other. Multiple diverticula within the frontal lobes may also be shown and in many cases these are considered to arise as a result of previous ventricular punctures. Recurrent attacks of meningitis in children are sometimes associated with congenital deafness and in such cases an abnormally large vestibule may be demonstrated on radiography of the inner ear. Contrast medium such as Myodil may be shown to pass from the cerebellopontine angle through the vestibule into the middle ear cavity and nasopharynx, and thus it outlines the route by which the meningeal infection may spread.

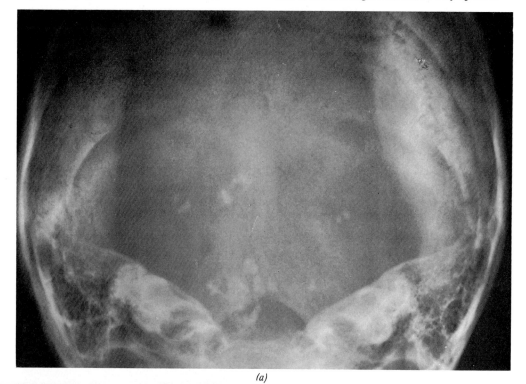

(a)

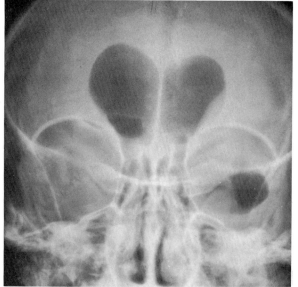

(b)

Figure 8.20. Tuberculous Meningitis: (a) Calcification around the base of the brain and tentorium following tuberculous meningitis several years previously. (b) Pneumo-encephalogram showing symmetrical dilatation of the lateral ventricles following tuberculous meningitis

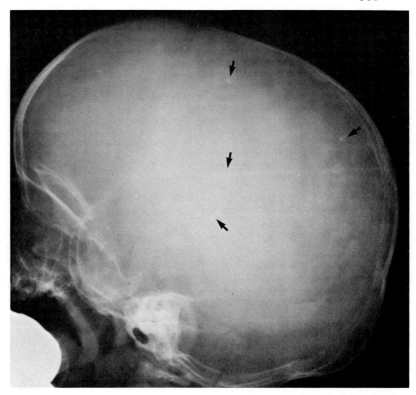

Figure 8.21. Toxoplasmosis: Calcification arranged in plaques and linear streaks due to toxoplasmosis. The size of the cranial vault is increased, indicative of associated hydrocephalus (By courtesy of Dr. J. L. G. Thomson, Frenchay Hospital, Bristol)

TUBERCULOUS MENINGITIS

Radiology is again only of importance in assessing the severity of the sequelae and the prognosis of this condition. Intracranial calcification is by no means uncommon following tuberculous meningitis and it occurs mainly around the base of the brain and around the region of the pituitary fossa (*Figure 8.20a*). The incidence is estimated at between 30 and 45 per cent and it develops from 2 to 8 years after the onset of the disease. Intracranial calcification is associated with a high incidence of postmeningeal fits or other neurological lesions, but may be compatible with a complete recovery from the disease (Lorber, 1961a). There may also be a correlation between extensive calcification and pituitary or hypothalamic sequelae such as sexual precocity or Frohlich's syndrome. Evidence of raised intracranial pressure or of hydrocephalus on pneumoencephalography was present in 62 per cent of Lorber's series (*Figure 8.20b*). These signs have a serious prognostic implication. The mortality rate is between 50 and 70 per cent. There is also a high incidence of physical and mental disability in the survivors. As in cases of pyogenic meningitis, cysts within the brain tissue may occasionally be present and they result from previous ventricular punctures. Gas may fail to enter the ventricles or part of the subarachnoid space. Although this may occur in normal individuals, it is nevertheless suggestive of obstruction to the flow of cerebrospinal fluid due to meningeal adhesions and it may precede the development of hydrocephalus. Evidence of healed or active tuberculous lesions in chest films may give an indication of the cause of neurological disease in children, but it has been pointed out that chest films may be quite normal in nearly half the cases of tuberculous meningitis. A normal chest film or calcified tuberculous foci in the lungs or mediastinal glands are thus no guarantee that tuberculous meningitis is not present.

TOXOPLASMOSIS

Hydrocephalus and calcification within the substance of the brain are the common radiological features in toxoplasmosis. The latter may be very variable in both its site and appearance. However, the parietal region is the most common situation and it seldom occurs below the tentorium. Plaque-like areas of calcification which, when seen end-on, appear as curvilinear streaks, are characteristic (*Figure 8.21*). In infancy, before calcification from tuberculous meningitis has had time to appear, toxoplasmosis is the commonest cause of intracranial calcification, but there are numerous less common conditions from which it has to be distinguished. These include tuberose sclerosis, cysticercosis, trichinosis, malaria, torulosis, histoplasmosis and blastomycosis.

CYTOMEGALOVIRUS AND OTHER FORMS OF VIRAL ENCEPHALITIS

These are conditions which may also give rise to intracranial calcification in infancy. Cytomegalovirus infection is considered to be especially liable to produce a necrosis which outlines the ventricular walls when it calcifies. This type of calcification may also occur in

312

toxoplasmosis, though less commonly. However, micro-cephaly, and not enlargement of the cranial vault, is usual in cytomegalovirus encephalitis. Changes in the long bones similar to those seen in congenital rubella have been described. The microcephaly and intracranial calcification are regarded as signs of bad prognostic import, indicative of severe neurological disability, mental impairment and behaviour disorders. Rubella during the early months of pregnancy commonly causes microcephaly in the infant born following maternal infection. It has been suggested that the small size of the head in the postnatal period may only reflect the small size of the infant as a whole. As growth proceeds, the size of the cranial vault becomes progressively smaller relative to that of the rest of the body. In cases in whom pneumo-encephalography has been carried out, severe generalized cerebral atrophy has been shown to occur.

CEREBRAL ABSCESS

Although cerebral abscesses are more common in adole-scents, they may occur in young children and even in infants, in whom they present a difficult diagnostic problem. Plain skull films are often normal. Pneumo-encephalography and arteriography are usually successful in demonstrating abscesses, but as these methods depend upon showing the presence of a space-occupying mass they may be negative in the early stages or when the abscess is infratentorial in site. It has been suggested by Tefft *et al.* (1966) that isotope scintigraphy may be able to give positive evidence of the presence of a cere-bral abscess at an earlier stage than is possible with pneumo-encephalography or arteriography. This results from the isotope accumulating in the region of the abscess due to the breakdown of the blood—brain barrier from the 'cerebritis'. An anteroposterior scan should be carried out first to determine the side of the lesion and this should be followed by a lateral scan to localize it to a particular part of the brain. The scan will continue to show the presence of the isotope for many weeks, in contrast to the behaviour of a sterile infarct in which the scan returns to normal after a week or two. The method is most likely to be diagnostic in supra-tentorial lesions and it should be supplemented by pneumo-encephalography or arteriography to demon-strate that a mass has formed before surgical drainage is undertaken. Following surgery, the use of contrast medium injected into the abscess cavity will allow assessment of the effectiveness of shrinkage and healing of the lesion (*Figure 8.22*).

HYDROCEPHALUS

The value of radiology in the investigation of cases of hydrocephalus lies in the identification of the abnor-mality, in the assessment of its severity and in the determination of its cause. There are rare instances in which a significant increase in head size, as estimated by measurement of head circumference or cranial capacity, is not due to hydrocephalus but to an increase in the size of the body as a whole or an increase in the mass of the brain. The latter is known as macrencephaly and it is associated with fits and mental retardation.

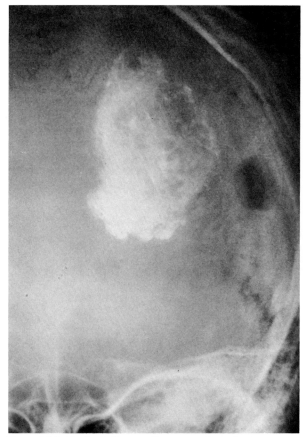

Figure 8.22. Cerebral Abscess: Contrast medium has been intro-duced into an abscess cavity in the left cerebral hemisphere to demonstrate its site and extent

The underlying cause is a diffuse gliosis with a reduction in the number of neurones. Pneumo-encephalography will enable the cause of the cranial enlargement to be determined because the size of the ventricles will be normal relative to that of the cranial capacity.

Radiological features

Of the general signs of hydrocephalus, the direct demon-stration of the size of the cranial vault and of the ventricles may be made on a qualitative basis when the dilatation of the ventricles is gross. In less severe cases, measurement of the cranial capacity and of the relative size of the ventricles and of the thickness of the cerebral hemispheres may be required. The methods by which such measurements can be made are discussed elsewhere (*see* pages 347 and 350). The thickness of the cerebral cortex has been used to divide the severity of hydro-cephalus into three grades: (1) thickness more than 3 cm; (2) between 3 and 1 cm; (3) less than 1 cm. However, it has been pointed out that correlation between such grading and ultimate intelligence is very poor (Lorber, 1961b). In-crease in the size of the cranial vault presupposes that the sutures are still unfused. The sutures become widened and the fontanelles enlarged as the ventricles dilate. These features, together with erosion of the tip of the dorsum sellae and of the lamina dura of the pituitary fossa and the development of indentations on the inner table of the cranial vault, are non-specific signs of increased intracranial pressure. They are considered in more detail elsewhere (*see* page 318). The indentations on the inner table of the vault, however, are sometimes confused with craniolacunia. This latter condition is primarily a defect in ossification, which may be distinguished from convolutional markings by the sharper borders of the translucent areas and the greater relative density of the intervening 'trabeculae' (*see* page 28) seen in craniolacunia. This condition, moreover, has a specific association with the type of hydrocephalus which develops in cases of meningomyelocele and the Arnold—Chiari malformation of the medulla and upper spinal cord; it is stated to occur in 40—50 per cent of cases.

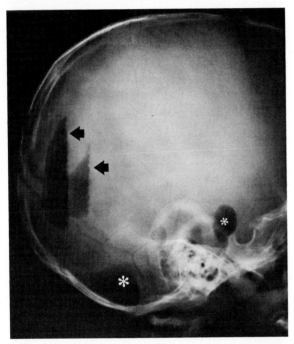

Figure 8.23. Communicating Hydrocephalus: Lateral pneumo-encephalogram in the prone position in which gas is present both in the basal cisterns (**) and in the markedly dilated lateral ventricles (arrowed) demonstrating free communication between the subarachnoid space and the ventricular system

Pneumo-encephalography or *ventriculography* enable the severity of the hydrocephalus to be determined by direct demonstration of the size of the ventricles and the thickness of the cortex. Patients with obstructive hydrocephalus can also be distinguished from those who have the communicating type. However, the procedure is not without risk, especially when the intracranial pressure is raised and in these cases ventriculography is the safer method. In small infants this last examination may readily be performed by ventricular puncture through the fontanelle (*see* page 289). It has been pointed out that there is a risk of cerebral damage resulting from such a procedure (Lorber and Grainger, 1963). Cerebrospinal fluid under pressure will leak along the needle track and form cysts or diverticula within the substance of the brain. These may grow progressively and contribute to the ultimate damage to the brain which results from the hydrocephalus. Successful filling of the ventricles in pneumo-encephalography will afford a direct

demonstration of the presence of communicating hydrocephalus (*Figure 8.23*). Failure to fill the ventricles may be suggestive, but not always conclusive, evidence of an obstructive type. However, when the ventricles fail to fill, the size and position of the pericallosal sulci lying above the corpus callosum may afford reliable evidence of an obstructive hydrocephalus. Normally, these sulci run horizontally and are less than 3 mm deep. In obstructive hydrocephalus, they lie at 45 degrees to the horizontal, are dilated and are more than 3 mm in depth (*Figure 8.24*).

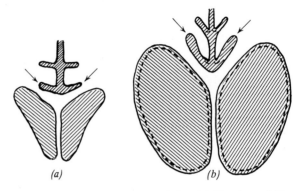

Figure 8.24. Obstructive Hydrocephalus: (a) The size and direction of the pericallosal sulci (arrowed) in the normal child and (b) in hydrocephalus where they are longer and run obliquely at 45 degrees to the vertical

Angiography may also give a characteristic pattern in the presence of hydrocephalus and it avoids the dangers from 'coning' or the risk of reactivating an arrested hydrocephalus. Such a pattern comprises stretching and splaying of the vessels around the dilated ventricles, especially the anterior cerebral and pericallosal arteries, which also lose their normal tortuosity (*Figure 8.25*). In the venous phase, the internal cerebral vein is flattened and the 'venous angle' becomes widened. Apart from the cases of hydrocephalus due to obstruction to cerebrospinal fluid flow by localized lesions such as tumours, and those due to shrinkage of brain substance (compensatory hydrocephalus) which are considered elsewhere, certain forms of primary hydrocephalus have radiological features which may help in their recognition.

OBSTRUCTIVE HYDROCEPHALUS

Occlusion of one foramen of Monro causes hydrocephalus of one lateral ventricle. It is most commonly secondary to cysts or tumours in this region, but may occasionally be due to developmental atresia or intrauterine infection. Such cases show absence of filling of the obstructed ventricle on pneumo-encephalography. Difficulty may be encountered in distinguishing the unobstructed lateral ventricles, which may also be dilated, from a porencephalic cyst or from the single midline ventricle seen in holoprosencephaly (*see* page 305). The position and characteristic shape of the ventricle should be sufficient to prevent such errors in interpretation. The obstructed ventricle may only be filled by direct ventricular puncture

314

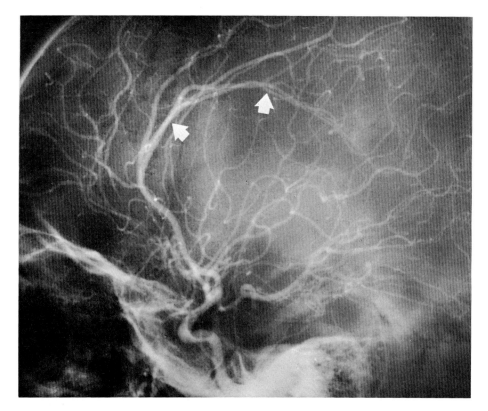

Figure 8.25. Hydrocephalus: Lateral view of the arterial phase of a carotid angiogram, showing displacement and stretching of the anterior cerebral artery (arrowed) by the dilated ventricles. These vessels are straighter than those at a greater distance from the ventricles, which retain their normal tortuosity

and gas may not pass from it into the rest of the ventricular system.

Stenosis of the aqueduct of Sylvius can be congenital or acquired. An unequivocal diagnosis of this condition depends upon a direct demonstration of the site of the block and this may be difficult (*Figure 8.26*). A combination of Myodil introduced into the third ventricle and aqueduct above the stenosis and gas introduced below the block via the lumbar route should be used in order to show not only the site of obstruction but also its type. This may take the form either of a membranous septum or of a longer stenosis. It may, however, not be possible to demonstrate the lower limit of the block if an Arnold—Chiari malformation or basal foraminal obstruction coexists, and this is frequently the case (Schechter and Zingesser, 1967).

Certain signs in the plain skull film, in particular changes in the shape of the pituitary fossa and clinoid processes, are suggestive of aqueduct stenosis (du Boulay and Trickey, 1970). These signs are: shortening of the dorsum sellae, a long steep anterior wall making a right angle with the rest of the sphenoid; and large anterior clinoid processes. On angiography, the basilar artery may be displaced backwards and the posterior communicating arteries stretched and elongated due to a protrusion of the floor of the dilated third ventricle into the cisterna interpeduncularis.

Obstruction of the basal foramina will produce a dilatation of the fourth ventricle known as a Dandy—

Walker cyst. This may fill most of the posterior fossa. The condition is associated with other developmental anomalies of the brain such as agenesis of the corpus callosum, porencephalic cysts and cerebellar defects. There may also be a pattern of congenital defects elsewhere in the body mainly affecting the alimentary tract and genito-urinary system. Dandy—Walker cysts may produce changes in the shape of the posterior fossa. It becomes enlarged and there is bulging of the occiput and widening of the lambdoid sutures. The Torcular Herophili is abnormally high in position and the lateral sinuses run obliquely downwards and outward to form an inverted 'Y' in the antero-posterior view. The average angle between the two lateral sinuses is 110 degrees compared with the normal angle which is 162 degrees. This feature may be detected in plain skull films, but is more strikingly demonstrated by dural sinus venography as seen either in the venous phase of a carotid arteriogram or by direct injection of contrast medium through the anterior fontanelle into the superior longitudinal sinus. Various measurements have been proposed which may help in the differentiation between Dandy—Walker cysts and other types of hydrocephalus, particularly aqueduct stenosis. The ratio of the distance between the nasion and the inion (internal occipital protuberance) and the distance from the inion to the foramen magnum is one of the simplest. This ratio is less than 4 in the Dandy—Walker syndrome and more than 7 in hydrocephalus due to aqueduct stenosis and

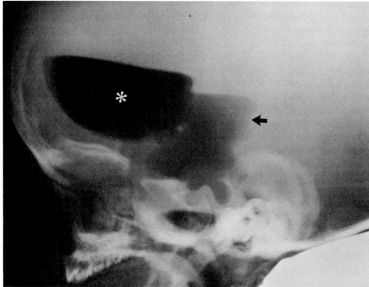

(a)

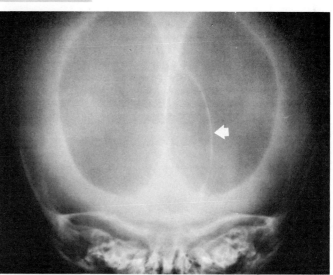

Figure 8.26. Hydrocephalus: (a) Lateral ventriculogram in an infant, performed by injecting gas directly into the lateral ventricles through the open anterior fontanelle. The film is taken with a horizontal beam and with the head inverted. In this position the gas outlines the inferior part of the enormously dilated lateral (*) and third ventricles, (arrowed) but has failed to pass through the aqueduct of Sylvius into the fourth ventricle. (b) Anteroposterior view of the same child in the supine position with the dilated third ventricle (arrowed) lying between, and superimposed on, the lateral ventricles. (c) Positive contrast medium in the third ventricle outlines its posterior part and is obstructed at the upper end of the aqueduct of Sylvius (arrowed). A small quantity of gas outlines the frontal horn of the lateral ventricle (By courtesy of Dr. J. L. G. Thomson, Frenchay Hospital, Bristol)

(b)

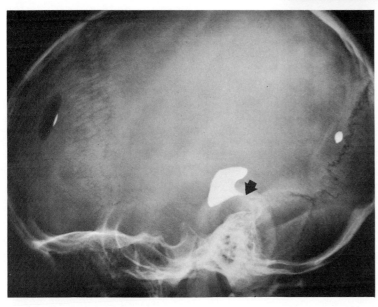

(c)

other supratentorial lesions (Wolpert, 1969) (*Figure 8.27c*). The area of skull lying below a line joining the lambda to the innominate synchondrosis between the exoccipital and supra-occipital bones is very much greater in Dandy–Walker cysts than in normal skulls. These measurements may be particularly helpful in the small infant in whom the grooves produced by the venous sinuses are poorly marked. On pneumo-encephalography, no ventricular filling is obtained. On

ventricular puncture, the large air-filled cavity in the posterior fossa may be readily demonstrated in the inverted lateral projection. It may be seen to extend through the foramen into the cervical part of the spinal canal and the occipital horns of the lateral ventricles are elevated.

In hydrocephalus associated with an *Arnold–Chiari malformation,* as with Dandy–Walker cysts, the ventricles fail to fill on pneumo-encephalography. In this

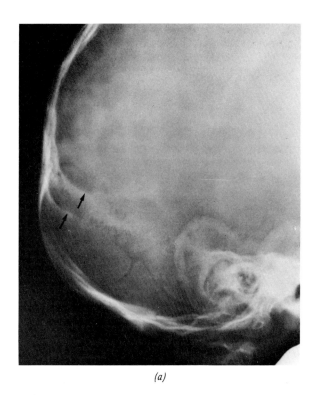

(a)

Figure 8.27. Dandy–Walker Cyst: (a) Plain film of posterior part of the skull. The grooves for the lateral sinuses (arrowed) are elevated and run parallel to the lambdoid sutures. The occipital bone below them bulges posteriorly. (b) A large 'cystic' cavity filled with gas and fluid is present, probably resulting from the rupture of the dilated fourth ventricle into the cisterna magna. The posterior horns of the lateral ventricles (arrowed) are elevated and shortened. (c) Differentiation of a Dandy–Walker cyst from other types of hydrocephalus can be assisted by estimating the ratio between the distances IN and IF, which is smaller in a Dandy–Walker cyst (ii) than in the normal skull (i). The elevation of the internal occipital protuberance (I) and its relation to the lambda (L), the posterior margin of the foramen magnum (F) and the innominate synchondrosis (S) are also shown (see text)

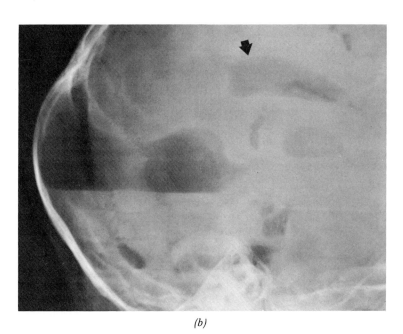

(b)

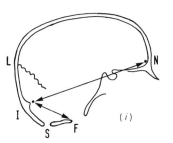

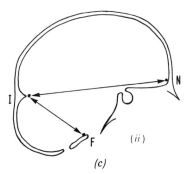

(c)

condition, the posterior fossa is not enlarged and it may even be abnormally small. There may also be an abnormally large foramen magnum and a scalloped outline of the postero-medial aspect of the petrous temporal bone. These features may be shown best in the submento-vertical or basal projection. The upper end of the cervical spine may also show congenital abnormalities. These consist of fusion between the occiput and the atlas and between the upper cervical vertebrae of the type seen in the Klippel–Feil syndrome. The

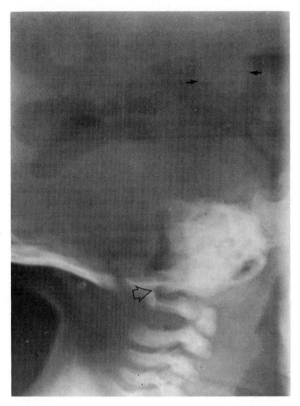

Figure 8.28. Arnold–Chiari Malformation: Ventriculography has filled the dilated third ventricle and lateral ventricles; the massa intermedia of the third ventricle (solid arrows) is abnormally large. The fourth ventricle (outline arrow) is shown to be low in position and to protrude through the foramen magnum into the upper end of the spinal canal. The small poorly marked posterior fossa is also a feature of this condition (By courtesy of Dr. J. L. G. Thomson, Frenchay Hospital, Bristol)

spinal canal in the cervical region may be widened in the anteroposterior diameter and it may exceed 2.2 cm. Craniolacunia, as has been already mentioned, is not infrequent in this type of hydrocephalus. The frequency of hydrocephalus in association with Arnold–Chiari malformation is about 75 per cent in cases of lumbar meningocele, but less frequent in meningoceles elsewhere in the spine. The size of the cranial vault in over a third of such cases is normal in spite of a demonstrable hydrocephalus (Lorber, 1961b).

Ventriculography has also been reported to show characteristic features in this type of hydrocephalus. These consist of an abnormally low position of the 4th ventricle and a consequent elongation of the aqueduct of Sylvius (*Figure 8.28*). The third ventricle may also be abnormal in a high proportion of cases. The commonest abnormality is a forward projection of its anterior end, forming a diverticulum above and separate from the anterior recess. There is also a large massa intermedia.

Demonstration of the abnormal medulla and cervical spinal cord by myelography may be readily achieved provided the patient is examined supine. A bilobed filling defect in the upper cervical region due to the herniated cerebellar tonsils is present; the cervical nerve roots run obliquely upwards and a widening of the upper cervical region of the spinal cord may also be shown. It has been stated that this is the most useful method for demonstrating the nature and severity of the malformation. Vertebral arteriography may also show a characteristic downward displacement of the vertebral, basilar and posterior inferior cerebellar arteries.

COMMUNICATING HYDROCEPHALUS

As has already been pointed out, the communicating type of hydrocephalus may be readily distinguished from the obstructive type by pneumo-encephalography (*Figure 8.23*). When hydrocephalus is due to an absorptive defect in the region of the superior longitudinal sinus, it is associated with widening of the subarachnoid space. As long as the cerebrospinal fluid pressure remains high the diagnosis is not difficult. It has recently been emphasized that these cases may attain a state of equilibrium, and that the intracranial pressure becomes normal. In this event the radiological appearances are indistinguishable from cerebral atrophy with an associated compensatory hydrocephalus. The distinction is however an important one, because such a 'low pressure' type of hydrocephalus may lead to disabling symptoms, such as loss of memory, ataxia, mental and emotional disturbances, which could be confused with cerebral degeneration or frontal lobe lesions; they may, however, be relieved by ventricular shunting procedures. It has been suggested that a disproportionate widening of the basal cisterns, the pericallosal sulci and interhemispheric and Sylvian fissures compared with the rest of the subarachnoid space is a helpful feature. This favours a communicating hydrocephalus and not cerebral atrophy. Convexity of the upper border of the fourth ventricle and an increase in the size of the anterior horns of the lateral ventricles are also suggestive of communicating hydrocephalus. Nevertheless, the distinction may often be difficult and the diagnosis of cerebral atrophy in young children should be made with caution, particularly where widening of the subarachnoid space over the hemispheres is the predominant feature ('external hydrocephalus'). Such findings may disappear in subsequent examinations and be associated with normal mental development (Lehrer, 1968).

Effects of treatment

The treatment of hydrocephalus consists predominantly in the creation of an artificial shunt by which the cerebrospinal fluid is drained from the ventricles to some other part of the body where it can be absorbed. This is usually into the venous side of the heart. The efficient

318

function of such shunts depends to a great extent upon correct placement of the catheters and upon the maintenance of their patency and integrity. Radiology may play a useful part in demonstrating the position of both ends of the catheter and in detecting breakages. In cases in whom the shunt is blocked, the site of the obstruction can be determined by injection of aqueous contrast medium into the valve barrel with a fine needle. Failure of the shunt may result in a recurrence of the signs of raised intracranial pressure. Chest radiography may also be of use when heart failure and pulmonary oedema have resulted from overloading of the circulation or when pulmonary emboli are produced as a result of thrombosis around the end of the atrial catheter.

Rapid decompression of the hydrocephalus may also lead to changes in the bones of the skull, or to subdural or extradural haematoma from rupture of bridging veins between the outer surface of the hemisphere and the meninges. Thickening of the bones of the vault may be seen in radiographs of the skull and may occur either directly as a result of the reduction in intracranial pressure (hyperostosis *ex vacuo*) analogous to that seen in cerebral atrophy, or as a result of ossification within an extradural haematoma (*Figure 8.29a*). A reduction in the size of the pituitary fossa and of the basal foramina has also been reported, and these are reversible if the shunt is removed. A complication which is not reversible and which may be potentially serious in its results is craniostenosis. This may supervene within a few months of a shunt procedure and may

lead to a relative reduction in the cranial capacity below the normal range for the child's age. There is a consequent liability to compression of the brain or at the least to an unsightly abnormality in the shape of the head. Fortunately this is a rare sequel to shunt operations, and it is stated by various authors to occur in from 0.5 to 3 per cent; it appears to be commoner where a low pressure type of valve has been used. The shape of the head resulting from the fusion of the sutures may be different from that produced by the congenital types of craniostenosis. The skull may be tall and narrow due to a reduction in the width of the vault, which can be fairly easily recognized in the anteroposterior projection (*Figure 8.29b*).

CYSTS AND TUMOURS

GENERAL CONSIDERATIONS

Space-occupying lesions within the skull or the spinal canal, if large enough, will produce radiographic signs by virtue of the increase of pressure which they cause, acting on the bony envelope which surrounds the brain and spinal cord. Such signs are well recognized, particularly in the case of the skull, but it should be emphasized that in children they may be absent or may differ in some respects from those which are present in adults. Thus it has been estimated that 46 per cent of children with cerebral tumours have normal skull films

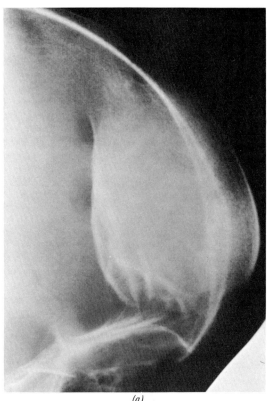

(a)

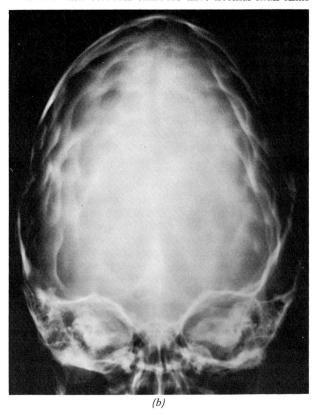

(b)

Figure 8.29. Changes in the Skull following Shunt Procedures for Hydrocephalus: (a) Hyperostosis thought to have resulted from ossification of a frontal subdural haematoma. There is also thickening of the bone externally. (b) Craniostenosis with fusion of the sagittal and lambdoid sutures. The shape of the cranial vault is abnormal due to a reduction in width and an increase in height. 'Convolutional markings' are indicative of an increase in intracranial pressure when they first present but this observation should never discourage further radiological investigations if the clinical signs and symptoms are suggestive (Grossman *et al.,* 1971). Below the age of 10 years, sutural separation of more than 2 mm is a valuable and early sign of increased intracranial pressure and it may be the only sign for a considerable period (*Figure 8.30c*). After the age of 10 years, it is later in appearing, occurs from 6 to 16 months after the onset of symptoms and is preceded by sellar changes (*Figure 8.30b*). These sellar changes may occur at any age, but below the age of 10 years are almost never seen as the sole finding, unless they are due to a local lesion such as a craniopharyngioma or glioma of the optic chiasma. Indentations on the inner vault (convolutional markings, beaten silver appearance) are an unreliable sign, unless they are gross and accompanied by other signs. They are common in normal children, particularly between the ages of 4 and 9 years. They are more likely to be significant, however, when they occur in the frontal and parietal regions than when they are present in the occipital or temporal areas (*Figure 8.30a*). The absence of such markings is perhaps a more valuable indication of abnormality, and this is frequently the case in cerebral atrophy (*see Figure 8.11*).

ARACHNOID CYSTS

These are commonly congenital in origin, though sometimes they may follow previous infection, injury or haemorrhage. They have also been described in association with the Hurler and Scheie types of mucopolysaccharidosis (*see* pages 5 and 7). Their course is that of a slowly growing space-occupying lesion and their early recognition is important. If untreated, they may lead to irreversible mental and neurological changes which arise from pressure on the brain or spinal cord. Localized asymmetry of the vault with local bulging and thinning of the bone over the site of the lesion, especially when this is over the convexity of the cerebral hemispheres, are suggestive changes which may be detected on plain skull films. Elevation, or erosion, of the lesser wing of the sphenoid and separation of the anterior clinoid processes may also occur. In addition, there may be unspecific signs of increased intracranial pressure. Pneumo-encephalography may show dilatation or displacement of the ventricles, especially in those cysts occurring in the paracollicular region or in the cisterna ambiens. As a rule, gas will not enter the cyst itself, but in the rare cases in whom it does so, the appearances may be diagnostic. Angiography may delineate the cyst by outlining the vessels displaced around it, appearances similar to those seen in slow-growing tumours or subdural effusions. Spinal arachnoid cysts may be outlined on myelography but they are difficult to distinguish from tumours.

INTRACRANIAL TUMOURS

Information as to the site, the size and the nature of intracranial tumours may be afforded by plain skull films, air studies, angiography, scintiscanning after the injection of radioisotopes and computerized axial tomography. These different methods of investigation should be regarded as complementary to each other, though some are likely to be particularly useful in certain types of tumour. The fact that about 60 per cent of all intracranial tumours in children are infratentorial makes it desirable that vertebral as well as carotid angiograms are performed (*Figures 8.31* and *8.32*). On the other hand, owing to the proximity of many such tumours to the cerebrospinal fluid pathways, signs of increased intracranial pressure may occur early and such evidence on the plain films may, in conjunction with the length of the history, give some indication as to the probable site of the tumour. Calcification is not very common, occurring in only 15 per cent of a series described by Grossman *et al.* (1971), but when it is present it may be a valuable indication as to the site and probable nature of the lesion. Thus, ependymoma may not uncommonly calcify and the calcification is characteristically dense. The presence of localized enostosis in the neighbourhood of meningiomas, and of prominent vascular channels in the cranial vault are well recognized signs in the plain skull film in both meningioma and haemangioma. The presence of marked sutural diastasis in intracranial neuroblastoma is a well established radiological sign. It has been suggested recently that this is due, not to the effects of increased intracranial pressure, but to direct extension of tumour into the suture itself. These lesions are known to have a tendency to extend in plaques between the inner table and the dura and they seldom occur deep to the meninges.

The radiological features of tumours in certain sites may be characteristic and these are therefore reviewed separately below.

Brain stem tumours

Diagnosis of this group of tumours may be difficult, because obstruction to cerebrospinal fluid flow is late and the clinical picture may suggest encephalitis, demyelinating diseases or vascular lesions. Plain skull films are relatively unhelpful; they may only show signs of raised intracranial pressure and these do not occur if the tumour is in the early stages of development. A combination of lumbar pneumo-encaphalography and positive contrast ventriculography is most likely to be of use because they will demonstrate the position and shape of the fourth ventricle, of the aqueduct and the pontine and interpeduncular cisterns and these are crucial signs. Displacement backwards or to one side of the midline is the usual finding (*Figure 8.33*). Vertebral angiograms alone, while often abnormal, are not usually diagnostic. Isotope scanning is unhelpful, because the tumour uptake is obscured by background activity from other structures in the neck and face.

Cerebellar tumours

Certain signs shown on plain films of the skull may be of assistance in distinguishing between the relatively benign cerebellar astrocytoma and the malignant cerebellar medulloblastoma. The former tumour, being slow-growing, tends to produce the following signs:

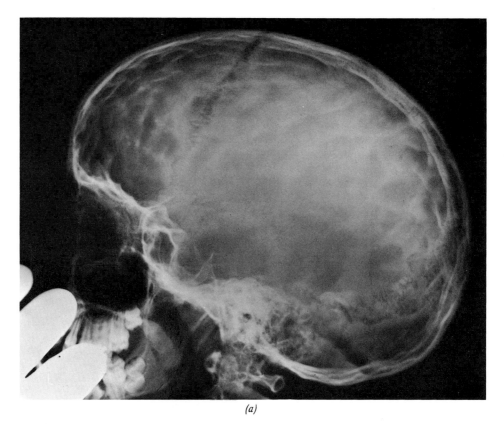

(a)

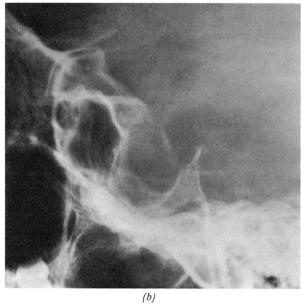

(b)

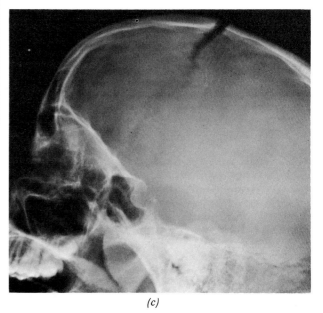

(c)

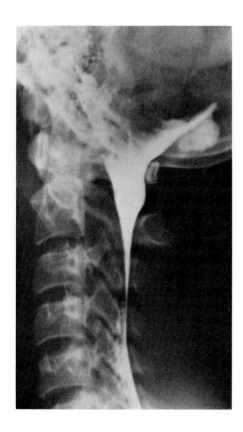

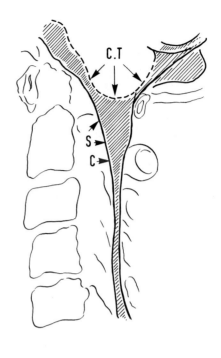

(d)

Figure 8.30. Increased Intracranial Pressure: (a) Sutural separation, increased convolutional markings and sellar changes in a child with obstructive hydrocephalus. (b) Localized view of the pituitary fossa in the same case as in (a). There is increase in all the dimensions of the fossa with destruction of the upper end of the dorsum sellae which is pointed rather than rounded in shape. The floor of the sella is depressed unequally on the two sides, giving rise to a double contour. (c) Sutural separation as the only sign of increased intracranial pressure. Enlarged adenoids are present within the nasopharynx, narrowing the airway. (d) A lateral myelogram with contrast medium in the region of the foramen magnum and cisterna magna, but obstructed anteriorly by the downward displacement of the medulla and cerebellum ('coning') (arrowed). CT—Cerebellar tonsils; SC—spinal cord. (e) Anteroposterior view of same case as in (d) showing the cerebellar 'tonsils' (arrowed) outlined by the contrast medium below them. These have been displaced downwards through the foramen magnum by the increased pressure within the skull ('coning')

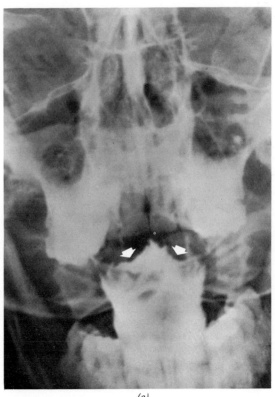

(e)

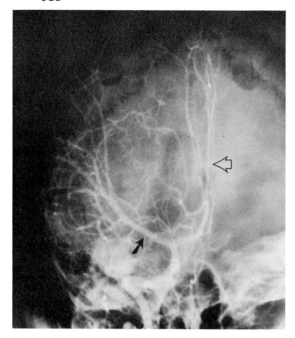 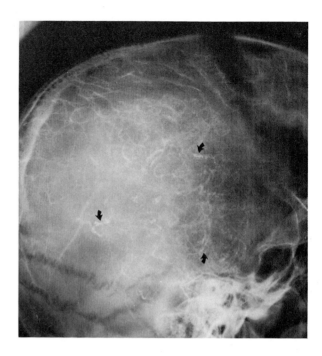

Figure 8.31. Angiographic Signs of Cerebral Tumour: In addition to displacement of major vessels by the expanding tumour, the smaller vessels supplying the tumour are abnormal. They are increased in number, excessively tortuous and of irregular calibre with local widening and narrowing. An overall increase in opacity may be present due to contrast medium in very small vessels ('tumour blush'). Carotid arteriogram: (a) Anteroposterior view. Elevation and straightening of the middle cerebral artery (solid arrow) and displacement of the anterior cerebral artery (outline arrow) across the midline by a glioma of the right cerebral hemisphere (compare with Figure 8.4). (b) Lateral view of same case. Contrast medium in the smaller arteries and capillaries within the tumour (arrowed)

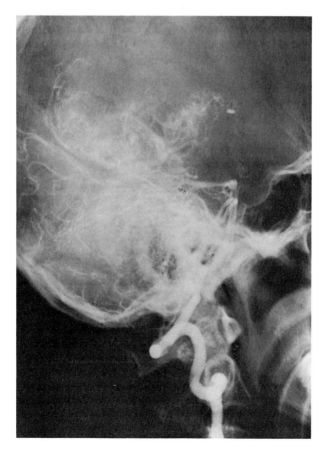

sutural diastasis, erosion of parts of the sella, enlargement of occipital emissary veins, lateral displacement of the jugular tubercles seen in the submentovertical projections and a basi-occipital concavity such that the clivus no longer forms a straight line. These changes do not appear in the case of medulloblastoma because the rapid growth of the tumour does not allow sufficient time for them to develop.

Parasellar and hypothalmic tumours

These are relatively common in comparison with other types of supratentorial tumour in childhood, and they may fail to give a diagnostic clinical picture. Radiology may therefore be of importance in the investigation of such lesions. Signs of increased intracranial pressure are not uncommon, and they are not specific. Changes in the region of the pituitary fossa, however, may reflect the presence of hydrocephalus in which case the signs consist of a generalized enlargement of the whole sella, with or without erosion of the dorsum sellae and lamina dura. On the other hand they may be due to the direct action of the expanding tumour, and intrasellar tumours of pituitary origin will cause 'ballooning' of the sella with erosion of the lamina dura. Gliomas of the optic

Figure 8.32. Tumour of Pineal Gland: Vertical angiogram demonstrating abnormal vessels and a 'tumour blush' (By courtesy of Dr. J. L. G. Thomson, Frenchay Hospital, Bristol)

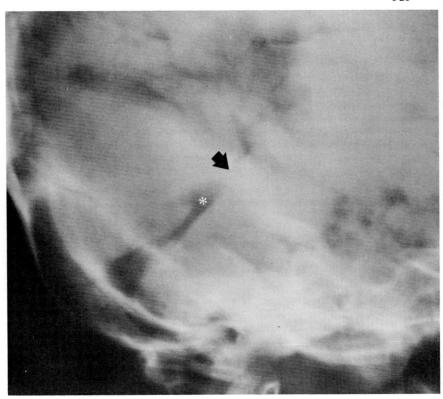

Figure 8.33. Brain Stem Tumours: 'Autotomogram' in which the fourth ventricle (*) and the aqueduct of Sylvius (arrowed) are shown to be dilated and displayed posteriorly by a tumour lying anteriorly in the brain stem. This technique enables the midline structures to be maintained 'in focus' while those lying laterally are blurred by rotation of the head around its central axis (By courtesy of Dr. J. L. G. Thomson, Frenchay Hospital, Bristol)

nerve or chiasma produce enlargement of the optic foramen on the affected side (*Figure 8.34b*) or of the chiasmatic sulcus, and the under-surface of the anterior clinoid processes is thinned and elevated (*Figure 8.34a*). Local bone sclerosis affecting the medial wall of the orbit or the lesser wing of the sphenoid is seen in meningiomata. Calcification is a common feature of craniopharyngioma and it may be variable in type, (*Figure 8.35*). Calcification may be more useful in indicating the size of the lesion than in detemining its exact nature, and this applies to many of the signs shown in plain skull films. Air studies should reveal the presence of the tumour mass in all cases, but pneumo-encephalography is often more valuable than ventriculography. This is because there is displacement and invasion of the aqueduct and third ventricle and there is also obliteration of the interpeduncular and suprachiasmatic cisterns (*Figure 8.36*). The third ventricle is commonly displaced upwards, but in meningiomas it may be pushed backwards and downwards. Displacement and indentation of the frontal and temporal horns of the lateral ventricles may also occur. On angiography the carotid siphon is opened out and the origin of the anterior and middle cerebral arteries elevated. A tumour circulation may sometimes be detected. Differentiation of these tumours from other causes of hydrocephalus is important and it is essential to exclude them before shunt procedures are undertaken.

Owing to their proximity to the hypothalamus and pituitary, these tumours may sometimes give rise to a highly characteristic illness in small infants, which is known as the *diencephalic syndrome* (*Figure 8.36*). The child fails to thrive and indeed may become severely emaciated in spite of a voracious appetite. In addition to the local signs of the tumour as enumerated above, x-rays of the limbs may reveal a striking loss of subcutaneous fat layers which may be confirmed by measurements of body tissue thickness (*see* page 360). Some tumours in this region may stimulate body growth and lead to sexual and skeletal precocity similar to that of the idiopathic form of cerebral gigantism (Soto's syndrome). In such cases skeletal maturation is accelerated.

Tumours of the choroid plexus

These tumours are not common; they present in childhood and are often curable. In addition to the signs of increased intracranial pressure common to other types of tumour, their intraventricular site ensures that they are visible as an irregular polypoid filling defect within the lumen of the ventricle on pneumo-encephalography. Those tumours that are pedunculated may be very mobile; they may therefore be overlooked if insufficient gas is used, because they fall to the lowest part of the ventricle. The hydrocephalus associated with these tumours is not always obstructive, but it may be of a communicating type, possibly due to overproduction of cerebrospinal fluid. In tumours of the lateral ventricles, the ventricle containing the lesion tends to be larger than the one on the other side. Dilated portions of the ventricle adjacent to the tumour may be confused with porencephalic cysts. Positive contrast ventriculography may sometimes be helpful in confirming the

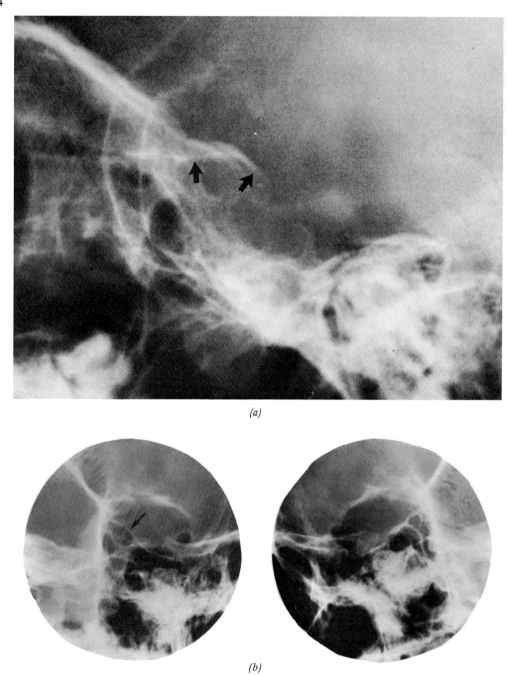

(a)

(b)

Figure 8.34. Glioma of Optic Chiasma: (a) Enlargement of the pituitary fossa with elevation and excavation of the under-surface of the anterior clinoid processes (arrowed). (b) Enlargement of the right optic foramen (arrowed) as compared with the normal left side

intraventricular site of tumours near the floor of the fourth ventricle. Calcification may occur in choroid plexus tumours, especially in ependymomas, which are common in childhood. It may also occur in papillomas situated in the temporal horns where it may resemble a calcified cast of this part of the ventricle. The area of calcification may also be displaced when the head is moved into different positions. It is difficult to differentiate a tumour from simple enlargement of the choroid plexus but these tumours do not present until significant hydrocephalus occurs and this is never seen in the case of simple hypertrophy. Difficulty in establishing the intraventricular site of the lesion may cause confusion with paraventricular gliomas or ependymomas and with tuberose sclerosis, which also project into the ventricular lumen. However, the radiological appearances may be more reliable than the clinical picture (Crofton and Matson, 1960).

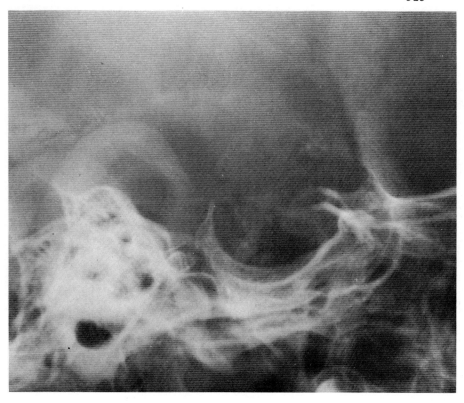

Figure 8.35. Craniopharyngioma: Enlargement of the pituitary fossa, especially in length, with restriction of the posterior clinoid processes and shortening of the dorsum sellae but without elevation of the anterior clinoid process. The cyst lying above the pituitary fossa is outlined by faint calcification within it (by courtesy of Dr. J. L. G. Thomson, Frenchay Hospital, Bristol)

Paraventricular and midline tumours

These form another group in which the clinical signs and symptoms are ill defined but which may give striking appearances on pneumo-encephalography or ventriculography. Of the tumours of the basal ganglia, those

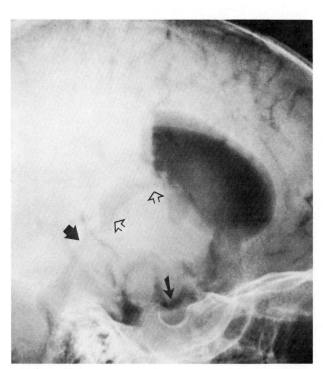

arising in the thalamus cause a crescentic deformity and displacement of the third ventricle. Pinealomas may be calcified and project into the suprapineal recess. Tumours of the septum pellucidum and corpus callosum separate the two lateral ventricles from each other and obliterate the upper part of the third ventricle (*Figure 8.37a*). The former are distinguished from midline cysts by their more irregular outline and by the fact that they never contain gas. Lipoma of the corpus callosum gives a highly characteristic appearance due to the translucency caused by the fat content and by a symmetrical crescentic calcification lying in the midline (*Figure 8.37b*). Other types of tumour may, however, occur in this site, including gliomas, angiomas and ependymomas, and these may be less diagnostic in their appearance.

SPINAL TUMOURS

Neoplasm of the spinal cord or nerve roots are lesions which it is important to diagnose early if successful treatment is to be undertaken. They are less common than intracranial tumours. Two-thirds of spinal tumours show evidence of their presence on plain films of the

Figure 8.36. Hypothalmic Tumour: Part of the third ventricle is obliterated by the tumour extending upwards from its base. The curved outline of the tumour (open arrows) is shown by the air in the rest of the ventricle. The aqueduct of Sylvius (thick black arrow) is displaced backwards and much of the interpedicular and chiasmatic cisterns obliterated by the tumour (thin black arrow). This child was severely wasted in spite of an apparently adequate intake of food and therefore was an example of the 'diencephalic syndrome'

326

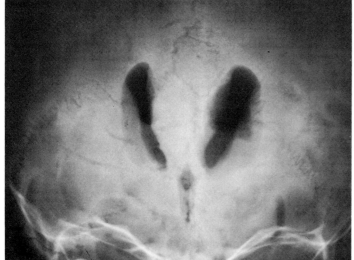

Figure 8.37. Midline Tumours: (a) A glioma of the septum pellucidum which separates the two lateral ventricles from each other. The third ventricle is in its normal position in distinction from agenesis of the corpus callosum, the appearance of which it may otherwise resemble (see Figure 8.14). (b) A lipoma of corpus callosum showing a thin rim of calcification surrounding a more translucent central portion containing fat (By courtesy of Dr. J. L. G. Thomson, Frenchay Hospital, Bristol)

spine, but the appearances are often relatively inconspicuous. They may easily be missed if not carefully looked for on adequate films of the whole spine. Erosion, demineralization or destruction of the pedicles, vertebral bodies, laminae and posterior ends of ribs afford the most direct evidence of the presence of a tumour but

these signs are often relatively late in appearance. Localized widening of the spinal canal as shown not only by increased interpedicular distances, but also by an increased anteroposterior diameter of the spinal canal (*Figure 8.38*), is a very important early sign, which may be difficult to detect without careful measurements

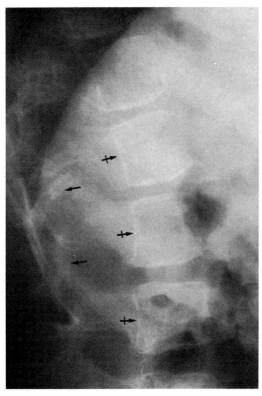

Figure 8.38. Intramedullary Tumour of Spinal Cord: (a) Plain film of the spine showing enlargement of the spinal canal (both types of arrows) in its anteroposterior diameter with scalloping of the posterior surfaces of the vertebral bodies (crossed arrows) (b) Myelogram showing the expanded spinal cord filling most of the theca and a number of tortuous vessels on the surface of the cord. The narrowing of the pedicles and the increase in the interpedicular distances in the region of the tumour are also well shown (By courtesy of Dr. J.L.G. Thomson, Frenchay Hospital, Bristol)

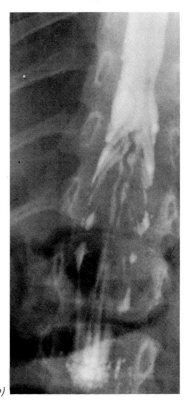

(*see* page 352). Calcification within the tumour itself and in a paravertebral soft tissue mass are also helpful signs. A localized deformity, either kyphoscoliosis or loss of the normal cervical or lumbar lordosis, may also sometimes point to the presence of a spinal tumour, as can the presence of spina bifida or other congenital anomalies. These latter features are non-specific and of little use unless accompanied by other signs. In any case in which the presence of a spinal tumour is suspected, either from the above radiological signs or on clinical grounds, myelography is essential to delineate the tumour itself and to determine its exact upper and lower limits (*Figure 8.38*). If a spinal block is present, injection of the contrast medium by cisternal puncture as well as by the lumbar route will be required. A repeat examination may be needed, if the evidence is equivocal. There is not considered to be any particular contraindication to this procedure. Spinal arteriography may also be useful in cases of vascular tumours, in whom not only may the tumour itself be shown, but the number and site of the arteries which supply the tumour and of the veins which drain it may be determined.

Spinal tumours may be mistaken for conditions such as poliomyelitis, cerebral palsy, torticollis and idiopathic scoliosis, largely because the possibility is not considered and myelography is therefore not undertaken. Other space-occupying lesions within the spinal canal may also give rise to difficulty. Among these should be mentioned syringomyelia, which may cause spinal block and resemble an intramedullary tumour, because of the dilatation of the central cystic space within the cord. A helpful feature, however, is the length of the dilated segment which may involve most of the length of the spinal cord leading to a very long gap between the upper and lower limits of the lesion. Spinal epidural haematomas have also been recently reported in infants. In these cases plain films are normal but there is evidence of a relative spinal block on myelography due to an extradural mass extending over a relatively long segment of the spine. The possible importance of such lesions has been emphasized by the suggestion that they could be responsible for a proportion of cot deaths.

TUBEROSE SCLEROSIS

Although this disease is genetically determined and is generalized in its effects throughout the body, involvement of the brain is of particular interest from a radiological standpoint. Furthermore, in cases when the clinical aspects are atypical the radiological features of the intracranial lesions may confirm the diagnosis. These lesions are not true tumours; they are commonly regarded as of a hamartomatous nature, but in spite of this it is convenient to refer to them in this section, because their appearance, particularly on encephalography may require to be distinguished from subependymal neoplasms.

In the plain skull film, calcification may be seen. It is found in 58 per cent of a large series of cases from the Mayo Clinic (Lagos *et al.*, 1968). The calcification, which is often bilateral, almost always occurs in the form of scattered discrete opacities, predominantly in the region of the basal ganglia and around the ventricles. It also occurs in the subcortical white matter. It should be emphasized that the presence and extent of the intracranial calcification has no necessary correlation with the degree of mental retardation which may be present,

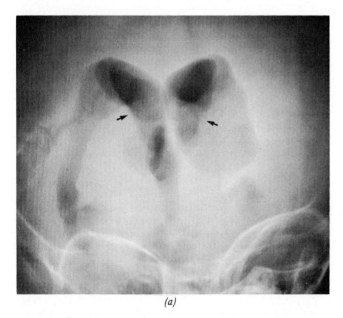

(a)

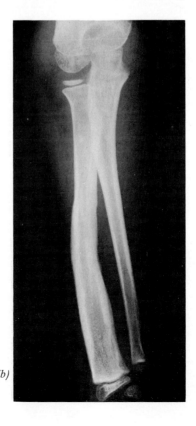

(b)

Figure 8.39. Tuberose sclerosis: (a) Anteroposterior pneumo-encephalogram taken in the supine position showing irregularity of the walls of the lateral ventricles due to subependymal masses projecting into the ventricular cavities ('candle guttering') (arrowed). (b) Cortical thickening of the shafts of the radius and the proximal parts of the ulna of another boy with tuberose sclerosis

and it is stated that 44 per cent of patients with the disease are of normal intelligence. On pneumo-encephalography, the lesions of tuberose sclerosis may be demonstrated because they are largely subependymal in situation (*Figure 8.39a*). They project into the lumen, especially from the walls of the lateral ventricles, as a nodularity described as 'candle guttering' from its resemblance to the melted wax solidifying down the side of a candle. Only 18 per cent of the Mayo Clinic cases showed this feature, but it has been suggested that it may be much more frequent than this in young children with the disease. Indeed it has been demonstrated as the sole finding which was suggestive of the diagnosis in an infant who presented with infantile spasms of the type associated with hypsarrhythmia, and who later developed the characteristic skin changes. Sometimes the lesions may obstruct the cerebrospinal fluid pathways and lead to hydrocephalus with signs of increased intracranial pressure in the plain film. Alternatively, the ventricles may be dilated due to cerebral atrophy.

For the sake of completeness, the other radiological features of this protean disease will be reviewed here, though they do not form part of the radiology of the nervous system. Areas of localized bone sclerosis may occur, often round or oval in shape, or sometimes irregular and flame-shaped. They vary from a few millimetres to a centimetre or more in diameter and may resemble osteopoikile, but they are larger and less numerous than in the latter condition. They tend to occur predominantly in flat bones such as the pelvis and vault of the skull, but may occur in vertebrae. In the cranial vault they may be confused with the intracranial calcification described above, but they never occur in such young children. Localized cortical thickening of the long bones (*Figure 8.39b*) and punched-out cystic erosions of the cortex of the metacarpals and metatarsals are also features which have occasionally been described in children. Rhabdomyomatous lesions of the heart may produce a localized deformity or protuberances of the heart outline. A reticular pattern of linear opacities in the lungs, resembling 'honeycomb lung', or miliary nodulation are features found in the chest films of cases of long-standing tuberose sclerosis; they are in consequence more often seen in adults than in children with the condition. Finally, involvement of the kidneys may lead to distortion and displacement of th renal pelves and calyces on urography, the appearances resembling those of polycystic disease, but they are more irregular and ill defined, with less elongation of the calyceal necks than in the latter condition.

TRAUMATIC LESIONS

HEAD INJURIES

Fractures of the skull are important mainly because of the associated injury to the brain which is likely to accompany them, and do not often require treatment in their own right. It is therefore proposed to discuss the radiological aspects in this section.

Indications for radiological examination

Considerable diversity of opinion is expressed on the question of whether all cases of head injury in children should have a skull x-ray to exclude a fracture and when this should be carried out. In many cases this is done largely for medico-legal reasons to obviate a possible charge of negligence, especially if complications should ensue at a later date. It is of interest, therefore, that it can be shown that there is little or no correlation between the presence of a skull fracture and the liability to develop serious sequelae. These are equally likely to occur whether a fracture is present or not. Indeed, it may plausibly be argued that, if no fracture is present on the x-ray, a false sense of security is induced, and this may prevent the adoption of adequate treatment for the head injury. When cerebral damage is present, the effect of this may be more serious if there is no fracture, because decompression of the associated raised intracranial pressure is not then possible. Therefore, a negative skull x-ray should never be a criterion for determining the line of treatment. This should always be assessed on clinical grounds. It follows that there are few occasions when radiological examination need be carried out as an emergency and it is often found that better results are obtained after the patient has been allowed to recover from the immediate effects of the injury.

The indications for a skull x-ray may be enumerated as follows (Burkinshaw, 1960):

(1) To obtain evidence that the head has been injured when no external signs are present.

(2) To confirm a clinical suspicion of a depressed fracture.

(3) When immediate surgical treatment is required, to determine the exact site and extent of the injury, particularly in relation to the known site of major blood vessels that may be involved.

Radiological features

The diagnosis of fractures of the skull may be a matter of some difficulty, especially in the newborn or very young infant. At this age they are usually simple linear fractures. These can be confused with normal variants in the ossification of the bones of the vault, with sutures, such as the metopic or mendozal, which normally fuse early and with sutures or fissures which are only present in a small proportion of normal individuals. The latter are particularly liable to cause confusion in the parietal region where independent interparietal bones occur in 10 per cent of normal infants and radial fissures are often present at the margins of the parietal bone. Fractures of the parietal bones usually run from the margin towards the centre of the bone and those of the frontal bones towards the supra-orbital ridges. The majority are either in the midline or extend to either side of the midline. Depressed fractures, if not radiographed tangentially, may be confusing because they may appear as lines of increased density (*Figure 8.40*). In the newborn, the vault may be depressed without actually being fractured. This may occur in the 'ping-pong ball' type of injury where the head is compressed against the sacral promontory or ischial spines during delivery. Other

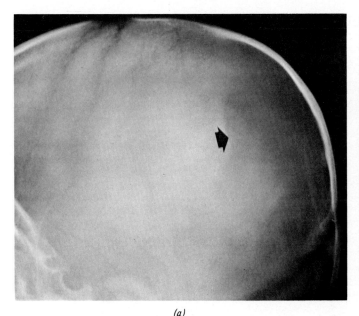
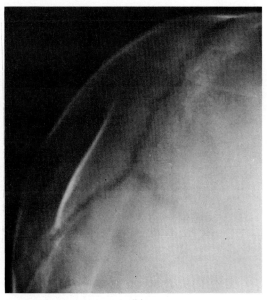

(a)   (b)

Figure 8.40. Depressed Fracture of Cranial Vault: (a) Lateral view of skull in which the fracture line is not clearly visible, but where the depressed fragment appears 'en face' as an area of translucency (arrowed). (b) Tangential view of the same case in which the depressed fragment is shown 'end-on' as a linear density (By courtesy of Dr. J. L. G. Thomson, Frenchay Hospital, Bristol)

sources of confusing translucencies are vascular channels and 'ripple marks' due to folds in the loosely attached tissues of the scalp in the newborn infant (*see Figure 8.1a*).

While overlooking a fracture may have serious consequences, it is arguable that these may be less unfortunate than diagnosing a fracture which is not present. The latter may have emotional and legal sequelae, especially when there is suspicion that the injury may be part of a 'battered baby' syndrome, or it may lead to unnecessary surgery. In cases of serious doubt, further observation may help to resolve the difficulty in the light of the child's progress.

Cephalhaematoma

This condition in the newborn infant is accompanied by a fracture in 25 per cent of cases and it may be a helpful additional sign in determining whether a translucent line in the cranial vault is significant. In most cases cephalhaematomas resolve without sequelae, but occasionally they may develop calcification which becomes incorporated into the underlying bones as an area of sclerosis or a protuberance which persists for several months. Infection of a cephalhaematoma occasionally leads to osteomyelitis, though this may be difficult to distinguish from local osteoporosis beneath a haematoma which is being absorbed.

Fractures of the base of the skull

These are difficult to detect without special projections and tomography. They may be of considerable importance because of the possibility of spread of infection from the sinuses or middle ear and of damage to cranial nerves or the auditory and vestibular organs. Air within the cranial cavity following an injury may be a valuable indirect sign, indicative of a fracture involving the sinuses or air cells. It is also important to detect fractures of the orbits and facial bones, because they may be associated with damage to the eyes or olfactory apparatus and lead to serious disfigurement. Fractures of the orbital floor may give rise to a soft tissue mass protruding into the antrum from the region of the fracture in its roof.

Growing skull fracture

Fractures of the skull often take a long time to heal completely. In some cases, the fracture line, so far from becoming less obvious, actually becomes wider during subsequent months and such cases may present later on with an extensive defect in the cranial vault. The frequency with which this occurs is estimated to be about 4 per cent, but this may be higher if only those cases in whom the injury occurred before the age of 3 years are included. The edges of such defects are often everted and the remains of the original fracture line may frequently be seen extending from the edge of the defect (*Figure 8.41*). Such 'growing skull fractures' are of importance because they imply that there is an area of unprotected brain beneath the defect. It is also likely that the original injury was severe and that it was associated with brain damage extensive enough to lead to fits or hemiplegia. There is usually some initial diastasis of the fracture and a tear in the dura beneath it is a constant feature. This allows the leptomeninges to herniate through the dural tear and to transmit the pulsations of the cerebrospinal fluid to the skull, which is then progressively eroded. The extent of the brain damage in such cases may be assessed by the demonstration of local cerebral atrophy or of porencephalic cysts on pneumo-encephalography.

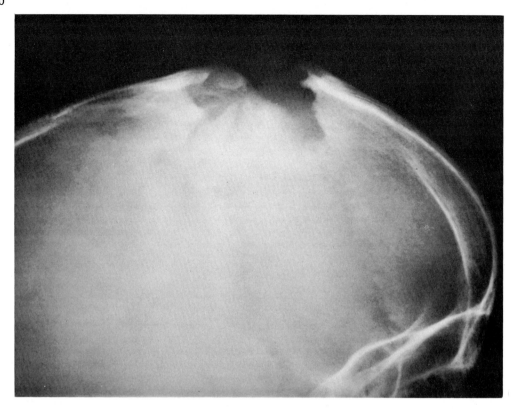

Figure 8.41. Growing Skull Fracture: The skull of a child who has sustained a fracture of the vault some years previously. The defect at the fracture site has resulted from the pulsations of the cerebrospinal fluid in the subarachnoid space being transmitted through a tear in the dura and exerting an erosive effect on the margins of the fracture (By courtesy of Dr. J. L. G. Thomson, Frenchay Hospital, Bristol)

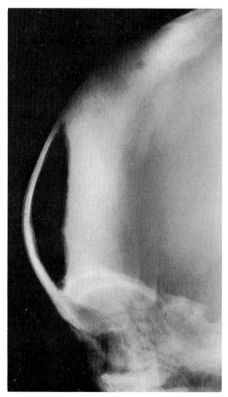

(a)

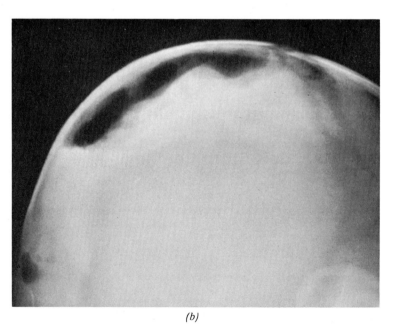

(b)

Figure 8.42. Subdural Effusion: The extent of a subdural effusion can be shown by the injection of air at a subdural tap, films being taken in different positions to allow the air to outline the anterior and posterior limits of the cavity. (a) Supine lateral with the air over the frontal pole of the hemisphere. (b) Prone lateral with the air overlying the parietal lobe

SUBDURAL HAEMATOMA AND EFFUSION

In the acute stages, these lesions present with a distinctive clinical picture and their existence may be confirmed by subdural puncture via the anterior fontanelle. Gas may be injected at the time of the puncture in order to outline the cavity and to determine its size and extent (*Figure 8.42*). It has been suggested that isotope studies following the injection of radioiodinated serum albumen into the subdural space may be a better method of doing this because it will diffuse throughout the whole extent of the effusion. It is particularly helpful in differentiating between the smaller unilateral effusions in which the result of treatment is good, and the large bilateral communicating type associated with severe brain damage in which the prognosis is worse. Plain skull films will often show evidence of the presence of subdural haematomas, in the form of sutural diastasis or an increase in the size of the cranial vault. Cerebral arteriography, however, is the most generally useful technique for demonstrating the lesion, especially in cases presenting after the fontanelle has closed. On angiography an 'avascular' area is shown which separates the inner table from the outer limit of the hemisphere. A diffuse area of opacification may also sometimes be present, and this is due to the presence of a layer of compressed brain tissue beneath a large haematoma or effusion. This latter feature is said to occur in about a third of cases, usually with frontal or parietal effusions and it indicates the likelihood of brain damage (Leeds

et al., 1968). Calcification in a subdural haematoma is a relatively late finding. It occurs usually as an oval cystic area with calcification in its margins overlying one of the cerebral hemispheres. Calcification may sometimes be present in subdural effusions as well as in haematomas, but such cases are rare. Enlargement of the cranial vault may sometimes be associated with dilatation of the ventricular system. The latter may be unilateral, but in this case, the enlarged ventricle is not necessarily related to the side of the subdural haematoma or effusion. It is considered to be caused by obstruction to absorption of cerebrospinal fluid by adhesions or compression of the subarachnoid space. Nevertheless, air encephalography may sometimes be a useful additional investigation. A significant relationship has been reported between subdural haematoma or effusion and the presence of subdural air following lumbar encephalography (Boudreau and Crosby, 1958). It is well recognized that gas may pass into the subdural space in spite of an apparent free flow of cerebrospinal fluid from the lumbar puncture needle, and this occurs when the needle lies half in and half out of the subarachnoid space (*see* page 291). However, when the air collects in significant amounts over the convexity of the hemispheres and can be made to pass freely from the frontal to the occipital pole on change of position, especially in a child under the age of 2 years, it may point to the possibility of an unsuspected subdural effusion.

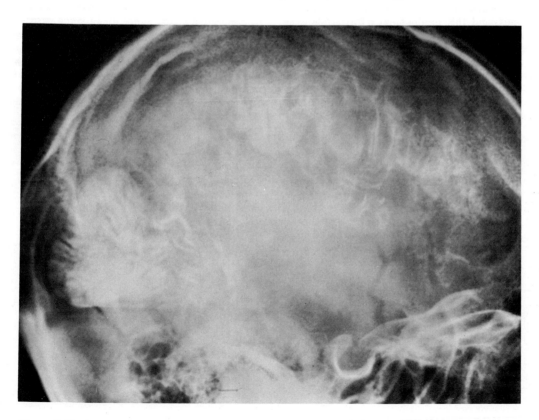

Figure 8.43. Sturge—Weber Syndrome: Calcification on the surface of the cerebral hemisphere. The curvilinear pattern and parallel lines are due to convolutions and sulci which are outlined by the superficial layer of calcium deposits

bone at the epiphyseal growth plate, accounting for the incidence of slipped femoral epiphysis and Scheuermann's disease of the spine at this age. Steroids given over long periods produce a retarding effect on growth and on maturation. In these cases, determination of skeletal age or the detection of osteoporosis and the consequent spinal fractures or deformities may call for radiography of the appropriate bones.

In cases in which growth is abnormal as a result of pituitary disorders, radiology of the skull and pituitary fossa, including the use of pneumo-encephalography to delineate cysts and tumours in the region of the base of the brain or parasellar region, may reveal the nature of the condition. Similarly, the characteristic pattern of bone lesions in hypothyroidism and the demonstration of adrenal cortical tumours or hyperplasia may point to these endocrine glands as the cause of the abnormal growth.

Growth defect due to lack of growth hormone is first apparent at about 1 to 2 years of age, and therefore the size of the child is normal at birth. This defect is commoner in males. It has recently attracted particular interest because of the possibility of specific therapy, and its diagnosis has therefore assumed importance. The ratio between height age and bone age is below unity, the average value being 0.69 as compared with an average of 1.28 in panhypopituitarism, in which there is also a defect in thyrotrophic hormone (Trygstad, 1969). Administration of growth hormone increases height to a greater degree than bone age, and the latter never advances beyond the chronological age. Hence there is no tendency to produce ultimate stunting from premature fusion of the epiphyses, as may occur after treatment with thyroid hormone or anabolic steroids.

The size of the pituitary fossa (*see* page 348) may be of value in differentiating cases of growth hormone deficiency from secondary hypopituitarism, because the fossa will often be enlarged in pituitary or brain tumours but it may be either normal or reduced in size in the former group. Most authors who have studied series of cases of hypopituitarism in which the sellar size has been estimated find that in about half the pituitary fossa is small. The thickness of both bone and muscle are reduced in growth hormone deficiency (3 times the standard deviation below the mean), whereas the thickness of the fat and subcutaneous tissue is increased (Tanner *et al.*, 1971). Not only is the total bone width reduced but the cortex is disproportionately thin relative to the medulla. These authors regard the dramatic reversal of these measurements following administration of growth hormone as a valuable test of the effectiveness of this form of treatment.

Pressure and traction

Mechanical forces also exert a marked effect on bone growth. Pressure applied to the growth plate inhibits growth by stopping further proliferation of cartilage cells. The effect of this is graphically demonstrated by the change in the shape of the vertebral bodies of children who are recumbent for long periods as a result of paralytic or muscular dystrophies. The absence of normal weight-bearing allows unimpeded growth in the height of the vertebral body which then becomes

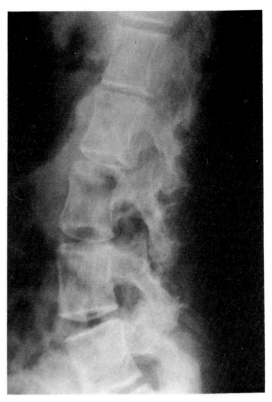

Figure 9.7. Lateral View of the Spine of a Child: The effect of prolonged recumbency on the shape of the vertebral bodies is shown. The height of the body is disproportionately great compared to the antero-posterior diameter

abnormally tall and narrow (*Figure 9.7*). Some deformities such as scoliosis and bowing of the long bones are recognized to be progressive during the period of active growth. This effect is due in large measure to inhibition of growth on the concave side where pressure is greatest, whereas growth continues to occur at a normal rate on the convex side. Traction across a growth plate does not, however, lead to stimulation of growth but produces degenerative effects.

Irradiation

Irradiation of epiphyseal growth plates, by x-rays or gamma-rays will inhibit growth. This is primarily a direct action on the proliferating chondrocytes which are affected by relatively small doses of 300 to 400 rads. It is also due to interference with the blood supply, a result which occurs only with higher doses (above 1300 rads). At the latter level, the effect is likely to be permanent and there may be premature epiphyseal fusion. Periosteal bone growth is considerably more resistant to irradiation than endochondral growth and bone width is therefore often unaffected. Similarly the cranial vault is unaffected by irradiation for cerebral tumours, unlike the jaws which will remain small and the eruption of teeth on the irradiated side will be delayed. Every effort compatible with efficient eradication of the neoplasm should thus be made to ensure that irradiation of actively growing bone is avoided during the treatment of tumours. This is because the spinal deformities and unequal limb length may lead to permanent disability.

Other factors affecting bone growth

Growth defects may also be produced by defective nutrition and emotional deprivation (Silver and Finkelstein, 1967). Stimulation of bone growth results from mainly two factors, the action of pituitary growth hormone and hyperaemia. Examples of the latter are enlargement of the ends of the long bones adjacent to joints which are inflamed or subject to repeated haemarthroses as occurs in disorders of the blood clotting mechanism (see Figure 3.19). Children with large haemangiomata of the limbs often develop inequality in limb length due to overgrowth of the abnormal side. Bone growth is also dependent on inherited genetic factors. The tendency for families to be abnormally tall or abnormally short in stature is well recognized.

Growth and bone disease

In addition to the measurement of limb length in cases of asymmetrical growth, an important contribution of radiology to the investigation of growth disorders consists in the demonstration of bone disease where this is responsible for the abnormal stature. Such generalized diseases of bone include those in which endochondral bone growth is directly affected, as is the case in achondroplasia. In this group the pattern of the skeletal changes is usually so characteristic as to make diagnosis a relatively easy matter. Abnormality of stature may also result from deformities or fractures due to the bone disease, as occurs in osteogenesis imperfecta or rickets, and again the radiological appearances are easily recognizable. In other types of congenital short stature the bones may, in general, appear radiographically normal except for their small size, as in Turner's syndrome (Tanner et al., 1971). However, in such chromosomally determined diseases, there is often a pattern of local bone abnormalities which enables the diagnosis to be suspected from the radiological appearances (see Figure 1.19). Furthermore, in this group of conditions, the growth defect is characteristically present at birth.

Other causes of short stature

A few other types of abnormally short stature may show radiological features which point to the cause of the condition.

(1) Babies who are 'small for dates' at birth may continue to have a small stature through later childhood (Tanner et al., 1971). They may often be distinguished from cases of genetic or constitutional short stature and from hypopituitarism by abnormal facies, short incurved little fingers and asymmetry of the two sides of the body. Such cases, some of which fall into the category of the Russell—Silver syndrome, have a bone age which is only slightly retarded and, though both bone and muscle thickness is reduced, so is the thickness of the fat and subcutaneous tissues.

(2) Short stature due to psychosocial causes comes on during the first few years of life and may therefore be confused with growth hormone deficiency. As in the latter group, bone age is retarded but this is less marked than in the case of height age. The thickness of bone and muscle is reduced and there is no corresponding increase in fat width.

(3) Hypothyroidism leads to considerable shortness of stature and in addition to the severely retarded bone age, it may show epiphyseal dysgenesis, characteristic abnormalities in bone shape and cardiomegaly. It has also been suggested that the pituitary fossa may be relatively large. These changes respond to treatment with thyroxine, and not to growth hormone or to steroids (see page 8).

Gigantism

Less common than shortness of stature, abnormally rapid growth may lead to increased height or, if localized, to asymmetry of the body. An advanced bone age may occur, as is the case in the adrenogenital syndrome, which may be of such a degree as to lead to premature fusion of the epiphyses and ultimate stunting. This may also be present in some other forms of gigantism, but not in the hyperpituitary type, in which ultimate stature is increased, because the height age is always in advance of the bone age. Increased bone growth may occur in relation to brain disease—Sotos' syndrome—and in such cases pneumo-encephalography will show generalized dilatation of the ventricles due to cerebral atrophy; there is also an association with the presence of a cavum septi pellucidi, a feature occasionally seen in otherwise normal children, but which is much more common in Sotos' syndrome. Excessive height is also associated with lipodystrophy, in which there is loss of subcutaneous fat. Because the muscles may also be increased in size, the ratio between fat and muscle thickness is grossly abnormal. The bone age is often advanced and dilatation of the third ventricle and basal cisterns has been reported on pneumo-encephalography and this is presumably related to a hypothalamic—pituitary abnormality. Fetal visceromegaly (Beckwith's syndrome) constitutes a form of gigantism, in which radiological determination of limb size may disclose an asymmetry between the two sides of the body. Because affected children always have considerable nephromegaly, measurement of renal size may suggest the condition. Rarely they may develop nephroblastoma or carcinoma of the adrenal cortex.

Prediction of adult height

In any case in which growth is abnormal, it may be desirable to form an estimate of the final height which is likely to be attained in the absence of effective treatment. This is required, not only for prognostic reasons, but also to assess how far there may be a need for such treatment; this may be required over a prolonged period and is usually expensive. It is possible to achieve such an estimate by consideration of the relationship between the degree of abnormality in height and the retardation or advancement in skeletal maturation. It is the latter which determines the point at which growth ceases as a result of fusion of the epiphyses. A further factor which may influence the result of such estimations is the rate of both growth and skeletal maturation; changes in this may lead to considerable inaccuracies in the predictions. Nevertheless, such predictions may have some value and when serial estimations of height and bone age are available, the trend of the predicted final heights may give an additional assessment of the effectiveness of treatment in terms of its ultimate result.

A rough estimate of the final height may be obtained by a comparison between height age and bone age. If the latter exceeds the former, growth may be expected to continue longer and some improvement in terms of height percentiles may be obtained before growth finally ceases. A more sophisticated, and possibly more accurate, value for predicted final height may be obtained by the use of tables which allow final heights to be read off from the existing values for height and bone age (Bayley and Pinneau, 1952). However, their accuracy has recently been criticized and it is suggested that estimations should be based on skeletal maturity values combined with other factors such as the state of previous health and nutrition, secondary sexual characteristics and parental growth history (Tanner *et al.*, 1975).

ESTIMATION OF SKELETAL MATURITY

The evaluation of skeletal maturity is one of the more important functions of radiology in the study of growth disorders in childhood, particularly those due to abnormalities of the endocrine glands, in which growth and maturation are often dissociated from each other. Maturation may, of course, also be abnormal as a result of malnutrition or chronic diseases of various types but, in such cases, growth and maturation are usually affected to the same extent. Several methods are available for the estimation of skeletal maturity and the fact that none of these has so far obtained general acceptance is probably an indication that, as yet, no entirely satisfactory method has been devised.

APPEARANCE AND FUSION OF OSSIFICATION CENTRES

The simplest and most objective method consists in the observation of the time of appearance of certain

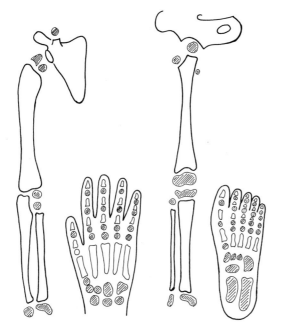

Figure 9.8. Elgenmark's Method for Estimation of Skeletal Maturity: Secondary centres of ossification used in this method in one arm and one leg

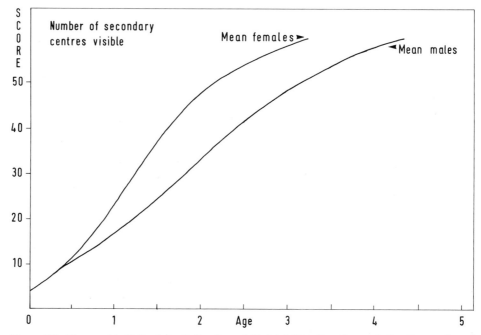

Figure 9.9. Elgenmark's Method for Estimation of Skeletal Maturity: Curve relating the number of secondary ossific centres present to chronological age of the patient

secondary centres of ossification and of the time at which epiphyses fuse with the primary centres. This is still useful in certain limited fields, but it is too crude and unreliable for general use. It suffers from the disadvantage that the time span over which it is operative is short. However, in the estimation of maturation in intra-uterine life and over the first 2 years of postnatal life it still has a part to play. It is desirable that a sufficiently wide distribution of secondary centres be used, as in the method described by Elgenmark (1946), in which all the secondary centres on one side of the body are enumerated (*Figure 9.8*). Because these amount to 68 in all, the results can be analysed statistically to give the average number of centres ossified at any given age, together with the range of normal variation on each side of the mean. The curve obtained shows a straight line relationship over the first 2 years of life, after which it begins to flatten out as the number of centres ossified approaches the total number present in the body (*Figure 9.9*). This method is probably the only reliable one at present available for estimation of skeletal maturity below 2 years of age, but has the disadvantage of requiring irradiation of the whole of one arm and one leg and also the hemipelvis and shoulder girdle.

ATLAS METHODS

The method which is in most general use at the present time makes use of an atlas of standard radiographs of a selected part of the body, such as the hand and wrist, with which the radiograph of the corresponding area of the patient may be compared. Separate standards are used for boys and girls, because there is a significant difference in maturation rates in the two sexes. The age of the standard series which corresponds most closely to that of the patient's radiograph is taken as the skeletal age or 'bone age', and this serves as a measure of the patient's skeletal maturity when expressed as a percentage of the patient's chronological age. The concept of bone age may be employed whatever method of assessing maturity is used, but it is most directly applicable to this one. Such a series of standards for the hand and wrist has been compiled by Greulich and Pyle (1959) and statistical analyses of the results are available to define the range of normal variation. Standards for other parts of the body, such as the knee or foot, are also available and may be used in the same way. Whatever method is used, the standard deviation for bone age approximates to 1 year above or below the mean except during the first few years of life when it is less. This implies that during most of childhood, a total variation in bone age of between 3 and 4 years, may be regarded as normal. This method is widely accepted as the best available by virtue of its simplicity and rapidity for estimating skeletal maturation, particularly in centres in which the demand for such information is infrequent or intermittent. Several criticisms of it have been made which can be summarized as follows:

(1) The method has a high degree of subjectivity which leads to considerable observer error. This, however, applies to all the methods in use at the present time with the exception of simple observation of the appearance or fusion of secondary centres as described above. It may, moreover, be minimized by averaging the readings obtained by several observers, or by ensuring that serial observations on the same patient are made by the same observer.

(2) It assumes a fixed pattern of development applicable to all the secondary centres in the region studied, whereas in practice very considerable variations occur in different individuals. This is not in our opinion a serious drawback, because each centre may, if necessary, be compared with its equivalent in the standard series and the total skeletal age determined by averaging the skeletal age obtained for each centre individually. Furthermore, such a procedure overcomes the discontinuity resulting from the fact that the standards are placed at 6 months or a year's interval from each other.

(3) The standard series currently available is derived from a sample of normal American children, who are all of Caucasian racial origin and from a limited social class. That social and racial differences have a significant effect on the degree of skeletal maturation attained is well recognized, and if the Greulich and Pyle atlas is used to estimate the maturity of children of British origin the resultant skeletal age obtained will be on average about 6–8 months too low. In the case of children of immigrant parents who may be of very different racial stock, this inaccuracy may be even more marked.

(4) Finally, the method has been criticized for estimating skeletal maturation in terms of time rather than in its own units. The use of such units is considered to be desirable, because there may often be dissociation from both growth and ageing of the skeleton, and because they will allow detection of variations in the degree of maturation in different areas of the body. Moreover, the use of 'skeletal age' has the effect of masking any normal variations in the rate of maturation, such as might be expected to occur at different periods of the growth process, by anology with other parameters of bodily development. This is inevitable, because the mean normal skeletal age must take the form of a straight line corresponding to the equivalent chronological age.

SCORING METHODS

The question of the type of unit in which maturation should be expressed is a difficult one, because the use of size or age has to be avoided. Acheson (1957) has put forward the concept of 'indicators', which he has defined as features of individual centres, shown in serial radiographs to occur in a regular, definitive and irreversible order, marking the progress of ossification of that centre to full maturity (*Figure 9.10*). This concept forms the basis of the various 'scoring' methods which have been devised. In these, successive stages in the ossification process are precisely defined and a score is assigned to each stage. The sum of the scores for each centre in the region which are used for the assessment constitutes the 'maturational index'. This may be compared with percentile curves showing the variation of this index with age and expressed as a percentile deviation from the mean for age, in the same way as for height or weight. Separate curves are necessary to allow for the differences between boys and girls.

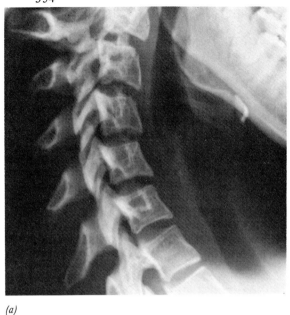

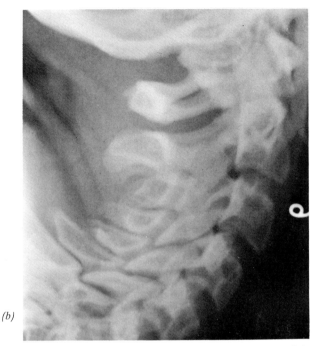

(a)   (b)

Figure 9.24. Normal Movement of Cervical Vertebrae on Flexion of the Neck in Children: (a) There is a forward displacement of the bodies of a number of cervical vertebrae relative to those below them on flexion. (b) This is corrected or even reversed when the neck is extended

body as a measure of its shape. This may be abnormal in recumbency or paralytic conditions, in Down's syndrome in which the height is increased relative to the depth, and in certain other types of skeletal dysplasia in which marked 'platyspondyly' occurs. The normal value for this ratio varies with age from about 1.0 in the first few months of life to between 0.7 and 0.8 in later childhood. A difference in the two sexes is also noted, when the ratio is correlated with height and not with chronological age.

A 'disc–body ratio' may be obtained by dividing the maximum height of the intervertebral disc by the maximum height of the adjacent vertebral body. This figure also varies with age, and it declines from about 0.40 at birth to 0.25 in later childhood and 0.20 in adults. Much higher values, even over 1.0, are found in certain types of skeletal dysplasia, such as achondroplasia (Brandner, 1970).

SCOLIOSIS AND KYPHOSIS

Assessment of the degree of deformity in patients with scoliosis may be assisted by measurement of the angles subtended by the curvature of the spine; these values may be a useful check on the progress of the condition or the effectiveness of treatment. Two methods are in general use for this purpose (*Figure 9.25a*). Ferguson's method is to draw lines between the centres of the vertebral bodies at each end of the curve and the centre of the body at the apex of the curve and measure the angle between these lines. Cobb's angle is measured between lines drawn parallel to the end-plates of the bodies or pedicles of vertebrae just beyond the limits of the primary curve. Ferguson's method is more accurate for mild curves which subtend an angle of less than 50 degrees and Cobb's angle for severe curves subtending an angle of over 50 degrees (Kittleson and Lim, 1970).

Measurements may be made from films taken of the patient in a supine or erect position, with or without a brace or support, or bending to left or right. Assessment of the degree of associated rotation of the vertebral bodies in scoliosis may be achieved from observation of the position of either the spinous processes or the pedicles relative to the lateral borders or midline of the vertebral body at the apex of the curve. The spinous process is displaced in a direction opposite to that of the body.

When a young child presents with a mild scoliosis, it is of considerable importance to determine whether the deformity will resolve spontaneously, or if it is likely to be progressive. Mehta (1972) claims that measurement of the difference between the rib–vertebral angles (*Figure 9.25b*) on the two sides of the apex of the curve will enable a reliable distinction between these two groups to be made. The majority of cases in which the difference is less than 20 degrees resolve spontaneously, whereas those in which the difference is more than 20 degrees are progressive. Serial estimations after an interval of 3 months will confirm these results, because the difference should become smaller in those cases in which the scoliosis is resolving.

MEASUREMENTS RELATING TO PELVIS AND HIP JOINTS

NORMAL OSSIFICATION

At birth, ossification of the pelvis is well advanced. The three primary centres for the ilia, ischia and pubes are still separated by cartilage. Cartilage also forms the iliac crests and the rim of the acetabula. The head of the femur is also entirely cartilaginous, the centre for the capital epiphysis appearing on average at between 4 and 6 months of age (*Figure 9.26*).

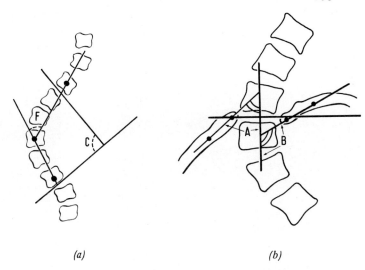

Figure 9.25. (a) Measurement of the Severity of a Scoliosis: Ferguson's angle (F) and Cobb's angle (C). (b) Rib vertebral angles. These are measured, on both the convex and the concave side of the scoliosis, between a line drawn perpendicular to the end plates of the vertebrae at the apex of the scoliosis and lines drawn between the mid-points of the ribs at the head and at the junction between the neck and the shaft

(a)

(b)

Fusion between the three pelvic bones is complete by about age 13 years, but the symphysis pubis remains cartilaginous throughout adult life. The synchondrosis between the pubis and ischium fuses between the ages of 7 and 9 years and the bone around it may become expanded during the process of normal ossification, an appearance which should not be mistaken for disease (*Figure 9.27*). The iliac crest ossifies relatively late. Its epiphysis begins to ossify from the outer end at between 12 and 14 years of age and fusion with the rest of the ilium may not be complete until 19 years of age. Previous to the appearance of this epiphysis the upper border of the ilium assumes an undulating contour with which the epiphysis interdigitates as it ossifies. This feature is seen in relation to other epiphyses which form at the site of muscular or ligamentous attachments, but it is particularly well shown at the iliac crest. The roof of the acetabulum is cartilaginous throughout early childhood but it may occasionally ossify as a separate epiphyseal centre, persisting as an os acetabuli.

ABNORMALITIES IN SHAPE

The shape of the ilium is often characteristic of different types of skeletal dysplasia. Such abnormalities are dependent on localized failure of growth, which often results in a reduction in the craniocaudal diameter of the ilium and a shortening of that part of the bone below the sacro-iliac joint. The ilium may then become square in shape and the sacrosciatic notch narrow and acute, a shape seen in achondroplasia. Rotation of the blade outwards produces a flaring of the ilium and the acetabular roof becomes more horizontal as seen in Down's syndrome and the other types of Trisomy (*see* page 22).

Measurement of the acetabular and iliac angles has been used to define such changes in the shape of the pelvis and the acetabulum (*Figure 9.28*). Caffey and Ross (1958) note that both the acetabular and iliac angles are reduced in Down's syndrome. In this condition an iliac or pelvic index derived from a combination of the two angles is stated by Nicolis and Sacchetti (1963) to give a better separation between cases of

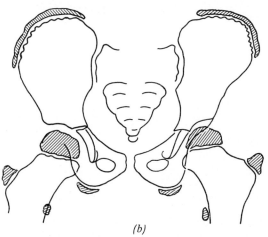

(a)

(b)

Figure 9.26. Ossification of the Pelvis: (a) At birth. (b) After puberty with secondary ossific centres (shaded)

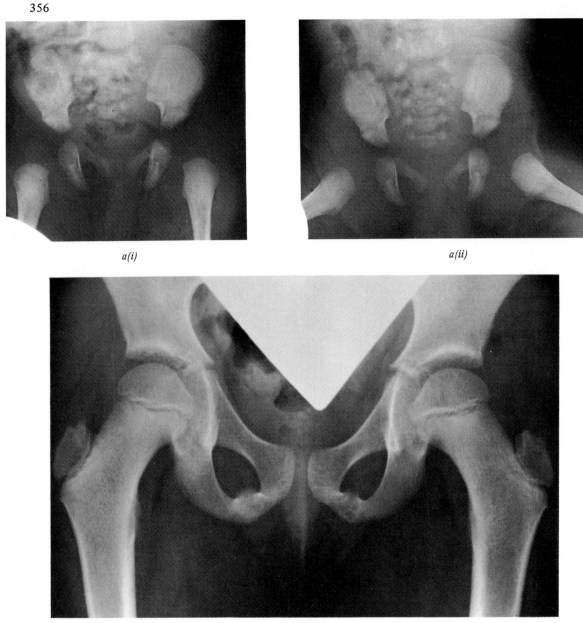

a(i)

a(ii)

(b)

Figure 9.27. Ossification of Pelvis and Hip Joints: (a) Pelvis of girl aged 5 months: (i) Antero-posterior projection with legs together; (ii) Andren-von Rosen projection with femora abducted to 45° and internally rotated. (b) Pelvis of girl aged 5 years; the appearance of the ischio-pubic synchondrosis is a normal variant

Down's syndrome and normal infants than the use of either angle alone. In other types of skeletal dysplasia such as achondroplasia and allied conditions, the acetabular angles are also reduced, but the iliac angles are increased. In Hurler's syndrome, the reverse is the case and the two angles become more nearly equal to one another. Normal values for these pelvic angles are age-dependent because the progressive ossification of the acetabular roof leads to a decrease in the angle. Caffey and Ross (1958) give normal values for the newborn infant of between 18 and 37 degrees for the acetabular angles, and between 44 and 66 degrees for the iliac angles. As the child grows older the normal values for the acetabular angles become smaller. The normal range is from 14 to 28 degrees for a child aged 1 year. The acetabular angle was originally devised as a means of differentiating those newborn infants who were liable to develop congenital dislocation of the hips from normal infants. The overlap between normal and abnormal values proved to be too wide for this to be a useful procedure, except in the small minority in whom the value was over 40 degrees. The radiological diagnosis of congenital dislocation of the hip at birth is notoriously difficult and this fact has led to a wide variety of measurements based on the distance of the neck of the femur from various landmarks around the acetabulum being proposed in order to make the diagnosis (*Figure 9.28*). These are discussed on page 35.

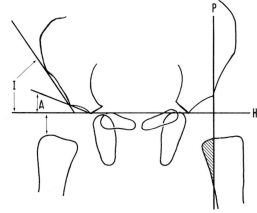

Figure 9.28. Measurement of the Pelvic Shape and Position of the Femoral Heads in the Newborn Infant: The acetabular angle (A) and the iliac angle (I) define the shape of the lateral border of the ilium in relation to Hilgenreiner's line (H). The position of the neck of the femur can be related either to Hilgenreiner's line or to Perkins' line (P). The highest point on the femoral neck should normally lie 8–10 mm below Hilgenreiner's line and up to one third of the neck should lie medial to Perkins' line (shaded)

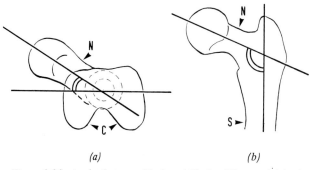

(a)   *(b)*

Figure 9.29. Angles between Neck and Shaft of Femur: (a) Angle of torsion. (b) Angle of inclination. C. Condyles. N. Neck. S. Shaft

RELATIONSHIP BETWEEN THE NECK AND SHAFT OF THE FEMUR

Measurement of the angles between the long axes of the neck and shaft of the femur are used in the evaluation of coxa vara and coxa valga (angle of inclination), and in the assessment of anteversion or retroversion of the femoral neck (angle of torsion) (*Figure 9.29*). Coxa vara is a relatively common deformity at all ages and is defined as being present when the angle of inclination is abnormally small. Normal values for this angle vary with age; the mean value is 146 degrees at birth, declining to 132 degrees in adolescence, and there is a range of normal variation of about 10 degrees above and below these values. Errors in measurement of this angle of inclination are liable to occur and result from the radiographic foreshortening of the neck that occurs when the femur is externally rotated. Ideally the neck should be placed parallel to the x-ray film. In order to achieve this a variable degree of medial rotation depending on the value of the angle or torsion between the neck and shaft must be employed when the radiograph is taken. Dunlap *et al.* (1953) are of the opinion that these two angles can only be accurately measured together. They advise the use of a postero-anterior view of the femur taken with the patient prone, the knees flexed and the ankles in contact, in order to ensure a reproducible degree of rotation. A view of each hip with the patient supine, the thigh flexed at 90 degrees and abducted 10 degrees, in order to bring the neck parallel to the film, should also be taken (*Figure 9.30*). The apparent angles of inclination and torsion are measured from these two films and the true angles calculated by applying a correction factor (Dunlop *et al.*, 1953). Normal values of the angle of torsion vary from 40 degrees of anteversion in the newborn infant to 16 degrees of anteversion in the adolescent. Estimation of this angle has a limited usefulness in planning corrective operations in cases of hip disease.

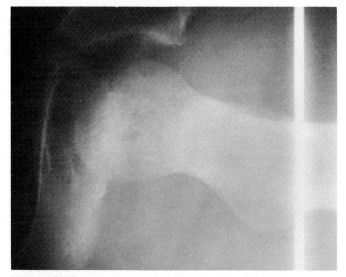

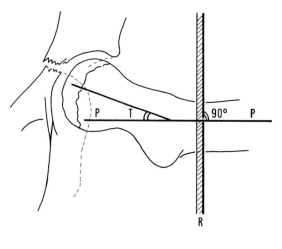

Figure 9.30. Measurement of the Angle of Torsion between the Neck and the Shaft of the Femur: The patient lies supine with the thigh flexed to 90° and abducted 10°. The tibia is supported in the horizontal position and a metal rod (R) is placed on the film parallel to long axis of the tibia. The transcondylar plane (P) lies at right angles to the metal rod. The angle of torsion (T) is measured between the line drawn through the long axis of the femoral neck and the transcondylar plane

MEASUREMENT OF THE HANDS AND FEET

Changes in the size and shape of the bones of the hands and feet have been extensively used to estimate skeletal maturation, and this is because a number of bones of different types are conveniently arranged in a relatively small area. This is discussed in detail elsewhere (*see* page 344).

METACARPAL INDEX

Abnormalities in the shape of the metacarpals, metatarsals and phalanges may be part of a more generalized disturbance in body proportions as occurs in Marfan's syndrome (*see* page 37). Sinclair, Kitchen and Turner (1960) have used a ratio between the length and the width of the metacarpals as a means of separating cases of Marfan's syndrome or isolated arachnodactyly from normal individuals. These measurements are made on a postero-anterior radiograph of the hand and the ratios calculated for the index, middle, ring and little finger metacarpals and these are then averaged. These authors state that the normal range varies from 5.4 to 7.9. In 80 per cent of normal cases the ratio lay between 7.0 and 7.9. In 20 cases of Marfan's syndrome it was between 8.4 and 10.4. Joseph and Meadow (1969) have, however, suggested that these normal values are too high for young children, because they do not allow for the ratio increasing with age. The ratio is also larger in girls than in boys. These authors give mean values for boys of 5.23 at 6 months increasing to 5.40 at 2 years and for girls of 5.60 at 6 months increasing to 5.84 at 2 years with a standard deviation of about 0.40 in all cases. In many cases of arachnodactyly the phalanges are more abnormally shaped than the metacarpals or metatarsals. Normal values for 'relative slenderness' have been estimated for the proximal phalanges, a measurement corresponding to the metacarpal index by Parish (1966).

MEASUREMENTS APPLIED TO THE BONES OF THE FEET

Measurements of the angles between the tarsal bones, especially the talus and calcaneum and the metatarsals, have been used to assess the degree of the deformity in cases of club foot of various types (*Figure 9.31*).

Templeton *et al.* (1965) have reviewed some of these measurements and they describe two *talo-calcaneal angles*. The first, defining varus and valgus of the hindfoot, is measured in the dorsoplantar projection. The value of this angle which diverges anteriorly, varies from a mean value at birth of 40 degrees, declining to 20 degrees at the age of 5 to 6 years and remaining constant after that age. The second talo-calcaneal angle, defining equinus and calcaneus, is measured between the long axes of the two bones in the true lateral projection and this angle normally converges anteriorly. There is a normal range of from 25 to 50 degrees, and this is not age-dependent. The angle between the *long axis of the talus and of the first metatarsal* may be useful as a measure of adduction or abduction of the forefoot. Normally the two axes should be parallel.

PES PLANUS AND PES CAVUS

An estimate of the height of the medial longitudinal arch of the foot can be obtained from the lateral view taken with the child standing on a firm wooden block. The distances between the head of the talus and the surface of the block and between the tubercle of the calcaneum and the neck of the first metatarsal are measured and the former expressed as a percentage of the latter. The normal range lies between 25 and 35 per cent; in cases of flat foot the ratio is below 25 per cent and in cases of pes cavus above 35 per cent (*Figure 9.32*).

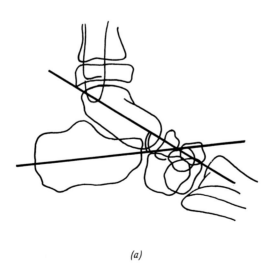

(a)

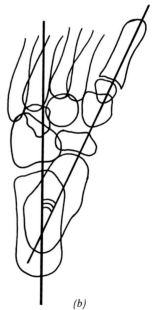

(b)

Figure 9.31. The talo-calcaneal angles measured between the long axes of the talus and the calcaneum in the (a) lateral and (b) dorsoplantar projections of the foot. The long axis of the calcaneum in the latter projection should also be parallel to the long axis of the first metatarsal

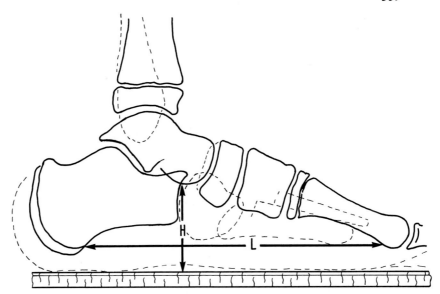

Figure 9.32. Measurement of the height of the medial plantar arch from a lateral view of the foot taken standing on a wooden block. The plantar index consists of the distance from the lowest point on the head of the talus to the surface of the block (H) expressed as a percentage of the distance from the tubercule of the calcaneum to the neck of the first metatarsal (L).

These measurements require careful position of the foot and angulation of the x-ray tube if they are to be accurate and it may be far from an easy matter to achieve this in children who have severely deformed feet. For this reason the chief value of these measurements is to afford a basis for comparison between serial films and to allow assessment of how effective treatment has been in correcting the deformity. The diagnosis of the deformity in the first place can usually be made by inspection of the films without the use of measurements (Beatson and Pearson, 1966)

MEASUREMENT OF BONE DENSITY AND SOFT TISSUE THICKNESS

BONE DENSITY OR MINERAL CONTENT

A number of different techniques are available for measurement of the mineral content of bone, many of which have been applied to children successfully. A qualitative assessment may be made by observing changes in the shape of bones subject to constant pressure, such as the vertebral bodies, or in the thickness of the cortex of the long bones in relation to the amount of their spongiosa. The latter may also show a change in trabecular pattern, in that the individual trabeculae are reduced in number and appear to stand out by contrast with the widened marrow spaces in the presence of osteoporosis. Such an assessment is necessarily inexact and subject to errors due to variations in radiographic technique.

A more precise estimation may be achieved by measuring the thickness of the cortex of the long bones, and in particular that of the metacarpals. Barnett and Nordin (1959) have proposed a 'metacarpal index' which they derive by dividing the sum of the thicknesses of the two cortices at the midpoint of the index finger metacarpal, by the total width of the bone at this level. McCrae and Sweet (1967) have applied this to children and give a mean value increasing from 0.33 in the first 2 years to 0.48 by the age of 10 years. There is, however,

a very wide range of normal variation and the chief value of this method is to allow the effect of disease and its treatment to be followed on serial examinations.

Densitometric methods, depending upon an estimation of the degree of absorption of x-rays by bone, may be applied to both cortical and spongy bone. Some device, such as the use of a water bath, is necessary to offset variations in soft tissue thickness. The density, measured from the radiograph by a recording microdensitometer, is compared with that of a standard step-wedge exposed at the same time under the same conditions. The midpoint of a metacarpal is used for assessment of cortical bone and the base of a proximal phalanx for trabecular bone. The ratio between the readings at two such sites in the ulna is considered by Doyle (1966) to be a more sensitive index of the amount of trabecular bone than a single reading over the distal end of the bone. A more accurate technique is one in which radioactive isotopes are used. The radiation is provided by a monochromatic gamma-ray source such as ^{125}I which has a high bone–soft–tissue contrast. This is combined with another source of gamma-rays such as [57]Co which has low contrast in order to allow for variations in soft tissue density. The intensity of radiation passing through the bone is measured by a scintillation counter and is calibrated in terms of mg of calcium per ml. The measurement is made at a constant site. Normal values for children vary with age from 115 mg/ml in infancy to a peak value of 230 mg/ml between 7 and 8 years of age (Schuster *et al.*, 1970).

The true bone density may also be calculated by using standard aluminium equivalents or other estimates of the amount of bone mineral in the path of the beam and by dividing these values by the cortical thickness. Such estimates are found to show a different pattern of age variation from cortical thickness or aluminium density equivalents when these are considered alone.

SOFT TISSUE THICKNESS

Radiological methods afford a simple and reasonably accurate means of estimating the thickness and hence the mass of the various soft tissues in the limbs, because when the radiographs are suitably exposed, the skin, subcutaneous tissues and muscle cylinder are easily differentiated from each other (*Figure 9.33*). A standard site for making such measurements and a knowledge of the normal values at this site at different ages are required. The results obtained may be used to study growth patterns or changes in tissue thickness in diseases in which there is variation or imbalance in the quantity of fat, muscle and bone.

Normal values are given for the calf at the point of greatest thickness of the muscle mass in the antero-posterior projection by Reynolds (1948), Reynolds and Grote (1948) and my Maresh (1961). Similar data are available for the thigh (Maresh, 1961), the upper arm (Heald *et al.*, 1963) and the forearm (Maresh, 1966). Measurements can be made over the trunk, either perpendicular to the tenth rib or over the bulge of the hip (Garn and Haskell, 1960; Maresh, 1966). The measurements may be recorded as absolute values or as percentages related to the total limb thickness. They are found to correlate well with clinical estimations of skin fold thickness. There is a characteristic variation in the values obtained for each tissue during growth, and this differs in the two sexes. Both muscle and bone thickness show a greater increase in boys during adolescence than they do in girls. Both muscle and bone thickness follow a curve which corresponds to that for body growth as a whole, and there is a prepubertal spurt. Fat thickness, on the other hand, behaves quite differently, It doubles in value in the first year of life, then shows a gradual

decrease until the age of 7 or 8 years is reached. Thereafter in girls it increases again and in boys it continues to decline. Such a unidimensional measurement of fat thickness was compared by Garn (1957) with estimates of total body fat made by chemical methods and the relationship was found to be nearly linear. It is therefore possible to use this measurement as an acceptable estimate of changes in body fat with age or disease. Correlation of fat, muscle and bone width with other body parameters has also been studied. Height was found to correlate best with bone width and to a lesser extent with fat thickness. Bone age correlates fairly well with fat thickness, and children who have an increase in fat width of 1 standard deviation above the mean have, on average, a bone age about 0.4 years in advance of their chronological age.

Effect of disease on soft tissue thickness

Litt and Altman (1967) have reviewed the results of tissue thickness measurements in various disease processes. They divide such conditions on the basis of a ratio between the muscle thickness and the total limb thickness, values between 0.64 and 0.72 being regarded as normal. Of the group with a ratio of less then 0.64, the muscle mass may be diminished by diseases with muscle wasting or flaccidity or by those in which the muscles are congenitally poorly developed, such as arthrogryposis multiplex. In these conditions an increase in the fat and subcutaneous tissues may mask the

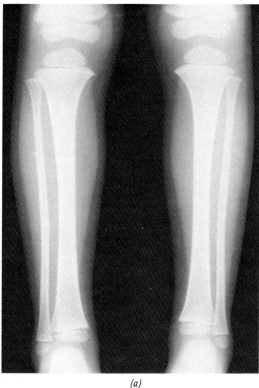

(a)

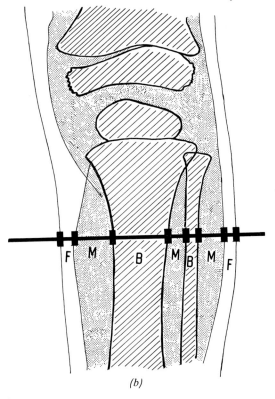

(b)

Figure 9.33. Anteroposterior View of the Calf for Estimation of Tissue Thickness According to the Method of Reynolds (1948): A horizontal line is drawn across the limb at the level of maximum thickness of the calf muscle. The width of the subcutaneous tissues (F), muscle (M) and bone (B) along this line are summated to give the total thickness of each tissue which can then be expressed as a percentage of the total limb thickness and compared with standard values for the age of the child. (a) Radiograph of limb showing subcutaneous tissues, muscle and bone. (b) Line drawing showing site for measurement

clinical evidence of muscle wasting, and the latter would only be revealed by radiological examination. Alternatively, the fat and subcutaneous tissues may be increased as in Cushing's syndrome. In exogenous obesity on the other hand the ratio is usually normal because fat is deposited within the muscles as well as subcutaneously. The group with a ratio of over 0.72 can similarly be divided into two groups. In the first of these the subcutaneous fat is diminished; this may be due to malnutrition, the diencephalic syndrome or total lipodystrophy. In the other group there is an increase in muscle mass such as occurs in the pseudohypertrophic muscular dystrophies and de Lange's syndrome of mental retardation and muscle hypertrophy.

Skin thickness

Estimations of this parameter require a special technique, because it is necessary to ensure that a sufficient length of skin is parallel to the x-ray beam and that the tangential effect of a curved skin surface is avoided. This is achieved by the use of a wooden block of sufficient size and weight to compress the skin, without obscuring the margins it is essential to measure. The total thickness of the pad of tissue beneath the under surface of the calcaneum on a lateral film of the ankle has also been used for a similar purpose. Such measurements have only a limited application in children, but they are possibly of use in the control of growth hormone therapy. They are increased in acromegaly and Cushing's syndrome.

MEASUREMENT OF HEART SIZE

Accurate radiological assessment of the size of the heart in children, especially in those under the age of 5 years, is more difficult than in adults (see Chapter 4). Not only has growth to be taken into account, but also the effect of crying and changes in respiratory phase, which cannot be easily controlled. These factors, combined with the presence of the thymus, all contribute to diminish the accuracy of the radiological estimation of heart size.

Effect of growth of thoracic cage

The position of the heart and of the diaphragm are related to the growth of the thorax. It is wide and short from top to bottom in the infant, but it undergoes changes in shape because of faster growth in the craniocaudal dimension than in width. As a result the heart becomes more vertical in position with increasing age, and the transverse diameter becomes relatively smaller compared to the other cardiac diameters. The cardiothoracic ratio (see page 362) decreases to some extent with age, but this is less marked than the decrease in the transverse diameter of the heart, because the thorax also becomes relatively less wide as age increases (Figure 9.34).

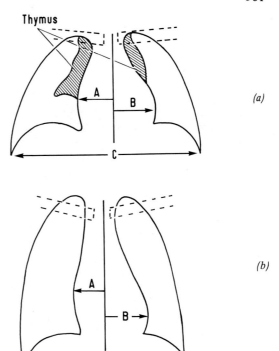

Figure 9.34. Variations in the Size and Shape of the Heart with Age: (a) In infancy the diaphragm is high in position so that the transverse diameter (A + B) is relatively greater; the upper part of the heart is overlapped by the thymus and this can also increase the apparent size of the heart. (b) In the older child the heart becomes more vertical in position and the diaphragm is not so high. The transverse diameter is relatively less, but the cardiothoracic ratio (A + B)/C remains fairly constant and can be used as a measure of heart size at both ages. The transverse diameter of the thorax (C) should be measured at its widest point

Effect of crying and diaphragmatic level

The effect of crying and respiratory phase on the apparent heart size in the neonatal period has been well studied by Burnard and James (1961) using cinefluoroscopic studies. They showed that the shadow of the heart and mediastinum do not vary much during quiet breathing. They considered that an adequate indication of the size of the heart could be obtained from films exposed under such conditions, no matter what the phase of respiratory movement or of the cardiac cycle was. The observed differences did not exceed 4 mm and this was within the range of error inherent in the method. During crying, however, this was no longer the case, and observed differences were outside the limits of error in a majority of the cases. They consider that the main factor controlling the variations in the size of the transverse diameter of the heart in the newborn infant is the blood flow into the right side of the heart and not the position of the diaphragm. It is however important to realize that diaphragmatic level substantially affects the flow of blood returning to the heart through the inferior vena cava.

Effect of thymus

The thymus may extend low enough in the anterior mediastinum to obscure the cardiac borders and the effect of this is exaggerated by the use of the supine position. Even so, the borders of a widened upper mediastinum may not uncommonly be formed by the superior vena cava on the right side and by the pulmonary artery and left atrial appendage on the left.

Measurements

The measurements most commonly used to assess heart size in infants, older children and adults, are the transverse diameter, the cardiothoracic ratio and the cardiac volume. The *transverse diameter* has the disadvantage of being age-dependent (*Figure 9.34*). There is a linear correlation between age and transverse diameter from the ages of 18 months to 5 years, but this is not the case below 18 months of age. Nevertheless, the use of the transverse diameter alone has been recommended in the newborn period. Burnard and James (1961) give a normal range of from 49 to 58 mm at birth for full-term normal infants. There is a fairly constant difference between males and females. The range of normal variation is not reduced by relating the transverse cardiac diameter to body length or body weight instead of age. However, birth weight and prematurity do influence heart size to a considerable extent and need to be considered in evaluating the degree of abnormality. The measurement of the transverse diameter alone is therefore of rather limited value, but the hypothesis that normal variations of the transverse diameter in newborn infants are more often due to differences in the blood volume within the heart than to changes in the shape of the thorax or the position of the diaphragm may justify its use.

The *cardiothoracic ratio* has the double advantage of simplicity and of not being age-dependent to more than a very slight degree. However, the conical shape of the infant's thorax makes it essential to measure the thoracic diameter at its widest point rather than at a level depending on the position of the diaphragm. The range of normal variation is quite wide, but an upper limit of 0.52–0.54 for children under age 5 years has, in our experience, proved reliable. It must be emphasized, however, that the radiograph used for making the measurement must be technically satisfactory and not taken on expiration. Small variations in the value of the cardiothoracic ratio are of no clinical or radiological significance.

Estimation of *cardiac volume* may be made according to the formula published by Lind (1950). This involves measurement of the long diameter, the broad diameter and the horizontal depth diameter of the heart (*Figure 9.35*). These are multiplied together and the product multiplied by a factor of 0.462. The cardiac volume obtained in this way is related to the surface area of the body which may be calculated from the height and weight according to du Bois' formula. Keats and Euge (1965) have constructed nomograms which allow du Bois' formula to be applied to young infants. They also suggest that the conversion factor of Lind's formula be varied according to the focus-film distance at which the radiograph is taken. Thus, for films taken at 100 cm, a

CARDIAC VOLUME

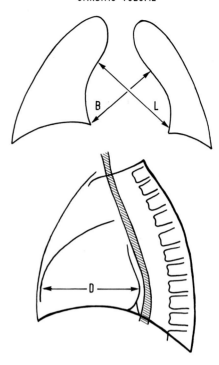

Figure 9.35. Estimation of Cardiac Volume (Lind, 1950): The long diameter (L), the broad diameter (B) and the horizontal depth diameter (D) are measured and the cardiac volume calculated from the formula L × B × D × 0.462

factor of 0.38 is used, and for those taken at 180 cm, a factor of 0.42 is used. Normal values are age-dependent and vary from 200 ml/m² of body surface at birth to 400 ml/m² at 14–16 years. The estimation of cardiac volume is a time-consuming procedure and it is not practical as a routine in a busy department.

For routine estimation of heart size in children, the cardiothoracic ratio is preferred, especially when it is desired to compare serial values in order to assess changes in cardiac size. It has been suggested that the transverse diameter might be related to the height of the thorax as well as to its width, so as to allow for variations in the position of the long axis of the heart due to abnormal thoracic shape or to elevation of the diaphragm, but this is not possible to apply in small children. In cases in whom the cardiothoracic ratio or transverse diameter give results which are at variance with the clinical findings, fluoroscopy may often be of great value and will enable a rapid assessment of the effect of respiratory phase and will always reveal the true cardiothoracic ratio.

MEASUREMENT OF THE SIZE OF THE KIDNEYS

The recent interest in the effects of chronic inflammatory disease on the kidney has led to the need for standards of the normal variations in renal size during normal growth. Serial estimations may also throw useful light on the distinction between congenital hypoplasia, in which the kidney has been small from birth and has not grown at the normal rate, and the effect of acquired renal disease. The latter may either inhibit growth of the kidney or lead to a reduction in its size from the effects of atrophy and scarring.

The simplest dimension used to assess renal size is the *bipolar length (Figure 9.36)*, and Hodson *et al.* (1962) have provided tables by which the normal variations may be assessed both in relation to age and to height. The latter is claimed to be a better parameter than age because it gives a linear relationship to renal size. It also takes account of the effect of the development of the body as a whole and this may affect renal size without necessarily being related to renal disease. Differences in the length of the two kidneys of less than 5 mm are found to occur frequently in normal children.

Other dimensions such as the *width* or *area* of the kidney as calculated by various formulae or by planimetry have been investigated but in general they are less

breadth of both the renal outline and of the pelvicalyceal system and dividing the produce of the latter by the product of the former measurements. They state that the mean value of this ratio is 0.35, but the range of normal variation is wide. There is a considerable overlap between the ratios in normal individuals and those in renal disease. Furthermore reduction in cortical thickness is often localized and it may be simpler and more informative to make measurements of the distances between the upper, lower and most lateral calyces and the nearest point on the renal surface as suggested by Gatewood *et al.* (1965). Such measurements however, have the disadvantage of being age-dependent and vary from 1.3 cm at birth to 3.1 cm at the age of 15 years.

REFERENCES

GENERAL

Bayley, N. and Pinneau, S. R. (1952). 'Tables for predicting adult height from skeletal age revised for use with the Greulich–Pyle hand standards.' *J. Pediat.* **40,** 423

Caffey, J., Madell, S. H., Royer, C. and Morales, P. (1958). 'Ossification of the distal femoral epiphysis.' *J. Bone Jt Surg.* **40A,** 647

Maresh, M. M. (1959). 'Linear body proportions; a roentgenographic study.' *Am. J. Dis. Child.* **98,** 27

Poznanski, A. K., Garn, S. M., Nagy, J. M. and Gall, J. C. (1972). 'Metacarpophalangeal pattern profiles in the evaluation of skeletal malformations.' *Radiology* **104,** 1

Rubin, P. (1964). *Dynamic Classification of Bone Dysplasias.* Chicago; Year Book Medical Publishers

Shopfner, C. E. (1966). 'Periosteal bone growth in normal infants.' *Am. J. Roentgl.* **97,** 154

Silver, H. K. and Finkelstein, M. (1967). 'Deprivation dwarfism.' *J. Pediat.* **70,** 317

Tanner, J. M., Whitehouse, R. H., Hughes, P. C. R. and Vince, F. P. (1971). 'Effect of human growth hormone treatment for 1 to 7 years on growth of 100 Children.' *Archs Dis. Childh.* **46,** 745

Marshall, W. A. and Carter, B. S. (1975). 'Prediction of adult height from height, bone age and occurrence of menarche, at ages 4 to 16 with allowance for midparent height.' *Archs Dis. Childh.* **50,** 14

Trygstad, O. (1969). 'Human growth hormone and hypopituitary growth retardation.' *Acta Paediat. Scand.* **58,** 407

Whalen, J. P., Winchester, P., Krook, L. Dische, R. and Nunez, E. (1971). 'Mechanisms of bone resorption in human metaphyseal remodelling.' *Am. J. Roentgl.* **112,** 526

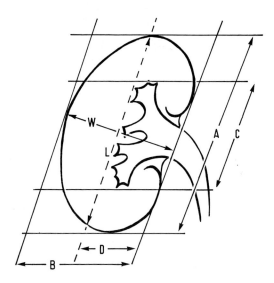

Figure 9.36. Estimation of Renal Size and of the Relative Thickness of the Renal Cortex: Renal size can be measured most simply from the bipolar length (L) either alone or in combination with the maximum width (W). Renal cortical thickness can be estimated by means of the renal cortical index as described by Vuorinen et al (1960). The dimensions of the renal pelvis (C × D) taken from parallel lines drawn at the level of the tips of the calyces are compared with the dimensions of the outer border of the kidney (A × B). The index I is calculated from the formula

$$I = (C \times D)/(A \times B)$$

well correlated with age than renal length. Ludin (1967), however, disagrees with this view and considers renal area to be the most accurate dimension to use. Correlation with other parameters such as the body surface area and the length of the upper four lumbar vertebrae have been suggested in an attempt to obtain a measure of renal size independent of total body size and age.

Cortical thickness is also of important in assessing the effect of renal disease on function and therefore in determining prognosis. Vuorinen *et al.* (1960) have devised a 'renal cortical index' for this purpose (*Figure 9.36*). This is obtained by measuring the length and

SKELETAL MATURATION

Acheson, R. M. (1954). 'A method of assessing skeletal maturity from radiographs.' *J. Anat.* **88,** 498

Acheson, R. M. (1957). 'The Oxford method of assessing skeletal maturity.' *Clin. Orthop.* **10,** 19

Campbell, S. and Newman, G. B. (1971). 'Growth of the fetal biparietal diameter during normal pregnancy.' *J. Obstet. Gynaec. Br. Commonw.* **78,** 513

Elgenmark, O. (1946). 'The normal development of the ossific centres during infancy and childhood.' *Acta Paediat, Scand.* **33,** Suppl. 1.

Greulich, W. W. and Pyle, S. I. (1959). *Radiographic Atlas of Skeletal Development of the Hand and Wrist* (2nd edn) Stanford, Calif., Stanford University

Tanner, J. M., Whitehouse, R. H., Marshall, W. A., Healy, M. J. R. and Goldstein, H. (1975). *Assessment of Skeletal Maturity and Prediction of Adult Height (T.W.2. Method)*. New York and London; Academic Press

— — Hughes, P. C. R. and Vince, F. P. (1971). 'Effect of Human Growth Hormone treatment for 1 to 7 years on growth of 100 children with growth hormone deficiency, low birth weight, inherited smallness, Turner's syndrome and other complaints.' *Archs Dis. Childh.* **46**, 745

MEASUREMENTS OF SKULL AND BRAIN

Burwood, R. J. (1970). 'The cranio-cervical junction.' Thesis for degree of M. D. Bristol University

— Gordon, I. R. S. and Taft, R. D. (1973) 'The Skull in mongolism.' *Clin. Radiol.* **24**, 475

Carlsson, L. B. and Lodin, H. (1969). 'Size of interpeduncular, pontine, ponto-cerebellar cisterns and cisterna magna in childhood.' *Acta Radiol.* **(Diagn.)** **8**, 65

Cronqvist, S. (1968). 'Roentgenologic evaulation of cranial size in children; a new index.' *Acta Radiol.* **(Diagn.)** **7**, 97

Evans, W. A. (1942). 'An encephalographic ratio for estimating the size of the cerebral ventricles.' *Am. J. Dis. Child.* **64**, 820

Fisher, R. L. and di Chiro, G. (1964). 'The small sella turcica.' *Am. J. Roentgl.* **91**, 996

Gerald, B. E. and Silverman, F. N. (1965). 'Normal and abnormal interorbital distances with special reference to mongolism.' *Am. J. Roentgl.* **95**, 154

Gordon, I. R. S. (1966). 'Measurement of cranial capacity in children.' *Br. J. Radiol.* **39**, 377

Hansman, C. F., (1966). 'Growth of interorbital distance and skull thickness as observed in roentgenographic measurements.' *Radiology* **86**, 87

Hinck, V. C., Hopkins, C. E. and Savara, B. S. (1961). 'Diagnostic criteria of basilar impression.' *Radiology* **76**, 572

Illingworth, R. S. and Lutz, W. (1965). 'Head circumference of infants related to body weight.' *Archs Dis. Childh.* **40**, 672

Jackson, H. (1956). 'Asymmetry and growth of the skull.' *Br. J. Radiol.* **29**, 521

Jorgensen, J. B., Paridon, E. and Quaade, F. (1961). 'The correlation between external cranial volume and brain volume.' *Am. J. phys. Anthropol.* **19**, 317

Lodin, H. (1968a). 'Size and development of the cerebral ventricular system in childhood.' *Acta Radiol.* (Diagn.) **7**, 385

— (1968b). 'Normal topography of the cerebral ventricular system in childhood.' *Acta Radiol. (Diagn.)* **7**, 512

Lorber, J. (1961). 'Systematic ventriculographic studies in infants born with meningomyelocele and encephalocele; the incidence and development of hydrocephalus.' *Archs Dis. Childh.* **36**, 381

Neilson, R., Peterson, O., Thygesen, P. and Willanger, R. (1966). 'Encephalographic ventricular atrophy; relationship between size of ventricular system and intellectual impairment.' *Acta Radiol. (Diagn.)* **4**, 240

Schuster, W. and Tamaela, L. A. (1966). 'Das Verhalten des Schadelnahte beim Neugeborenen and Saugling unter physiologischen und pathologischen Bedingungen.' (The behaviour of the cranial sutures in newborns and infants under physiologic and pathologic conditions). *Ann. Radiol.* **9**, 232

Silverman, F. N. (1957). 'Roentgen standards for size of the pituitary fossa from infancy through adolescence.' *Am. J. Roentgl.* **78**, 451

SPINE

Brandner, M. E. (1970). 'Normal values of the vertebral body and intervertebral disk index during growth.' *Am. J. Roentgl.* **110**, 618

Cattell, H. S. and Filtzer, D. L. (1965). 'Pseudosubluxation and other normal variations in the cervical spine in children; a study of one hundred and sixty children.' *J. Bone Jt Surg.* **47A**, 129

Hinck, V. C., Hopkins, C. E. and Savara, B. S. (1962). 'Sagittal diameter of the cervical spinal canal in children.' *Radiology* **79**, 97

— Clark, W. M. and Hopkins, C. E. (1966). 'Normal interpediculate distances (minimum and maximum) in children and adults.' *Am. J. Roentgl.* **97**, 141

Houston, C. S. and Zaleski, W. A. (1967). 'The shape of vertebral bodies and femoral necks and relation to activity.' *Radiology* **89**, 59

Kittleson, A. C. and Lim, L. W. (1970). 'Measurement of scoliosis.' *Am. J. Roentgl.* **108**, 775

Knutsson, F. (1961). 'Growth and differentiation of the postnatal vertebra.' *Acta Radiol.* **55**, 401

Locke, G. R., Gardner, J. I. and Van Epps, E. F. (1966). 'Atlas–Dens interval (ADI) in children; a survey based on 200 normal cervical spines.' *Am. J. Roentgl.* **97**, 135

Mehta, M. H. (1972). 'The rib–vertebra angle measurement in the early differential diagnosis of resolving and progressive infantile scoliosis.' *J. Bone J Surg.* **54B**, 230

Naik, D. R. (1970). 'Cervical spinal canal in normal infants.' *Clin. Radiol.* **21**, 323

Simril, W. A. and Thurston, D. (1955). 'The normal interpediculate space in the spines of infants and children.' *Radiology* **64**, 340

PELVIS AND LIMBS

Beatson, T. R. and Pearson, J. R. (1966). 'A method of assessing correction in club feet.' *J. Bone Jt Surg.* **48B**, 40

Caffey, J. and Ross, S. (1958). 'Pelvic bones in infantile mongoloidism; Roentgenographic features.' *Am. J. Roentgl.* **80**, 458

Dunlap, K., Shands, A. R., Hollister, L. C., Gaul, J. S. and Streit, H. A. (1953). 'A new method for determination of torsion of the femur.' *J. Bone Jt Surg.* **35A**, 289

Joseph, M. C. and Meadow, S. R. (1969). 'The metacarpal index of children.' *Archs Dis. Childh.* **44**, 515

Nicolis, F. B. and Sacchetti, G. (1963). 'A nomogram for the x-ray evaulation of some morphological abnormalities of the pelvis in the diagnosis of mongolism.' *Pediatrics, Springfield* **32**, 1074

Parish, J. G. (1966). 'Radiographic measurements of the skeletal structure of the normal hand.' *Br. J. Radiol.* **39**, 52

Sinclair, R. J. G., Kitchen, A. H. and Turner, R. W. D. (1960). 'The Marfan syndrome.' *Q. Jl Med. N. S.* **29**, 19

Templeton, A. W., McAlister, W. H. and Zim, I. D. (1965). 'Standardization of terminology and evaluation of osseous relationships in congenitally abnormal feet.' *Am. J. Roentgl.* **93**, 374

BONE DENSITY AND SOFT TISSUE THICKNESS

Barnett, E. and Nordin, B. E. C. (1960). 'The radiological diagnosis of osteoporosis: a new approach.' *Clin. Radiol.* **11**, 166

Doyle, F. H. (1966). 'Some quantitative radiological observations in primary and secondary hyperparathyroidism.' *Br. J. Radiol.* **39**, 161

Garn, S. M. (1957). 'Roentgenogrammetric determinations of body composition.' *Hum. Biol.* **29**, 337

— and Haskell, J. A. (1960). 'Fat thickness and developmental status in childhood and adolescence.' *Am. J. Dis. Child.* **99**, 746

HEART AND KIDNEY MEASUREMENTS

Heald, F. P., Hunt, E. E., Schwartz, R. Cook C. D., Elliott, O. and Vajda, B. (1963). 'Measures of body fat and hydration in adolescent boys.' *Pediatrics, Springfield* **31**, 226

Litt, R. E. and Altman, D. H. (1967). 'Significance of the muscle cylinder ratio in infancy.' *Am. J. Roentgl.* **100** 80

Maresh, M. M. (1961). 'Bone, muscle and fat measurements; longitudinal measurements of the bone, muscle and fat widths from roentgenograms of the extremities during the first six years of life.' *Pediatrics, Springfield* **28**, 971

Maresh, M. (1966). 'Changes in tissue widths during growth.' *Am. J. Dis. Child.* **111**, 142

McCrae, W. and Sweet, E. M. (1967). 'Diagnosis of osteoporosis in children.' *Br. J. Radiol.* **40**, 104

Reynolds, E. L. (1948). 'Distribution of the tissue components in the female leg from birth to maturity.' *Anat. Rec.* **100**, 621

— and Grote, P. (1948). 'Sex differences in the distribution of tissue components in the human leg from birth to maturity.' *Anat. Rec.* **102**, 45

Schuster, W., Reiss, H. and Kramer, K. (1970). 'The objective assessment of disorders of bone mineralisation in congenital and acquired skeletal diseases in childhood.' *Annls Radiol.* **13**, 255

Burnard, E. D. and James, L. S. (1961). 'The cardiac silhouette in newborn infants: a cinematographic study of the normal range.' *Pediatrics, Springfield* **27**, 713

Gatewood, O. M. B., Glasser, R. J. and van Houtte, J. J. (1965). 'Roentgen evaluation of renal size in pediatric age groups.' *Am. J. Dis. Child.* **110**, 162

Hodson, C. J., Drewe, J. A., Karn, M. N. and King, A. (1962). 'Renal size in normal children; a radiographic study during life.' *Archs Dis. Childh.* **37**, 616

Hoffman, R. B. and Rigler, L. G. (1965). 'Evaluation of left ventricular enlargement in the lateral projection of the chest.' *Radiology* **85**, 93

Keats, T. E. and Euge, I. P. (1965). 'Cardiac mensuration by the cardiac volume method.' *Radiology* **85**, 850

Lind, J. (1950). 'Heart volume in normal infants, a roentgenological study.' *Acta Radiol.,* Suppl. 82

Ludin, H. (1967). 'Radiologic estimation of kidney weight.' *Acta Radiol.* (Diagn.) **6**. 561

Vuorinen, P., Pyykonen, L. and Anttila, P. (1960). 'A renal cortical index obtained from urography films.' *Br. J. Radiol.* **33**, 622

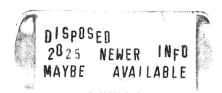

INDEX